Third Edition

Platinum Notes

Preclinical Sciences (2012–13)

Volume –1

- ❑ Anatomy
- ❑ Biochemistry
- ❑ Microbiology
- ❑ Pharmacology
- ❑ Physiology
- ❑ Forensic
- ❑ Pathology
- ❑ Social and Preventive Medicine

Ashfaq Ul Hassan MBBS MS

Lecturer Anatomy
SKIMS Medical College Bemina,
Srinagar, Jammu and Kashmir
India

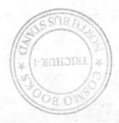

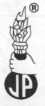

JAYPEE BROTHERS MEDICAL PUBLISHERS (P) LTD

New Delhi • Panama City • London

Published by
Jaypee Brothers Medical Publishers (P) Ltd

Corporate Office
4838/24 Ansari Road, Daryaganj, **New Delhi** - 110002, India
Phone: +91-11-43574357, Fax: +91-11-43574314

Offices in India
- **Ahmedabad**, e-mail: ahmedabad@jaypeebrothers.com
- **Bengaluru**, e-mail: bangalore@jaypeebrothers.com
- **Chennai**, e-mail: chennai@jaypeebrothers.com
- **Delhi**, e-mail: jaypee@jaypeebrothers.com
- **Hyderabad**, e-mail: hyderabad@jaypeebrothers.com
- **Kochi**, e-mail: kochi@jaypeebrothers.com
- **Kolkata**, e-mail: kolkata@jaypeebrothers.com
- **Lucknow**, e-mail: lucknow@jaypeebrothers.com
- **Mumbai**, e-mail: mumbai@jaypeebrothers.com
- **Nagpur**, e-mail: nagpur@jaypeebrothers.com

Overseas Offices
- **Central America Office, Panama City, Panama,** Ph: 001-507-317-0160
  e-mail: cservice@jphmedical.com, Website: www.jphmedical.com
- **Europe Office, UK,** Ph: +44 (0) 2031708910, e-mail: info@jpmedpub.com

Platinum Notes: Preclinical Sciences (2012-13) (Volume–1)

© 2012, Jaypee Brothers Medical Publishers

First Edition: **2010**
Second Edition: **2011**
Third Edition: **2012**
ISBN : 978-93-5025-916-0
Typeset at JPBMP typesetting unit
Printed in **India**

Contributors

Ghulam Hassan MBBS MS
Ex-Prof and Head
Anatomy, GMC, Srinagar

Zahida Rasool MBBS
Medical Consultant
IUST Awantipora, Kashmir

Muneeb Ul Hassan MBBS
Assistant Surgeon
Directorate of Health Services Kashmir

Shabinul Hassan BDS
Resident SKIMS Soura

Life so short, the art so long...-Hippocrates

Preface

The news of **NEET** and changing pattern of the Examinations of **AIPG, AIIMS, DNB** and state level exams prompt me to introduce new changes with new ideas and new topics for the third edition of Platinum notes.

I am hence once again pleased to present a newer, more simplified, interesting, easy, palatable, lucid and High yield book for the Medical students.

After an excellent positive feedback and unexpected success of the First Edition and Second Edition of Platinum Notes, I am pleased to again update Platinum notes and present the Third Edition of Platinum Notes.

It gave me immense pleasure and satisfaction to read the comments for my book from students all over the country.

The book because of its contents and the amount of concentrated knowledge contained in it has been not only been able to compete but also surpass its counterparts. This gives me immense satisfaction taking into account that Platinum has been able to achieve a great place during its first edition only and I would provide my little amount of wisdom hopefully annually updating Platinum on yearly basis to tailor the book to the needs of Medical students.

A Substantial feedback from students especially preparing for AIPGE Examinations has prompted me to bring this third edition best suited for this examination and I would thank the appreciators of my book for all their comments. But at the same time I would be more thankful to the critics who pointed out certain deficiencies in my first edition and due to their healthy criticism I have been able to add what was deficient.

I thank medical students from all over India especially the students of Maharashtra, Rajasthan, Delhi, Karnataka, Tamil Nadu, Uttar Pradesh, Bihar, Kerala, Kolkata and Jharkhand for their feedback. In the first instance I would not have expected the response but thanks to Almighty for everything.

I would like to express great satisfaction at my personal level as to the feedback of students appearing for AIIMS, PGI, DNB, UPSC for their continuous feedback via emails.

I would like to express my apology to all those students to whose queries I could not respond via email. I hope you will continue guiding me similarly in future as well.

Wishing you a good academic career.

Ashfaq Ul Hassan

Acknowledgments

No word would be sufficient to thank the **Almighty** for all the necessary guidance and courage he provided me throughout my life and especially for preparation of this project and blessings to **Prophet Muhammad** [(PBUH)].

I would firstly like to express my special gratitude to my parents particularly my father **Prof Ghulam Hassan,** Ex-Prof and Head, Anatomy, GMC Srinagar who has been a role academic model to me and provided me guidance, necessary facilities and most of all good wishes. Without his guidance and support I would not have been able to accomplish this task. As a consequence of constant interaction with him, I have learnt the maximum in my life.

I would like to take this as an opportunity to thank my academically brilliant and favorite teachers from whom I have imbibed a lot. I would wholeheartedly like to express my thanks to my seniors, academically brilliant colleagues who have laid a major emphasis on my life. I personally and whole heartedly acknowledge the following:

- Prof Ghulam Hassan MS Ex-Prof and Head, Department of Anatomy, GMC Srinagar
- Prof Showqat Zargar Prof and Head Gastroenterology Department/Director SKIMS, Soura
- Prof AR Trag Vice Chancellor, IUST, Awantipora
- Prof GQ Allaqaband MD Ex-Principal, Ex Head Deptt of Medicine, GMC/SMHS Srinagar
- Dr Sheikh Aijaz Additional Professor Surgery, SKIMS Soura
- Prof Mehraj Din Ex Director SKIMS Soura
- Prof Saleh Al Damegh, Director Al Raji Group of Colleges, KSA
- Prof Abdullah Al Gasham Dean Al Qasim University, KSA
- Prof Khursheed Iqbal Dean DM Cardiology, SKIMS Soura
- Prof AH Ahanger HOD CVTS SKIMS, Soura
- Prof Syed Amin Tabish, Head Hospital Adminstration, SKIMS Soura
- Prof AH Zargar Prof and Head Endocrinology, Ex-Director SKIMS, Soura
- Prof Pervez Shah DM Neurology, SMHS Hospital Srinagar
- Dr Tanveer Masood MD Professor, Medicine, SMHS Srinagar
- Prof Riyaz Unthoo MBBS MS, Head of The Department Opthomology, SKIMS Bemina
- Dr Arshad Farooq MBBS MD Paediatrics, SKIMS Bemina
- Dr Masood Kirmani MBBS MS Head of The Department, ENT, SKIMS, Bemina
- Dr Khursheed MBBS MD Head Microbiology, SKIMS Bemina
- Dr Rashid MBBS MD Head Pathology, SKIMS, Bemina
- Dr Manzoor, Consultant Dermatology, SKIMS Bemina
- Dr Rifat MBBS MD, Head Obstetrics/Gynaecology, SKIMS Bemina
- Prof Anil Bhan MS Mch CVTS Surgeon, Med City, Gurgaon, Delhi
- Prof Sameer Kaul Consultant Oncologist, New Delhi
- Dr Sajjad Reshi MRCP Interventional, Cardiologist, Cardiff, UK
- Dr Sunil Munshi MRCP Consultant Leicster General Hospital, Leicester, UK
- Dr AY Izideen MRCS Consultant Surgeon, Prince Charles Hospital, UK
- Dr Manzoor Dar MS MRCS, UK
- Dr Maki Alvi Ashraf, MRCOG Consultant Gynaecologist, UK
- Prof Altaf MS MRCS, Prince Charles Hospital, UK
- Prof RN Bargotra, Ex-Prof and Head, GMC, Jammu
- Dr RD Mehra Prof, Department of Anatomy, AIIMS, New Delhi
- Prof Showqat Jeelani Head Surgery Department, SMHS, Srinagar

- Dr Asif MBBS MS, Consultant ENT, SKIMS Bemina
- Dr Riyaz Malik MBBS MD, Lecturer, Paediatrics, SKIMS Bemina
- Dr Nusrat MBBS MS Lecturer, Opthomology, SKIMS Bemina
- Dr Ashfaq Bhat MBBS MD Lecturer SPM, SKIMS, Bemina
- Dr Afiya MBBS MD Pathology, Lecturer SKIMS Bemina
- Dr Sajid Wani MBBS Tutor Demonstrator, Microbiology, SKIMS Bemina
- Dr Talib Khan Lecturer Anesthesiology, SMHS Srinagar

Special Mention of My Favorite, Academically Brilliant Teachers
- Prof Ghulam Hassan Ex-Prof and Head Anatomy GMC Srinagar
- Prof Pervez Shah MD DM Neurology, SMHS Srinagar
- Dr Tanveer Masood MD Associate Prof, Medicine, SMHS Srinagar
- Dr Rouf Ahamed MS Prof ENT Department SMHS Srinagar
- (Late) Dr Tajamul Assistant Surgeon Medicine, SMHS Srinagar
- Mr TN Kaul Teacher CMS, Tyndale Biscoe School, Srinagar

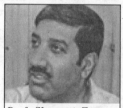
Prof. **Showqat Zargar**

"I am extremely obliged to Prof Showqat Zargar MBBS MD DM Director and Head Department of Gastroenterology SKIMS, Soura for his help, support and moral boosting approach, guidance for this project and allowing me to be a Member and a part of SKIMS fraternity."

No words to express my gratitude to **Dr Zahida Rasool**, Medical Consultant for her help in contributing their academic skills and all needed support help for every part during the preparation of this book. Her idea and effort at adding vital information and latest topics has been a real help.

The acceptance of my work by **Shri Jitendar P Vij** (Chairman and Managing Director) and overall incharge of Jaypee Brothers Medical Publishers (P) Ltd. and his interest and overall supervision of the whole project deserves special thanks.

I would specially like to express my renewed gratitude and thanks to **Mr Bhupesh Arora** (General Manager) Jaypee Brothers Medical Publishers (P) Ltd. for his improved suggestions for third edition. His constant help, guidance and exhaustive interaction throughout the course of preparation of this book has been of immense help. It has taken long, interactive and detailed sessions between both of us which have helped in making the project a success. I admire the working ability and highly professional attitude of this gentle man.

I would like to thank **Manas Yadav & Tahira Parveen** for all expertise at printing and giving the final look of the book and working really hard on the project. His effort at final formatting of the book has been commendable.

Author /Editor in Chief:

Ashfaq Ul Hassan

I would like suggestions from the readers of this book, not only for improving the quality of the book but also for aiding all future candidates in their career.
Contact: *ashhassan@rediffmail.com*

From the Publisher's Desk

We request all the readers to provide us their valuable suggestions/errors (if any) at:
jaypeemcqproduction@gmail.com

so as to help us in further improvement of this book in the subsequent edition.

Abbreviations

1°	Primary		A/W or a/w	Associated with
2°	Secondary		BBB	Bundle branch block
#	Fracture		bid	Twice a day
ACE	Angiotensin converting enzyme		BMR	Basal metabolic rate
ACE-I	Angiotensin converting enzyme inhibitor		BP	Blood pressure
ACTH	Adrenocorticotropic hormone		BPH	Benign prostatic hypertrophy
ACh	Acetylcholine		BUN	Blood urea nitrogen
Adr	Adrenaline		B/L	Bilateral
AD	Autosomal dominant		BM	Bone marrow, basement membrane
ADH	Anti-diuretic hormone		b/n or b/w	Between
AF	Atrial fibrillation		C/S	Culture and sensitivity
AFB	Acid-fast bacilli		Ca2+	Calcium
AFP	Alpha-fetoprotein		CABG	Coronary artery bypass graft
A.k.a	Also known as		CAD	Coronary artery disease
ALL	Acute lymphocytic leukemia		CCF	Congestive cardiac failure
AML	Acute myelogenous leukemia		CT	Computerized tomography
ANA	Antinuclear antibody		CHF	Congestive heart failure
ANS	Autonomic nervous system		CHO	Carbohydrate
AP	Anteroposterior		CML	Chronic myelogenous leukemia
AR	Autosomal recessive		CMV	Cytomegalovirus
ARDS	Acute respiratory distress syndrome		CN	Cranial nerves
ARF	Acute renal failure		CNS	Central nervous system
AS	Aortic stenosis		CO	Cardiac output
ATP	Adenosine triphosphate		C/O	Complaining of
ASD	Atrial septal defect		COLD	Chronic obstructive lung disease
AV	Atrioventricular		COPD	Chronic obstructive pulmonary disease
A/E	All except		CPK	Creatine phosphokinase
Acc/ to	According to		CRF	Chronic renal failure
Ad/E, ad/e	Adverse effects		CRP	C-reactive protein

CSF	Cerebrospinal fluid		EUA	Examination under anesthesia
CVA	Cerebrovascular accident		FBS	Fasting blood sugar
CVP	Central venous pressure		FEV	Forced expiratory volume
CVS	Cardiovascular system		FFP	Fresh frozen plasma
CXR	Chest X-ray		FRC	Functional residual capacity
Ca	Carcinoma/Cancer		FTT	Failure to thrive
C/c	Complication		FVC	Forced vital capacity
C_T	Chemotherapy		FA	Fatty acid
C/I	Contraindication		FFA	Free fatty acid
CI/f	Clinical features		GFR	Glomerular filtration rate
CTD	Connective tissue disease		GH	Growth hormone
Cont./L	Contralateral		GIT	Gastrointestinal tract
Cx	Cervix		GTT	Glucose tolerance test
D and C	Dilation and curettage		GU	Genitourinary
DI	Diabetes insipidus		HAV	Hepatitis A virus
DIC	Disseminated intravascular coagulopathy		HCG	Human chorionic gonadotropin
DIP	Distal interphalangeal joint		HDL	High density lipoprotein
DKA	Diabetic ketoacidosis		Hb	Hemoglobin
dL	Deciliter		HIV	Human immunodeficiency virus
DM	Diabetes mellitus		HLA	Histocompatibility locus antigen
DTR	Deep tendon reflexes		H/O	History of
DVT	Deep venous thrombosis		HR	Heart rate
d/to	Due to		HSV	Herpes simplex virus
D/g	Diagnosis		HTN	Hypertension
DOC	Drug of choice		HS	Hereditary cpherocytosis
Ds, d/s	Disease, disease		HCC	Hepato cellular carcinoma
DM	Diabeties mellitus		HD	Hodgkin's cisease
ECG	Electrocardiogram		I and D	Incision and drainage
ECT	Electroconvulsive therapy		IDDM	Insulin dependent diabetes mellitus
ECHO	Echocardiography		Ig	Immunoglobulin
EMG	Electromyogram		IM	Intramuscular
EOM	Extraocular muscles		INR	International normalized ratio
ESR	Erythrocyte sedimentation rate		ITP	Idiopathic thrombocytopenic purpura
ERCP	Endoscopic retrograde cholangio-		IV	Intravenous
	pancreatography		IVP	Intravenous pyelogram

IVU	Intravenous urogram	OCG	Oral cholecystogram
ICT	Intracranial tension	PA	Posteroanterior
IOC	Investigation of choice	PDA	Patent ductus arteriosus
ILD	Interstitial lung disease	PMN	Polymorphonuclear leukocyte (neutrophil)
IOT	Intraocular tension	PP	Patient profile
Ipsi/L	Ipsilateral	PT	Prothrombin time, or physical therapy
JVP	Jugular venous pressure	PTCA	Percutaenous transluminal coronary angioplasty
K+	Potassium	PTH	Parathyroid hormone
K/as	Known as	PTT	Partial thromboplastin time
LAE	Left atrial enlargement	P/g	Prognosis
LBBB	Left bundle branch block	P_x	Prophylaxis
LDH	Lactate dehydrogenase	PBC	Primary bilary cirrhosis
LMN	Lower motor neuron	RA	Rheumatoid arthritis
LE	Lupus erythematosus	RBBB	Right bundle branch block
LP	Lumbar puncture	RBC	Red blood cell
LV	Left ventricle	RIA	Radioimmunoassay
LVH	Left ventricular hypertrophy	RNA	Ribonucleic acid
LN	Lymph node	RTA	Renal tubular acidosis
MAO	Monoamine oxidase	RVH	Right ventricular hypertrophy
MEN	Multiple endocrine neoplasia	Rx	Treatment
MI	Myocardial infarction or mitral insufficiency	R, or T/t	Treatment
mL	Milliliter	R_T	Radiotherapy
MMR	Measles, mumps, rubella	SBE	Subacute bacterial endocarditis
MRI	Magnetic resonance imaging	SGOT	Serum glutamic-oxaloacetic transaminase
MRSA	Methicillin resistant staph aureus	SGPT	Serum glutamic-pyruvic transaminase
MG	Myasthenia gravis	SIADH	Syndrome of inappropriate antidiuretic hormone
Mc or MC	Most common	SLE	Systemic lupus erythematous
MN	Malnutrition	SCLC	Small cell lung carcinoma
M/m	Management	SM	Smooth muscle
Ms, m/s	Muscle	Supf.	Superficial
Na	Sodium	SqCC	Squamous cell carcinoma
NIDDM	Non-insulin dependent diabetes mellitus	TIBC	Total iron binding capacity
NSAID	Non-steroidal anti-inflammatory drugs	tid	Three times a day
n.or nv	Nerve	TSH	Thyroid stimulating hormone
NHL	Non-Hodgkin's lymphoma	TT	Thrombin time

TTP	Thrombotic thrombocytopenic purpura	**vWD**	von Willebrand's virus
TURP	Transurethral resection of prostate	**VZV**	Varicella zoster virus
TOC	Treatment of choice	**V/s**	Vessel
UC	Ulcerative colitis	**Vs**	Versus (= against)
UMN	Upper motor neuron	**WBC**	White blood cell
URI	Upper respiratory infection	**WPW**	Wolff-Parkinson-White
US, U/S	Ultrasound	**WG**	Wegner's granulomatosis
UTI	Urinary tract infection	**WT**	Wilm's tumor
UVA	Ultraviolet A light	**XLR**	X linked recessive
U/L	Unilateral	**Yr**	Year
VF	Ventricular fibrillation	**Zn**	Zinc
VDRL	Venereal disease research laboratory	**ZES**	Zollinger Ellison Syndrome
	(test for syphilis)	——	Reaction block by, inhibited by
V/Q	Ventrilation-perfusion	~	Denotes heading
VT	Ventricular tachycardia	!	Increase

Contents

1. Anatomy .... 1 - 122

2. Physiology .... 123 - 206

3. Biochemistry .... 207 - 278

4. Forensic .... 279 - 314

5. Microbiology .... 315 - 398

6. Pathology .... 399 - 496

7. Pharmacology .... 497 - 616

8. Social and Preventive Medicine .... 617 - 712

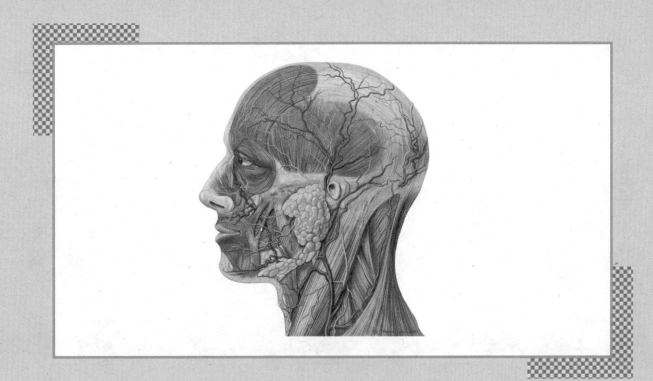

ANATOMY

"The text contains Highly Concentrated Topics which are highly likely to be asked in the Examinations. A student is suggested to read the below text with high degree of concentration and depth. Multiple revisions are advised."

Father of Modern Anatomy: Vesalius	TN 2007

➲ Important Vessels and Source of Bleeding:

☐	Hemoptysis:	Bronchial artery ☞☞	
☐	**Duodenal** ulcer:	Gastroduodenal artery☞	**AIIMS 2011**
☐	**Gastric** ulcer:	Left Gastric artery	
☐	SDH:	Bridging veins ☞☞	
☐	EDH:	Middle meningeal artery ☞☞☞	**UPSC 2000**
☐	Tonsillectomy:	Paratonsillar **vein** ☞☞	**AI 1990**
☐	Menstruation:	Spiral arteries	

➲ Structure Eroded in Posterior Duodenal Perforation: Gastroduodenal Artery

Posterior wall perforation leads to bleeding due to involvement of **gastroduodenal artery** that lies posterior to the 1st part of duodenum.	**AIIMS 2011**

➲ Important Membranes in Body (High Yield for 2011/2012)

☐	Huxles Membrane	**Inner layer** of cells of root sheath of hair	**AIIMS 1995**
☐	Henles Membrane	**Outer layer** of cells of root sheath of hair☞☞	**AIIMS 1995**
☐	Bowmans Membrane	"**Anterior**" limiting membrane of **Cornea**☞☞	
☐	Decemet's Membrane	"**Posterior**" limiting membrane of **Cornea**	
☐	Bruchs Membrane	**Pigment** membrane in **Retina**☞☞	
☐	Elschings Membrane	Astroglial membrane covering **Optic Disk**☞☞	
☐	Heusers Membrane	**Exocelomic** Membrane	
☐	Sharpnells Membrane	Pars Flaccida of the tympanic membrane	**MP 2007**

➲ Eponym Ducts:

☐	Parotid duct:	Stensons duct☞☞
		(*opens opposite upper 2nd molar in vestibule of mouth*). MAH 2012
☐	Submandibular duct:	**Whartons duct.**☞
☐	Pancreatic duct:	**Wirsungs duct** ☞☞
☐	**Accessory** pancreatic duct:	**Santoniris duct**☞
☐	Gartners duct:	**Remanant of Mesonephric duct (WOLLFIAN)**	DNB 2008
☐	Thoracic duct:	**Pecquets duct**☞	PGI 1999

1

ANATOMY

➲ Important Anatomical Lines Commonly Asked:

- **Hiltons line:** At level of interval between subcutaneous part of external sphincter and lower border of internal anal sphincter. Felt as a groove on digital examination
- **Pectinate line:** Circular line of attachment of anal valves.
- **Holdens line:** Lateral to pubic tubercle about 8 cms. prevents extravasation of urine into lower limb
- **Reids base line:** Horizontal line between infraorbital margin and centre of external acoustic meatus.

➲ High Yield for 2011-2012 Types of Cells:

Continuously dividing cells or Labile cells:

- Epithelial cells
- Cells of bone marrow & hemopoietic tissue.

Quiescent cells or Stable cells:

- Can undergo division in response to stimuli.
- Are in Go phase but can go into Gl.
- Cells include
- **Parenchymal cells of liver,** kidney, pancreas,
- Mesenchymal cells,
- Fibroblasts,
- Smooth muscles & vascular endothelium.

Non-diving cells or Permanent cells

- Nerve cells
- Skeletal & cardiac muscle cells.

➲ Important Canals in Histology:

- **Herrings Canal:**
  Fine terminal ductules lined by cuboidal epithelium lining Intralobular bile canaliculi with bile ducts in portal canals
- **Petit Canal:**
  Space between zonules of Zinn and Viterous humor
- **Rosenthals Canal:**
  Spiral canal of Cochlea
- **Schelmms Canal:**
  Canal at sclerocorneal junction   UPSC 2003
- **Volkmans Canal:**
  Osseous canal carrying **blood supply from periosteum**
- **Haversian Canal:**
  Neurovascular channel around which the **lamella arranged in concentric cylinders in a bone**

1

➲ Other Important Canals: (High Yield for 2011/2012)

☐ **Haversian canals:** central vascular channels in Haversian systems;

☐ **Guyon's canal:** canal for the **ulnar nerve and vessels**; defined medially by the pisiform, and posteriorly by the flexor retinaculum.

☐ **Hunter's canal:** Canalis adductorius. The adductor canal.

☐ **Alcock's canal:** canalis pudendalis

☐ **Dorello's canal:** An opening sometimes found in the temporal bone through which the abducens nerve and inferior petrosal sinus together enter the cavernous sinus.

☐ **Canal of Nuck:** A diverticulum of the peritoneal membrane extending into the inguinal canal, accompanying the round ligament in the female, or the testis in its descent into the scrotum in the male; usually completely obliterated in the female.

☐ **Stilling's canal :** A minute canal running through the vitreous from the discus nervi optici to the lens

☐ **Palatovaginal canal:** Transmits **pharyngeal branch from pterygopalatine ganglion and pharyngeal branch from maxillary artery**

☐ **Vomerovaginal canal :** Transmits **pharyngeal vessels and nerves**

➲ Important Cells in Histology: (High Yield for 2011/2012)

☐ **Stave cells:** special cells linning spleeinc sinusoids

☐ **Tanycytes:** Special cells linning ventricles of brain

☐ **Littoral cells:** phagocytic cells lining **capillaries**

☐ **Rouget cells:** Phagocytic cells lining **sinusoids**

➲ Usually Asked in AIIMS/PGI/AIPGME

☐	Bergmann Cells		→	Glial cells of Cerebellum
☐	Gitter cells	KERALA 2001	→	Microglia
☐	Intersititial cells of Cajal		→	Nerve cells of superficial layers of cerebral cortex
☐	Supporting cells of Claudius		→	Cells in floor of Cochlear canal of inner ear
☐	Dieters Cells ☞		→	Outer hair cells of organ of Corti
☐	Hensens cells		→	Supporting cells in organ of Corti external to Dieters cells
☐	Houfbauers Cells	AMU 1991	→	Ellipsoidal cells in chorionic villi of placenta
☐	JG cells	ROHTAK 1987	→	Smooth muscle cells of affarent arteriole. (Kidney)
☐	Ito Cells ☞☞	PGI 1999	→	Stellate cells in liver
☐	Langerhans cells ☞☞ ✳		→	Antigen presenting epithelial dendritic cells
☐	Langhans Cells ☞☞ ✳		→	Cytotrophoblastic cells of chorionic villi
☐	Basket Cells		→	Myoepithelial cells in salivary/mammary/sweat glands
☐	Gitter cells	KERALA 2001	→	Microglia of brain
☐	Basket Cells of Cerebellum		→	Neurons of molecular layer of Cerebellum
☐	Merkel Cells		→	Sensory nerve endings
☐	Muller's Cells ☞	COMED 2005	→	Neuroglial cells in Retina
☐	Hilus cells☞		→	Rare cells found in Medulla of Ovary at Hilum of Ovary
☐	Lacis Cells☞☞		→	Extra glomerular Mesengial Cells outside Glomerulus
☐	Peg Cells ☞		→	Secretory cells in mucosa of uterine tube
☐	Glomus Cells ☞	COMED 2002	→	Present in Carotid Bodies

Eponyms	Description
Bowman's capsule	Glomerular capsule of the kidney seen on histology slides
Bowman's membrane	Layer in the cornea below epithelium seen on histology slides
Brunner's glands	Glands in the duodenum seen on histology slides
Bundle of His	Atrioventricular bundle
Cords of Billroth	Splenic cords of the spleen seen on histology slides
Crypts of Lieberkuhn	Epithelial glands in the small intestine seen on histology slides
Descemet's membrane	Limiting layer of the cornea seen on histology slides
Ducts of Bellini	Papillary duct of the kidney seen on histology slides
Ducts of Luschka	Small ducts found in the connective tissue between the gallbladder and the liver
Golgi aparatus	Intracellular organelle
Golgi tendon organ	Sensory nerve ending embedded in a tendon for proprioception
Graafian follicle	Tertiary follicle of an ovary seen on a histology slide
Haversian canal	Central canal of an osteon of bone seen on a histology slide
Haversian system	Osteon of bone seen on a histology slide
Islets of Langerhans	Pancreatic islets of the pancreas seen on histology slides
Leydig cells	Interstitial cells of the testis
Loop of Henle	U shaped loop in the nephron of the kidney
Krause end bulbs	Cylindrical/oval sensory receptor
Malpighian corpuscle	Renal corpuscle of the kidney seen on histology slides
Meissner's corpuscle	Mechanoreceptor
Meissner 's plexus	Submucosal plexus
Merkel's disc	Tactile receptor
Moll's gland	Glands of the conjunctiva
Nissl bodies	Rough endoplasmic reticulum of a neuron
Node of Ranvier	Rrea between two Schwann cells covering nerve fibers with axon which is not covered by myelin
Organ of Corti	Small organ of sound transduction; spiral organ
Pacinian corpuscle	Lamellar corpuscle
Peyer's patches	Aggregates of lymphatic tissue in the ileum seen on histology slides

cont...

cont...

Purkinje fibers	Part of the conducting system of the <u>heart</u>
Renal columns of Bertin	Renal columns seen on histology slides
Ruffini's corpuscle	<u>Sensory receptor</u>
Space of Disse	Perisinosoidal space of the <u>liver</u> seen on histology slides
Volkmann's canals	Perforating canals of <u>bone</u>
Wharton's jelly	Mucous connective tissue seen in umbilical cord

➲ Valves of Body:

☐ Hasners valve	☐ Nasolacrimal duct JKBOPEE 2012
☐ Thebesian valve.	☐ Valve of the coronary sinus
☐ Heisters valve	☐ Valves of the duct of gallbladder cystic duct
☐ Valves of Kerckring	☐ Valves at The mucosal surface of the small intestine contains numerous circular mucosal folds

➲ Diaphragms of Body:

- ▶ Diaphragm of **oral cavity**: Mylohyoid ☞   JKBOPEE 2012
- ▶ Diaphragm of **Superior thoracic aperture**: Sibsons Fascia ☞ ☞
- ▶ **Pelvic** diaphragm: Levator ani and coccygeus ☞ ☞
- ▶ **Urogenital** diaphragm: Deep transverse perinei and sphincter urethrae, perineal membrane.   AI 2010
- ▶ **Diaphragm sella**: fold of duramater overlying pituitary fossa ☞ ☞
- ▶ **Iris diaphragm**: in eye ☞

➲ Eponym Fascias (Repeated in exams)

▶ Toldts fascia:	✓ **Anterior** renal fascia ☞
▶ Zuckerkandl fascia:	✓ **Posterior** renal facia ☞
▶ Bucks fascia:	✓ **Deep** fascia of **penis** AMU 1986
▶ Denonvillers fascia:	✓ Fascia separating <u>Rectum from Prostate</u> ☞ ☞ KAR 2008 DNB 2011 KCET 2012
▶ Waldeyers fascia:	✓ fascia separating <u>Rectum from Coccyx</u> ☞ ☞
▶ Campers fascia	✓ **Superficial fatty layer** of superficial fascia
▶ Scarpas fascia	✓ **Deep membranous layer** of Superficial fascia
▶ Fascia Colli	✓ Investing layer of **deep cervical fascia of neck** ☞ ☞
▶ Fascia transversalis	✓ Forms **anterior wall** of femoral sheath
▶ Fascia iliaca	✓ Forms **posterior wall** of femoral sheath
▶ Pelvic fascia	✓ Forms hypogastric sheath AI 2010

1

⊃ Important Triangles in Anatomy (Frequently asked)

⇨ Triangle of Koch ✳✳✳

Is bounded by	PGI 2005
✓ Tricuspid valve,	
✓ Margin of coronary sinus opening,	
✓ Tendon of Todaro.	AIIMS 2003

It is a part of **fibrous skeleton of the heart**.

The **tendon of Todaro** is a continuation of the Eustachian Valve of the Inferior vena cava and the **Thebesian valve** of the coronary sinus. Along with the opening of the coronary sinus and the **septal cusp of the tricuspid valve** it makes up **the triangle of Koch**. The centre of the triangle of Koch is the location of the **atrioventricular node**. It makes up **the triangle of Koch**. The centre of the triangle of Koch is the location of the **atrioventricular node**.

⇨ Triangle of Auscultation: ✳

Only part of back not covered by muscles.	JK BOPEE
Respiratory sounds are best heard here.	
Boundaries:	
✓ **Medial border of scapula laterally**	DNB 2008
✓ **Lateral border of trapezius medially**	DNB 2008
✓ **Upper border of latissmus dorsi inferiorly**	

Is a small triangular space on the back where the relatively thin musculature allows for respiratory sounds to be heard more clearly with a stethoscope.

The floor is formed by

7th rib

6th & 7th intercostal spaces

Rhomboideus major

On the left side, the **cardiac orifice of the stomach** lies deep to the triangle, and in days before X-rays were discovered the sounds of swallowed liquids were auscultated over this triangle.

⇨ Triangle of Petit: ✳

✓ **Superiorly: 12 th rib**
✓ **Inferiorly: Iliac crest**
✓ **Laterally: Posterior border of External oblique muscle**

⇨ **Lessers Triangle:✱✱**

✓ Hypoglossal nerve above
✓ Two bellies of digastric on either sides

⇨ **Hasselbachs Triangle:✱✱✱**

Bounded by	PGI 1985
✓ Lateral margin of Rectus Abdominis Medially,	
✓ Inferior epigastric artery laterally and	
✓ Inguinal ligament inferiorly	

⇨ **Triangle of Doom:**

✓ Gonadal vessels laterally	AIIMS 2008
✓ Vas deferens medially	

⇨ **Mc Ewans Suprameatal Triangle:**

Triangular depression posterior to external acoustic meatus.	JK BOPEE 2011
✓ It is bounded by posterosuperior margin of external acoustic meatus,	
✓ Supramastoid crest and	
✓ A vertical line tangent to posterior border of external acoustic meatus	

⇨ **Triangle of Pain:**

Lateral to triangle of doom.
✓ Gonadal vessels medially
✓ Iliopubic tract laterally
✓ Inferiorly by inferior edge of skin incision.

⇨ **Circle of Death:**

Called corona mortis. It is a vascular ring formed by an arterial network ,
✓ Common iliac artery,
✓ Internal iliac artery,
✓ External iliac artery,
✓ Obturator artery,
✓ Accessory obturator artery and
✓ Inferior epigastric artery.

⇨ **Trautman Triangle:**

➠ Anterior: bony labyrinth
➠ Posteriorly: sigmoid sinus
➠ Above: superior petrosal sinus

1

ANATOMY

⇨ Delto pectoral triangle: infraclavicular fossa

⊃ **Important Angles: (High Yield for 2011/2012)**

→ Neck shaft angle of <u>femur</u> in adults: 125°. More in females

→ Angle of femoral torsion: 15°

→ **Carrying angle**: Angle made by long axis of arm with long axis of forearm. 170°

→ Angle of <u>humeral</u> torsion: 164°

→ **Renal angle**: junction of 12 th rib with erector spinae muscle

→ **Lovibonds angle**: angle between nail plate and proximal nail fold

→ **Sternal angle**: angle of Louis

→ **Citteles angle**: Sino dural angle

→ **Alpha angle** : (in eye) between visual axis and optical axis

→ **Kappa angle**: (in eye) between pupillary axes

→ **Cobbs angle**: used in scoliosis

➥ **Cubitus valgus** is increase in carrying angle. Feature of Turners syndrome.

➥ **Coxa vera**: reduction in neck shaft angle of femur

➥ **Coxa valga**: increase in neck shaft angle of femur

⊃ **Lengths of Important Structures Commonly Asked: (High Yield for 2011/2012)**

❑ Female urethra:	✓ 4 cms	
❑ Male urethra:	✓ 18-20 cms	Kerala 2008
❑ Spinal cord,	✓ 18 inches or 45 cms	
❑ Femur,	✓ 18 inches or 45 cms	
❑ Vas defrens,	✓ 18 inches or 45 cms	
❑ Thoraxic duct:	✓ 18 inches or 45 cms	
❑ Ureter:	✓ 10 inches	
❑ Esophagus:	✓ 10 inches	UPSC 2005
❑ Trachea:	✓ 4-6 inches	

Remember:

⇨ **Tortuous arteries**✶

❑ Facial artery➤➤	
❑ Splenic artery➤	
❑ Uterine artery➤➤	DNB 2011, KCET 2012
❑ Vaginal artery➤	
❑ Ophthalmic artery➤	
❑ Lingual artery➤	
❑ PICA (Post Inferior <u>Cerebellar</u> Artery)➤	

⇨ **END ARTERIES:**

☐ Central artery of retina

☐ Central branches of cerebral artery

☐ Coronary artery

☐ Segmental branches of renal/spleenic artery

⇨ **Foramina asked in Exams:**

—	Foramen of **Morgagni** refers to an opening in: **The Diaphragm**	DNB 2006
—	Foramen of Winslow is: **Between greater and lesser sac**	DNB 2006
—	Foramen of **Magendie, Lushka** are related to fourth ventricle	
—	Foramen of **Monro** is Interventricular foramen.(Brain)	
—	Foramen of **Vesalius** (Emisary Sphenoidal Foramen)	

➲ **Important Arteries and Their Branches: High yield for 2011-2012**

Axillary artery

✓ Is continuation of **subclavian** artery.

✓ Pectoralis **minor** divides it into three Branches:-

▶ Ist part:

    o **Superior thoracic artery.**   **AIIMS 1998**

▶ 2nd part:

    o **Thoracoacromial artery.**

    o **Lateral thoracic artery.**

▶ 3rd part:

    o **Subscapular artery.**

    o **Anterior circumflex humeral artery.**

    o **Posterior circumflex humeral artery.**

⇨ **Internal carotid artery:**

➥ *No branches in neck*

➥ Caroticotypanic

➥ Pterygoid

➥ Cavernous branch to trigeminal ganglion

➥ Superior and inferior hypophyseal

➥ Opthalmic

➥ Anterior cerebral

➥ Middle cerebral

➥ Posterior communicating

➥ Anterior choridal

1

ANATOMY

⇨ **External carotid artery:**

- Superior thyroid
- Lingual
- Facial
- Occipital
- Posterior auricular
- Ascending pharyngeal
- Maxillary
- Superficial temporal

⇨ **Subclavian artery:**

- Vertebral artery,
- Internal thoraxic artery,
- Thyrocervical trunk (Inferior thyroid, suprascapular, superficial cervical)
- Costocervical trunk (Superior intercostal, Deep cervical)

⇨ **Vertebral artery:**

- Spinal
- Muscular
- Meningeal
- Anterior spinal
- Posterior spinal
- Posterior inferior cerebellar
- Medullary

⇨ **Basilar artery:**

- **Formed by union of two vertebral arteries:**
- Posterior cerebral arteries
- Superior cerebellar
- Pontine
- Labrynthine
- Anterior inferior cerebellar

⇨ **Internal iliac artery:**

- ✓ Is **smaller** terminal branch of common iliac artery.
- ✓ It is about one and half inches long (3-3.5cm).
- ✓ It begins in front of **sacroiliac joint.**
- ✓ It divides into ant. and post. Divisions at upper margin of greater sciatic notch.

Branches from <u>Anterior Division</u>: - (Six in males and seven in females.)
- ✓ Superior vesical artery.
- ✓ Inf vesical.   COMED 2003
- ✓ Obturator
- ✓ Middle rectal
- ✓ Inf. Gluteal.
- ✓ Internal pudendal
- ✓ In females, inferior vesical is replaced by vaginal artery
- ✓ Uterine artery is the 7th branch in females.   UPSC 2001

Branches from <u>Posterior Division</u>:
- ✓ Superior gluteal.
- ✓ Ilio lumbar.
- ✓ Lateral sacral.

⇨ **Questions asked in various examinations:**

▶ Inferior thyroid artery is a branch of:	Throcervical trunk	✓	PGI 2003
▶ Ascending pharyngeal artery is a branch of	External carotid artery	✓	TN 2004
▶ Internal pudendal artery in females is a branch of	Internal iliac artery	✓	DELHI 1992
▶ Left gastroepiploic artery is a branch of	Spleenic artery	✓	AI 1989
▶ Spleenic artery is a branch of	Celiac trunk	✓	PGI 1988
▶ Uterine artery is a branch of	Internal iliac artery	✓	PGI, UPSC 1989
▶ Cystic artery is a branch of	Right hepatic artery	✓	PGI 2001
▶ Cilio retinal artery is a branch of	Choridal artery	✓	TN 2002
▶ Middle meningeal artery is a branch of	Maxillary artery	✓	UPSC 1986
▶ Anterior spinal artery is a branch of	Veretebral artery	✓	PGI 1993
▶ Opthalmic artery is a branch of	Internal carotid artery	✓	PGI 1993

⇨ **Female gametogenesis**

▶ Oogonia are derived from yolk sac	MAHE 1998
▶ Germ cells are derived from yolk sac	ICS 2005
▶ Polar bodies are formed during oogenesis	AI 2006
▶ Polar bodies are extruded *24 hrs prior to ovulation*.	AI 2008

⇨ **Male gametogenesis**

▶ Spermatogenesis occurs at temperature lower than body temperature.	AI 2008
▶ Y chromosome is ACROCENTRIC.	AIIMS 2007
▶ In absence of Y chromosome ovaries develop.	AIIMS 2007
▶ Sperms are stored in epididymis.	AIIMS 1993
▶ Length of mature human sperm is 50-60 microns.	DNB 1992

⇨ **Chromosomal configuration of important cells in Gonads:**

Number of chromosomes in cells during Gametogenesis	
⓪ Primordial germ cell, oogonia, spermatogonia	► 46, 2N
⓪ Primary oocyte, Primary Spermatocyte	► 46, 4N
⓪ Secondary oocyte, Secondary Spermatocyte	► 23, 2N
⓪ Oocyte, Spermatid, Sperm	► 23, 1N

⊃ **Important Events and Their Time Sequence: (days)**

► Implantation occurs at :	► 6 days
► Uteroplacental circulation establishes at:	► 11-12 days
► Primitive streak appears on :	► 13- 15 th day
► Formed from:ectoderm RJ 2009	
► Angiogenesis:	► 15th day
► Closure of anterior neuropore	► 24 days ORISSA 2004
► Embryo develops by:	► 8 week
► Fetus is	► > 8 weeks

⇨ **Common Signaling Pathways Used during Development**

The differentiation of many different cell types is regulated through a relatively restricted set of molecular signaling pathways:

- **Morphogens.** These are diffusible molecules that specify which cell type will be generated at a specific anatomic location and direct the migration of cells and their processes to their final destination.
- These include

  - ✓ Retinoic acid,
  - ✓ Transforming growth factor bone morphogenetic proteins (BMPs), and
  - ✓ The hedgehog and the Wnt protein families

- **Notch/Delta.** This pathway often specifies which cell fate precursor cells will adopt.
- **Transcription factors.** This set of evolutionarily conserved proteins activates or represses downstream genes that are essential for many different cellular processes. Many transcription factors are members of the homeobox or helix-loop-helix (HLH) families. Their activity can be regulated by all of the other pathways described in this chapter.
- **Receptor tyrosine kinases (RTKs).** Many growth factors signal by binding to and activating membrane-bound RTKs. These kinases are essential for the regulation of cellular proliferation, apoptosis, and migration as well as processes such as the growth of new blood vessels and axonal processes in the nervous system.

⇨ **Fetal landmarks (weeks):**

▶ Within 1 week	▪ Implantation⭠	
▶ Within 2 week	▪ **Bilaminar** disc⭠✳	
▶ Within 3 week	▪ **Trilaminar** disc(Gastrulation)✳⭠	AI 2002
▶ Within 3 week	▪ Primitive streak begins to form,	
	▪ Notochord forms ⭠	NIMHANS 2001
▶ Within 3-8 week	▪ Organogenesis,	
	▪ Teratogen susceptibility maximum	
▶ Week 10	▪ Genitalia with male and female characters	

⇨ **Remember derivatives of**

Primitive streak :	Sacrococcygeal teratoma⭠⭠

Primitive streak
- ➡ The first sign of gastrulation is the appearance of the primitive streak
- ➡ ▪ At the beginning of the third week, an opacity formed by a thickened linear band of epiblast-the **primitive streak**-appears caudally in the median plane of the dorsal aspect of the embryonic disc. Remnants of the primitive streak may persist and give rise to a sacrococcygeal teratoma.

Remanants of Notochord:	Chordoma⭠⭠

➲ **Important Embryological Structures (Repeated in PG examinations):**

Meckel's Diverticulum✳

This true diverticulum is a remnant of the **vitelline duct** and often contains ectopic gastic mucosa which can cause bleeding and perforation. The bleeding is often painless.   AIIMS 2005

⇨ **The Ductus venosus ✳**

is a shunt that bypasses the liver and carries blood from the umbilical vein directly to the IVC. Its remnant is the **ligamentum venosum.**   TN 1988

⇨ **The Ductus arteriosus ✳**

is a shunt that bypasses the lungs to carry blood from the pulmonary artery to the aortic arch. Its remnant is the **ligamentum arteriosum.**   TN 1993

⇨ **The Urachus ✳**

becomes the **median** umbilical ligament.⭠⭠⭠   UP 2005
The **2 umbilical arteries** becomes the **medial** umbilical ligaments.⭠⭠
Urachal fistula from persistent allantois.   MAH 2000

⇨ **The Vitelline duct ✳**

is a connection with the yolk stalk and bowel, but normally obliterates during week 7 of development.

1

ANATOMY

1

ANATOMY

⇨ Umbilical cord:

- ► Connects fetus and placenta.
- ► Is rich in whartons jelly.
- ► Has 2 arteries and one vein. ☛☛   DNB 2007 AIIMS 89, TN 1989, PGI 1987
- ► <u>Rt umbilical vein disappears</u>, left is left.
- ► In case of single artery only, congenital anomalies should be excluded. ☛☛
- ► Umbilical arteries carry <u>deoxygenated blood</u>. ☛☛
- ► Umbilical arteries don't possess internal elastic lamina.
- ► Vas vasorum are absent in cases of umbilical vessels.

⇨ Stem cells ✱✱

Stem cells must be able to:

- ▪ Divide to produce sufficient cells;
- ▪ Differentiate into the cell types needed;
- ▪ Survive after transplant;
- ▪ Mesh into the surrounding tissues;
- ▪ Function properly for long enough to extend the recipient's life or to improve it significantly;
- ▪ Avoid harming the recipient.

⇨ Karyotyping

In 1961 an international meeting was held at the University of Colorado Medical School in Denver, Colorado to standardize the format for a normal human karyotype. The format that evolved is known as the "Denver System." ✱ Each chromosome has its own individuality as shown by its size, shape, and position of its kinetochore. Using the "**Denver System,**" the chromosomes are put into similar groups designated by letters. Then numbers are used to subdivide the chromosomes within the groups designated by numbers based on the position of the kinetochore and the length of the chromatids. The homologous chromosomes are paired based on their banding.

<u>X Chromosome belongs to group C</u>☛☛
<u>Y chromosome belongs to group G</u>☛☛

Group A	Ch 1,2,3
Group B	Ch 4,5
Group C	Ch 6,7,8,9,10,11,12,X
Group D	Ch 13,14,15
Group E	Ch 16,17,18
Group F	Ch 19,20
Group G	Ch 21,22,Y

⇨ **Placentation:**

1.	PLACENTA develops from chorion frondosum.		DNB 2011
2.	Weight of full developed placenta: 500 gms		MAH 2012
3.	Biscoidal placenta:	Placenta has two discs.✎✎	
4.	Lobed placenta:	Placenta divides into lobes.✎	
5.	Diffuse placenta:	Chorionic villi persist all around the blastocyst.✎	
6.	Placenta succenturaita:	Small part of placenta separated from the rest.✎	
7.	Fenestrated:	Placenta has hole in centre.✎	
8.	Circumvallate:	Edge of placenta covered by circular fold of decidua.✎	

⇨ **According to umbilical cord attachment:**

1.	**Marginal:** Marginal as well as battle dore placenta refers to placenta with cord attached to margins.✎
2.	**Furcate:** Blood vessels divide before reaching the placenta.✎
3.	**Velemantous insertion:** blood vessels are attached to amnion where they ramify before reaching the placenta.✎
4.	Two arteries and one vein are present in umblical cord.
5.	Right umblical vein disappears.

AIIMS 1991
AIIMS 1992

⇨ **Twinning**

Dizygotic twins (Fraternal):

— Develop from 2 zygotes,

— Have 2 placentae,

— 2 chorions,

— 2 amniotic sacs

Monozygotic twins (Identical):

— 1 placenta,

— 1 chorion,

— 2 amniotic sacs

▶ **Oligohydraminos:** Low Level of Amniotic fluid (< 400 ml) in Renal agenesis✱✎

▶ **Polyhydraminos:** High Level Of Amniotic fluid (>2000 ml)

   Ⓞ In Anencephaly,

   Ⓞ Esophageal atresia,

   Ⓞ Maternal Diabetes✎✎✎

▶ **Amniotic Band syndrome:** when bands of amniotic membrane encircle and constrict parts of fetus causing limb amputations and Craniofacial anomalies✎

⇨ **Remamants of important Fetal Structures:**

Fetal Structure	Adult remanant
▶ R and L Umblical artery	▪ Medial Umblical Ligament☞☞
▶ L Umblical vein	▪ Ligamentum Teres☞
▶ Ductus venosus	▪ Ligamentum Venosum☞
▶ Foramen ovale	▪ Fossa Ovalis☞
▶ Ductus arteriosus	▪ Ligamentum arteriosum

➲ **Derivatives of Germ Layers: (Important topic)☞☞☞☞ (asked innumerable times)**

Ectoderm	Mesoderm	Endoderm
❒ **Skin** and **most of** **appendages**	❒ **Musculoskeletal** system	❒ **Epithelial** lining of GIT
❒ **Lens** of eye	❒ **Cardiovascular** system	❒ **Epithelial** lining of Biliary tract. **MP 2K**
❒ Epithelial linning of **Lower half** of Anal canal	❒ **Kidney, ureter,**	❒ **Epithelial** lining of Respiratory tract
	❒ **Trigone** of bladder (mesonephric duct absorption) **UP 2006**	
❒ Epithelial lining of external **auditory meatus**	❒ **Posterior** wall of female urethra	❒ **Epithelial** lining of vagina
	❒ **Posterior** wall of prostatic part of male urethra.	
	❒ Reproductive tract except labia majora, minora and major part of prostate	❒ **Epithelial** lining of auditory tube, middle ear
❒ Epithelial lining of **distal part of male urethra**	❒ **Mesothelium** of pleural, pericardial and peritoneal cavities	
❒ **Adenohypophysis**	❒ **Dentine** of teeth	
	❒ **Cornea, sclera, choroid**, ciliary body and iris of eye	
	❒ **Somites** from paraxial mesoderm. **TN 1995**	
	❒ **H mole** is deficent in mesoderm. **AIIMS 1999**	
Tympanic membrane is formed from all three layers		**UP 2003**

➲ **Derivatives of Neural Crest:☞☞☞ (High Yield for 2011/2012)**

▶ Neurons of **spinal posterior nerve root ganglia.**	**AIIMS 1986**
▶ Neurons of **sensory ganglia.**	**PGI 1986**
▶ Neurons of **autonomic ganglia (sympathetic ganglia)**	**AI 2002**
▶ **Schwann** cells	**KERALA 1987**
▶ **Melanocytes**	**PGI 2003**
▶ **Piamater and arachnoid matter.**	
▶ **Mesenchyme** of **dental papillae**	**MP 2K**
▶ **Cartilage cells of branchial arches**	
▶ **Chromaffin** tissue	

⊃ Defective Migration of Neural Crest Cells Results in:

► Albinism

► Melanoma

► Hirschsprungs disease   KERALA 2001, UP 2000

► Oropharyngeal teratoma

► Neurocristopathies (Cleft Lip, Cleft palate, Digeorges syndrome, Waarden burgs syndrome, CHARGE syndrome

⊃ Neural Migration Disorders:

► Lissencephaly   AIIMS 2011

► Schizencephaly

► Porencephaly   AIIMS 2011

► Agyria

► Macrogyria

► polymicrogyria

⊃ Tumors of Neural Crest Origin:

✓ Neuroblastoma

✓ Phaeochromocytoma

✓ Carcinoid Tumor

✓ Neurofibromatosis

✓ Medullary carcinoma Thyroid

⊃ Embryology of Lungs:

➥ By the fourth week, a **laryngotracheal diverticulum** develops from the floor of the primordial pharynx.

➥ The laryngotracheal diverticulum **becomes separated from the foregut** by tracheoesophageal folds that fuse to form a tracheoesophageal septum. This septum results in the formation of the esophagus and the laryngotracheal tube.

➥ **The endoderm of the laryngotracheal tube gives rise to the epithelium of the lower respiratory organs and the tracheobronchial glands.** The splanchnic mesenchyme surrounding the laryngotracheal tube forms the connective tissue, cartilage, muscle, and blood and lymphatic vessels of these organs.

➥ **The distal end of the laryngotracheal diverticulum gives rise to a respiratory bud that divides into two bronchial buds.** Each bronchial bud soon enlarges to form a main bronchus, and then the main bronchus subdivides to form lobar, segmental, and subsegmental branches.

➥ Each tertiary bronchial bud (segmental bronchial bud), with its surrounding mesenchyme, is the primordium of a bronchopulmonary segment. Branching continues until *approximately* 17 orders of branches have formed. Additional airways are formed after birth, until *approximately* 24 orders of branches are present.

cont...

1

ANATOMY

cont...

- Lung development is divided into four stages:
- ✓ Pseudoglandular (6-16 weeks),
- ✓ Canalicular (16-26 weeks),
- ✓ Terminal sac (26 weeks to birth), and
- ✓ Alveolar (32 weeks to *approximately* 8 years of age).
- By 20 weeks, type II pneumocytes begin to secrete pulmonary surfactant. Deficiency of surfactant results in respiratory distress syndrome (RDS) or hyaline membrane disease (HMD).
- A tracheoesophageal fistula (TEF), which results from faulty partitioning of the foregut into the esophagus and trachea, is usually associated with esophageal atresia

➲ Embryology of Heart

Embryonic structure	Adult structure
Truncus arteriosus	- Aorta - Pulmonary Trunk
Bulbus cordis	- **Smooth** part of R ventricle - **Smooth** part of L ventricle
Primitive ventricle	- **Rough** part of R ventricle - **Rough** part of L ventricle
Primitive atrium	- **Rough** part of R atrium - **Rough** part of L atrium
Sinus venosus MP 2004	- **Smooth** part of R atrium - **Coronary sinus (Lt horn of sinus venosus)** - **Oblique vein of Left Atrium**

➲ Extra Edge:

- ✓ **The primitive atrium** gives rise to the *trabeculated* part of the right and left atria.
- ✓ **The primitive ventricle** gives rise to the *trabeculated* part of the right and left ventricles.
- ✓ The truncus arteriosus gives rise to the proximal portions of the <u>ascending aorta and the pulmonary trunk.</u>
- ✓ The 3rd, 4th, and 6th aortic arches and the right and left dorsal aortae contribute to the remainder of the aorta.
- ✓ The bulbus cordis gives rise to the right ventricle and the aortic outflow tract.
- ✓ **The left horn of the sinus venosus** gives rise to the coronary sinus.
- ✓ The right common cardinal vein gives rise to the superior vena cava.
- ✓ **The right horn of the sinus venosus** gives rise to the smooth part of the right atrium

➲ **Embryology of Thoracic Vessels: (High Yield for 2011/2012)**

Embryonic structure	Adult Structure
▶ Aortic arch 1	
▶ Aortic arch 2➴	
▶ Aortic arch 3➴	➥ Common Carotid artery
	➥ Internal carotid artery (proximal part)
▶ Aortic arch 4➴	➥ Rt. Subclavian artery(proximal part)
	➥ Part of Aortic arch
	➥ Persistence leads to double aortic arch **DNB 2006**
▶ Aortic arch 5➴	➥ Regresses
▶ Aortic arch 6➴ ✳	➥ Pulmonary artery
	➥ Ductus arteriosus

⇨ **Remember:**

Ventral Mesogastrium➴➴	Lesser Omentum, Hepatoduodenal, Hepatogastric, Falciform, Coronary and Triangular Ligament of Liver➴➴
Dorsal Mesogastrium➴	Greater Omentum, Mesentry of small intestine, Mesoappendix, Sigmoid Mesocolon, Transverse Mesocolon

➲ **Embryology of Urinary Tract:**

Embryo	Adult structure	
Ureteric Bud➴➴	➥ Collecting duct	**AIIMS 1995**
	➥ Major/Minor Calyx	
	➥ Renal pelvis	
	➥ Ureter	
	➥ **Epithelium of ureter from mesonephros.**	**AIIMS 2007**
Metanephric Mesoderm➴	➥ Renal Glomerulus	
	➥ Bowmans capsule	
	➥ PCT	
	➥ DCT	
	➥ Loop Of Henle	
	➥ Collecting Tubule	

➲ **Embryology of Genital tract:**

Gonads	Ovary		Testis
Paramesonephric duct or **Mullerian duct**➴➴ **RJ 2009** *Non fusion of theses ducts leads to uterus diadelphus.* **MAH 2012**	➥ Uterine tubes	➥ **Uterus** ➥ Cervix ➥ Hydatid of morgagni	Appendix testis

1

ANATOMY

Mesonephric "duct" or Wollfian duct	Appendix vesiculosa	Epididymis, ductus deferens
	Duct of Garnier	Seminal vesicles
	JKBOPEE 2012	Ejaculatory ducts
		Appendix epididymis
Mesonephric "tubules"	Epoophoroon JKBOPEE 2012	Efferent ductules
	Paraphooron JKBOPEE 2012	Paradidymis
Phallus	Clitoris	Glans penis
Urethral folds	Labia minora	
Genital swellings	Labia majora	Scrotum

- ➡ The Urachus becomes the <u>median</u> umbilical ligament.   **JK BOPEE 2010**
- ➡ The **2 umbilical arteries** becomes the <u>medial</u> umbilical ligaments.
- ➡ **Obliterated umblical arteries** form **lateral umblical ligament.**
- ➡ Urachal fistula from persistent allantois.

Embryonic structure	Female	Male
▶ Genital ridge✳	Ovary (**6 week**) AIIMS 1991	Testis
▶ Genital swelling✳	L. majora	Scrotum **KERALA 1995**
▶ Genital fold✳	L. minora	Ventral aspect of penis
▶ Genital tubercle✳	Clitoris **MAH 2002**	Glans penis

⇨ **SRY gene**

- ➡ SRY (for **sex-determining region Y**) is a gene located on the short (p) arm just outside the pseudoautosomal region.
  It is the master switch that triggers the events that converts the embryo into a male.
- ➡ Without this gene, you get a female instead. So femaleness is the "default" program.
- ➡ On very rare occasions aneuploid humans are born with such karyotypes as XXY, XXXY, and even XXXXY. Despite their extra X chromosomes, all these cases are male.
- ➡ *(A test based on a molecular probe for SRY was used to ensure that potential competitors for the women's Olympic events in Atlanta had no SRY gene.)*

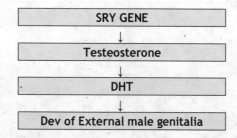

```
        SRY GENE
           ↓
      Testeosterone
           ↓
           DHT
           ↓
Dev of External male genitalia
```

⇨ Pharyngeal Apparatus✳✳✳

- ▶ Pharyngeal <u>Arches</u> are derived from Mesoderm☞
- ▶ Pharyngeal <u>clefts</u> are derived from Ectoderm☞
- ▶ Pharyngeal <u>Pouches</u> are derived from Endoderm☞

⊃ Pharyngeal Arch 1 Derivatives:☞(High Yield for 2011/2012)

▶ Meckels Cartilage:	MAH 2010
▶ Mandible,	
▶ Malleus,	
▶ Incus,	
Spheno Mandibular Ligament	UP 2007, DELHI 1991, DELHI 1993
▶ Muscles: Muscles of Mastication (Medial Pterygoid and Lateral Pterygoid, Masseter,Temporalis)	
▶ **Two Tensors** (Tensor Tympani Tensor Palati)	
▶ Mylohyoid, **anterior** belly of digastrics	

⊃ Pharyngeal Arch 2 Derivatives (Word S)☞ (High Yield for 2011/2012)

▶ Reicherts Cartilage:	
▶ Stapes,	DNB 2008
▶ Styloid process,	
▶ Smaller cornu of Hyoid Bone,	
▶ Superior surface of Hyoid Bone,	
▶ Stylohyoid ligament,	KAR 1999
▶ Muscles of facial expression, Stapedius, Stylohyoid, **Posterior** Belly of Digastric	MAH 2001
▶ Platysma	MAH 2001
▶ Stapedial artery is a remanent of 2nd arch	MAH 2010

⊃ Pharyngeal Arch 3 Derivatives☞

▶ **Greater cornu** of Hyoid Bone	AP 1998, JIPMER 1987
▶ Stylopharyngeus muscle	

Think of Stylo pharyngeus when thinking about Glosso pharyngeal Nerve

⊃ Pharyngeal Arch 4 and 6 Derivatives☞

▶ Cartilages of larynx ,	
▶ Intrinsic muscles of Larynx and pharynx	MAH 2012

ANATOMY

➾ Pharyngeal Arch 5 does not contribute to Development

⇨ Nerve Supply of Pharyngeal Arches is: My Father Gaveme Some Rupees

▶ Mandibular Nerve	1st arch	
▶ Facial Nerve	2nd arch	
▶ Glossopharyngeal Nerve	3rd arch	AI 1994, UP 2003
▶ Superior laryngeal Nerve	4th arch	
▶ Reccurent laryngeal Nerve	6th arch	MAH 2011

Pharyngeal Pouch		Adult Structure	
✓ Pharyngeal Pouch 1		Epithelial linning of **Auditory tube/ Middle ear**	
✓ Pharyngeal Pouch 2		Palatine tonsil	PGI 1988
✓ Pharyngeal Pouch 3		**Inferior** parathyroid and **Thymus**	DNB 2011
✓ Pharyngeal Pouch 4	TN 2006	**Superior** parathyroid and **Ultimobranchial body**	
		Para follicular cells are derived from ultimobranchial body	KERALA 1987
Pharyngeal Cleft/Groove		**Adult Structure**	
1	UP 2005	External linning of **External auditory meatus**	
2, 3, 4		Obliterated	

➾ Meatuses and their openings: (High Yield for 2011/2012)

Meatus	Opening	
❑ Superior meatus	→ Posterior ethmoidal sinus	
❑ Middle meatus	→ Maxillary sinus	
	→ Middle ethmoidal sinus	
	→ Frontal sinus	
❑ Inferior meatus	→ Nasolacrimal duct	JKBOPEE 2012

➾ Treacher-Collins Syndrome / Mandibulofacial Dysostosis (High Yield for 2011/2012)

- ➡ Abnormal formation of pharyngeal arch
- ➡ Faulty migration of neural crest cells.

⇨ Patients are mostly characterized by the following abnormalities:

- ▶ **Hypoplasia of the facial bones.** An underdeveloped mandibular and zygomatic bone leading to a small and malformed jaw.

- ▶ **Ear anomalies.** consist small, rotated or even absent ears with or without bilateral stenosis or atresia of the external auditory cannels

cont...

cont...

► **Eye problems**, varying from colobomata of the lower eyelids and aplasia of lid lashes to short, downslanting palpebral fissures and missing eyelashes. Vision loss can occur and is associated with strabismus, refractive errors, and anisometropia.

► **Cleft palate**

► **Airway problems**, who are often a result of mandibular hypoplasia.

► **Dental anomalies** consist in tooth agenesis, enamel disformaties and malplacement of the maxillary first molars.

⇨ **Less frequent defects are:**

— Nasal deformity

— High-arched palate

— Coloboma of the upper lid

— Ocular hypertelorism

— Choanal atresia

— Macrostomia

— Preauricular hair displacement

➲ **Cleft Lip and Cleft Palate (Detailed overview) (High Yield for 2011/2012)**

Unilateral cleft lip. Also called **Hare lip**	Failure of fusion of medial nasal process with maxillary process
Midline defect of **upper lip**	Defect in development of lowermost part of frontonasal process
Midline defect of **lower lip**	Defective fusion of mandibular processes
Microstomia	Excessive fusion of maxillary and mandibular processes
Macrostomia	Inadequate fusion of maxillary and mandibular processes
Oblique facial cleft	Non fusion of maxillary and lateral nasal process

At birth following structures are of **adult size: mastoid antrum, Ear ossicles, tympanic cavity**   **AIIMS 2009**

► **Cleft Lip:**

— Failure of Fusion of **Maxillary and Medial Nasal Process**

— Usually associated with cleft palate. (Commonest)   **PGI 2001**

— Midline cleft lip is due to failure of fusion of two medial nasal processes.   **KERALA 2001**

► **Cleft Palate:** Failure of Fusion of Lateral Palatine Process, Nasal Septum and Median Palatine Process (Occasional)

1

➲ Important Points About Ear:

►	Pinna is supplied by **Vagus and auriculo temporal nerve.**	**PGI 2007**
►	External auditory canal is suplied by auriculotemporal nerve.	
►	Tympanic plexus is formed by **tympanic branch of glossopharyngeal nerve.**	**PGI 1996**
►	**Toynbees muscle** is: Tensor tympani	
►	**SECOND Smallest muscle in body** is stapedius	**PGI 2005**
►	Smallest is erector pili	**DELHI 2006**
►	Nerve supply of stapedius is **facial nerve.**	
►	Function of stapedius is to **prevent hyperacusis**	

➲ Tongue Development High Yield for AIPGME/AIIMS/PGI 2013

➜	**1st pharyngeal arch** forms ant2/3	
➜	**3rd and 4th arch** forms post 1/3	
➜	**Muscles** of tongue develop from **occipital myotomes**	**AIIMS 2007**
➜	**Muscles** of tongue are both smooth and skeletal muscles	**MP 2009**
	Remember: IMPORTANT points about the tongue.	
➥	Use your tongue less and brain more Though	**Not Asked In Any Exam**
➥	Muscles of tongue are supplied by <u>hypoglossal nerve</u>.	
➥	Safety muscle of tongue is <u>genioglossus.</u>	**TN 1988**
➥	Tip of tongue drains to <u>sub mental lymph nodes</u>.	
➥	Posterior 1/3 of tongue is supplied by glossopharyngeal nerve	
➥	Pain of cancer base of tongue is also referred to ear through glossopharyngeal nerve.	**ERALA 1994**
➥	Circum vallate pappilae of tongue are supplied by glossopharyngeal nerve.	**MAH 2000**

The muscles of tongue are made up of **Skeletal and smooth muscle**	**MP 2009**
Intrinsic muscles of tongue are derived from occipital somites.	**AIIMS 2007**

SENSATION	AREA
o Sweet	o Tip
o Salt	o Dorsum anteriorly.
o Sour	o Edges.
o Bitter	o Posterior 1/3rd

➲ General Features of Tongue: ✶ ✶

⇨ Anterior 2/3

Anterior 2/3 of tongue develops from **lingual swellings and tuberculum impar.**☞	**RJ 2008**
Anterior 2/3 of tongue is supplied by chorda tympani (FACIAL) (Taste)☞	**UP 2004**
Anterior 2/3 of tongue is supplied by lingual nerve (General)☞	
Anterior 2/3 of tongue drains into **submandibular lymph nodes.**	

⇨ **Posterior 1/3**

Posterior 1/3 of tongue develops from **hypobranchial eminence**.	RJ 2008
Posterior 1/3 of tongue is supplied by glossopharyngeal nerve **(Taste)**➤➤	
Posterior 1/3 of tongue is supplied by glossopharyngeal nerve **(General)**➤➤	
Posterior 1/3 of tongue drains into **juguloomohyoid lymph nodes**.	
Tip drains into **submental lymph nodes**.	

⇨ **Tonsil**

▶ Has <u>non keratinized</u> squamous epithelium

▶ Is an <u>endodermal</u> structure.   PGI 2003

▶ Rests on <u>superior constrictor</u> muscle of pharynx

▶ Vagus supplies tonsil.

▶ Main nerve supply is the glossopharyngeal nerve.   UP 1996

▶ Lymph drains into <u>jugulo digastric nodes.</u>   JIPMER 1996

▶ Arterial supply :

✓ Ascending palatine,

✓ Descending palatine and

✓ Ascending pharyngeal artery supply tonsils   PGI 2004

⊃ **Diaphragm Development**

▶ Septum transversum

▶ Pleuroperitoneal folds   AIPGME 2011

▶ Body wall

▶ <u>Dorsal</u> Mesentry of esophagus

⊃ **Development of Intraabdominal Organs Frequently Asked:(High Yield for 2011/2012)**

Spleen is unique in respect to its development within the gut. While most of the gut viscera are endodermally derived (with the exception of the neural-crest derived suprarenal gland), the spleen is derived from **mesenchymal tissue**. Specifically, the spleen forms within, and from, the dorsal mesentery.

Pancreas The pancreas develops between the layers of the mesentery from **dorsal and ventral pancreatic buds of endodermal cells**, which arise from the caudal or dorsal part of the foregut. Most of the pancreas is derived from the dorsal pancreatic bud. The larger dorsal pancreatic bud appears first and develops a slight distance cranial to the ventral bud.

The liver, gallbladder and the biliary duct system arise as a ventral outgrowth (hepatic diverticulum) from the caudal foregut in the 4th week.

cont...

1

ANATOMY

cont...

▶ This hepatic diverticulum extends into septum transversum, a mass of splanchnic mesoderm between the developing heart and the midgut.

▶ The septum transversum forms the **ventral mesentery** in this region. This double-layered membrane gives rise to the lesser omentum and the falciform ligament.

▶ The superior layers of the coronary and left triangular ligaments meet and continue as a **ventral mesentery** attached to the ventrosuperior aspect of the liver.   **AIIMS 2010**

Gall bladder arises from **pars cystica** (from the hepatic bud).

➲ Developmental Anomolies of Tongue High Yield for AIPGME/AIIMS/PGI 2013

▶ **Ankyloglossia:** The lingual frenulum normally connects the inferior surface of the tongue to the floor of the mouth. Sometimes the frenulum is short and extends to the tip of the tongue. **This interferes with its free protrusion and may make breastfeeding difficult.** A short frenulum usually stretches with time, making surgical correction of the anomaly unnecessary.

▶ **Macroglossia:** An **excessively large** tongue is not common.

▶ **Microglossia:** An **abnormally small tongue** is extremely rare and is usually associated with micrognathia (underdeveloped mandible and recession of the chin) and limb defects **(Hanhart's syndrome).**

▶ **Bifid Tongue**

▶ **Fissured tongue**

➲ Developmental Anomalies of larynx High Yield for AIPGME 2013

▶ **Laryngeal Atresia:** This anomaly results from failure of recanalization of the larynx, which causes obstruction of the upper fetal airway. Distal to the region of atresia (blockage) or stenosis (narrowing), the airways become dilated, the lungs are enlarged and echogenic

▶ **Laryngeal web**: results from incomplete recanalization of the larynx during the 10th week. A membranous web forms at the level of the vocal folds, partially obstructing the airway.

▶ **Laryngoptosis:** Larynx is situated lower down in neck.

▶ **Laryngeocele:** excessive enlargement of saccule of larynx.

➲ Developmental Anomalies of Trachea High Yield for AIPGME/AIIMS/PGI 2013

▶ **Tracheoesophageal Fistula:** A fistula between the trachea and esophagus. **Most affected infants are males.** In more than 85% of cases, the tracheoesophageal fistula (TEF) is **associated with esophageal atresia.** A TEF results from incomplete division of the cranial part of the foregut into respiratory and esophageal parts during the fourth week. Incomplete fusion of the tracheoesophageal folds results in a defective tracheoesophageal septum and a TEF between the trachea and esophagus.

▶ TEF is the **most common anomaly of the lower respiratory tract.** Four main varieties of TEF may develop. **The usual anomaly is for the superior part of the esophagus to end blindly (esophageal atresia) and for the inferior part to join the trachea near its bifurcation. Polyhydramnios is often associated with esophageal atresia.** The excess amniotic fluid develops because fluid cannot pass to the stomach and intestines for absorption and subsequent transfer through the placenta to the mother's blood

○ Developmental Anomalies of Cardiovascular System High Yield for AIPGME/AIIMS/PGI 2013

► **Ectopia cordis:** Non union of sternal plates exposing the heart to surface

Dextrocardia: If the heart tube bends to the left instead of to the right, the heart is displaced to the right and there is transposition-the heart and its vessels are reversed left to right as in a mirror image. Dextrocardia is the most frequent positional abnormality of the heart. In isolated dextrocardia, the abnormal position of the heart is not accompanied by displacement of other viscera.

► **Atrial Septal Defects:** An atrial septal defect (ASD) is a common congenital heart anomaly and occurs more frequently in females than in males. The most common form of ASD is patent oval foramen. A small isolated patent oval foramen is of no hemodynamic significance; however, if there are other defects (e.g., pulmonary stenosis or atresia), blood is shunted through the oval foramen into the left atrium and produces cyanosis.

► **Common atrium**: is a rare cardiac defect in which the interatrial septum is absent. This situation is the result of failure of the septum primum and septum secundum to develop (combination of ostium secundum, ostium primum, and sinus venosus defects).

► **Ventricular Septal Defects:** VSDs are the most common type of CHD. VSDs may occur in any part of the IV septum but membranous VSD is the most common type frequently, small VSDs close spontaneously. Most people with a large VSD have massive left-to-right shunting of blood. Muscular VSD is a less common type of defect and may appear anywhere in the muscular part of the interventricular septum. Sometimes there are multiple small defects, producing what is sometimes called the "Swiss cheese" VSD.

► **Cor biloculare: Two chambered heart**

► **Cor Triloculare: Three chambered heart**

► **L. cor triloculare biatriatum: (Two atria, one ventricle):** Absence of the IV septum-single ventricle.or common ventricle-resulting from failure of the IV septum to form, is extremely rare and results in a three-chambered heart (L. cor triloculare biatriatum).

► **Persistent Truncus Arteriosus:** Persistent TA results from failure of the truncal ridges and aorticopulmonary septum to develop normally and divide the TA into the aorta and pulmonary trunk. In this defect, a single arterial trunk, the TA, arises from the heart and supplies the systemic, pulmonary, and coronary circulations.

► **Aorticopulmonary Septal Defect:** Aorticopulmonary septal defect is a rare condition in which there is an opening (aortic window) between the aorta and pulmonary trunk near the aortic valve. The aorticopulmonary defect **results from localized defect in the formation of the aorticopulmonary septum.** The presence of pulmonary and aortic valves and an intact IV septum distinguishes this anomaly from the persistent truncus arteriosus defect.

► **Transposition of the Great Arteries:** TGA is the most common cause of cyanotic heart disease in newborn infants. TGA is often associated with other cardiac anomalies (e.g., ASD and VSD). In typical cases, the aorta lies anterior and to the right of the pulmonary trunk and arises from the morphologic right ventricle, whereas the pulmonary trunk arises from the morphologic left ventricle. The aorticopulmonary septum fails to pursue a spiral course during partitioning of the bulbus cordis and TA. This defect is thought to result from failure of the conus arteriosus to develop normally during incorporation of the bulbus cordis into the ventricles. Recent studies suggest that defective migration of neural crest cells may also be involved.

▶ **Tetralogy of Fallot :** This classic group of four cardiac defects
  - ❑ **Pulmonary stenosis (obstruction of right ventricular outflow)**
  - ❑ **VSD**
  - ❑ **Dextroposition of aorta (overriding or straddling aorta)**
  - ❑ **Right ventricular hypertrophy**

▶ **Coarctation of the Aorta:** Aortic coarctation (constriction) occurs in approximately 10% of children and adults with CHDs. Coarctation is characterized by an aortic constriction of varying length. **Most coarctations occur distal to the origin of the left subclavian artery** at the entrance of the DA (juxtaductal coarctation). The classification into preductal and postductal coarctations is commonly used.Coarctation of the aorta occurs **twice as often in males** as in females and is associated with a bicuspid aortic valve in 70% of cases.

➲ Developmental Anomalies of Lymphatic System High Yield for AIPGME/AIIMS/PGI 2013

Cystic hygroma: large swellings usually appear in the inferolateral part of the neck and consist of large single or multilocular, fluid-filled cavities. Hygromas may be present at birth, but they often enlarge and become evident during infancy. Most hygromas appear to be derived from **abnormal transformation of the jugular lymph sacs.** Hygromas are believed to arise from parts of a jugular lymph sac that are pinched off or from lymphatic spaces that fail to establish connections with the main lymphatic channels.   **KCET 2011**

➲ Developmental Anomalies of GIT

▶ **Esophageal Atresia:** Esophageal atresia is **associated with tracheoesophageal fistula in more than 85% of cases**. Atresia may occur as a separate anomaly, but this is less common. Esophageal atresia results from deviation of the tracheoesophageal septum in a posterior direction as a result, there is incomplete separation of the esophagus from the laryngotracheal tube. A fetus with esophageal atresia is unable to swallow amniotic fluid; consequently, this fluid cannot pass to the intestine for absorption and transfer through the placenta to the maternal blood for disposal. This results in polyhydramnios **VATER association,** an acronym for a nonhereditary concurrence of anomalies including vertebral or vascular defects, anal anomalies, TE fistula, esophageal atresia, and radial limb or renal anomalies. **An alternative acronym is VACTERL (vertebral, anal, cardiac, tracheal, esophogeal, renal, and limb).**   **AIPGME 2011**

▶ **Esophageal Stenosis:** Narrowing of the lumen of the esophagus can be anywhere along the esophagus, but it usually occurs in its distal third, either as a web or as a long segment of esophagus with a threadlike lumen. Stenosis usually results from incomplete recanalization of the esophagus

▶ **Short Esophagus (Congenital Hiatal Hernia):** Initially the esophagus is very short. Its failure to elongate sufficiently as the neck and thorax develop results in displacement of part of the stomach superiorly through the esophageal hiatus into the thorax-congenital hiatal hernia. Most hiatal hernias occur long after birth, usually in middle-aged people.

▶ **Dysphagia Lusoria:** Abberant vessels compressing esophagus leading to dysphagia. Usually Abnormal right subclavian artery is implicated.   **MAH 2009**

▶ **Duodenal Atresia:** Complete occlusion of the lumen of the duodenum. If recanalization of the lumen fails to occur a short segment of the duodenum is occluded. The blockage occurs nearly always at the junction of the bile and pancreatic ducts (hepatopancreatic ampulla) but occasionally involves the horizontal (third) part of the duodenum.

▶ In infants with **duodenal atresia, vomiting begins a few hours after birth. The vomitus almost always contains bile;** Duodenal atresia may occur as an isolated anomaly, but other congenital anomalies are often associated with it, e.g., anular pancreas cardiovascular abnormalities, anorectal anomalies, and malrotation. Importantly, approximately one third of affected infants have Down syndrome and an additional 20% are premature. Duodenal atresia is associated with bilious emesis (vomiting of bile) because the blockage occurs distal to the opening of the bile duct. Polyhydramnios also occurs because duodenal atresia prevents normal intestinal absorption of swallowed amniotic fluid. The diagnosis of duodenal atresia is suggested by the presence of a **"double bubble" sign** on plain radiographs or ultrasound scans. This appearance is caused by a distended, gas-filled stomach and proximal duodenum.   **AIIMS 2011**

▶ **Riedels Lobe:** A **tongue like extension** of right lobe of liver

▶ **Phrygian cap: Fundus of the gall bladder folded upon itself** giving rise to an appearance of cap worn by people of an ancient Asian community of Phrygia.

▶ **Moynihans Hump:** Normally the arterial supply of gall bladder is from cystic artery which is a branch of Right hepatic artery. Sometimes an accessory cystic artery is also seen to arise from either Gastroduodenal or right hepatic artery. **The Right hepatic artery takes a tortuous course called "caterpillar turn" or "Moynihans hump."** This can be a source of profuse bleeding.   **JK BOPEE**

▶ **Extrahepatic Biliary Atresia:** This is the most serious anomaly of the extrahepatic biliary system and occurs in one in 10,000 to 15,000 live births. The most common form of extrahepatic biliary atresia is obliteration of the bile ducts at or superior to the porta hepatis-a deep transverse fissure on the visceral surface of the liver. Biliary atresia could result from a failure of the remodeling process at the hepatic hilum or from infections or immunologic reactions during late fetal development. Jaundice occurs soon after birth and stools are acholic (clay colored).

▶ **Accessory Pancreatic Tissue :** Accessory pancreatic tissue is most often located in the wall of the stomach, Wall of duodenum, in an ileal diverticulum (e.g., a Meckel diverticulum)

▶ **Anular Pancreas:** may cause duodenal obstruction. The ringlike or anular part of the pancreas consists of a thin, flat band of pancreatic tissue surrounding the descending or second part of the duodenum. An anular pancreas may cause obstruction of the duodenum either shortly after birth or later. Infants present with symptoms of complete or partial bowel obstruction. Blockage of the duodenum develops if inflammation (pancreatitis) develops in the anular pancreas. An anular pancreas may be **associated with Down syndrome, intestinal atresia, imperforate anus, pancreatitis, and malrotation.**

▶ **Congenital Omphalocele:** This anomaly is a persistence of the herniation of abdominal contents into the proximal part of the umbilical cord. Herniation of intestines and herniation of liver and intestines occurs. The abdominal cavity is proportionately small when there is an omphalocele because the impetus for it to grow is absent. Surgical repair is required and is often delayed if the defect is very large. Infants with these large omphaloceles often suffer from pulmonary and thoracic hypoplasia and a delayed closure is a better clinical decision. The covering of the hernial sac is the epithelium of the umbilical cord, a derivative of the amnion.

High Yield for AIPGME/AIIMS/PGI 2013

▶ **Umbilical Hernia:** When the intestines return to the abdominal cavity during the 10th week and then herniate through an imperfectly closed umbilicus, an umbilical hernia forms. This common type of hernia is different from an omphalocele. In an umbilical hernia, the protruding mass (usually the greater omentum and part of the small intestine) is covered by subcutaneous tissue and skin. The defect through which the hernia occurs is in the linea alba The hernia protrudes during crying, straining, or coughing and can be easily reduced through the fibrous ring at the umbilicus. Surgery is not usually performed unless the hernia persists to the age of 3 to 5 years.

▶ **Gastroschisis:** This anomaly is a relatively uncommon congenital abdominal wall defect. Gastroschisis results from a defect lateral to the median plane of the anterior abdominal wall. **The linear defect permits extrusion of the abdominal viscera without involving the umbilical cord.** The viscera protrude into the amniotic cavity and are bathed by amniotic fluid. The defect usually occurs on the right side lateral to the umbilicus and is more common in males than females.

▶ **Anomalies of the Midgut**

▶ **Nonrotation** occurs when the intestine does not rotate as it reenters the abdomen. As a result, the caudal limb of the midgut loop returns to the abdomen first and the small intestines lie on the right side of the abdomen and the entire large intestine is on the left.and the cecum lies just inferior to the pylorus of the stomach. The cecum is fixed to the posterolateral abdominal wall by peritoneal bands that pass over the duodenum *these bands and the volvulus (twisting) of the intestines cause duodenal obstruction. When midgut volvulus occurs, the superior mesenteric artery may be obstructed, resulting in infarction and gangrene of the intestine supplied by it. Infants with intestinal malrotation are prone to volvulus and present with bilious emesis*

▶ **Reversed Rotation:** In very unusual cases, the midgut loop rotates in a clockwise rather than a counterclockwise direction. As a result, the duodenum lies anterior to the superior mesenteric artery rather than posterior to it, and the transverse colon lies posterior instead of anterior to it. In these infants, the transverse colon may be obstructed by pressure from the superior mesenteric artery

▶ **Congenital Megacolon or Hirschsprung Disease:** This disease is a **dominantly inherited** multigenic disorder with incomplete penetrance and variable expressivity. An absence of ganglion cells **(aganglionosis)** in a variable length of distal bowel. Infants with congenital megacolon or Hirschsprung's disease lack autonomic ganglion cells in the myenteric plexus distal to the dilated segment of colon. The **enlarged colon-megacolon** has the normal number of ganglion cells. The dilation results from failure of relaxation of the aganglionic segment, which prevents movement of the intestinal contents, resulting in dilation.

AIPGME 2011

▶ **Imperforate Anus and Anorectal Anomalies:** Imperforate anus occurs approximately once in every 5000 newborn infants and is more common in males Most anorectal anomalies result from abnormal development of the urorectal septum, resulting in incomplete separation of the cloaca into urogenital and anorectal portions. There is normally a temporary communication between the rectum and anal canal dorsally from the bladder and urethra ventrally but it closes when the urorectal septum fuses with the cloacal membrane.

▶ **Anal Agenesis, with or without a Fistula:** The anal canal may end blindly or there may be an ectopic anus or an anoperineal fistula that opens into the perineum. The abnormal canal may, however, open into the vagina in females or the urethra in males.

▶ **Anal Stenosis:** The anus is in the normal position, but the anus and anal canal are narrow. This anomaly is probably caused by a slight dorsal deviation of the urorectal septum as it grows caudally to fuse with the cloacal membrane. As a result, the anal canal and anal membrane are small.

➲ Developmental Anomolies of Urinary Tract

▶ **Horseshoe Kidney:** In 0.2% of the population, the poles of the kidneys are fused; usually the inferior poles fuse. **The large U-shaped kidney usually lies in the hypogastrium, anterior to the inferior lumbar vertebrae.** Normal ascent of these fused kidneys is prevented because they are caught by the root of the inferior mesenteric artery. A horseshoe kidney usually produces no symptoms because its collecting system develops normally and the ureters enter the bladder. If urinary flow is impeded, signs and symptoms of obstruction and/or infection may appear. Persons with **Turner's syndrome** have horseshoe kidneys.

▶ **Ectopic Ureter:** An ectopic ureter does not enter the urinary bladder. In males, ectopic ureters usually open into the neck of the bladder or into the prostatic part of the urethra, but they may enter the ductus deferens, prostatic utricle, or seminal gland. In females, ectopic ureters may open into the bladder neck, urethra, vagina, or vestibule of the vagina. Incontinence is the common complaint resulting from an ectopic ureter because the urine flowing from the orifice does not enter the bladder; instead it continually dribbles from the urethra in males and the urethra and/or vagina in females.

▶ **An ectopic ureter:** results when the ureter is not incorporated into the trigone in the posterior part of the urinary bladder. Instead it is carried caudally with the mesonephric duct and is incorporated into the middle pelvic portion of the vesical part of the urogenital sinus.

▶ **Cystic Kidney Diseases**

▶ **In autosomal recessive polycystic kidney disease**, diagnosed at birth or in utero by ultrasonography, both kidneys contain many hundreds of small cysts which result in renal insufficiency.

▶ **Multicystic dysplastic kidney** disease results from dysmorphology during development of the renal system. The outcome for children with multicystic dysplastic kidney disease is generally good because the disease is unilateral in 75% of the cases. In multicystic dysplastic kidney disease, fewer cysts are seen than in autosomal recessive polycystic kidney disease and they range in size from a few millimeters to many centimeters in the same kidney.

1

▶ **Congenital Adrenal Hyperplasia: (CAH)** An abnormal increase in the cells of the suprarenal cortex results in excessive androgen production during the fetal period. In females, this usually causes masculinization of the external genitalia. Affected male infants have normal external genitalia, and the syndrome may go undetected in early infancy. Later in childhood in both sexes, androgen excess leads to rapid growth and accelerated skeletal maturation. CAH is a group of autosomal recessive disorders that result in virilization of female fetuses.

➲ Developmental Anomolies of Genital System

▶ **Mesonephric Duct Remnants in Males**

The cranial end of the mesonephric duct may persist as an **appendix of the epididymis**, which is usually attached to the head of the epididymis Caudal to the efferent ductules, some mesonephric tubules may persist as a small body, **the paradidymis.**

▶ **Mesonephric Duct Remnants in Females**

The cranial end of the mesonephric duct may persist as an **appendix vesiculosa**. A few blind tubules and a duct, the **epoophoron**, correspond to the efferent ductules and duct of the epididymis in the male. The epoophoron may persist in the mesovarium between the ovary and uterine tube. Closer to the uterus, some rudimentary tubules may persist as the **paroophoron**. Parts of the mesonephric duct, corresponding to the ductus deferens and ejaculatory duct, may persist as **Gartner's duct cysts** between the layers of the broad ligament along the lateral wall of the uterus and in the wall of the vagina

▶ **Paramesonephric Duct Remnants in Males**

The cranial end of the paramesonephric duct may persist as a **vesicular appendix of the testis,** which is attached to the superior pole of the testis.

The prostatic utricle, a small saclike structure that opens into the prostatic urethra, is homologous to the vagina.

▶ **Paramesonephric Duct Remnants in Females**

Part of the cranial end of the paramesonephric duct that does not contribute to the infundibulum of the uterine tube may persist as a **vesicular appendage.**

➲ Cryptorchidism or Undescended Testes High Yield for AIPGME/AIIMS/PGI 2013

▶ Cryptorchidism (Greek, kryptos, hidden) occurs in up to 30% of premature males and in approximately 3% to 4% of full-term males. This reflects the fact that the testes begin to descend into the scrotum by the end of the second trimester. Cryptorchidism may be unilateral or bilateral. Cryptorchid testes may be in the abdominal cavity or anywhere along the **usual path of descent of the testis**, but they are usually in the inguinal canal

▶ **Ectopic Testes:** After traversing the inguinal canal, the testis may **deviate from its usual path of descent** and lodge in various abnormal locations

➜ **Interstitial (external to aponeurosis of external oblique muscle)**

➜ **In the proximal part of the medial thigh**

→ Dorsal to the penis

→ On the opposite side (crossed ectopia)

▶ **Exstrophy of the bladder** results from a rare ventral body wall defect through which the posterior wall of the urinary bladder protrudes onto the abdominal wall. Epispadias is a common associated anomaly in males; the urethra opens on the dorsum of the penis.

⊃ Embryology of Nervous System: High yield for 2011-2012

→ **The nervous system** develops from the **neural plate** which appears at the beginning of the third week as thickening of the ectoderm.

→ Its lateral edges soon elevate to form the **neural folds.**

→ With further development, the neural folds continue to elevate, and form a tube known as **neural tube,**

→ The neural tube has an enlarged cranial part that forms the brain, and a narrow caudal part that becomes the spinal cord.

→ The wall of the neural tube at first has a single layer of cells. They multiply and form three layers- **ependymal, mantle and marginal layer.**

⇨ **Neural tube closure begins at cephalic end.**   AI 2009

The mantle layer divides into a
- ➡ **Ventral part, the basal lamina, and**
- ➡ **Dorsal part, the alar lamina, separated by a groove, the sulcus limitans.**

Alar plate gives rise to sensory areas of the spinal cord and the sensory nuclei

Basal plate forms the motor areas of the spinal cord and motor nuclei.

The cerebellum and its nuclei develop from the dorsal parts of the alar plate.

Inferior olivary and Substantia nigra are sensory nuclei and thus derived from the alar plate.

Hypoglossal is a motor nuclei and develops from the basal plate.

THE WALL OF THE SPINAL CORD

Neuroepithelial layer	Mantle layer	Marginal layer
1) These cells extend over the entire thickness of the wall & form a thick PSEUDOSTRATIFIED EPITHELIUM	1) Once the neural tube closes, neuroepithelial cells begin to give rise to another cell type.	1) The outermost layer of the spinal cord, the marginal layer, contains nerve fibers emerging from neuroblasts in the mantle layer.
2) Junctional complexes at the lumen connect them	2) These cells are characterized by a large round nucleus with pale nucleoplasm and a dark-staining nucleolus. These are primitive nerve cells, or NEUROBLASTS.	2) As a result of myelination of nerve fibers, this layer takes on a white appearance & therefore is called the White matter of the spinal cord.
3) After closure of neural tube, they divide rapidly, producing more & more neuroepithelial cells	3) They form the mantle layer, a zone around the neuroepithelial layer. The mantle layer later forms the gray matter of the spinal cord.	

ANATOMY

Remember:

Forebrain		
(*Prosencephalon*)	Telencephalon	Cerebral hemispheres
	Diencephalon	Thalamus
		Hypothalamus
		Posterior Pituitary
		Pineal body
Mid Brain		
(*Mesencephalon*)	No division	Tectum
Hind brain		
(*Rhombencephalon*)	Metancephalon	Pons
	Cerebellum	
	Myelencephalon	Medulla JKBOPEE 2012
Remainder of neural Tube	No division	Spinal cord

3 rd ventricle develops from **diencephalon**.	Orissa 2005
4 th ventricle develops from **rhombencephalon**	Orissa 2005

⇨ **MYELINATION:**

- ▶ Myelin is formed in the **central nervous system by oligodendrocytes.**   UPSC 01
- ▶ There **are no myelinated fibers in the CNS before the end of the fifth fetal month.**
- ▶ There is no myelination of the forebrain until the seventh fetal month. Most myelination in the telencephalon occurs in the third trimester and postnatally.
- ▶ The first neurones to acquire myelin sheaths are the olfactory, optic and acoustic cortical areas and the motor cortex (pyramidal cells).
- ▶ The last to be myelinated are the projection commissure and association neurones of the cerebral hemispheres
- ▶ Myelination is a critical process for the development of the brain because it enhances the speed of neural communication. It occurs most rapidly during the first 2 years of life, but continues until early adulthood

⇨ **In CNS myelin is produced by oligodendrocyte.**

A single oligodendrocyte myelinates as many as 20 or 30 different CNS axonal segments, each over a length of 1 mm or less.   **DNB 2011**

Oligodendrocyte membrane extensions wrap around the axons in a concentric fashion to form the myelin sheath. Myelin proteins include proteolipid protein, myelin basic protein, myelin-associated glycoprotein, and a number of less abundant proteins detectable by electrophoretic separation.

Active myelin synthesis starts in utero and continues for the first 2 years of life; slower synthesis continues during childhood and adolescence.

⊃ **Congenital Anomalies associated with spinal cord:** ✻ ✻ ✻

⇨ **High Yield for AIPGME/AIIMS/PGI 2013**

- ❑ **Spina bifida:** The original defect lies in the **vertebrae** when their laminae fail to cover the spinal cord dorsally. Spina bifida may be simple or complicated. Complicated Spina bifida is associated with involvement of the cord and its membranes.☛☛

- ❑ Rarely do the two halves of the vertebral body fail to fuse and the spinal cord protrudes anteriorly through the gap. This rarity is called as **anterior spina bifida**☛

- ❑ **Spina bifida occulta:** Here the spinal cord is normal .The **defect is not manifest externally** and usually a **tuft of hair is present on the skin** over the affected area.

- ❑ **Meningocele:** The **Arachnoid and the Piamater** covering the spinal cord protrude through the opening of the bifid spine and form a cystic swelling.☛☛

- ❑ **Meningomyelocele:** Here the **spinal cord along with its meninges** and the spinal nerves are seen to protrude. It is a more **serious condition** owing to development of infection of the cord itself.☛

- ❑ This condition is associated with **displacement of medulla and a part of cerebellum which cause obstruction of the foramen magnum producing hydrocephalus.** An association of hydrocephalus and Meningomyelocele is called **Arnold Chiari malformation.**☛☛

- ❑ **Syringomyelia:** Once the central canal of the spinal cord is distended with excessive fluid it is called Syringomyelia☛☛

- ❑ **Myelomalacia:** Abnormal softening of spinal cord. Usually seen after trauma to spinal cord.

⊃ **Neural Tube Defects: High yield for 2011-2012**

- ➙ They are two types of Open and Close

Open neural tube defects:

- ➙ Occur when the brain and/or spinal cord are exposed at birth through a defect in the skull or vertebrae Examples

- ✻ Anencephaly,
- ✻ Encephaloceles,
- ✻ Hydranencephaly,
- ✻ Iniencephaly,
- ✻ Schizencephaly,
- ✻ Spina bifida.

Closed neural tube defects:

- ➙ Occur when the spinal defect is covered by skin. Common examples of closed

- ✻ Lipomyelomeningocele,
- ✻ Lipomeningocele,
- ✻ Tethered cord.

Detection is by:

- ➥ **Ultrasound examination**
- ➥ **Measurement of maternal serum alpha-fetoprotein (MSAFP).**
- ➥ **Amniotic fluid acetylcholinesterase (AFAChE)**

⊃ Syringomyelia:

> ▶ In Syringomyelia there is softening of the spinal cord and the central canal becomes very wide at lesion in this position will **interrupt the pain and temperature fibres** which pass in front of the central canal as they cross from one side to another.
>
> ▶ Syringomyelia usually occurs in the lower cervical and the upper thoracic regions of the spinal cord and the <u>loss of pain and temperature.</u>☛☛
>
> ▶ Only the fibres of the pain and temperature which pass in from of the central canal are injured: the <u>lateral spinothalomic tracts</u> "themselves" remain normal and there is no loss of pain and temperature in the lower limbs.☚☚
>
> ▶ Touch can be felt in the area of the skin in which pain and temperature are lost: this condition in which pain and temperature is lost while touch is nearly normal called <u>Dissociated sensory loss.</u>

⊃ Types of Neurons Based on Poles:

Unipolar Neurons:✷

They have only one pole.

Both Axon and Dendrons arise by a common stem.

Present in

> ✓ **Foetal life.**
> ✓ **Posterior root ganglion.**
> ✓ **Sensory nucleus of the fifth cranial nerve.**

Bipolar Neurons:✷

They have two poles.

Axon and Dendron lie at opposite poles.

Present in

> ✓ **Coachlear ganglion of the eight nerves.**
> ✓ **Vestibular ganglion of the eight nerves.**
> ✓ **Retina.**
> ✓ **Olfactory nerve.**

Multipolar Neurons:✷

They have multiple poles.

The Axon and all other Dendrons form multiple poles.

Present in

> ✓ **The Spinal Cord**
> ✓ **Cerebral Cortex**
> ✓ **Cortex of cerebellum**

Important changes in Phases of Cell Cycle

▶ Leptotene:	Chromosomes become visible	
▶ Zygotene:	Pairing of Chromosomes	
▶ Pachytene:	Tetrad formation, Crossing over, Chiasmata formation	JK BOPEE 2009
▶ Diplotene:	Chromosomes break	
▶ Metaphase:	Spindle formation	
▶ Anaphase:	Chromosomes move from equator to poles	
▶ Telophase:	Chromosomes move completely to opposite sides	

⊃ Sex Chromatin or Barr Body✱ (High Yield for 2011/2012)

Of the two X- chromosomes in a Female only one is functionally active. The other (Inactive) X- chromosome forms a mass of heterochromatin that lies just under the nuclear membrane. This mass of heterochromatin can be identified in suitable preparations and can be useful in determining whether a particular tissue belongs to a male or a female. Because of this association with sex this mass of heterochromatin is called the SEX CHROMATING. It is also called a BARR-BODY after the name of the scientist who first discovered it.

In NEURONS it forms a rounded mass lying very close to the nucleolus and is therefore called a NUCLEOLAR SATELLITE.✱✱

In NEUTROPHIL LEUCOCYTES it may appear as an isolated round mass attached to the rest of the nucleus by a narrow band, thus resembling the appearance of a DRUM-STICK.✱ Rarely, some individuals may have more than two X-chromosomes. In these cases only one X-chromosome is active (and hence euchromatic) while others are represented by masses of heterochromatin.

▶ In normal females XX :	✓ there is one barr body.
▶ In normal males XY :	✓ there is no barr body.
▶ In Turners Syndrome XO:	✓ there is no barr body.
▶ In males with Klienfilters syndrome XXY:	✓ there is one barr body.
▶ In super female XXX,	✓ there are two barr bodies. MAHE 1998
▶ The number of Barr bodies is (X-1)	

Epithelium

⇨ Simple Squamous Epithelium

▶ Alveoli of lungs	
▶ Mesothelium of Pleura, Peritoneum and Pericardium	PGI 1995
▶ Endothelium of Heart and Blood Vessels	

⇨ **Simple Cuboidal Epithelium**

> ▶ Lining of the Thyroid follicles
>
> ▶ Germinal epithelium of ovary
>
> ▶ Anterior surface of lens of eye

⇨ **Simple Columnar Epithelium**

> ▶ the lining of Stomach
>
> ▶ Intestines
>
> ▶ Gall bladder

⇨ **Simple Columnar Ciliated**

> ▶ Fallopian tubes and the Uterus
>
> ▶ Central canal of Spinal cord
>
> ▶ Osseous part of Eustachian tube

⇨ **Pseudo stratified Columnar (Pseudo: False, Stratified: Layered)**

It is a simple type of columnar cells resting on a clear wavy basement membrane. The cells are crowded over each other and appear multi layered. The nuclei are arranged at different levels, some situated basal and others centrally as a result of which a false impression of multi layered cells is created. However, most of the cells reach the basement membrane. The cells may be ciliated or non ciliated.

With cilia

- Nasal cavity, nasal air sinuses, nasopharynx, larynx, trachea and bronchi   RJ 2000
- Eustachian tube in its cartilaginous parts.

Without cilia

- Vas deferens
- Part of male urethra

⇨ **Stratified squamous epithelium**

The surface of the cells may be **keratinized (Protective function)** as in case of

> ▶ Epidermis of Skin
> ▶ External ear
> ▶ External nose

> The surface of the cells may be without keratin called **Non Keratinized** as in case of
> ▶ Esophagus
> ▶ Tongue
> ▶ True vocal cords   JK 2009
> ▶ Cornea   AP 1991
> ▶ Tonsil   UP 2008

⇨ **Stratified Columnar Epithelium**

▶ Conjuctival fornicies
▶ Penile part of male urethra
▶ Ano-rectal junction

⇨ **Transitional Epithelium:**

— It is a type of epithelium composed of multiple cell layers.

— They have extra reserve of cell membrane. **JIPMER 1995**

— **The Top cell layers** are broader.

— **The intermediate cell layers** are polyhedral without intercellular bridges separated by mucus like substance. The cells can undergo transition in relaxed and contracted state. In the relaxed state the number of layers is 6-8 while as in the contracted state it is 2-3 layers.

— The Basal cell layers are Cuboidal.

It is present in :

▶ Calyces	**AIIMS 2007**
▶ Ureter	**UP 2008**
▶ Urinary bladder	**AIIMS 2007, UP 2007**
▶ UV junction	**JIPMER 1993**
▶ Male Urethra	

Urothelium

Lines much of the urinary tract, extending from the ends of the collecting ducts of the kidneys, through renal calyces, pelvis, urethras and bladder to the proximal portion of the urethra. In males it covers the urethra as far as the ejaculatory ducts, then becomes intermittent, finally being replaced by *stratified columnar epithelium in the membranous urethra*. In females it also extends as far as the urogenital membrane.

Urothelium or Transitional epithelium has the ability to stretch greatly without loosing its integrity. Thus the urinary organs lined by urothelium can undergo considerable distention and contraction.

▶ <u>Gap junctions</u> allow exchange between cells.	**AI 2003**
▶ Sensory type of neuroepithelium is present in	
✓ Visual system,	
✓ Olfactory and	
✓ Gustatory system.	**AIIMS 2005**

⇨ **Important Stains used in Histology**

❖ **H&E Stain** (Haematoxylin and Eosin). **Haematoxylin,** a natural dye product, acts as a basic dye that stains blue or black. Nuclear heterochromatin stains blue and the cytoplasm of cells rich in ribonucleoprotein also stains blue. ✳

❖ The aniline dye, **Eosin,** is an acid dye that stains cytoplasm, muscle, and connective tissues various shades of pink and orange. This difference in staining intensity is useful in differentiating one tissue from another.

❖ **Vital Stain:** such as **Neutral red, Trypan blue** are used for staining living cells such as Reticulo endothelial cells.✳

❖ **Metachromatic Stains:** are used for staining mast cells with **Touidine blue.** The stains react with granules of mast cells (metachromasia) to give a new color to the cells✳

❖ **Periodic Acid-Schiff Method** (PAS) principally used to demonstrate structures **rich in carbohydrate macromolecules such as glycogen, glycoprotein, and proteoglycans** found in ground substance of connective tissues, basement membranes and mucus. ✳

❖ **Phosphotungstic Acid Haematoxylin** (PTAH). This is an ideal stain for the demonstration of **striated muscle fibers and mitochondria,** which stain blue. ✳

❖ **Silver Stains** Certain tissue components called Argyrophilic have a natural affinity for silver salts. **Reticular fibers and the granules in diffuse endocrine cells are argyrophilic.** ✳

❖ **Sudan Stains** Sudan dyes are used to stain lipids. The Sudan dyes, e.g., **Sudan IV**, dissolve in droplets containing triglycerides and color them intensely. ✳

Points	Smooth muscle	Skeletal muscle	Cardiac Muscle	
SITE	in the viscera	around skeleton	in the heart	
SHAPE	spindle	cylindrical	Cylindrical	
STRIATIONS	non straited	straited	less marked	
SARCOLEMMA	thin	thick	very thin	
SARCOPLASM	pale	red and pale	Red	
SIZE	small	large	Medium	
BRANCHING	no	yes	yes and anastomosing	
DIAMETER	Up to 10 microns	Up to 80 microns	Up to 20 microns	
NUCLEI	single, central	multiple peripheral	Central	UPSC 2001
Intercalated DISCS	absent	absent	Present	COMED 2003
ACTION	involuntary	voluntary	Involuntary	

⮑ **Salivary Glands: High yield for 2011-2012**

Gland	Duct	Type of Gland	Duct opening
☐ Parotid	☐ Stensons duct	✓ Serous	Vestibule of mouth opposite second upper molar
☐ Submandubular	☐ Whartons duct	✓ Mixed but **predominantly serous**	On the floor of mouth on summit of sublingual papplila at the side of frenulum of tongue
☐ Sublingual	☐ Bartholins duct	✓ Mixed but **predominantly mucus**	On the floor of mouth on summit of sublingual papplila

Structures within parotid gland:

- External carotid artery
- Retromandibular vein
- Facial nerve

⇨ **Questions frequently asked from Histology of Liver:**

☐ **Classic Hepatic Lobule.** This model is based on the direction of blood flow. In sections, liver substructure exhibits a pattern of interlocking hexagons; each of these is a classic lobule. Whereas lobules in pigs are defined by a sheath of connective tissue, there is less connective tissue in humans and the lobule boundaries are indistinct. The central vein at its center, and the alternating hepatocyte plates and sinusoids that lie between them.

☐ **Portal Canal /triad.** One triad occupies a potential space (portal space) at each of the 6 corners of the lobule. Each triad contains 3 main elements surrounded by connective tissue: **a portal venule** (a branch of the portal vein), **a hepatic arteriole** (a branch of the hepatic artery), and **a bile ductule** (a tributary of the larger bile ducts). A lymphatic vessel may also be seen. In the portal canal blood vessels and bile ductules are separated by a space called as **Space of Mall**

☐ **Portal lobule.** This model is based mainly on the direction of bile flow, which is opposite to that of blood. From this perspective, the liver parenchyma is divided into interlocking triangles, each of which has a portal triad at the center and a central vein at each of its 3 comers.

☐ **Hepatic lobule:** It is the structural unit of liver. It has a Central vein. A single vein marks the center of each lobule. This vessel is easily distinguished from those in the portal triad by its larger opening and lack of a connective tissue investment.

▶ Kuffer cells are Reticuloendothelial cells of liver.   Kerala 2000

▶ Itto cells are fat storing cells in liver.

▶ "Space of Dissie" and "Space of Mall" are seen in Liver.   JK BOPEE 2006

⊃ **Important Histological Features:**

➡ **Hassals corpuscles**	☐ Thymus	MAH 2012
➡ **Corpora amaylacea**	☐ Prostate	
➡ **Corpora atretica**	☐ Ovary	
➡ **Germinal centre**	☐ Lymph node	
➡ **Corpora aranacea**	☐ Pineal gland	
➡ **Herring bodies**	☐ Pituitary gland	
➡ **Cords of Billiroth**	☐ Spleen	

⊃ Cells of Stomach

The Mucus neck cells:

JKBOPEE 2012

- ✓ Called so as they are present in the necks of glands.
- ✓ They secrete **mucin** which serves as a protective layer against HCL.
- ✓ They appear **pale** because of dissolved mucin.
- ✓ They are low columnar with basal flat nuclei.

The Chief cells (The Peptic cells or the Zymogen cells)

- ✓ Called as chief because they line the main part of the **body of the gland.**   AI 2009
- ✓ They are low columnar with basal round nuclei.
- ✓ They secrete **pepsinogen.**

Oxyntic cells (parietal cells)

- ✓ They are scattered in between peptic cells.
- ✓ They are highly acidophilic.
- ✓ **Intrinsic factor of Castle** is secreted by parietal cells   AI 2009
- ✓ They secrete **HCL.**
- ✓ They contain secretory canaliculi and are rounded.

The Argentaffin cells:

- ✓ They are chromaffin Positive and stain positive with Silver salts.
- ✓ They also contain acidophilic granules and are oval in shape.

⊃ Cells of Intestine:

Simple Columnar cells
- ✓ Line the villi and crypts
- ✓ Have free brush border due to presence of microvilli to increase surface area.

Goblet Cells
- ✓ Are also present in the villi and crypts
- ✓ They are unicellular glands
- ✓ They are flask shaped
- ✓ They secrete mucin

Paneth Cells
Are acidophilic
- ✓ Secrete intestinal enzymes
- ✓ Rich in **Rough ER**   AI 2009

Argentaffin cells
- ✓ These are cells with silver staining properties
- ✓ They secrete serotonin.

⊃ Cells of Trachea:

The trachea is composed of

- ➡ **Pseudostratified columnar ciliated cells**, goblet cells, and basal cells.
- ➡ Basal cells are capable of differentiating into goblet or ciliated cells.
- ➡ Other cells making up the epithelium include
- ➡ **Brush cells,**
- ➡ **Serous cells, and**
- ➡ **Kulchitsky cells.**

⊃ Diffuse Lymphatic Tissue, Isolated Lymphatic Nodules: (High Yield for 2011/2012)

The Diffuse lymphatic tissue is a collection of lymphatic tissue in

- ▪ **Alimentary tract**
- ▪ **Respiratory tract**
- ▪ **Genitourinary tract**

The lymphoid tissue is deposited randomly in the **sub epithelial layers** and placed **strategically** so as to **detect and destroy** the pathogenic agents instantaneously and effectively. **Located in adventitia.**   AI 2009

Functioning in close collaboration is other set of **localized concretions** of lymphocytes in the form of **follicles and nodules** such as

- ▪ **Pharyngeal tonsils**
- ▪ **Palatine tonsils**
- ▪ **Lingual tonsils**
- ▪ **Peyers patches** In the small intestine especially in the ileum
- ▪ **Lymphoid follicles in appendix/abdominal tonsil**

In the alimentary canal the diffuse and the local lymphatic systems combine synergistically to form the **GUT ASSOCIATED LYMPHOID TISSUE (GALT).** The main function of this system is to act along with the main lymphatic organs

UPPER LIMB

⇨ Brachial Plexus:

❑	C5 and C6 roots join to form the upper trunk
❑	C7 root alone forms the middle trunk
❑	C8 and T1 roots join to form the lower trunk

Each trunk divides into an anterior and posterior division

- ▶ **All the posterior divisions join to form the posterior cord**
- ▶ **The upper two anterior divisions join to form the lateral cord**
- ▶ **The lowest anterior division alone forms the medial cord**

1

⇨ **Branches of the brachial plexus**

Branches from the roots

- ▶ Nerve to **serratus anterior** (C5,C6,C7) ✱☛☛
- ▶ **Dorsal scapular nerve** (C5) ☛
- ▶ Muscular branches to the 3 scalene muscles

Branches from the trunks

- ▶ **Suprascapular** nerve (C5,C6) ☛   AIPGME 2011
- ▶ **Subclavius** nerve (C5,C6) ☛   AIPGME 2011

Branches from the cords

Medial cord

- ▶ Medial head of median nerve (C8,T1) ☛
- ▶ Medial pectoral (C8,T1) ☛
- ▶ Ulnar nerve (C8,T1) ☛
- ▶ Median cutaneous nerve of forearm (C8,T1) ☛
- ▶ Median cutaneous nerve of arm (T1) ☛

Lateral cord

- ▶ Lateral pectoral (C5,C6,C7) ☛
- ▶ Lateral head of median (C5,C6,C7)☛
- ▶ Musculocutaneous (C5,C6,C7) ☛   TN 2007

Posterior cord

- ▶ Radial (C5,C6,C7,C8,T1) ☛☛
- ▶ Axillary (C5,C6) ☛
- ▶ Nerve to latissimus dorsi (C6,C7,C8) ✱☛
- ▶ Subscapular Upper (C5,C6) ☛   DNB 2001
- ▶ Subscapular lower

➲ **High Yield Facts About Scapula: (High Yield for 2011/2012)**

❏ **Winging scapula**	→ *Injury to thoraxic nerve of Bell. Prominence of medial border of scapula.*
❏ **Pulsating scapula**	→ *In coarctation of aorta, dilatation and tortusity of collaterals around scapula occurs*
❏ **Fracture scapula**	→ *Due to violent trauma*
❏ **Sprengels deformity**	→ *Scapula remains elevated. Failure of descent.*
❏ **Klippel feil deformity**	→ *Bilateral failure of descent of scapula. Webbing of neck and limitation of neck movements due to failure of fusion of occipital bone and cervical spine defects is a feature*

⇨ **Anastomosis around the scapula:**

A rich anastomoses exists around the scapula between branches of subclavian artery (first part) and the axillary artery (third part). This anastomoses provides a collateral circulation through which blood can flow to the limb when the distal part of subclavian artery or the proximal part of axillary artery is blocked.

Anastomosis around the scapula:
Formed by branches of:

> **Subclavian artery- First part**
> - Suprascapular artery
> - Deep branch of transverse cervical artery
>
> **Axillary artery-third part**
> - Subscapular artery & its circumflex scapular branch

Anastomoses over the acromion process:
Formed by-

> - Acromial br. of thoraco-acromail artery
> - Acromial br. of suprascapular artery
> - Acromail br. of posterior circumflex humeral artery
>
> The subscapular artery also forms anastomoses with intercostals arteries.

⇨ Movements at shoulder joint:

Remember: Shoulder joint is weak inferiorly. Kerala 2009

✳ Flexion	➔ Clavicular head of pectoralis major, anterior fibres of deltoid	UPSC 2008
✳ Extension	➔ Posterior fibres of detoid, latismus dorsi	
✳ Adduction	➔ Pectoralis major, latismus dorsi	
✳ Abduction	➔ Deltoid, supraspinatus, serratus anterior, trapezius	
✳ Medial rotation	➔ Pectoralis major, anterior fibres of deltod, latismus dorsi, teres major	
✳ Lateral rotation	➔ Posterior fibres of deltoid, infraspinatus, teres minor.	

⇨ Nerve Supply of:

➔ Dorsal scapular nerve	✳ Rhomboids	
➔ Long thoraxic nerve	✳ Serratus anterior	
➔ Suprascapular nerve	✳ Supraspinatus, infraspinatus	DNB 2007
➔ Lateral pectoral nerve	✳ Pectoralis major	
➔ Medial pectoral nerve	✳ Pectoralis major, pectoralis minor	

⇨ Actions of:

✳ Lumbricals and interossei	➔ Flexion at MP joints, extension at IP Joints
✳ Palmar interossei	➔ Adductors
✳ Dorsal interossei	➔ Abductors

> — **Erbs palsy/Policemans tip hand /Porter's tip** position of upper limb is the result of injury to **Upper trunk of brachial plexus**
> — Erb's point is at union of: **C5-C6**   MP 2006
> — **Klumpkes palsy** is the result of injury to **lower trunk of brachial plexus**   MP 2009

1

ANATOMY

> **Remember:**
>
> The anterior rami of five spinal nerves, C5, C6, C7, C8, and T1 (C4 and T2 may also contribute to the brachial plexus), exit through the intervertebral foramina and form trunks that pass through the scalene triangle and then divide behind the clavicle. The divisions of the trunks reunite to form cords that surround the axillary artery as it passes behind the pectoralis minor tendon. The division of these cords into the major motor and sensory nerves of the upper extremity usually occurs distal to the pectoralis minor tendon.
>
> Rami from C8 and T1 form the lowest trunk, which lies on the first rib behind the subclavian artery and is responsible for the groove in the rib (which is often attributed to the artery). **The peripheral distribution <u>of C8 and T1 fibers</u> provides sensory perception from the fifth finger and medial half of the fourth finger and from the medial aspect of the forearm.**   AIPGME 2012

⇨ **Questions frequently asked from nerves of upper limb**

Ulnar nerve "Musicians nerve"

► Ulnar nerve supplies medial 1/3 of palm. (Hypothenar area)	AIIMS 2007
► Ulnar nerve in hand supplies:	
→ 3,4 Lumbricals,	
→ Palmar and dorsal interosei,	UP 2006
→ Adductor pollicis,	UP 2006
→ Hypothenar muscles.	

> ► Ulnar nerve in hand supplies **flexor carpi ulnaris and medial half of flexor digitorum profundus.**
>
> Lesion of ulnar nerve causes
>
> → **Weakness of ulnar deviation**
>
> → **Weakness of wrist flexion**
>
> → **Adductor pollicis paralysis with loss of thumb adduction**   PGI 2007

⇨ **In ulnar nerve palsy there is:**

☐ Positive Card test	
☐ Positive Book test/Froment sign	PGI 2007
☐ Positive Egawas test	
☐ Ulnar Claw hand	UP 2006

⇨ **Median nerve: "Labourers nerve", Eye of hand**

> • Does not supply arm.
> • Supplies all flexors except Flexor carpi ulnaris and medial half of flexor digitorum profundus in forearm
> • Supplies thenar eminence.   AIIMS 2002

→ Lumbrical 1 and 2,

→ Opponens pollicis,

→ Abductor pollicis brevis,

→ Flexor pollicis brevis in hand. (LOAF).

Implicated in :

Lunate dislocation.   PGI 2000

⊃ Median Nerve Deformity Causes:

❑ Ape thumb deformity,☛☛	AI 2000
❑ Carpal tunnel syndrome, ☛	
❑ Pointing index,☛	
❑ Pen test is positive in median nerve injury	
❑ Loss of opposition and abduction of thumb☛	

⇨ Radial Nerve:

Supplies

- Extensor compartment of arm, forearm,
- Triceps,
- Anconeus and extensors of forearm. Extension of MCP joint   AIIMS 2K
- Injury to RN Causes
  ▶ Wrist drop.☛
  ▶ Saturday night palsy/ crutch palsy☛
- Commonly injured in Radial groove

In Saturday night palsy,

The nerve is damaged during sleep in a drunkard in whom the arm has been placed over the back of a chair. The triceps is usually spared but the weakness conspicuous in the wrist and finger extensors, brachioradialis and supinator. Sensory loss is slight.

⇨ Common Questions in Surgical Anatomy (Hot Questions)

▶ In "supra condylar fracture" of humerus triangular relationship of three bony prominences is not disturbed. In elbow dislocation it is disturbed.☛

▶ The" shoulder joint" is the most commonly dislocated major joint in the body.☛

▶ MC dislocation is inferior   MP 2008

▶ In subacromial bursitis, person feels pain when arm is abducted. "Dawbarns sign" is seen in subacromial bursitis.☛☛

▶ PIN (Posterior interosseous nerve) is a branch of radial nerve. No wrist drop is seen in injury to PIN.

▶ If posterior medial aspect of elbow is banged against a hard object, it mat cause temporary ulnar nerve damage. This may result in painful tingling sensations along ulnar aspect of forearm and hand.Because of these sensations, this area of elbow is called "Funny bone/ Crazy bone".☛

▶ Eye of hand: median nerve. Enables the indiviual to feel thinness and texture of cloth.☛

▶ Pronator syndrome: compression of Median nerve between two heads of pronator teres.☛

▶ Infection of pulp spaces is Felon/ Whitlow.☛

⇨ **Pronator Syndrome**

This is the uncommon entrapment neuropathy of median nerve.
Can occur as nerve passes
1. **Deep to biceps aponeurosis**
2. **Between two heads of pronator teres**
3. **Through a fibrous arch of flexor digitorum superficialis**
Clinical features
- 1. Pain & tenderness in proximal aspect of anterior fore-arm
- 2. Symptoms often follow activities that involve repeated elbow movements.
- 3. Weakness of all muscles innervated by median nerve including abductor pollicis brevis and long finger flexors.
- 4. Sensory impairment on palm.

⇨ **Posterior Interosseous Nerve Palsy**

Entrapment neuropathy of Posterior interosseous nerve

It is seen within forearm extensors.

No sensory impairment as superficial radial nerve arises above this level.

1. Radial wrist extensors & brachioradialis are normal.

2. Extensor carpi ulnaris is usually affected – Attempted wrist extension causes radial deviation.

   Branches to ECRB & supinator may arise from main trunk of radial nerve (above **arcade of Frohse**) where

   entrapment occurs.

   This is characterized by weakness of

1. Finger extension

2. Thumb extension & abduction

⇨ **Injury to Suprascapular Nerve**

Causes:

1. Neuralgic amyotrophy

2. Entrapment neuropathy in scapular notch

3. Damage due to trauma to scapula and shoulder

Features:

1. Pain in shoulder

2. Wasting and weakness of supraspinatus & infraspinatus.

⇨ **Important Nerves Involved in:**

❑ **Wrist drop:** ✱	▪ Radial nerve palsy	**PGI 2001**
❑ **Foot drop:** ✱	▪ Common peroneal nerve palsy	
❑ **Meralgia parasthetica:** ✱	▪ Lateral cutaneous nerve of thigh	
❑ **Winging of scapula:** ✱	▪ Long thoracic nerve of bell	**AIIMS 2003**
❑ **Erbs Palsy:** ✱	▪ Upper trunk of brachial plexus	**AIIMS 2004**
❑ **Klumpkes palsy:** ✱	▪ Lower trunk of brachial plexus	
❑ **Sluders neuralgia** ✱	▪ Middle turbinate pressing anterior ethmoidal nerve	

- **The Axillary nerve** is a branch of the posterior cord of the brachial plexus.

  It is particularly susceptible to the injury in **shoulder dislocations** that displace the humeral head or in fracture of the surgical neck of the humerus.

- A poorly placed crutch **(Crutch Palsy)** may also damage this nerve causing paralysis of the **Teres minor and Deltoid** muscles.   **PGI 2006**

  Arm abduction is impaired and there is associated loss of sensation over the lower half of the deltoid.

  KCET 2012

- The **Lower Subscapular nerve** innervates the **Teres major**, which is responsible for **adducting and medially rotating** the arm, it is a branch of the posterior chord (C5 C6) of the brachial plexus. **MAH 2005**

- The **Suprascapular nerve** innervates the **Supraspinatus and Infraspinatus muscle,** that are responsible for **abduction and lateral rotation** of the arm the nerve is derivated from the C5 & C6 nerve roots.

- In shoulder abduction :

- Humerus elevates

- Clavicle rotates

- Lateral rotation of scapula occurs along with acromioclavicular joint movement.   **AI 2010**

- The **Throacodorsal nerve** innervates the **latissimus dorsi** muscle, that is responsible from **adduction and extension** of the arm. The nerve arises from the posterior chord (C5,C6,C7) of the brachial plexus

- **Musculocutaneous nerve** supplies (BBC) biceps, brachialis, corocabrachialis.   **PGI 2006**

- **Brachioradialis is supplied by radial nerve.**

➲ Action of Various Muscles of Upper Limb: (High Yield for 2011/2012)

► Flexors of forearm: Biceps, brachialis, brachioradialis.	**PGI 2006**
► Extensors of arm: Triceps, Anconeus.	
► Muscles attached to greater tubercle: Supraspinatus, infraspinatus, teres minor.	**PGI 2005**
► Muscles attached to lesser tubercle: subscapularis.	
► Muscles attached to coracoid process: short head of biceps.	**PGI 2005**
✓ Abductors of shoulder joint: Deltoid, serratus anterior, trapezius	**PGI 1997**
✓ Adductors of shoulder joint: pectoralis major, lattismus dorsi	

⇨ Remember: (High Yield for 2011/2012)

☐ Musculocutaneous nerve	Muscles of anterior compartment of arm Supplies Biceps, corocabrachialis, brachialis. ➤ *Injury causes loss of elbow flexion and weakness in supination*.

cont...

cont...

☐ Median nerve	Muscles of anterior compartment of forearm Injury to median nerve at wrist causes: ↪ *Ape thumb deformity.* ↪ *Pen test for abductor pollicis brevis* ↪ *Inability to count on fingers with thumb.*	
☐ Axillary nerve	Deltoid and teres minor Injury causes ↪ *Loss of abduction of shoulder.* ↪ *Rounded contour of shoulder is lost.* ↪ *Sensory loss over lower half of deltoid.*	Fracture surgical neck of humerus dislocation of shoulder
☐ Radial nerve	Posterior muscles of arm and forearm Injury causes ↪ *Saturday night palsy* ↪ *Crutch palsy* ↪ *Wrist drop*	Fracture of humeral shaft

⇨ **The 'Anatomical snuffbox' (High Yield for 2011/2012)**

↪ Triangular depression formed on the **posterolateral side of the wrist** and metacarpal I by the extensor tendons passing into the thumb.

↪ Historically, ground tobacco (snuff) was placed in this depression before being inhaled into the nose.

The base of the triangle is at the wrist and the apex is directed into the thumb. The impression is most apparent when the thumb is extended:

✳ The **lateral border is formed by the tendons of the abductor pollicis longus and extensor pollicis brevis;** the **medial border is formed by the tendon of the extensor pollicis longus;**

✳ The floor of the impression is formed by the scaphoid and trapezium, and distal ends of the tendons of the extensor carpi radialis longus and extensor carpi radialis brevis. **Structures inside:**

⇨ **Remember essentially**

↪ **The radial artery** passes obliquely through the anatomical snuffbox

↪ **Terminal parts of the superficial branch of the radial nerve** pass subcutaneously over the snuffbox

↪ Origin of the **cephalic vein** from the dorsal venous arch of the hand.

⇨ **Ape thumb Deformity:**

↪ Injury of median nerve at wrist leads to wasting of thenar muscles and the thumb is adducted and laterally rotated.

↪ Abduction is lost, opposition is lost, flexion is lost.

↪ **Ape hand deformity** is a deformity in humans who cannot move the thumb outside of the plane of the palm.

↪ It is caused by inability to oppose the thumb and the limited abduction of the thumb.

⇨ **Arcade of Frohse:**

- ↪ Supinator arch
- ↪ Is the most superior part of the superficial layer of the supinator muscle, and is a fibrous arch over the posterior interosseous nerve.
- ↪ The arcade of Frohse is the **most frequent site of posterior interosseous nerve entrapment**, and is believed to play a role in causing progressive paralysis of the posterior interosseous nerve, both with and without injury.

⇨ **Syndromes:**

Pronator syndrome: entrapment of **median nerve** as it passes between two heads of pronator teres.

Cubital tunnel syndrome: entrapment of **ulnar nerve** as it passes between two heads of flexor carpi ulnaris.

Carpal tunnel syndrome: entrapment **of median nerve** as it passes in carpal tunnel

⇨ **Cleidocranial dysostosis:**✹

- ☐ Congenital absence of clavicle.
- ☐ Patient can approximate both shoulders close to each other in front of chest.
- ☐ Faulty ossification of membranous bones.
- ☐ Additional skull bone deformities are also seen.

⇨ **Four rotator cuff muscles are:**

Supraspinatus,	UP 2006
Infraspinatus,	UP 2006
Teres minor,	
Subscapularis	

⇨ **Remember:**

▪ Frozen shoulder☛	▶ is adhesive capsulitis or periarthritis	
▪ Dropped shoulder	▶ paralysis of trapezius	UP 2006
▪ Chronic supraspinatus tendinitis	▶ is painful arc syndrome.	
▪ Tennis elbow ☛	▶ is lateral epicondylitis.	
▪ Golfers elbow ☛	▶ is medial epicondylitis.	
▪ Base pitchers elbow☛	▶ is damage to soft tissues/ bones around elbow.	
▪ De quevarians disease	▶ is tenosynovitis of Extensor pollicis brevis and abductor pollicis longus.	
▪ Trigger finger ☛	▶ is thickening of tendon sheaths at metacarpophalyngeal joint.	
▪ Mallet finger ☛	▶ is avulsion of extensor tendon of distal interphalengeal joint.	

ANATOMY

1

ANATOMY

1

⊃ Frozen Shoulder (Adhesive Capsulitis or Periarthritis)

It is due to tendinitis involving **rotator cuff**. All shoulder movements are restricted due to adhesions. Its cause is unknown.

Spontaneous recovery is seen in six to twelve months.

⇨ Mallet Finger

This is caused by hyperflexion that disrupts the extensor mechanism of the distal phalanx. It is common in baseball players.

Three types of injury occur:

1. Stretching of the extensor tendon
2. Complete disruption of the extensor tendon
3. Avulsion fracture of the base of the distal phalanx

⇨ Ganglion

The most common site is the dorsum of the wrist just lateral to the common extensor of the fingers.

It is considered that a ganglion results from cystic degeneration of connective tissue near joints or tendon sheaths.

The only finding may be a slowly growing, localized swelling. Most patients report intermittent aching & mild weakness.

⇨ Painful arc syndrome (Supraspinatus Syndrome)

It is characterized by

1. Pain in 60-120 degree abduction
2. Chronic thickening of supraspinatus tendon causing impingement of tendon against coraco-acromial arch.

Causes of the syndrome
1. Violent dislocation of the shoulder
2. Tear of supraspinatus tendon
3. Calcified deposit in supraspinatus tendon
4. Injury of greater tubercle

⊃ The Carpal Bones:

⇨ The 8 carpal bones are arranged in 2 rows.

- **The proximal row**, which contains the scaphoid, lunate, triquetrum, and pisiform, articulates with the radius and triangular cartilage to form the carpus.
- **The distal row** contains the trapezium, trapezoid, capitate, and hamate.
- **The ulnar nerve** runs deep to the flexor carpus ulnaris tendon through the **canal of Guyon.**
- **The median nerve** lies between the flexor carpus radialis and the palmaris longus tendon in the carpal tunnel. Blood is supplied via the radial and ulnar arteries, which form the dorsal palmar arch.

- **The scaphoid bone** receives its blood supply from the distal part of this arch, which is prone to injury. **(Especially Avascular Necrosis).** The scaphoid is usually fractured secondary to hyperextension of the wrist, often from falls onto the outstretched hand.

- **Carpal bone dislocation** is usually the result of extreme flexion or extension injuries of the wrist. The type of dislocation or fracture-dislocation produced by these mechanisms depends on the direction and intensity of the acting force or the position of the hand in relation to the forearm at the moment of impact. The integrity of the lunate-capitate relationship is the most crucial factor in all dislocations of the wrist. **Lunate is the bone most commonly to undergo dislocation and dislocation of lunate can cause median nerve injury.**

⇨ Rotator Cuff Tears

The rotator is composed of the tendons of the

- Supraspinatus,
- Infraspinatus,
- Subscapularis &
- Teres minor.

These are attached to the anterior, superior & posterior aspect of upper end of humerus.

⟳ Nerves of Lower Limb: (High Yield for 2011/2012)

✳ **Femoral nerve (posterior division of L2,L3,L4)**	<u>Anterior</u> compartment of high	
✳ **Obturator nerve (anterior division of L2,L3,L4)**	<u>Medial</u> compartment of thigh	**AIIMS 2000**
✳ **Tibial nerve**	<u>Posterior compartment</u> of thigh	
	<u>Posterior compartment</u> of leg	
✳ **Common peroneal nerve**	Short head of biceps femoris	
✳ **Superficial peroneal nerve**	<u>Lateral compartment</u> of leg	
	Injury causes loss of eversion of foot.	
✳ **Deep peroneal nerve**	<u>Anterior compartment</u> of leg	
	Injury causes foot drop.	

Superior gluteal nerve **(Very important)**	Gluteus minimus, gluteus medius, tensor fascia <u>lata</u> <u>NOT Gluteus maximus</u>. **AIIMS 2010**
	injury Causes
	loss of abduction of limb
	Impairment of gait
	Patient cannot keep pelvis level when standing on one
	leg. Tredlenburgs sign+
Inferior gluteal nerve	Gluteus maximus. Injury causes:
	Weakened hip flexion
	Difficulty rising from sitting position.

⇨ **Trendelenburg test**

A positive Trendelenburg is relatively non-specific and may indicate:

- Pain (e.g. due to osteoarthritis of the hip joint)
- Weak hip abductors (gluteus medius, gluteus minimus)
  - ➡ Short femoral neck
  - ➡ Fracture of neck
  - ➡ Dislocation or subluxation of the hip.
  - ➡ Neuropathy
  - ➡ Gluteus medius and minimus are supplied by Superior Gluteal nerve.

⇨ **Trendelenburg test**

Normally when a person is made to stand on one leg, the hip abductors of the ipsilateral side raise the opposite and the unsupported side of the pelvis, **If the abductor mechanism is defective,** the unsupported side of the pelvis drops and this is known as positive Trendelenburg test. Failure of any of the component of the abductor mechanism may result in positive Trendelenburg test.

➲ **Compartment Syndromes of Lower Limb**

- → **Deep posterior compartment syndrome-** there will be pain on passive **dorsiflexion of the foot** and on **toeextension** (since muscles in the deep post compartment are plantar flexors and phalangeal flexors)
- → **Anterior compartment syndrome-** there will be pain on passive **plantar flexion of the foot** and toe flexion.
- → **Lateral compartment syndrome-** there will be pain on passive **foot inversion.**
- → **Superficial posterior compartment syndrome-** pain is on passive **dorsiflexion of foot.**
- → Definitive diagnosis of a chronic CS can be made with an **Intracompartmental pressure test.** A catheter is inserted into the offending compartment to measure its pressure.

⇨ **Action of various muscles of lower limb:**

Hip joint	
• **Medial rotator** of thigh: Gracilis	
• **Lateral rotators** of femur are: Obturator internus, Obturator externus, Sartorius, Pyriformis,	 TN 2008
Superior gamelus, inferior gamellus	DNB 2001
• **Abductors of the hip** include the gluteus medius and gluteus maximus.	AI 2000
• **Adductors of the hip** include the adductors longus, brevis, and magnus.	
• **Extensors and lateral rotator of the hip** include gluteus maximus.	
• **Iliopsoas is flexor of hip**	

Remember
- Tensor fascia lata is extensor of knee, Abductor and medial rotator of hip. (Imp)
- Ilio tibial tract is flexor, external rotator, abductor of hip.(Imp)

Knee joint
- Extensor of knee: Quadriceps femoris.   AIIMS 1991
- Flexion of knee: Biceps femoris. Semimembranosus, semitendonosus
- Medial rotation: Semimembranosus, semitendonosus, popliteus
- Lateral rotation: Biceps femoris

⇨ **Psoas Abscess**

Tuberculous disease of body of any of the thoracic or lumbar vertebrae gives rise to a cold abscess (**no signs of inflammation**). This abscess trickles under psoas sheath up to the insertion of psoas major. This painless swelling may be mistaken for a femoral hernia & flexion deformity of hip it due to spasm of psoas.

⊃ **Important Points: (High Yield for 2011/2012)**

- ▶ **Meralgia Parasthetica** Lateral cutaneous nerve of Thigh✱
- ▶ **Anterior Tarsal Tunnel Syndrome**: Deep peroneal nerve ✱
- ▶ **Tarsal Tunnel Syndrome**: Tibial nerve✱
- ▶ **Joggers Foot**: Medial plantar nerve✱
- ▶ **Hip Pointer**: Iliac Crest✱
- ❖ **Tennis Leg**: Gastrocnemius Soleus strain✱

⇨ **Iliotibial Tract Friction Syndrome**

It is caused by the tense iliotibial tract rubbing the lateral femoral condyle during running. It induces an inflammatory response. The resulting lateral knee pain is felt above the joint.

Iliotibial tract friction syndrome usually occurs in
1. Bowlegged runners (joggers) with pronated feet
2. Wearing shoes with worn lateral soles

Hip
- ▶ Ileo femoral ligament is <u>ligament of Bigelow</u>.
- ▶ It is the <u>strongest ligament</u>.
- ▶ It <u>prevents hyperextension</u> of hip.   AI 1997
- ▶ Pain of hip is referred to knee joint.

Knee
- ▶ <u>Coronary ligament</u> is present between menisci and tibial condyle.   AI 2008
  <u>There is other Coronary ligament in liver.</u>
- ▶ <u>Posterior dislocation of Femur </u>is prevented by anterior cruciate ligament.   UP 2008
- ▶ Posterior cruciate ligament prevents <u>posterior dislocation of Tibia</u>.   AIIMS 2006
- ▶ Ligament of Humphery and Wrisberg are anterior and posterior meniscofemoral ligaments

⇨ **Meniscal Tear**

► Medial meniscus is 20 times more prone to injury than lateral meniscus. The medial meniscus is firmly adherent to the deep part of tibial collateral ligament. In forceful strains (adduction and lateral rotation of the femur over the tibia with the foot firmly placed on the ground) the medial meniscus gets torn. It is because:

► The medial collateral ligament does not allow the meniscus to move away from under the femoral condyle.

► It gets compressed crushed between femoral and tibial condyles that are moving with great force.

► Part of torn cartilage may get displaced. This small piece floats in the joint cavity. It may get lodged between femoral and tibial condyles causing locking of knee joint in flexed position.

⇨ **Nerves related to lower limb compartments (Revise)**

► Adductor compartment of thigh : AIIMS 2000	Obturator nerve
► Flexor compartment of thigh:	Femoral nerve
► Posterior compartment of thigh (hamstrings);	Tibial part of sciatic nerve
► Gluteal region:	Superior and inferior gluteal nerves
► Anterior compartment of leg:	Deep peroneal nerve
► Lateral compartment of leg:	Superficial peroneal nerve
► Posterior compartment of leg:	tibial nerve

❖ **Q angle**: quadriceps angle is formed by line of pull of quadriceps femoris muscle and that of ligamentum patellae as they intersect at centre of patella. more pronunced in females

❖ **Genu valgum** (knock knee) angle< 165°

❖ **Genu varum** (bow legs) angle > 180°

⇨ **The Common Peroneal nerve**

Branches into the superficial and deep peroneal nerves, which supply the muscles of the anterior compartment of the leg and cutaneous areas of the distal anterior leg, dorsum of the foot, and most of the digit

⇨ **The Tibial nerve**

Supplies all the muscles in the posterior compartment of the leg (e.g, tibialis posterior, flexor digitorum longus, gastrocnemius, and soleus).

⇨ **Movements at different joints:✱**

► Ankle:	Dorsiflexion, Plantar flexion	
► Subtalar joint:	Inversion, eversion	UP 2008
► Mid tarsal joint:	Forefoot adduction and abduction	

◗ **Movements at Hip Joint and Muscles Producing these Movements High Yield for 2011-2012**

Flexion	Psoas major, iliacus, sartorius
Extension	Gluteus maximus, hamstrings
Adduction	Adductor longus, brevis, magnus
Abduction	Gluteus medius, minimus, tensor facia lata
Medial rotation	Tensor facia lata
Lateral rotation	Two obturators, two gamelli and quadrates femoris

⇨ **Arterial supply of hip joint:**

- ✓ Obtuator artery
- ✓ Medial circumflex artery
- ✓ Lateral circumflex artery
- ✓ Superior gluteal artery
- ✓ Inferior gluteal artery

⇨ **Nerve supply of hip joint:**

- ✓ Femoral nerve through nerve to rectus femoris
- ✓ Anterior division of obturator nerve
- ✓ Nerve to quadrates femoris
- ✓ Superior gluteal nerve

⇨ **Movements at knee joint and muscles producing these movements**

❑	Flexion	→	Biceps femoris, semimembranosus, semitendonosus
❑	Extension	→	Quadriceps femoris
❑	Medial rotation	→	Popliteus, semimembranosus, semitendonosus
❑	Lateral rotation	→	Biceps femoris

◗ **Arterial Supply of Knee Joint: (High Yield for 2011/2012)**

- ✓ Genicular branches of popliteal artery
- ✓ Genicular branches of femoral artery
- ✓ Genicular branches of lateral circumflex femoral artery
- ✓ Branches of anterior tibial artery
- ✓ Branches of posterior tibial artery

◗ **Nerve Supply of Knee Joint:**

- ✓ Femoral nerve through nerve to vasti
- ✓ Posterior division of obturator nerve
- ✓ Sciatic nerve through tibial and common peroneal nerves

1

ANATOMY

⇨ **Remember:**

> ► **Largest & most complex joint** of the body = knee joint
>
> ► **Locking** of the knee joint is brought about by = Quadriceps
>
> ► **Unlocking** of the knee joint is done by = Popliteus
>
> ► **Meniscus** which is more vulnerable to injury = medial meniscus because of its fixity to the tibial collateral ligament & greater extension during rotatory movements.

⇨ **Ankle joint:**

Dorsiflexion	► Tibialis anterior
	► Extensor digitorum longus
	► Extensor hallucis longus
	► Peroneus tertius
Plantar flexion	✓ Gastrocneimus
	✓ Soleus
	✓ Plantaris
	✓ Tibialis posterior
	✓ Flexor hallucis longus
	✓ Flexor digitorum longus
Inversion	► Tibialis posterior
	► Flexor hallucis longus
	► Flexor digitorum longus
Eversion	✓ Peroneius longus
	✓ Peroneus brevis
	✓ Peroneus tertius

Ligaments at ankle joint

DELTOID LIGAMENT (medial collateral ligament)✱

Consists of superficial and deep fibres.

Superficial fibres:

✓ Anterior tibionavicular
✓ Middle tibiocalcaneal
✓ Posterior tibiotalar

Deep fibres:

Anterior tibiotalar

Lateral collateral ligament:

> ✓ Anterior talofibular
>
> ✓ Posterior talofibular
>
> ✓ Calcaneofibular

⇨ Footballer's Ankle

> Football goalkeeper kicks the ball mostly from close to proximal part of dorsum of foot in a plantar-flexed position.
>
> Over a period of time, the repeated impact initiates formation of bony spicule on the front of neck of talus. This makes the ankle painful.

Root values:		
• Axillary nerve:	⊙ C5, C6✳	
• Ulnar nerve:	⊙ C7, C8, T1✳	
• Radial nerve:	⊙ C5, C6,C7, C8, T1✳	
• Pudendal nerve:	⊙ S2,S3, S4✳	MP 2009
• Femoral nerve:	⊙ L2, L3,L4✳ (DORSAL DIV)	
• Obturator nerve:	⊙ L2,L3,L4✳ (VENTRAL DIV)	UP 2005

⊃ Reflexes: (High Yield for 2011/2012)

▶ Biceps,	⊙ C5, C6
▶ Supinator	⊙ C5, C6
▶ Pronator	⊙ C5, C 6
▶ Triceps	⊙ C6, C7
▶ Cremaster	⊙ L1, L2
▶ Knee	⊙ L2, L3, L4
▶ Plantar	⊙ L5 S1
▶ Ankle	⊙ S1, S2
▶ Anal, Bulbocavernous	⊙ S3 S4

⇨ Breast

> ▶ The protuberant part of the human breast is generally described as overlying **the 2nd to the 6th ribs**, and extending from the **lateral border of the sternum to the anterior axillary line**. Actually, a thin layer of mammary tissue extends considerably farther from the clavicle above to the 7th or 8th ribs below, and from the midline to the edge of latissimus dorsi posteriorly.
>
> ▶ **The Axillary tail of Spence** ✳in the breast is of considerable surgical importance. In some normal cases it is palpable, and in a few it can be seen premenstrually or during lactation. A well-developed axillary tail is sometimes mistaken for a mass of enlarged lymph nodes or a lipoma.

1

ANATOMY

▶ The lobule✳ is the **basic structural unit of the mammary gland**. The number and size of the lobules vary enormously: they are most numerous in young women. From **10 to over 100 lobules** empty via ductules into a **lactiferous duct of which there are from 15 to 20**. Each lactiferous duct is lined by a spiral arrangement of contractile **myoepithelial cells** and is provided with a terminal ampulla — a reservoir for milk or abnormal discharges.

▶ The **ligaments of Cooper** ✳are hollow conical projections of fibrous tissue filled with breast tissue, the apices of the cones being attached firmly to the superficial fascia and thereby to the skin overlying the breast. These ligaments account for the **dimpling of the skin overlying a carcinoma**.

▶ The **areola** contains **involuntary muscle arranged in concentric rings** as well as radially in the subcutaneous tissue. The areolar epithelium contains numerous **sweat glands and sebaceous glands**, the latter of which enlarge during pregnancy and serve to lubricate the nipple during lactation **(Montgomery's tubercles). ✳**

▶ The **nipple** is covered by thick skin with corrugations. Near its apex lie the orifices of the lactiferous ducts. The nipple contains smooth muscle fibres arranged concentrically and longitudinally; thus is an erectile structure which points outwards. Lymphatics of the breast drain predominantly into the axillary and internal mammary lymph nodes. The **axillary nodes** receive approximately 75 per cent of the drainage and are arranged in the following groups:

⇨ **Blood supply is via:**

▶ Internal thoracic artery	PGI 2007
▶ Intercostal artery	PGI 2007
▶ Lateral thoracic artery.	

⇨ **Lymph nodes of Breast:**

• **Lateral**, along the axillary vein; ✳

• **Anterior**, along the lateral thoracic vessels; ✳

• **Posterior**, along the subscapular vessels; ✳

• **Central** embedded in fat in the centre of the axilla; ✳

• **Interpectoral,** a few nodes lying between the pectoralis major and minor muscles; ✳

• **Apical,** which lie above the level of the pectoralis minor tendon in continuity with the lateral nodes and receive the efferents of all the other groups. ✳

The apical nodes are also in continuity with the **supraclavicular nodes and drain into the subclavian lymph trunk** which enters the great veins directly or via the thoracic duct or jugular trunk. The sentinal node is that lymph node designated as the first axillary node draining the breast.

The internal mammary nodes are fewer in number and lie along the internal mammary vessels deep to the plane of the costal cartilages.

Mondor's disease✳ is thrombophlebitis of the superficial veins of the breast and anterior chest wall (although it has also been encountered in the arm).

Familial breast cancer✱ Recent developments in molecular genetics and the identification of a number of breast cancer predisposition genes (**BRCA1, BRCA2 and TPS3**). These women have a risk of developing breast cancer two to 10 times above baseline.

▶ Lymph nodes <u>below</u> Pectoralis Minor **Level 1**☞☞

▶ Lymph nodes <u>behind</u> Pectoralis Minor **Level 2**☞☞

▶ Lymph nodes <u>above</u> Pectoralis Minor **Level 3**☞☞

▶ ☞The principal nodes which drain the breast are: <u>Axillary Group</u> of Lymph nodes.

▶ ☞About <u>70 -75%</u> of lymph from breast drains into Axillary group of Lymph nodes, <u>20%</u> into internal mammary group of Lymph nodes and <u>5%</u> into posterior intercostal group of lymph nodes.

▶ ☞Among the Axillary Group Chief is the <u>Anterior group.</u>

▶ **Rotters nodes** are <u>interpectora</u>l nodes☜

▶ Absence of sternal head of pectoralis major: Polands syndrome☜

➲ Openings of Diaphragm: (High Yield for 2011/2012)

▶ Vena caval opening:
  — Thoraxic 8 level
  — Inferior vena cava,
  — Rt phrenic nerve

▶ esophageal opening:
  — Thoraxic 10 level
  — Esophagus,
  — Vagus nerves,
  — Esophageal branch of lt. gastric artery

▶ Aortic opening:
  — Thoraxic 12 level
  — Aorta,
  — Thoracic duct,   JKBOPEE 2012
  — Azygous vein.   PGI 2003

  ▶ Esophageal opening lies <u>in muscular part</u> of diaphragm☜
  ▶ Vena caval lies <u>in central tendon</u> of diaphragm☜
  ▶ Aortic opening is <u>not a true opening</u> but an osseo aponeurotic opening.☜

  ▶ Greater and lesser splanchnic nerves pierces <u>each crus</u> of diaphragm✱
  ▶ <u>Lt crus</u> is also pierced by hemi azygous vein.✱
  ▶ Sympathetic chain passes behind <u>medial</u> arcuate ligament
  ▶ Subcostal nerves vessels pass behind <u>lateral</u> arcuate ligament.
  ▶ Superior epigastric vessels and lymphatics pass through <u>Foramen of Morgagni (Larrys space)</u> PGI 2004
  ▶ Musculo phrenic vessels pierce the diaphragm

1

ANATOMY

▶ Hernia <u>does not</u> occur through vena caval opening.		AI 2002
▶ Bochaldeks hernia occurs through <u>posterolateral part of diaphragm</u>.		AI 1996
▶ Morgagni hernia occurs <u>anteriorly on right usually</u>.		AI 2007
▶ Remember Accessory phrenic nerve is commonly a branch from the nerve to subclavius		MP 2004

⇨ **Sites of esophageal constrictions:✳**

Distance from incisor	Landmark	
▶ 6 inches	Pharyngeoesophageal junction	
▶ 9 inches	Aortic arch crossing	
▶ 11 inches	Left bronchus	
▶ 15 inches	Pierces diaphragm	AIIMS 1992

⇨ **Esophagus**

▶ Length **25 cm**	PGI 2004
▶ Commences at **lower end of cricoid**	TN 2002
▶ Has **squamous** epithelium	PGI 2004
▶ Toughest layer is **muscularis**.	
▶ **No** serosa	

⇨ **The Trachea:**

- It Is a **fibromuscular tube**
- It is **10 to 12 cm. in length** and varying from 13 to 22 mm. in width.
- Approximately 20 U-shaped hyaline cartilages support the trachea laterally and ventrally.
- The trachea **originates at the level of the cricoid cartilage** and descends through the superior aperture of the thorax and the **superior mediastinum** to its bifurcation at the level of the sternal angle (lower border of the fourth thoracic vertebra). **JKBOPEE 2012**
- Here it divides into the right and left primary bronchi.
- The trachea is composed of **pseudostratified columnar ciliated cells**, goblet cells, and basal cells. Basal cells are capable of differentiating into goblet or ciliated cells. Other cells making up the epithelium include **brush cells, serous cells, and Kulchitsky cells.**

⇨ **Thorax:**

Heart

▶ **Right coronary** artery arises from **anterior aortic cusp✳**	AI 2002
▶ **Left Coronary** arises from **Posterior aortic cusp.✳**	
▶ Posterior interventricular artery determines coronary dominance.	
▶ In case it arises from right coronary artery, right dominance	AIIMS 2007
▶ In case it arises from left coronary, left dominance.	
▶ Rt Coronary artery mostly supplies SA node, AV node, AV bundle.	AI 2003

- ▶ The **SA node** is usually supplied by Right coronary artery and **Right Vagus**✳   MAH 2002
- ▶ The **AV node** is usually supplied by Right coronary artery and **Left vagus.**✳
- ▶ Sympathetic innervation is by **T2-T6**   DNB 2001
- ▶ Maximum (90%) of venous drainage of Heart goes to **Coronary Sinus**✳
- ▶ In fetal life left sided svc drains into coronary sinus   AI 2010
- ▶ **Great Cardiac Vein** follows Anterior Interventricular artery.☛
- ▶ **Middle Cardiac Vein** follows Posterior Interventricular artery.☛   AI 2003
- ▶ **Small Cardiac Vein** follows Rt. Marginal artery.☛

➲ Coronary Sinus

Is the largest venous channel of the heart about 3 cms. It located **in left posterior coronary sulcus.**

It is a remnant of **left horn of sinus venosus**   PGI 2011

While the right horn gets incorporated into right atrium.

It opens into the right atrium of the heart through an orfice of coronary sinus and has a valve called the

Thebesian valve. It receives :

- ✓ Great cardiac vein   PGI 2011
- ✓ Middle cardiac vein   PGI 2011
- ✓ Small cardiac vein   PGI 2011
- ✓ Right marginal vein
- ✓ Oblique vein of left atrium
- ✓ Right marginal vein

➲ Thoracic Duct:

- — Also called as **Pecquets duct.**   DNB 2006
- — **Beaded** in appearance.
- — **18 inches in length.**
- — **Is the largest** lymphatic pathway in body.
- — The duct commences in the abdomen as an elongated lymph sac of the cisterna chili is: **Thoracic duct.**   UP 2007
- — Begins from cisterna chylii at the level of T12 vertebrae
- — Injury to thoracic duct by trauma leads to chylothorax

- ▶ <u>Inferior surface</u> of heart is formed by Rt and Lt ventricle.   AI 1993
- ▶ <u>Base</u> of heart is formed by Rt and Lt atrium.   JIPMER 1983
- ▶ <u>Part of heart lying close to esophagus:</u> Lt atrium.   TN 1997

1

ANATOMY

Structures	Present In:	
• Musculi pectinati :	Atria of heart	
• Trabeculae carnea:	Rt. ventricle of heart	JKHND 2005
• Moderator band/Septomarginal trabeculae:	Right ventricle	
• Coronary sinus, SVC, IVC:	Open in Right atrium.	MAH 2003
• SA node is located in:	Rt. Atrium	
• Whole of conducting system is mostly supplied by rt coronary artery except Right bundle branch (supplied by left coronary artery)		
• Holmes heart:	Single ventricle	

⮩ Lungs

⇨ Bronchopulmonary segment:

► Vascular segment

► Independent

► Bronchial artery supplies till respiratory bronchiole   AI 2008

► Largest subdivision of lobe.

⇨ Peculiarities of Blood Supply of Lung ← ← ←

► Smallest functional unit of lung is **lobule**.   UP 2008

► Blood supply of lung tissue proper is by **Bronchial arteries**.

► Bronchial arteries are branches of **descending Thoracic Aorta**.

► They supply nutrition to bronchial tree and pulmonary tissue **upto respiratory bronchiole.**

► Segments **distal to respiratory bronchiole** are supplied by branches from **Pulmonary vessels.**

► On the **right side there is only one BA** arising **indirectly** from descending Thoracic Aorta.

► On the **Left side there are two BA** arising **directly** from descending Thoraxic Aorta.

► Bronchial arteries are responsible for Haemoptysis.

► Pulmonary arteries carry deoxygenated blood.

► Pulmonary veins carry oxygenated blood.

► Sequestered segments are supplied by systemic circulation.   UP 2008

⇨ Azygos Lobe of Lung

▪ Azyos means unpaired. Azygos lobe may be seen on the right lung.

▪ It is seen as a result of developmental anomaly related to lung bud and posterior cardinal vein.

▪ The posterior cardinal vein (future azygos vein) gets embedded in the substance of lung which passes as lung bud below the arch formed by posterior cardinal vein.

▪ The part of lung medial to the vein forms the azygos lobe.

⊃ Gems About Intra Abdominal Organs:

⇨ The Spleen

- Is a **haemolymphatic** organ.
- The **second largest organ of the reticuloendothelial system.**
- It is located in the posterior left upper quadrant of the abdomen **(left hypochondrium)** where its relationships to the diaphragm, stomach, pancreas, left kidney, and splenic flexure of the colon are maintained by suspensory ligaments. The splenophrenic, splenorenal, and splenocolic ligaments are usually relatively avascular and their transection allows the spleen to be displaced medially and anteriorly.
- The "Gastrosplenic ligament" extends from the greater curvature of the body and fundus of the stomach to the spleen, <u>contains the short gastric arteries and veins.</u>
- The "Splenorenal" ligament (Lienorenal) and attached to the spleen at the hilum: <u>splenic artery and vein, lymphatic structures, and often the tail of the pancreas</u>
- The arterial supply to the spleen is derived from the celiac artery from both the **splenic artery and the short gastric arteries,** which usually arise as branches of the gastroepiploic or the splenic arteries
- The **splenic vein** is formed by a coalescence of polar veins in the splenic hilum and courses with the splenic artery along the dorsal surface of the pancreas to **enter the portal system.**

⊃ The Stomach

Starts from **gastroesophageal junction to the pylorus.**

It is bounded on the left by the spleen and on the right by the liver

The blood supply to the stomach is extensive,

- ▶ **Left gastric artery,** which supplies the upper lesser curvature of the stomach from celiac trunk
- ▶ The **right gastric artery** branches off the hepatic artery, which originates from the celiac axis; it supplies blood to the distal lesser curvature.
- ▶ The **left gastroepiploic artery** is a branch off the short gastric vessels; it comes from the splenic and therefore originally from the celiac axis.
- ▶ The **right gastroepiploic artery** branches off the gastroduodenal artery, which comes originally from the hepatic artery and therefore from the celiac axis.

The **venous drainage of the stomach** empties in a variety of directions, including venous tributaries along the esophagus, veins that flow with the short gastrics to the splenic vein, and venous drainage that is carried toward the duodenum and toward the **portal vein.**

Nerve supply is predominantly by the vagus.

An **anterior (left) and posterior (right) vagus** nerve courses with the esophagus until the gastroesophageal junction.

The **"criminal" nerve of Grassi** is the first branch of the posterior vagal nerve innervating the greater curvature fundus. At the junction of the fundus and the antrum of the stomach, the vagal nerves branch and innervate the antrum. This vagal branch point is called the **crow's foot.**

The **lesser sac is** bounded ventrally by the stomach and is an important location during operation, in that it is a *frequent space for fluid collection and is an important plane for the exposure of gastric anatomy.*

1

ANATOMY

⊃ Duodenum

The duodenum **extends from the pylorus about 20 to 30 cm. and ends at the ligament of Treitz**, which is where the jejunum begins. This is marked by adhesive bands between the duodenal-jejunal junction and the retroperitoneum on the left side of the abdomen.

The duodenum is divided into **four anatomic regions:**

✓   The first portion or the cap or bulb;

✓   The second portion or the descending duodenum;

✓   The third or transverse portion; and the

✓   Fourth or ascending portion

⇨ Gems About Duodenum:

The duodenal cap lies just beyond the pylorus. **Ninety percent of ulcers occur in the duodenal cap region.**

The **gastroduodenal artery** *lies directly behind the duodenal cap, and penetrating ulcers into the pancreas initially erode through the gastroduodenal artery, accounting for the massive bleeding that occurs with these ulcers.*

The **second (descending) portion** of the duodenum: **The ampulla of Vater and the minor papilla both enter into the duodenum in this portion.** The second portion of the duodenum is approximately 10 cm. in length.

The third and fourth portions of the duodenum (transverse and ascending portions) are **mostly retroperitoneal.**

The third portion is attached to the uncinate process and crosses the abdomen and over the aorta.

Compression of the junction of the third and fourth portions of the duodenum by the angle of the SMA and the aorta is called the **SMA syndrome.**

The fourth portion of the duodenum blends into the jejunum at the **ligament of Treitz,** which attaches this junction to the retroperitoneum. Mobilization of the ligament of Treitz is necessary in duodenal resections. The ligament is often composed of small strands of striated muscle that eventually extend to the crus of the diaphragm.

"Kerckring's folds" *The mucosal surface of the small intestine contains numerous circular mucosal folds called <u>the plicae circulares (valvulae conniventes, or valves of Kerckring)</u>* of the duodenum begin just beyond the cap and continue throughout the duodenum. The concentric folds of Kerckring are approximately 1 to 2 mm. thick and 2 to 4 mm. high. They are taller and more numerous in the distal duodenum and proximal jejunum, becoming shorter and fewer distally.

⇨ Difference between Small and Large intestine ✳ ✳

✓ Small intestine	✓ Large intestine
✓ About **6 -7 metres** in length	✓ About **180 cms** in length
✓ **Small** diameter	✓ **Larger** diameter
✓ Mucosa has **villi and crypts**	✓ Mucosa has crypts but **no villi**
✓ Paneth cells **present**	✓ Paneth cells **absent**

✓ **Less** goblet cells	✓ **More** goblet cells
✓ Brunner's glands in duodenum **present** MAH 2005	✓ Both **absent**
✓ Peyers patches in ileum **present**	
(*Peyer's patches are lymph nodules aggregated in the submucosa of the small intestine. These lymphatic nodules are most abundant in the ileum, but the jejunum also contains them.*)	
✓ Sacculations **absent**	✓ Sacculations **present**
✓ Appendices epiploicae **absent**	✓ Appendices epiploicae **present**
✓ Taenia **absent**	✓ Taenia **present**

➲ Celiac trunk: PGI 2003,

▶ **Left Gastric Artery**→ esophageal branch, gastric branch ✳

▶ **Common Hepatic Artery**→ right hepatic , left hepatic, GASTRODUODENAL ARTERY→ supraduodenal, right gastroepiploic, superior pancreaticoduodenal artery

▶ **SPLEENIC ARTERY**→ short gastric, left gastroepiploic, pancreatic branches

⇨ Meckel's diverticulum

• A Meckel's diverticulum, a **true congenital diverticulum.**✳

• It is a **vestigial remnant of the omphalomesenteric duct** (also called the vitelline duct), and is the most frequent malformation of the gastrointestinal tract☛

• Meckel's diverticulum is located in the **distal ileum**, usually within about 60-100 cm of the ileocecal valve.

• It is typically **3-5 cm long**, runs **antimesenterically** and has its own blood supply.☛

• It is a remnant of the connection from the umbilical cord to the small intestine present during embryonic development.

⇨ A memory aid is the rule of 2's: ✳

▶ **2%** (of the population)

▶ **2 feet** (from the ileocecal valve)

▶ **2 inches** (in length)

▶ **2%** are symptomatic,

▶ **2 types** of common ectopic tissue (gastric and pancreatic)

▶ Most common age at clinical presentation is **2**,

▶ Males are **2** times as likely to be affected.

Anal canal above Dentate Line	Anal Canal Below Dentate Line
◍ Endodermal	◍ Ectodermal
◍ Cuboidal epithelium	◍ Stratified squamous
◍ Superior Rectal artery	◍ Inferior Rectal artery
◍ Superior Rectal Vein	◍ Inferior Rectal Vein
◍ Internal Iliac group of Lymph Nodes	◍ Superficial inguinal group of lymph nodes
◍ Pain insensitive	◍ Pain sensitive

⊃ The Liver

► Lies in the **right upper quadrant** of the abdomen.

► It is the **largest gland** in the body, it weighs approximately 1500 gm.

► The gallbladder lies on the **dorsal surface of the liver** in a transpyloric plane.

► A peritoneal membrane **(Glisson's capsule)** covers the liver.

► **The superior surface** of the liver conforms to the undersurface of the right diaphragm. The relations of the **inferior surface** of the liver are the duodenum, colon, kidney, adrenal gland, esophagus, and stomach. Peritoneum invests the entire liver except for a bare area under the diaphragm on the posterosuperior surface adjacent to the inferior vena cava and hepatic vein.

⇨ Ligaments of Liver:

1. **The falciform ligament**, which attaches the liver to the anterior abdominal wall from the diaphragm to umbilicus and incorporates the ligamentum teres hepaticus

2. **The anterior and posterior right and left coronary ligaments**, which in continuity with the falciform ligament connect the diaphragm to the liver. The lateral aspects of the anterior and posterior leaves of the coronary ligaments fuse to form the right and left triangular ligaments.

3. **The gastrohepatic and hepatoduodenal ligaments**, which consist of the anterior layer of lesser omentum and are continuous with the left triangular ligament. The hepatoduodenal ligament contains the hepatic arteries, portal vein, and extrahepatic bile ducts. It forms the anterior boundary of the **epiploic foramen of Winslow** and the communication between the greater and lesser peritoneal cavities.   MAH 2012

⇨ Four lobes of the liver are commonly described:

► Right

► Left

► Quadrate

► Caudate.

⇨ Portal Vein:

- ✓ The portal vein provides about **three fourths of the liver's blood supply.**

- ✓ The combination of the **superior mesenteric and splenic veins** forms the portal vein, behind the **neck of the pancreas.**

- ✓ The portal vein then passes superiorly, **posterior to the first part of the duodenum** at the level of the second lumbar vertebra.

- ✓ Portal vein is **1 to 3 cm. in diameter** and **5 to 8 cm in length** before dividing into right and left branches at the porta hepatis

- ✓ The portal vein usually passes behind the bile duct and hepatic artery in the hepatoduodenal ligament.

- ✓ The portal trunk divides into **left and right hepatic branches in the portal fissure. The left branch of the portal vein is longer.**

- ✓ The portal vein divides into small veins and venules, which **finally enter hepatic sinusoids.**

- ✓ The portal **vein has no valves.**

⇨ Portocaval Anastmosis:

Numerous tributaries of the portal vein connect outside the liver with the systemic venous system. Under normal circumstances these communications have little physiologic significance. However, if portal hypertension develops, these rudimentary portosystemic communications develop into large channels with increased collateral flow.

⇨ Sites of Portosystemic Anastomoses include:

- ▶ The submucosal veins of the proximal stomach and distal esophagus, which can receive blood from the coronary and short gastric veins to drain into the azygous veins (**high blood flow through this pathway produces gastric varices, esophageal varices, or both**);

- ▶ Umbilical and periumbilical veins, recanalized from the obliterated umbilical vein in the ligamentum teres hepaticus, and which may cause **caput medusae** or the loud Cruveilhier-Baumgarten bruit

- ▶ Tributaries of the inferior mesenteric vein, which include the superior hemorrhoidal veins that communicate with the middle and inferior hemorrhoidal veins of the systemic circulation and may cause large **hemorrhoids**; and

- ▶ Other retroperitoneal communications, including connections to the **renal and adrenal veins.**

⇨ Sphincter of Oddi.

The circular smooth muscle fibers in the ampulla of Vater area constitute the sphincter of Oddi, which *regulates the flow of bile from the liver into the duodenum.*

The three principal parts of the sphincter of Oddi are:

- The sphincter of the choledochus (i.e., the circular muscle fibers surrounding the intramural and submucosal bile duct);

- The pancreatic sphincter, which consists of the amuscular septum between the bile and pancreatic ducts;

- Ampullary sphincter: The ampullary sphincter, the most important component of the sphincter of Oddi, includes a layer of longitudinal muscle fibers that help prevent reflux of intestinal contents into the ampulla.

Relaxation of the ampullary sphincter may promote reflux into the pancreatic duct.

⊃ Gallbladder:

The gallbladder, a pear-shaped (pyriform), distensible appendage of the extrahepatic biliary system.

Capacity: 30 to 50 ml. of bile.

Parts: It has a fundus, body, and neck.

The duct of gallbladder cystic duct varies in length and usually contains spiral valves of Heister that regulate bile flow.

Enlargement of the neck of the gallbladder such as from a stone may form a pouch (Hartmann's pouch).

The triangle bounded by the cystic duct, common hepatic duct, and inferior border of the liver is the Triangle of Calot.

The gallbladder receives its blood supply from the cystic artery, which originates from the right hepatic artery.

Venous drainage of the gallbladder enters principally into the portal vein.

The lymphatics drain into cystic duct nodes near the superior aspect of the cystic duct. (Cystic Lymph node of Lund).

⊃ The Triangle of Calot:

Is a surgical landmark used to identify important structures during cholecystectomy, is bounded by the cystic duct, the common hepatic duct, and the inferior border of the liver.

The right hepatic and cystic arteries are located within it, and anomalous structures often pass through it.

"Moniyhans Hump": An abnormal bend in the course of the right hepatic artery, throwing it into the configuration of a caterpillar hump, (Moynihan's hump) invites injury unless it is carefully dissected free

⇨ The Pancreas (Pan: all creas: flesh)

- Is a retroperitoneal organ, lying posterior to the stomach and lesser omentum.

- It extends from the duodenal C loop to the hilum of the spleen.

- The gland has a distinctive yellow/tan/pink color and is multilobulated.

- The pancreas is covered by peritoneum anteriorly, and posteriorly it lies in proximity to the inferior vena cava, right renal vein, aorta at the level of the first lumbar vertebra, superior mesenteric vessels, and splenic vein.

- ➡ The gland is divided into **four portions:**
- ✓ **The head (which includes the uncinate process),**
- ✓ **The neck,**
- ✓ **The body, and**
- ✓ **The tail.**

- ➢ The head of the gland extends to the right of the neck, lying within the confines of the duodenal C loop; it includes the posteroinferior extension arising from the ventral primordium, designated the uncinate process. The uncinate process extends posterior to the superior mesenteric vein, ending at the right margin of the superior mesenteric artery. The body of the pancreas lies immediately to the left of the neck; the tail of the pancreas extends to the left of the body into the splenic hilum.

- ➢ The head of the pancreas is intimately associated with the second portion of the duodenum, and these two structures are jointly supplied by two arterial arcades known as the **anterior and posterior pancreaticoduodenal arteries.** These arteries originate from the **superior and inferior pancreaticoduodenal vessels** as branches of the *celiac axis and superior mesenteric artery, respectively.* The distal body and tail of the pancreas are supplied by short branches of the splenic and left gastroepiploic arteries. Within the posterosuperior and posteroinferior aspects of the body of the pancreas lie the superior and inferior pancreatic arteries, respectively.

- ➢ Veins draining the pancreatic parenchyma eventually terminate in the **portal vein,** which arises posterior to the neck of the pancreas at the junction of the splenic and superior mesenteric veins.

Multiple lymph node groups drain the pancreas.

- ➡ <u>From the head</u> of the gland, nodes in the **pancreaticoduodenal groove communicate with subpyloric, portal, mesocolic, mesenteric, and aortocaval nodes.**

- ➡ Lymphatics <u>in the body and tail of the pancreas</u> drain to retroperitoneal nodes in the **splenic hilum or to celiac, aortocaval, mesocolic, or mesenteric nodes.**

⊃ The Kidneys

- ▪ **Bean shaped**

- ▪ **Retroperitoneal**

- ▪ **Right kidney is lower** than left (but right suprarenal is higher than left.)

- ▪ Each kidney is **9 to 15 cm. long, 4 to 5 cm. wide, and approximately 3 cm. thick** They are located on each side of the vertebral column between the parietal perineum and the fascia and musculature of the posterior abdominal wall and are embedded in a variable amount of fat and surrounded by a layer of fascia **(Gerota's fascia)**

- ▪ They lie on the side of the psoas muscle.

- ▪ They are not parallel, with the upper poles being approximately 2 cm. from the midline and the lower poles approximately 3.5 cm. from the midline.

⇨ **Coverings of Kidney (From inside to out)**

✓   Fibrous capsule
✓   Perinephric fat
✓   Renal fascia with 2 layers.
Anterior layer of Toldts Fascia,
Posterior layer of fascia of Zuckerkandl.
✓   Pararenal Fat

⇨ **Posterior relations of Kidney:**

▪   3 parts of diaphragm: Medial arcuate ligament, Lateral arcuate ligament, Diaphragm
▪   3 muscles: Psoas major, quadrates lumborum, transverses abdominis
▪   3 nerves: Subcostal, iliohypogastric, ilioinguinal nerves.
▪   Right kidney: 12 th rib
▪   Left kidney: 11th and 12th rib.

⇨ **Ureter:**

— 25cm long	(PGI 2008)
— Totally retroperitoneal	
— It enters true pelvis after crossing iliac vessel	

➲ **Important Points About Ureter: (PGI 2005)**

•   Starts at the hilum
•   Changes its direction at the ischial spine
•   Penetrates the bladder wall without any valve
•   Enters the bladder at the lateral angle of the trigone
•   Enters pelvis in front of bifurcation of common iliac artery

⇨ **The Supra renals or the Adrenal glands**

▪   Are bilateral retroperitoneal organs located on the superior medial aspect of the upper pole of each kidney
▪   Each gland weighs approximately 4 gm. The left adrenal is larger and flatter
▪   The normal adrenal cortex is bright yellow and thicker than the red-brown medulla.

➲ **Blood Supply of Supra Renals:**   **JK BOPEE 2012**

▶ Superior suprarenal artery: branch of Inferior Phrenic artery	UP 2000
▶ Middle suprarenal artery: branch of Abdominal aorta	UP 2000
▶ Inferior suprarenal artery :branch of Renal artery	

⇨ **Venous Drainage :**

The left adrenal vein empties primarily into the left renal vein but may occasionally drain directly to the vena cava.

Lymphatic plexuses within the subcapsular portion of the adrenal cortex and the adrenal medulla drain to the adjacent para-aortic subdiaphragmatic and renal lymph nodes.

⊃ Important Anatomical Relations

Relations at hilum of kidney (Anterior to Posterior) "VAP"✳

- Renal vein   RJ 2009
- Renal artery
- Renal pelvis

Relations at Femoral Triangle (From Medial to Lateral) "VAN"✳

- Femoral vein
- Femoral artery
- Femoral nerve

Intercostal space (From Above Down Wards). " VAN"✳

- Intercostal vein
- Intercostal artery
- Intercostal nerve

Cubital Fossa (From Medial to lateral side). "MBBR"✳

- Median nerve (Medial aspect)
- Brachial artery
- Biceps tendon
- Radial nerve
- Lateral boundary by brachioradialis muscle.   DNB 2007

⊃ Male Reproductive Tract: High Yield for AIPGME/AIIMS/PGI 2013

Testes

- ✓ Is **male gonad**.
- ✓ Are two oval structures average **4 to 5 cm. in length** and **2.5 to 3.5 cm. in width** in the normal adult male.
- ✓ 10-15 gms in weight (Indians average)
- ✓ Testis arises from the genital ridge

⇨ Covered by

- ➡ Tunica vaginalis
- ➡ Tunica albugenia
- ➡ Tunica vasculosa

- **Blood supply** is by **testicular artery** which is a branch of abdominal aorta.

- **Venous drainage** of the testis is through the **pampiniform plexus** to the spermatic vein, which is usually single and emerges from the upper end of the cord and then follows the internal spermatic artery through the retroperitoneum. **On the right the spermatic vein empties into the vena cava below the right renal vein, whereas on the left the spermatic vein empties into the main renal vein.** Increased hydrostatic pressure, particularly on the left, may result in dilatation of the pampiniform venous plexus, producing a **varicocele.**

- **The lymphatic drainage** of the testis is through the spermatic cord and the inguinal canal and then to the **common iliac and pre aortic and paraortic nodes**, with the latter communicating across the midline at the level of the kidneys and also with the mediastinal and supraclavicular chains.

- Histologically, there are two principal portions of the testis: **The seminiferous tubules,** which are responsible along with the **Sertoli cells for spermatogenesis**, and the **interstitial or Leydig cells,** which elaborate androgenic hormones, predominantly testosterone.

Testicular descent

▶ Iliac Fossa:	3 rd month	
▶ Deep Inguinal Ring:	7 th month	
▶ Pass through Inguinal Canal:	7 th month	AIIMS 1997
▶ At Superficial Inguinal ring:	8 th month	
▶ Enter Scrotum:	9 th month	AI 1996

Epididymis:

Are coiled structures each containing a single epididymal tubule **12 to 19 feet long** and attached to the posterolateral surface of each testis.

Remember: From the tails of the epididymides sperm are **transmitted into the vasa deferentia**, which are direct continuations of the duct of the epididymides passing up the spermatic cord, across the inguinal canal, and then retroperitoneally to the ampulla of the seminal vesicles, with which **they conjoin to form an ejaculatory duct on each side.** The ejaculatory duct **then empties directly into the prostatic urethra.**

The principal blood supply for the epididymis is from the internal spermatic artery. Venous drainage corresponds to the arterial supply, and the lymphatic drainage of the epididymis parallels that of the testis. The prime function of the epididymis is not only as a conduit for spermatozoa but also for biochemical and functional maturation and ultimate storage.

ANATOMY

Ductus deferens / Vas Deferens

Is 18 inches inlength. The vas deferens is an easily discernible structure within the scrotum and spermatic cord because it is a **heavily muscled tubular** structure.

Spermatic Cord

The spermatic cord, **suspending each testis** and its attached epididymis, is composed of the *vas deferens, the internal spermatic artery, the external spermatic artery, the pampiniform plexus of veins, the lymphatic drainage system of the contents of the scrotum, and the autonomic nerve supply to the testis.* In addition, the cord is surrounded by fibers of the cremasteric muscle, which assist by contraction and relaxation in the maintenance of optimal testicular temperature and provide for testicular retraction with sexual excitation or in the primitive fright reaction.

⇨ **Contents of spermatic cord:-**

- The ducts deferens
- Testicular and cremastric arteries.
- Artery of vas
- The pampiniform plexus of veins.
- Lymph vessels from testis.
- Genital branch of Genitofemoral nerve.
- Remains of processus vaginalis.

Scrotum

⇨ **High Yield for AIPGME/AIIMS/PGI 2013**

The scrotal sac, consisting of two lateral compartments fused in the midline **encloses the testes, epididymides, and terminal portions of the spermatic cords.** The dartos, consisting of elastic fibers, connective tissue, and smooth muscle fibers, is attached to the corrugated skin of the scrotum, rich in sebaceous glands, and provides for muscular contraction of the scrotal sac in response to temperature changes or sexual excitation. The principal function of the scrotum is to aid in temperature control of the testes for optimal spermatogenesis, which takes place at temperatures several degrees lower than those in the intra-abdominal cavity.

The blood supply of the scrotum comes from the **deep pudendal branches of the femoral artery and branches of the internal pudendal artery.**

The lymphatics of the scrotal halves anastomose freely, surround the penis, and drain to the inguinal and femoral nodes. There are no connections between the lymphatics of the scrotum and the testes; the scrotal lymphatics do not accompany the pudendal vessels.

1

ANATOMY

Seminal Vesicles

Are **paired, monotubular, convoluted structures** lying beneath the base of the bladder and trigone. *Posteriorly they are invested by Denonvilliers' fascia, which separates them from the anterior wall of the rectum.*

DNB 2011

The two seminal vesicles fuse immediately with the ampullae of the vasa, forming the ejaculatory ducts, which open into the prostatic urethra at the level of the verumontanum. The seminal vesicles secrete a mucoid vehicle for the spermatozoa and also elaborate the body's only source of fructose, which is used as an essential nutrient for maintenance of spermatozoal viability.

Prostate Gland

Is a <u>fibromuscular, glandular organ</u> that surrounds the neck of the urinary bladder and the proximal portion of the male urethra. The gland is supported **anteriorly** by the puboprostatic ligaments, **inferiorly** by the genitourinary diaphragm (external urinary sphincter), and **posteriorly** by the rectal wall, which is separated from the prostate by an obliterated pelvic reflection of the peritoneum called **Denonvilliers' fascia.**

DNB 2011

The prostate consisting of two portions: **an anterior (inner) group** of glands intimately associated with the urethra and a **posterior (outer) portion** of more fibromuscular character.

Arterial supply: The inferior vesical and internal pudendal arteries provide the blood supply to the prostate, entering the gland posterolaterally at the vesical neck.

Venous drainage of the prostate is complex and diffuse, with plexuses over the anterior and lateral portions of the gland that drain into the internal iliac veins.

Intercommunicating lymphatics of the prostate, bladder, seminal vesicles, vasa deferentia, and rectum provide drainage into both the internal and external iliac systems as well as the sacral promontory nodes.

Zones of Prostate

These zones have **physiologic and surgical significance because Benign enlargement of the prostate (BHP)** <u>occurs in the transition or periurethral zone</u> and <u>Malignancy develops in the majority of cases in the Peripheral zone.</u>

Urethra

➲ **High Yield for AIPGME/AIIMS/PGI 2013**

18-20 cms in length with 3 parts

▪	Prostatic (3 cms semilunar)
▪	Membranous (2 cms stellate)
▪	Spongy/penile (15 cms slit shaped)

Prostatic part is widest and more dilatable part.

Contains:

- ✓ Veru montanum (urethral crest)

- ✓ Colliculus seminalis

- ✓ Prostatic sinuses

- ✓ Prostatic utricle (analogius to uterus /vagina of females)

Cowper's Glands. (Bulbourethral glands of Cowper) are small, paired glands lying between the layers of the urogenital diaphragm at the junction of the bulbous and membranous portions of the urethra. The ducts of the glands empty distally into the bulbous urethra traversing the corpus spongiosum. The secretions from this gland not only act as a lubricant but may also have factors that aid in seminal fluid coagulation after ejaculation.

Penile Tissue

- Organ of **copulation and excretion of urine.**

- It consists of two parallel erectile tissues as the **corpora cavernosa**, which are situated dorsolaterally, and the **corpus spongiosum**, which invests the urethra ventrally, terminating distally in the erectile glans penis.

- Each corpus cavernosum and the corpus spongiosum are enveloped in fascial sheaths, and all three corpora are surrounded by **Buck's fascia.**

- The **blood supply** of the penis is through the **dorsal arteries** derived from the **internal pudendal arteries,** which are **branches of the internal iliac artery.**

- **The venous drainage** is through the **dorsal veins, with the superficial dorsal vein** emptying into the saphenous vein, and the deep dorsal vein emptying into the prostatic plexus known as the plexus of Santorini.

- Penile erection is induced by the engorgement of the erectile tissues of the corpora, principally the corpora cavernosa.

- **Lymphatic drainage** of the penis is abundant. The lymphatics from the shaft of the penis, the corpora cavernosa, and the skin pass through the superficial and deep inguinal nodes, communicating with the iliac nodes.

- **Lymphatic drainage of the glans penis** drains into **deep inguinal nodes** and **rest** of the penis drains into **superficial inguinal nodes.**

- The skin of the penis differs considerably from other skin of the body in its **paucity of sebaceous glands, its elasticity, and its extensive blood supply.**

ANATOMY

1

1

Remember:

⇨ **High Yield Points**

▶ **The bulbourethral glands** secrete mucus for lubrication.

▶ **The epididymis** concentrates and stores sperm for ejaculation.

▶ **The prostate gland** secretes alkaline fluid to neutralize vaginal pH and induces clotting of the semen.

▶ **The seminal vesicles** produce fructose, citric acid, prostaglandins, and fibrinogen. These comprise about 60% of the volume of semen.

▶ **The ampulla** is the end of the vas deferens.

▶ **The bulbourethral glands** secrete mucus for lubrication.

▶ **The epididymis** concentrates and stores sperm for ejaculation.

▶ **The prostate gland** secretes alkaline fluid to neutralize vaginal pH and induces clotting of the semen.

The seminal vesicles produce fructose, citric acid, prostaglandins, and fibrinogen. These comprise about 60% of the volume of semen.

⊃ **Female Reproductive Tract:**

⇨ **The Vagina**

The vagina is a female copulatory organ. It is a muscular tube lined with stratified squamous epithelium the adult vagina measures 12 to 13 cm. in depth. In virgin lower end of vagina is closed partially by annular fold of mucus membrane called **hymen** which gets distorted after intercourse forming rounded elevations called **caruncle hymenale.**

⇨ **The Cervix**

▪ Is the **lower cylindrical portion** of the uterus.

▪ The cervix, is a fibromuscular organ covered with **stratified squamous epithelium.** The walls of cervix show mucosal folds called **arbor vitae.**

▪ The **squamocolumnar junction** is the most common site of origin of squamous cell carcinoma.

▪ The **endocervical canal** is lined by columnar epithelium, and **racemose glands,** lined with similar epithelium, are found in the fibromuscular stroma. Such glands, if obstructed, may form **nabothian cysts** on the cervical surface.

▪ The **nulliparous** cervical os is **round.**

⇨ **The Uterus**

- ➡ The uterus is a **hollow, fibromuscular-walled organ** between the bladder

- ➡ The normal position of uterus is **anteverted and anteflexed.**

- ➡ **Angle of anteversion** is 90°

- ➡ **Angle of anteflexion** is 120°

- ➡ The organ is **pear shaped** and in nonpregnant women measures approximately **8 cm. in length and weighs 30 to 100 gm.**

- ➡ The fallopian tubes and the cervical canal communicate with the uterine cavity, which is lined by the endometrium.

- ➡ The **uterine fundus** is covered by peritoneum except in the lower anterior portion, where the bladder is contiguous with the lower uterine segment and the peritoneum is reflected, and laterally where the folds of the broad ligament are attached. The uterus is supported by condensations of endopelvic fascia and fibromuscular tissue laterally at the base of the broad ligaments.

  Blood supply of uterus is by **uterine artery** which is **tortuous** and **branch of <u>anterior</u> division of internal iliac artery** lying on the **lateral aspect** of uterus in the **broad ligament.**

⇨ **Uterine prolapse, or procidentia and uterine descensus:**

- ✓ Occurs when the uterus and its adjoining structures herniate through the vaginal canal.

- ✓ Prolapse is described as first, second, or third degree in severity, the last being protrusion of the entire uterus from the vagina, with the entire vagina everted as a consequence.

- ✓ Although congenital weakness of the supporting tissues may occasionally cause uterine prolapse, the most frequent cause is childbirth. The signs of uterine prolapse are protrusion of the cervix or uterus through the introitus. Prolapse is frequently associated with cystocele or rectocele, and these defects may cause presenting symptoms. Symptoms include backache, significant pelvic pressure, and ulceration or bleeding of the prolapsed structures.

⇨ **The Fallopian tubes:**

- ► **Tortous ducts about 10 cms in length.**

- ► Arise from the superior portion of the lateral borders of the uterus, superior to the attachment of the round ligaments, and **are patent**. The distal ends, the fimbriae, open into the abdominal cavity and the proximal ends open into the uterine cavity. It is divided into **interstitial, isthmic, ampullar, and fimbriated portions.**

- ► The wall is thin with two muscular layers and an outer layer of peritoneum within the upper borders of the broad ligament.

⇨ The Ovaries

Lie in the **ovarian fossa**. Ovaries are **almond-shaped** structure measuring 2 × 3 × 3 cm. and is located on the posterior surface of the broad ligament and inferior to the fallopian tube. The ovary has a **cortex and a medulla**. **Germinal epithelium**, a single layer of cuboidal cells, covers condensed fibrous tissue called the tunica albuginea. Follicles originate within the ovarian cortex and are composed of the basic embryonic complement; **no new follicles are formed after birth.**

Mesovarium is a fold of peritoneum by which ovary is connected to the broad ligament.

The **Arterial blood supply** is predominantly by **ovarian artery** a branch of **Abdominal aorta.**

Venous drainage is by **Pampniform plexus**. The **left ovarian vein** empties into the left renal vein; the **right ovarian vein** empties into the vena cava just inferior to the renal vein.

⊃ The Adult Inguinal Canal

High Yield for AIPGME/AIIMS/PGI 2013

- It is approximately **4 cm. in length**
- Extends between the **internal (deep inguinal) ring and the external (superficial inguinal) ring opening.**
- The inguinal canal contains either the **spermatic cord or the round ligament of the uterus.**
- The inguinal canal is bounded **superficially** by the external oblique aponeurosis.
- The **superior wall** is composed of internal oblique muscle, transversus abdominis muscle, and the aponeuroses of these muscles.
- The **inferior wall** of the inguinal canal is formed by the inguinal ligament and lacunar ligament.
- The **posterior wall** (floor) of the inguinal canal is formed by the transversalis fascia and the aponeurosis of the transversus abdominis muscle.
- **Hesselbach's triangle:** The inferior epigastric vessels serve as the superolateral border of Hesselbach's triangle. The medial border of the triangle is formed by the rectus sheath, and the inguinal ligament serves as its inferior border.
- Hernias occurring within Hesselbach's triangle are considered **direct hernias**, whereas hernias occurring lateral to the triangle are **indirect hernias.**

Contents of Important Structures:

⇨ Contents of spermatic cord:-

- The ducts deferens.
- Testicular and cremastric arteries.
- Artery of vas.
- The pampiniform plexus of veins.
- Lymph vessels from testis.
- Genital branch of Genitofemoral nerve.
- Remains of processus vaginalis.

⇨ **Contents of rectus sheath:**

— Rectus abdominis and pyramidalis muscle
— Superior epigastric artery and inferior epigastric artery
— Superior epigastric vein and inferior epigastric vein
— Lower five intercostal nerves and subcostal nerve

⇨ **Contents of broad ligament:**

— Uterine tube	AI 1992
— Round ligament of uterus,Ligament of ovary	AI 1992
— Uterine vessels,Ovarian diseases	
— Uterovaginal ,ovarian nerve plexus	
— Epoophron ,Paraoophron	
— Lymph vessels, lymph nodes	

⇨ **Contents of Ischiorectal fossa:**

— Perianal space
— Ischiorectal space
— Lunate fascia
— Pudendal canal

⊃ **Ischiorectal Fossa:**

High Yield for AIPGME/AIIMS/PGI 2013

▶ It is a wedge spaced space situated one on either side of the anal canal below the pelvic diaphragm.

▶ The base is directed downwards towards the skin.

▶ It is 5 to 6 cm deep, anterioposteriorly 5 cm, and 2.5 cm side to side, lying below the levator ani muscles and on either side of anal canal. Post anal space connects the two fossae posteriorly by a horse shoe path. The space is filled with loose areolar tissue and loosely arranged large loculi of fat. The infection of this space leads to abscess formation and are least painful because swelling can occur without tension.

⇨ **Boundaries**

▶ **Base**- is formed by the skin.

▶ **Apex** - Is formed by meeting of Obturator fascia with the inferior fascia of the pelvic diaphragm (anal fascia). The line corresponds to the origin of levator ani from the lateral pelvic wall.

▶ **Anteriorly** - The fossa is limited by the posterior border of perineal membrane.

▶ **Posteriorly** - (a) lower border of the gluteus maximus and (b) Sacro tuberous ligament.

1

▶ **Lateral wall** is vertical and is formed by (a) **Obturator internus with Obturator fascia**, and medial surface of ischial tuberosity below the attachment of Obturator fascia. **(Choice given as answer)**

▶ **Medial wall** - Slopes upwards and laterally and is formed by (a) external anal sphincter with fascia covering it in the lower part and (b) levator ani with anal fascia in the upper part.

⊃ Contents of Adductor Canal are   MP 2008

— Femoral artery

— Saphanous nerve

— Nerve to vastus medialis

⊃ Fascia Colli: Deep Fascia in the Neck High Yield for 2011-2012

is divided into an

➡ Investing layer,

➡ Pretracheal layer,

➡ Prevertebral layer,

➡ Carotid sheath.

1. Investing layer:

Investing layer lies deep to the platysma, and surrounds the neck like a collar.

It splits to enclose

➡ **Muscles**- trapezius and sternocleidomastoid

➡ **Salivary glands**- parotid and submandibular

➡ **Spaces**-suprasternal supraclavicular

➡ **Forms pulleys for**-digastric and omohyoid

2. Pretracheal fascia:

Its importance is that it encloses and suspends the thyroid gland and forms its false capsule on either side forms **"Ligament of Berry"**

3. Prevertebral fascia:

It covers the anterior vertebral muscles and forms the floor of the posterior triangle of the neck.

The cervical and brachial plexuses lie behind the prevertebral fascia. As the subclavian artery and the brachial plexus emerge from behind scalenus anterior they carry the prevertebral fascia downwards and laterally as the **Axillary sheath.**   **(JKBOPEE 2010)**

4. Carotid sheath:

It is a condensation of deep cervical fascia around the common and internal carotid arteries, the internal jugular vein, and the vagus nerve. <u>**The external carotid artery lies outside the sheath.**</u>

Lemniscii

Lemniscus, tract and sensation	Thalamic nucleus	Part of the internal capsule	Sensory areas of the cerebral cortex
Medial lemniscus.✷ (proprioception & fine touch). **Spinal lemniscus.** (pain, temperature & crude touch).	P.L.V.N.T.	SENSORY RADIATION	Upper $^1/_3$ of sensory area in post-central gyrus (Arm & leg region).
Trigeminal lemniscus.✷ (pain, temperature, touch & proprioception from the «head», taste)	P.M.V.N.T.	in posterior ½ of post. limb of internal capsule (I.C)	Lower $^1/_3$ of sensory area in post-central gyrus (Face region).
Lateral lemniscus ✷ (hearing) **UP 2004**	Medial geniculate body [M.G.B.]	AUDITORY RADIATION in sublentiform part of I.C.	Auditory area in Heschl's gyrus in temporal lobe (area 41 & 42).

⮞ **Internal Capsule:**

High Yield for AIPGME/AIIMS/PGI 2013

Part of Internal Capsule	Types of fibres in it
▶ Anterior limb	Fibres from & to the prefrontal area of the cortex.
▶ Genu (MOTOR)	Corticobulbar fibres. Sensory fibres from thalamus to brain. **DNB 2007**
▶ Ant.½ of posterior limb (MOTOR)	Corticospinal fibres.
▶ Post.½ of posterior limb (SENSORY)	SENSORY radiation (From PLVNT & PMVNT to main sensory area in post central gyrus).
▶ Retrolentiform part (VISION)	OPTIC radiation **DNB 2008** (From L.G.B. to visual sensory area 17).
▶ Sublentiform part (HEARING)	AUDITORY radiation **DNB 2008** (From M.G.B. to auditory area in temporal lobe).

Remember: M-M(medial geniculate body/ hearing (music)	*RJ 2008*
Lateral L-L Lateral geniculate body / light)	*RJ 2009*

A small lesion at the level of internal capsule can result in a clinical scenario with widespread manifestations and most of them lethal depending on what part of internal capsule is damaged.

The internal capsule may be damaged by a cerebro vascular lesion mostly by Haemorrage (**rupture of Charcots artery**) leading to Hemiplegia on the opposite side of the body.

In this type of Hemiplegia motor functions are effected mostly and sensory functions later or not at all because motor fibres lie laterally and the arterial supply is more laterally as a result of which motor fibres are likely to be effected more.

1

ANATOMY

⊃ Summary of the Lesion in Brown Sequard Syndrome✱

On The «same» side of the lesion

► **Pyramidal tract** damage results in: U.M.N.L. and motor paralysis below the injury (spastic paralysis, hyperactive reflexes, loss of superficial reflexes and Babinski sign). **AIIMS 2011**

► **Proprioceptive tracts damage** (gracile & cuneate) results in: loss of sense of position, sense of passive movement, sense of vibration and touch discrimination below the injury. These are the signs of sensory ataxia.

On the «opposite» side of the lesion:

► **Lateral spinothalamic tract** damage results in: loss of pain & temperature sensation beginning one or two dermatomes below the lesion.

► **Ventral spinothalamic tract** damage results in: little or No change in the sense of simple touch.

Remember:

Midbrain: Usually the fibres of the third (oculomotor) nerve are affected ⟶ **alternating oculomotor hemiplegia**, this means;

Hemiplegia on opposite half of the body (U.M.N.L.).

Signs of oculomotor nerve paralysis on the same side (L.M.N.L.).

Pons: usually the fibres of the sixth (abducent) nerve are affected ⟶ **alternating abducent hemiplegia**, this means:

Hemiplegia on opposite half of the body (U.M.N.L.).

Signs of abducent nerve paralysis on the same side (L.M.N).

Medulla: usually the fibres of the hypoglossal nerve are affected ⟶ **alternating hypoglossal hemiplegia**, this means

Hemiplegia on opposite half of the body (U.M.N.L.).

Signs of hypoglossal nerve paralysis on the same side (L.M.N.L.).

⊃ Arterial Territories and Important Points in Blood Supply of Brain

✱ ✱ ✱ (High Yield for 2011/2012)

► **Left middle cerebral artery** Blockage of this vessel would cause, among other effects, right-sided hemiplegia and sensory deficits mainly of the face and arms, a right visual field defect with inability to gaze to the right, and aphasia. **UP 2008**

► **Right middle cerebral artery** Blockage of this vessel would cause, among other things, left-sided hemiplegia and sensory deficits mainly of the face and arms and left visual field neglect with inabilityy to gaze to the left. In addition, there may be neglect of the left side. **COMED 2007**

► **Left anterior cerebral artery** This vessel supplies the medial aspects of the left hemisphere. Blockage may cause a weak, numb right leg (and possibly arm symptoms in milder forms). The face is typically spared.

▶ **Right anterior cerebral artery** This vessel supplies the medial aspects of the right hemisphere. Blockage may cause a weak, numb left leg (and possibly arm symptoms in milder forms). The face is typically spared.

▶ **Left posterior cerebral artery** This lesion presents as a right-sided visual field deficit, alexia without agraphia (if the corpus callosum is spared), and possible defects in naming colors.

▶ **Right posterior cerebral artery** This lesion typically presents as a left-sided visual field deficit along with left-sided sensory loss if the thalamus is affected. There may also be left-sided neglect.   **TN 2007**

▶ **Visual cortex is supplied by posterior+middle cerebral artery**

▶ **Left posterior inferior cerebellar artery** This lesion would cause infarction of the lateral medulla and inferior cerebellar surface, causing vertigo with vomiting, dysphagia, and dysarthria. In addition, there would be nystagmus looking toward the left, left-sided Horner's syndrome, and loss of pinprick sensation on the left side of the face and on the right side of the trunk and extremities. This condition is also known as **Wallenberg's syndrome**.   **MAH 2012**

▶ **Right posterior inferior cerebellar artery** This lesion would cause infarction of the lateral medulla and inferior cerebellar surface, causing vertigo with vomiting, dysphagia, and dysarthria. In addition, there would be nystagmus looking toward the right, right-sided Horner's syndrome, and loss of pinprick sensation on the right side of the face and on the left side of the trunk and extremities. This condition is also known as **Wallenberg's syndrome**.

⭢ Various Important Areas of Cerebrum:✳✳✳

▬ Motor area:	▶ Precentral gyrus☞
▬ Premotor area:	▶ Anterior to motor area☞
▬ Brocas area:	▶ Motor speech area (Inferior frontal gyrus)☞☞
▬ Sensory area:	▶ Post central gyrus☞
▬ Visual area:	▶ Occipital lobe☞
▬ Werneckies area	▶ Superior temporal lobe☞
▬ Remember :	▶ Facial angle gives us impression about development of brain **DNB 2008**

⭢ Cranial Nerves:

High Yield for AIPGME/AIIMS/PGI 2013

▶ Optic nerve is not only a cranial nerve. It is a **tract** and direct extension of CNS.☞

▶ This nerve is about 4cm long

▶ The optic nerve is enclosed in 3 sheaths covering with meninges.   **MP 2004**

▶ It is crossed by ophthalmic artery   **MP 2004**

▶ Trigeminal nerve is the **largest** cranial nerve.☞

▶ Abducent nerve has the **longest** course.☞

▶ Trochlear nerve has **the longest intracranial** course.☞Thinnest as well   **MAH 2005**

1

▶ Cranial nerve 3 and 4 have their nuclei in **midbrain.**		MAH 2005
▶ Cranial nerve 5,6,7,8 have their nuclei in **pons.**		
▶ Cranial nerve 9,10,11,12 have their nuclei in **medulla.**		UP 2007

▶ Cranial nerve emerging from dorsal aspect of brain: Trochlear	UP 2003
▶ MC nerve involved in intracranial aneurysms: occulomotor.	AI 1996
▶ Common nucleus for VII, IX , X nerves is Nucleus Tractus Solitarius.(NTS)	AMU 2005
▶ Trochlear nerve has **the longest intracranial** course.	KERALA 1993

➲ **Branches of Facial Nerve:**

- ▶ **In facial canal:** Nerve to stapedius, Chorda tympani,Greater petrosal
- ▶ **At its exit from Stylomastoid foramina:** Branches to Posterior auricular, posterior belly of digastric, stylohyoid.
- ▶ **In the face:** Temporal, Zygomatic, Buccal, Mandibular and cervical **(Pes Anserinus)**

➲ **Blood Supply of Facial Nerve: PGI 2006**

- ➡ Ascending pharyngeal artery
- ➡ Stylomastoid artery

➲ **Summary of Distribution of Cranial Nerves:**

No.	Nerve	Type	Function
(1)	Olfactory	Sensory	SMELL
(2)	Optic	Sensory	VISION
(3)	Oculomotor	Motor	To all muscles of the eye **except two:** (superior oblique & lateral rectus)
(4)	Trochlear	Motor	To **one eye muscle** (superior oblique)
(5)	Trigeminal	Mixed mainly sensory with small motor part	**Sensory to** — mouth — face — ant. ½ of scalp
(6)	Abducent	Motor	To **one eye muscle** (lateral rectus)
(7)	Facial	Mixed Motor ——Sensory Parasympathetic	◆ Motor to muscles of the face ◆ Sensory : taste to anterior 2/3 of tongue ◆ Parasympathetic to certain glands.
(8)	Vestibulocochlear	Sensory	a) **Hearing** (cochlear part) b) **Equilibrium** (Vestibular part)
(9)	Glossopharyngeal	Mixed Motor ——Sensory	▪ Sensory for **pharynx and tongue** ▪ Motor to : **one muscle of pharynx**

(10)		Parasympathetic	• (stylopharngeus) • Parasympathetic to **parotid gland**
(11)	**Vagus (including Cranial accessory)**	Mixed Motor ———Sensory Parasympathetic	— Motor to : **muscles of pharynx, larynx & palate** Parasympathetic & sensory to: — **the structures in the thorax & abdomen**
(12)	**Spinal Accessory**	Motor	To 2 important muscles of the neck: a) **Sternomastoid** b) **Trapezius**
(13)	**Hypoglossal**	Motor	To **all muscles of the tongue** (except one)

◯ Cranial Nerves:

THE FIRST (OLFACTORY) NERVE PALSY ✷✷

The olfactory nerve branches penetrate through the cribriform plate, and collect in the olfactory bulb and nerve which passes under the frontal lobe to the temporal lobe and other centres.

EXAMINATION

Each nostril is examined separately. One nostril is closed while the patient sniffs with the other. Mild aromatic substances such as orange, coffee, or tobacco should be used as strong irritant smells stimulate the sensory endings of the fifth nerve. The result of affection will be **loss of smell** or **anosmia**.

THE THIRD (OCULOMOTOR) NERVE PALSY✷✷

It supplies all **extra ocular muscles except the superior oblique and the lateral rectus**

Complete paralysis results in:

External ophthalmoplegia: In a **complete lesion** inability to move the eye upward, inward and downward. ☛

External Squint: the eye is deviated laterally and downwards due to the unopposed action of the lateral rectus and superior oblique. ☛

Diplopia: A person sees double. ☛

Ptosis: drooping of the upper eyelids due to paralysis of levator palpabre superioris. ☛   AIIMS 2011

Dilated non-reactive pupil due to paralysis of the sphincter pupillae. The pupil also shows no reaction to light (direct or consensual), or to accommodation. ☛

THE FOURTH (TROCHLEAR) NERVE PALSY✱✱

▶ There is weakness or paralysis of the **superior oblique muscle which normally moves the eye downwards and inwards.**☞

▶ **Result:** defective depression of the adducted eye. The patient is unable to look at his shoulder.

▶ **Symptom presentation:** DIPLOPIA (double vision), when looking downwards e.g. when reading or descending the stairs. The head may tilt to the opposite side to minimize the diplopia.

THE SIXTH (ABDUCENT) NERVE PALSY✱✱

The sixth nerve supplies the **lateral rectus which normally rotates the eye laterally**. Its paralysis causes:

▶ **Internal Squint:** The eyeball is turned inwards due to unopposed adduction of the medial rectus.☞

▶ **Diplopia,** which is maximum on looking outwards.

THE FIFTH (TRIGEMINAL) NERVE PALSY✱✱

The sensory fibres are divided into 3 divisions:

1. **OPTHALMIC DIVISION.**
2. **MAXILLARY DIVISION.**
3. **MANDIBULAR DIVISION.**

SENSATION

Sensation is tested in the distribution of the 3 divisions of the nerve. Routinely, it is sufficient to test the Sensation at 3 sites : on the forehead, the cheek and over the lower jaw, together with anterior two-thirds of the tongue.

MOTOR FUNCTIONS

A. MASSETERS AND TEMPORALIS:

▶ Any wasting of the temporalis.

▶ The degree of contraction of the temporalis and masseter by palpation while asking the patient to bite hard.

THE SEVENTH (FACIAL) NERVE PALSY✱✱

Weakness in the facial muscles may result from:

▶ **Upper motor neuron lesion:**

Here only the muscles of the lower part of face are affected. The eye closure is normal.☞☞

This is because the muscles of the lower part (unlike those of the lower part) are activated through the upper motor neuron fibres of both sides.

Spontaneous emotional expression is unaffected.

▶ **Lower motor neuron lesion:**

All the muscles of the face (upper and lower) are affected on the same side. ☛☛

Facial nerve passes through parotid gland but does not supply it.

Facial nerve supplies Submandibular and lacrimal glands.   MP 1998

Arterial supply to facial nerve: ascending pharyngeal artery   PGI 2005

THE EIGHT (VESTIBULO-COCHLEAR) NERVE PALSY✹✹

The eighth nerve consists of 2 parts which have different functions Cochlear and vestibular nerves.

The **Cochlear part is concerned with hearing.** *An affection results is tinnitus and deafness.*

The **vestibular part is concerned with equilibrium.** *Its affection may result in vertigo.* ☛

THE NINTH (GLOSSOPHARYNGEAL) NERVE PALSY✹✹

Paralysis of Glossopharyngeal nerve causes:

▶ Anaesthesia of the pharynx; ☛

▶ Loss of taste on the posterior third of the tongue. ☛
Glossopharyngeal nerve is involved in:

▶ **Jugular foramen syndrome**: Involving IX, X, XI Cranial Nerves. ☛☛

▶ **Collet Sicard Syndrome**: involving IX, X, XI, XII Cranial nerves (ExtraCranially)

▶ **Villaret Syndrome**: Lesion in Retropharyngeal space involving IX, X, XI, XII Cranial nerves

THE TENTH (VAGUS) NERVE PALSY✹✹

Paralysis of vagus nerve causes:

Ipsilateral paralysis of the palate, ☛

Ipsilateral paralysis of the pharynx and ☛

Ipsilateral paralysis of the larynx with anaesthesia of the larynx on the affected side. ☛

THE ELEVENTH (ACCESSORY) NERVE PALSY✹✹

As a Result of damage to the Accessory nerve

Sternomastoids

Unilateral

Apparent wasting.

The muscle does not stand out on testing

Bilateral

Wasting of the neck which appears like that of a chicken.

Falling of head backwards.

Trapezius

Unilateral paralysis

- Drooping of the shoulder when arm is hanging.
- Weak movements on testing:

Supplies all palatal muscles except Tensor palati	Orissa 1998
Spasmodic torticollis is due to central irritation of this nerve(cranial part)	KOL 2002

THE TWELFTH (HYPOGLOSSAL) NERVE PALSY✷✷

Lesion of one hypoglossal nerve results in deviation of the tongue "towards the paralysed side". If you ask the patient to protrude his tongue the muscles of the same side of the lesion become paralysed and begin to atrophy (lower motor neurone lesion)☛	UP 1996
Safety muscle of tongue is genioglossus supplied by hypoglossal nerve.	TN 1989

Gems never to be forgotten:

⊃ Cavernous Sinus: (High Yield for 2011/2012)

▶ Paralysis of 3, 4, 6 cranial nerves indicates lesion of cavernous sinus.	AI 2005
▶ Occulomotor, trochlear and opthalmic nerves lie in <u>lateral wall</u> of cav. sinus.	KERALA 1995
▶ Abducent nerve is a <u>direct content</u> of cavernous sinus.	
▶ Infections from <u>dangerous area of face</u> can spread to cavernous sinus	

Facial nerve has

- ▶ The longest intraosseous course.
- ▶ Is the Mc paralysed cranial nerve.

Muscles supplied by facial nerve:

▶ Platysma	AIIMS 2007
▶ Stylohyoid	
▶ Muscles of facial expression	AIIMS 2003
▶ Buccinator	AIIMS 2007
▶ Stapedius	
▶ Posterior belly of digastric	
▶ Submandibular, Lacrimal, nasal gland	MP 1998
▶ Supplies gustatory sensation to soft palate	RJ 2009
▶ Kindly never forget that despite the fact that facial nerve <u>traverses the substance of parotid but does not supply it.</u> (keeps it high and dry)	

Facial nerve is related to

✓ Pterygopalatine ganglion   MP 2004

✓ Geniculate ganglion   MP 2004

✓ Submandibular ganglion

⊃ Sympathetic and Parasympathetic Systems

Organ	Sympathetic	Parasympathetic
Pupil	Dilates	Constricts
Lacrimal & salivary glands	Stops secretion	Produces secretion
Heart	accelerates	Slows
Bronchioles	Dilates	Constricts
Alimentary canal	Dilates	Contracts
Urinary bladder	Dilates	Contracts
Penis		causes erection [For this reason the pelvic nerve was called the nervus erigens].

⊃ Limbic System

▶ Subcallosal Gyri.

▶ Cingulate Gyri.

▶ Hippocampal formation comprising of Hippocampal Gyrus, Para hippocampal Gyrus and Dentate gyrus, Amygdaloidal Nucleus.

▶ Mammillary bodies.

▶ Anterior thalamic nucleus.

Briefly functions of the limbic system can be summarised by **five Fs**

▶ Feeding,

▶ Flight,

▶ Feeling,

▶ Fighting and

▶ Fun {sex}.

⊃ **Skull Foramina and Contents**

High Yield for JKBOPEE/KCET/DNB/AIPGME/AIIMS/PGI 2013

Foramen		Contents
▶ Optic canal✏ ✏	DNB 2006	▶ Optic (II) Nerve and ophthalmic artery
▶ Superior orbital fissure✏		▶ III, IV, VI and ophthalmic division of V cranial nerves, sympathetic nerves and ophthalmic veins
▶ Stylomastoid foramen✏		▶ VII cranial nerve
▶ Foramen Rotundum✏	UP 2007	▶ Maxillary division of V
▶ Foramen ovale✏	AI 1999	▶ Mandibular division of V and accessory meningeal artery
▶ Foramen spinosum✏	PGI 1992	▶ Middle meningeal artery, meningeal branch of the Mandibular nerve
▶ Foramen magnum✏	AIIMS 1991	▶ Accessory (XI) nerve, vertebral and spinal arteries. **NOT SPINAL CORD.** AI 2010
▶ Foramen lacerum✏		▶ Internal carotid artery, ▶ lesser petrosal Nerve (branch of IX), ▶ greater petrosal Nerve (branch of VII), ▶ deep petrosal
▶ Jugular foramen✏	MAH 2006	▶ Inferior petrosal sinus (anterior part) ▶ Internal jugular vein and IX, X, XI cranial nerves
▶ Hypoglossal foramen✏		▶ XII cranial nerve, meningeal branch of ascending pharyngeal artery
▶ Internal auditory meatus✏	PGI 2003	▶ VII and VIII cranial nerves, labyrinthine (internal auditory) artery
▶ Dorellos canal	PGI 1999	▶ Abducent nerve.

⊃ **Cerebrospinal Fluid (CSF):**

High Yield for AIPGME/AIIMS/PGI 2013

▶ Clear fluid.
▶ Colourless fluid.
▶ Choroid Plexus (formed by).
▶ Chloride content ↑,
▶ Cells minimal.
▶ Cushions the brain.
▶ Cirrculus arteriosus (branches) supply choroids plexus.

ANATOMY

1

➔	CSF is principally secreted by <u>choroid plexus</u>.	**JIPMER 1992**
➔	Choroid plexus is absent in anterior horn of lateral ventricle.	**MP 2009**
➔	Total volume of CSF. **150 ml.**	**PGI 1995**
➔	Normal adult CSF pressure: **6-12 mm Hg**	
➔	pH of CSF is: **7.33**	**PGI 1995**
➔	**Epidural space** is devoid of CSF.	
➔	Rate of CSF absorption is the main factor controlling CSF Pressure.	**AIIMS 2008, DNB 2008**
➔	<u>Persistent leekage</u> can cause headache.	
➔	<u>No neutrophils</u> in normal state seen.	**AIIMS 2007**

➲ Medial Medullary Syndrome

✳ **Occlusion of the vertebral artery may cause Medial Medullary Syndrome which is characterised by:**   **UP 2006**
— Paralysis or atrophy of tongue on the side of lesion (XII nerve involvement)
— Paralysis of arm and leg on opposite side
— Impaired tactile and proprioceptive sense on opposite side (involvement of pyramidal tract and medial lemniscus

➲ Lateral Medullary Syndrome

High Yield for AIPGME/ JKBOPEE/AIIMS/PGI 2013

✳**The posterior inferior cerebellar artery:**
— It is the **largest** and main branch of the vertebral artery.
It has a **tortuous S-shaped course.** Immediately after it arises from the vertebral artery, it runs backwards around the lower the lower end of the olive passing through the rootlets of the hypoglossal nerve, it then turns round the inferior cerebellar peduncle and finally divides into two terminal branches which supply: (a) **the inferior vermis (b) the posterior part of the inferior surface of the cerebellum.**   **Delhi 2006**

— **Impaired pain and temperature sense on opposite side.**
— Nystagmus (involvement of Vestibular nucleus).
— Dysphagia (involvement of Nucleus ambigus).
— Nystagmus (involvement of Cerebellum).
— Horner's Syndrome (involvement of sympathetic pathway).
— PTOSIS, MIOSIS, ANHYDROSIS, LOSS OF CILIOSPINAL REFLEX.   **DNB 2011**

➲ Occlusion of the Anterior Spinal Artery may cause:

▶ Loss of motor function below the level of the lesion (due to damage to the corticospinal tracts).
▶ **Loss of pain and temperature Sensation** below the level of the lesion (due to damage to the spinothalamic tracts).
▶ Weakness of limbs (due to damage of the anterior grey horns in the cervical or lumbar regions of the cord).
▶ Loss of Bowel and Bladder Control (due to damage of the descending autonomic tracts).

1

ANATOMY

⊃ **Occlusion of the Posterior spinal artery may cause:**

> ▶ **Loss of position sense, vibration sense and light touch** due to damage of the posterior white columns

⊃ **Parathyroid glands:**

High Yield for AIPGME/AIIMS/PGI 2013

> ▶ The vascular supply to the parathyroid glands is usually from the **inferior thyroid artery**, but it can arise from the superior thyroid artery, the lowest thyroid artery (thyroid ima), and arteries in the larynx, trachea, esophagus, or mediastinum or from anastomoses between these vessels.
>
> ▶ The **inferior, middle, and superior thyroid veins** drain the parathyroid glands.
>
> ▶ About 50% of all parathyroids are found adjacent to the area where the **inferior thyroid artery** enters the thyroid parenchyma.
>
> ▶ The superior parathyroid glands are usually embedded in fat and located on the **posterior surface of the middle or upper portion of the thyroid lobe** "close to the point where the recurrent laryngeal nerve enters the larynx."
>
> ▶ The lower parathyroid glands are more ventral, close to the lower pole of the thyroid gland and the thyrothymic ligament.
>
> ▶ The <u>Chief</u> Cells and the <u>Oxyphil</u> cells are arranged in trabeculae or islands. The main cell of primate glands and the only cell of many lower species is the chief cell

⊃ **Larynx :**

High Yield for AIPGME/AIIMS/PGI 2013

Larynx has 3 paired and 3 unpaired cartilages.	**UP 2003**
Extends from C3-C6.	
Anatomic basis of stridor is in larynx.	**PGI 2000**
The larynx serves as the **sounding source for speech**. A fundamental tone is produced by the movement of the vocal cords, which is brought about by the flow of exhaled air past lightly approximated vocal cords.	
➡ The internal laryngeal nerve is sensory to larynx <u>above</u> vocal cords. ☞	**KAR 1991**
➡ The Recurrent laryngeal nerve is sensory to larynx <u>below</u> vocal cords. ☞	
➡ All muscles of larynx except cricothyroid are supplied by Recurrent laryngeal nerve. ☞	
➡ Cricothyroid is supplied by External laryngeal nerve. ☞	**JKBOPEE**

⊃ **Muscles of Larynx and their action:✱**

Abductor of vocal cords:	Posterior Cricoarytenoid☞☞☞	**JKBOPEE 2012**
Adductor of vocal cords:	• Lateral Cricoarytenoid☞	**PGI 2007**
	▪ Transverse arytenoids	**PGI 2007**
	▪ Cricothyroid☞	**PGI 2007**
	▪ Thyroarytenoid	
Tensor of vocal cords:	Cricothyroid☞☞	
Relaxor of vocal cords:	• Thyroarytenoids	
	▪ Vocalis	

⊃ Muscles Acting at Temporomandibular joint:

— Depression:	Lateral Pterygoid ☜☜	AP 1996
— Elevation:	Temporalis, Massetter, Medial Pterygoid ☜	
— Protrusion:	Pterygoids ☜	MP 2K
— Retraction:	Posterior fibres of Temporalis ☜☜	AIIMS 2003
— Lateral movements:	Pterygoids ☜	
— Buccinator:	Not a muscle of mastication.	AI 2003

⊃ Ansa Cervicalis: ✳

Ansa cervicalis is a thin nerve loop that lies in the anterior wall of carotid sheath.

Superior root is a continuation of descending branch of **hypoglossal (XII) Cranial nerve.** Superior root supplies Superior belly of omohyoid. Its fibres are derived from first cervical nerve.

Inferior root is derived from spinal nerves C_2 and C_3.

Loop of Ansa supplies:

➡ Inferior belly of omohyoid

➡ Sternothyroid

➡ Sternohyoid

➡ **Dangerous area of face:** lower part of nose and upper lip ✳✳

➡ **Dangerous area of scalp:** loose areolar tissue layer of scalp ✳

➡ **Dangerous zone of eye:** ciliary body ✳

⊃ Sesamoid Bones:

▶ They develop in muscle tendons	MP 2007
▶ They are **devoid of periosteum.** ☜☜	MP 2007
▶ They ossify by multiple centres after birth	
▶ They are **devoid of haversian system** ☜☜	
▶ They **prevent friction** of tendons against bones and alter their direction of pull.	
▶ Largest sesamoid bone is patella	
▶ Fabella is present in **Lateral head of gastrocnemius**	KOL 2007

Myoid cells are present in Testis

Halo cells are present in Ductus Epididymis

Peg cells are present in Fallopian tubes

1

➲ Commonest Sites

► Commonest site of BHP: ☞☞	periurethral zone
► Commonest site of cancer prostate: ☞	peripheral zone
► Commonest site of varicocele: ☞	left side
► Commonest position of appendix: ☞	retrocecal
► Commonest site of internal hemorrhoids:☞	3, 7 and 11 o clock.

➲ Superficial Cutaneous Reflexes

Reflex	Stimulus	Response	Center - spinal segment involved
Scapular	Irritation of skin at the interscapular space	Contraction of scapular muscles & drawing in of scapula	C5 to T1
Upper abdominal	Stroking the abdominal wall below the costal margin	Ipsilateral contraction of abdominal muscle & movement of umbilicus towards the site of stroke	T6 to T9
Lower abdominal	Stroking the abdominal wall at umbilical & iliac level	Ipsilateral contraction of abdominal muscle & movement of umbilicus towards the site of stroke	T10 to T12
Cremasteric✱	Stroking the skin at upper & inner aspect of thigh	Elevation of testicles	L1, L2
Gluteal	Stroking the skin over glutei	Contraction of glutei	L4 to S1, S2
Plantar✱	Stroking the sole	Plantar flexion & adduction of toes	L5 to S2
Bulbocavernous✱	Stroking the dorsum of glans penis	Contraction of bulbocavernous	S3, S4
Anal ✱	Stroking the perianal region	Contraction of anal sphincter	S4, S5

➲ Important Points About Functional Anatomy of Cerebral Cortex:✱✱✱

Frontal lobe	Pre central cortex (Post. Part)	Primary motor area✱ (concerned with initiation of voluntary movements & speech)	Area 4 - center for movement
			Area 4S - suppressor area. Inhibits movements initiated by area 4.
		Pre motor area✱	Area 6 - concerned with coordination of movements initiated by area 4.
			Area 8 - frontal eye field.

Parietal lobe	Pre -frontal cortex (Ant. Part)	Supplementary motor area✳	Area 44 & 45 (broca's area) – motor area for speech. .
			Concerned with co-ordinated skilled movements.
		Silent area or association area	Area – 9 to 14, 23, 24, 29 & 32. Center for planned action.
		Center for higher functions – emotion, learning, memory.	Seat of intelligence. Personality of individual.
	Somesthetic area I		Area 1 – concerned with sensory perception
			Area 2 and 3 – integration of these sensations. Spatial recognition. Recognition of intensity, similarities & diff. B/W stimuli
	Somesthetic area II		Concerned with perception of sensation.
	Somesthetic association area		Synthesis of various sensations perceived by S.Area-I. Stereognosis.
Temporal lobe	Primary auditory area✳	MP 2008	Area 41, 42 & wernicke's area – concerned with perception of auditory impulses, analysis of pitch, determination of intensity & source of sound.
			Superior part of temporal gyrus. TN 2006
	Auditopsychic area		Area 22 – interpretation of auditory sensation
	Area of equilibrium		Maintenance of equilibrium
Occipital lobe	Primary visual area✳	RJ 2007	Area 17 – perception of visual impulse
			Lines of Gernari seen. TN 2006
	Visual association area✳		Area 18 - Interpretation of visual impulses
	Occipital eye field ✳		Area 19 - Movements of eye

▶ Loss of tactile localization and two point discrimination occurs in damage to somatosensory area 1   AI 2002

▶ Brocas area is present in inferior frontal gyrus   UP 2003

➲ Functions of Limbic System:

▶ Emotion   PGI 2006

▶ Memory   PGI 2006

▶ Higher functions

✓ **Consolidation** of long term memory occurs in **hippocampus**

✓ **Processing of short term memory to long term occurs in hippocampus**

✓ Amgdala is the **window of limbic system.**   WB 2003

✓ Damage to amgdala causes **Kluver Blucky syndrome**

✓ **Reward centre is in medial forebrain bundle.**

○ Herniations

✓ **Uncal or transtentorial herniation.**＊☞ The herniated uncus will compress *the oculomotor nerve, the posterior cerebral artery, and the brainstem*. The pathophysiologic consequences include oculomotor paralysis (manifesting with fixed and dilated pupil on the same side), ipsilateral infarction of the occipital lobe, and hemorrhages within the midbrain and pons. The latter may result in respiratory paralysis and death.

✓ **Cerebellar tonsillar herniation** ＊☞refers to downward displacement of the cerebellar tonsils through the foramen of magnum. This results from space-occupying lesions in the infratentorial compartment, such as bleeding and tumors. It leads to *compression of the medulla and death by cardiorespiratory arrest*.

✓ **Subfalcine (cingulate) herniation** ＊☞describes the lateral *displacement of the cingulate gyrus beneath the falx cerebri*. This event is caused by space-occupying masses in the cerebral hemisphere. It leads to compression of the anterior cerebral artery and infarction of dependent cerebral territories (mostly the medial portion of the frontal and parietal lobes).

✓ **Reverse cerebellar herniation**＊☞ is a rare form of herniation due to *midbrain lesions (again, hemorrhages and tumors) that push the midbrain upward through the incisura of the tentorium.*

✓ **Transcalvarial herniation** ＊☞may develop in *open (i.e., accompanied by calvarial bone fractures) head injuries* if brain parenchyma is displaced outside the cranial cavity through a calvarial defect.

Split brain syndrome: Disconnection syndrome of cerebral cortex resulting from transection or congenital absence of cerebral cortex.

○ The Pituitary Gland

High Yield for AIPGME/AIIMS/PGI 2013

Also known as **Hypophysis** cerebri. Pineal is **Epiphysis** cerebri.

The average adult pituitary measures 11 × 15 × 5 mm.

The gland is oval, bilaterally symmetrical, and brownish red.

The pituitary is approximately 20% larger in females than in males and **it enlarges about in females during pregnancy.**

It lies within the **sella turcica** *(Turkish saddle)*.

This fossa is bordered **anteriorly, posteriorly, and inferiorly by the sphenoid bone** and laterally by the cavernous sinus.

The floor of the sella forms the roof of the sphenoidal sinus.

The diaphragma sellae, a thick reflection of dura mater, covers the roof of the sella and closely encircles the pituitary stalk in 50% of individuals.

The arterial supply to the hypothalamic-pituitary region is complex and arises from three sources.

✓ **The inferior hypophyseal artery**, a branch of the carotid artery, supplies the posterior pituitary.

✓ **The superior hypophyseal arteries** branch from the circle of Willis to supply the median eminence.

✓ **The middle hypophyseal arteries** are of variable origin and supply the pituitary stalk.

Capillary portions of the superior hypophyseal arteries drain from the hypothalamus, the median eminence, and the superior portions of the pituitary stalk. These vessels drain into the hypophyseal portal system, which forms a secondary venous plexus in the anterior pituitary and ultimately empties into the cavernous sinus. <u>This portal venous system constitutes the principal blood supply to the anterior pituitary and serves as the medium through which releasing hormones from the hypothalamus reach the pituitary.</u>

<u>The pituitary has dual embryonic origin.</u>

► <u>The Anterior pituitary</u> arises from <u>embryonic ectoderm (Rathke's pouch)</u> and includes the pars distalis, pars intermedia (vestigial in humans), and pars tuberalis.

► <u>The Posterior pituitary</u> of the gland arises from the <u>diencephalon</u> and includes the neural stalk, infundibulum, and posterior lobe.

► Embryonic defects in invagination and obliteration of the pharyngeal extent of Rathke's pouch may lead to craniopharyngiomas or hormonally active ectopic pituitary adenomas.

⊃ Types of Fibres in CNS:

Association fibres: connecting different areas of same cerebral hemisphere.

► Superior longitudnal fasiculus — PGI 2007
► Inferior longitudnal fasiculus — PGI 2007
► Cingulum
► Uncinate fasiculus

Projection fibres: connecting cerebral cortex to other parts of CNS.

► Corticospinal tract
► Internal capsule — MP 2007

Commisural fibres: connecting corresponding parts of two cerebral hemispheres

► Corpus callosum
► Anterior commisure
► Posterior commisure
► Hippocampal commisure
► Habenular commisure
► Hypothalmic commisure

⊃ Effect of Upper Motor Neuron & Lower Motor Neuron Lesion: ✱✱

	Effects	Upper motor neuron	Lower motor neuron lesion
Clinical observation	Muscle tone	Hypertonic	Hypotonic
	Paralysis	Spastic type of paralysis	Flaccid type of paralysis
	Wastage of muscle	No wastage	Present
	Superficial reflexes	Lost	Lost
	Plantar reflex	Abnormal – babinski's sign	Absent
	Deep reflexes	Exaggerated	Lost
	Clonus	Present	Lost

1

ANATOMY

⊃ Anatomy of Eye:

➟ The "Extroter" of Eye Ball is **Inferior Oblique and Inferior Rectus**	AIIMS 1995
➟ The "Introter" of Eye ball is **Superior Oblique and Superior Rectus.**	PGI 2004, AIIMS 1995
➟ Action of Superior oblique is **Abduction, Intorsion and depression.**	PGI 1997
➟ Dilator Pupillae **dilates** pupil and is supplied by *Sympathetics.*	
➟ Sphincter Pupillae **constricts** pupil and is supplied by *Parasympathetics.*	
➟ LR$_6$SO$_4$	
▶ Lateral Rectus is supplied by **6 th Cranial Nerve** (Abducent)	
▶ Superior Oblique is supplied by **4 th Cranial Nerve** (Trochlear)	AIIMS 2004
▶ Rest other ocular muscles are supplied by **3 rd Cranial Nerve** (Occulomotor)	
▶ Muscle attached to posterior tarsal margin: **Mullers muscle**	KERALA 1994
▶ Ligament of Lockwood is found in Orbit.	AIIMS 1990

Structures passing through "**Superior Orbital Fissure**" are:	AIIMS 1994
Live Free To See NO Insult At All.	
➟ Lacrimal Nerve	PGI 2005
➟ Frontal Nerve	
➟ Trochlear Nerve	
➟ Superior Opthalmic Vein	
➟ Nasociliary Nerve	
➟ Inferior Opthlamic vein	
➟ Abducent Nerve	

⊃ Remember Genetic Transmission

▶ Male to Male:	Autosomal Dominant
▶ Male to female:	X linked Dominant
▶ Female to ALL:	Mitochondriopathies
▶ Only Males affected usually:	X linked Recessive

⊃ Eponym's Foramina

F. Caecum ➟➟	The foramen anterior to the Crista Galli in the base of the Skull.
F. Caecum ➟	Located at the junction of Ant 2/3 rds and Post 1/3 rd of tongue (in midline)
Epiploic Foramen➟	Communication between Greater and lesser sacs of peritoneal cavity.
F of Langer➟	A foramen in the axillary fascia through which the Axillary tail of Spence (Part of Breast) passes through

cont...

cont...

F of Monro (Interventricular F)	Opening of lateral ventricles into III ventricle.
F of Magendie	Median aperture in the Roof of fourth Ventricle.
F of Luschka	Openings of the Lateral recesses of fourth Ventricle.
F of Scarpa	Incisor Foramen in the mouth.
F of Vesalii	Transmits veins communicating between the Cavernous sinus to Pterygoid Plexus

⊃ Spinal Cord

- ▶ Spinal cord in adults ends at **L1- L2**
- ▶ Spinal cord in infants ends at **L3**
- ▶ Thoracix and sacral curves are **concave anteriorly**
- ▶ Sub arachnoid space/ Sub dural space ends at S2   AI 1992
- ▶ Dural sheath ends at S2
- ▶ Filum terminale and piamater extend upto tip of coccyx.
- ▶ Number of spinal nerve pairs: **31**.   KERALA 1990

⊃ Important Points About Spinal Cord: (PGI 2008)

- In adults spinal cord ends at lower border of L1 vertebra   JKBOPEE 2012
- In newborn may extend up to L3
- Cauda equina extends from lumbar vertebra to coccyx
- In embryonic period cord extends up to coccyx

⊃ Spinal Anaesthesia:

- is given at level: L_{2-4}
- Spinal anesthesia is usually performed at the level of the **L3 or L4 vertebrae** in the adult patient, because the spinal needle is introduced below the level at which the spinal cord ends.

⊃ Ascending Tracts of Spinal Cord:

High Yield for AIPGME/AIIMS/PGI 2013

Situation	Tract	Function
Anterior white funiculus	Anterior spinothalamic tract	"Crude" touch sensation
Lateral white funiculus	Lateral spinothalamic tract	Pain & temperature sensation
	Ventral spino cerebellar tract	Subconscious kinesthetic sensations
	Dorsal spino cerebellar tract	Subconscious kinesthetic sensations
	Spinotectal tract	Concerned with spinovisual reflex

cont...

ANATOMY

cont...

	Fasiculus dorsolateralis	Pain & temperature sensations
	Spinoreticular tract	Conciousness & awareness
	Spinoolivary tract	Proprioception
	Spinovestibular tract	Proprioception
Posterior white funiculus	Fasciculus gracilis JIPMER 2005	✓ Tactile sensation ✓ Tactile localization ✓ Tactile discrimination ✓ "Vibratory" sensation ✓ "Conscious kinesthetic sensation" ✓ "Stereognosis" AIIMS 1996
	Fasciculus cuneatus JIPMER 2005	

➲ Descending Tracts of Spinal Cord:

Situation	Tract	Function
Pyramidal tracts	Anterior corticospinal tract	▶ Control voluntary, skilled movements✻
	Lateral corticospinal tract	▶ Forms upper motor neurons✻
Extra Pyramidal tracts	Medial longitudinal fasciculus	▶ Coordination of reflex ocular movement ✻ ▶ Integration of movements of eyes & neck
	Anterior vestibulospinal tract	▶ Maintenance of muscle tone & posture✻
	Lateral vestibulospinal tract	▶ Maintenance of position of head & body during acceleration✻
	Reticulospinal tract	▶ Coordination of voluntary & reflex movements.✻ ▶ Control of muscle tone. ▶ Control of respiration & blood vessels.
	Tectospinal tract	▶ Control of movement of head in response to visual & auditory impulses. ✻
	Rubrospinal tract	▶ Facilitatory influence on flexor muscle tone. ✻
	Olivospinal tract	▶ Control of movements due to proprioception. ✻

➲ Important Points About Vessels

- ➡ Umbilical arteries carry venous blood
- ➡ Pulmonary vasculature also follows reverse pattern
- ➡ Coronary arteries have 3 elastic lamina : internal, middle and external
- ➡ Umbilical arteries have no elastic lamina
- ➡ The arteries of lower limb have more developed muscular tissue than those of upper limb

➲ Varicose Veins:

The term varicose is derived from the Latin word meaning dilated.

It implies a dilated, tortuous, and elongated vein.

Although varicosities may occur in any venous system,

More frequent sites are:

- Lower esophageal area,
- The anorectal area, or the
- Spermatic cord,
- They occur **most frequently in the lower extremity.**

➲ Important Nutrient Arteries: (High Yield for 2011/2012)

Nutrient artery of clavicle	▶ Suprascapular artery
Nutrient artery of humerus	▶ Profunda brachii artery
Nutrient artery of femur	▶ Second perforating artery. Sometimes by first and third perforating arteries
Nutrient artery of tibia. Largest in body	▶ Posterior tibial artery
Nutrient artery of fibula	▶ Peroneal artery

➲ Axis Arteries:

Axis artery of upper limb: seventh cervical intersemental artery persisting as
- Axillary,
- Brachial,
- Anterior interosseous artery and
- Deep palmar arch

Axis artery of lower limb: fifth lumbar intersemental artery persisting as

- Inferior gluteal artery,
- Companion artery of sciatic nerve,
- Popliteal artery,
- Peroneal artery and
- Plantar arch

The Marginal artery of Drummond is also known as the Marginal artery of the colon.

The anastomoses of the terminal branches of the ileocolic, right colic and middle colic arteries of the continuous arterial circle or arcade along the inner border of the colon known as the marginal artery of Drummond.

Components

- Ileocolic artery - colic branch
- Right colic artery – ascending and descending branches
- Middle colic artery – right and left branches
- Left colic artery – ascending and descending branches
- Sigmoid arteries – unnamed terminal branches

From this marginal artery, straight vessels (known as **vasa recta**) pass to the colon.

The marginal artery is an important connection between the SMA and IMA, and provides collateral flow in the event of occlusion or significant stenosis. The junction of the SMA and IMA territories is at the

Superior mesentric artery (SMA), and of the left colic and sigmoid branches of the IMA, form a splenic flexure. Anastomoses here are often weak or absent, hence the marginal artery at this point (known as **Griffiths' point**) is often focally small or discontinuous. For this reason, the splenic flexure is a watershed area prone to ischaemia and infarction.

One of the commonest area of colonic ischemia is called **Sudeck's point**   MP 2009

➲ Charcots Artery:

Charcots artery: lenticulostriate arteries arteries which arise at the commencement of the middle cerebral artery supply blood to part of the basal ganglia and posterior limb of the internal capsule. The lenticulostriate perforators are end arteries.The name of these arteries is derived from some of the structures it supplies: the lenticular nucleus and the striatum.

➲ Arc of Riolan

High Yield for AIPGME/AIIMS/PGI 2013

The cecum, ascending colon, hepatic flexure, and proximal portion of the transverse colon derive arterial blood supply from the ileocolic, right colic, and middle colic branches of the superior mesenteric artery. The inferior mesenteric artery supplies blood to the distal transverse colon, splenic flexure, descending colon, and sigmoid by means of the left colic artery and branches of the sigmoid and superior hemorrhoidal vessels. The rectum is supplied by a rich network of vessels from the middle hemorrhoidal and inferior hemorrhoidal arteries. As the main vessels course through the mesentery toward the bowel wall, they bifurcate and form arcades at 1 to 2 cm. from the mesenteric border and define a continuous chain of communicating vessels.

This vascular structure is called the marginal artery of Drummond.

The anastomosis or linking of arcades between the superior and inferior mesenteric vessels is known as the long anastomosis of Riolan. **Because of this arc even if Inferior mesenteric artery (IMA) is thrombosed the arc of Riolan can still contribute to the blood supply of gut supplied by IMA.**   AIIMS 2011

➲ Heubner's Artery: High Yield for AIPGME/AIIMS/PGI 2013

Heubner's artery: a branch of **anterior Cerebral artery**, supplies the anteromedial part of the head of the caudate and antero inferior internal capsule Its vascular territory is the anteromedial section of the caudate nucleus and the anterioinferior section of the internal capsule.

➲ Artery of Adamkiewicz (High Yield for 2011/2012)

Artery of Adamkiewicz : Arteria Radicularis Magna,"Great radicular artery of Adamkiewicz... provides the major blood supply to the lumbar and sacral cord.When damaged or obstructed, it can result in <u>anterior spinal artery syndrome</u>, with loss of <u>urinary</u> and <u>fecal continence</u> and impaired motor function of the legs; sensory function is often preserved to a degree.It is important to identify the location of the artery when treating a <u>thoracic aortic aneurysm</u> or a <u>thoraco-abdominal aortic aneurysm</u>.

⇨ The Dorsalis Pedis Artery

— The **dorsalis pedis artery** is the continuation of the **<u>anterior tibial artery</u>** after the artery anterior tibial artery crosses the ankle to reach the dorsum of the foot.

— Its pulse is the **most distal palpable pulse** in the lower limb and therefore is useful for evaluating the arterial supply to the limb.

— On the dorsum of the foot, the pulse may be felt as the artery passes over the **navicular bone** between the extensor hallucis longus tendon and the extensor digitorum longus tendon.

⇨ Batson's Vertebral Venous Plexus:

Batson's vertebral venous plexus: the valveless vertebral venous veins that communicate withthe prostatic venous plexus and explain the readiness with which carcinoma of the prostatespreads to the pelvic bones and vertebrae.

⇨ Important Points About Bones:

➡ Brachycephaly: **Premature closure of coronal suture.✹✹**

➡ Scaphocephaly: **Premature closure of saggital suture✹**

➡ Trigonocephaly: **Premature closure of metopic suture✹**

➡ Oxy cephaly: **Premature closure of all sutures.✹**

⇨ Pneumatic Bones:

➡ Contain air spaces. Usually present in skull.

➡ Make the skull light in weight.

➡ Act as air conditioners.

    ✓ Maxilla,   **PGI 2007**

    ✓ Sphenoid   **PGI 2007**

    ✓ Ethmoid,   **AIIMS 2003**

    ✓ Mastoid Bones   **AIIMS 2003**

⇨ Sesamoid Bones:

➡ Patella

➡ Pisiform

➡ Fabella

1

ANATOMY

⇨ **Bones Ossified at Birth:**

- Lower end of femur
- Upper end of tibia
- Calcaneum

⇨ **Important Points About Muscles**

- ▶ Synergist: aiding the action of prime mover
- ▶ Fixator: preventing any unnecessary movement, stabiloizes one part of body during movement of other part.
- ▶ Prime mover: active in initiating and maintaining movement
- ▶ Antagonist: muscle acting in opposition to movement generated by agonist

▶ Anti rape muscle /muscle virgineous:✎✎	Gracilis	
▶ Cheating muscle: ✎	Superior oblique of eye	
▶ Safety muscle of tongue: ✎	Genioglossus	
▶ Tailors muscle: ✎	Sartorius	
▶ Thermostat of testis	Cremaster	UP 2006
▶ Bladder muscles in whorls	Detrusor	

⇨ **Important Subcutaneous Muscles:**

- ✓ Dartos in Scrotum
- ✓ Platysma in neck
- ✓ Corrugator cutis ani
- ✓ Palmaris brevis
- ✓ Muscles of scalp
- ✓ Subareolar muscles of nipple

⇨ **Hybrid/ Composite Muscles:✎✎**

Adductor magnus	AI 2008
Biceps Femoris	AI 2008
Pectineus	
Digastric	
Flexor digitorum superficialis	AI 2010

⇨ **Digastric Muscles:✎✎**

Digastric: Anterior belly, posterior belly	
Omohyoid: Superior belly, inferior belly	AI 2008
Occipitofrontalis: Occipital belly, frontal belly	AI 2008
Gastrocnemius: Lateral head, medial head	
Ligament of Treitz: Skeletal part, smooth part	AI 2008

1

⟳ Muscles with dual nerve supply:

Brachialis	Musculonutaneous nerve, radial nerve
Adductor magnus	Obturator nerve, tibial part of sciatic nerve
Pectinius	Femoral nerve, obturator nerve
Digastric	Mandibular nerve, facial nerve
Flexor pollicis brevis	Median nerve, ulnar nerve
Flexor digitorum profundus	Median nerve, ulnar nerve

⟳ Intra Tympanic Muscles:

High Yield for AIPGME/AIIMS/PGI 2013

Stapedius:
— Attached to neck of stapes
— Nerve supply is facial nerve
— Muscle of second arch

Tensor tympani:
➡ Arises from cartilaginous part of pharyngotympanic tube and part of greater wing of sphenoid.
➡ Inserted into handle of malleus.
➡ Innervated by mandibular nerve (branch of trigeminal nerve)   AIIMS 2010
➡ Action is evident from name (tenses tympanic membrane)
➡ Muscle of first arc

Tensor tympani and stapedius reflex:
➡ Loud sounds elicit reflex contraction of tensor tympani and stapedius, which attenuates movement of tympanic membrane and middle ear ossicles.
➡ Afferent impulses travel via the cochlear part of 8th cranial nerve.
➡ Efferent fibres to tensor tympani arise in trigeminal motor nucleus and travel in mandibular division of trigeminal nerve.
➡ Efferent fibres to stapedius originate in facial nucleus and travel in the facial nerve.

⟳ Gems About Gastrocnemius:

➡ Is a strong plantar flexor of foot.
➡ **Fabella** is a sesamoid bone developing in **Lateral Head** of Gastrocnemius.
➡ Muscles used in normal walk during stance and swing: **Gastrocnemiu (DNB 2004)**
➡ **Long plantar ligament** is divorced tendon of gastrocnemius.
➡ An important Bursa (**Brodies Bursa** lies deep to **Medial head** of gastrocnemius)
➡ Tendon of Gastrcnemius fuses with tendon of soleus to form **Tendo Achillis.**
➡ **Sural nerve passes between two heads of gastrocnemius.**
➡ Two heads of gastrocnemius along with soleus are called **Triceps surae**

1

ANATOMY

⊃ Important Lymph Nodes:

▶ Glans Penis and clitoris:	✓ Cloquets node☞☞ PGI 2004
▶ Rest of Penis:	✓ Superficial inguinal node
▶ Labium majus	✓ Superficial inguinal node UP 2004
▶ Testis:	✓ Preaortic/ Para aortic nodes☞☞ UP 2006
▶ Ovaries:	✓ Preaortic/ Para aortic nodes☞☞
▶ Palatine tonsil:	✓ **Jugulo digastric** nodes☞☞
▶ Tip of Tongue:	✓ **Sub mental** nodes☞ COMED 2004
▶ Anal canal **above pectinate line:**	✓ **Internal iliac** nodes☞☞
▶ Anal canal **below pectinate line:**	✓ Superficial inguinal nodes☞
▶ Delphic nodes	✓ Pretracheal DNB 2008
▶ Spongiform urethra	✓ **Deep inguinal nodes** AI 2010

✓ **Lymph node of lund: cystic lymph node of gall bladder**

✓ **Cloquets node/Rossenmullers node:**

✓ **Mucocutaneous lymph node syndrome:**

✓ **Sister mary josephs node:**

✓ **Virchows node:**

✓ **Rotter's lymph nodes** are small interpectoral lymph nodes located between the pectoralis major and pectoralis minor muscles. They receive lymphatic fluid from the muscles and the mammary gland, and deliver lymphatic fluid to the axillary lymphatic plexus.

✓ **Schmorl's nodes** or **Schmorl's nodules:** "Not a lymph node" BUT are protrusions of the cartilage of the intervertebral disc through the vertebral body endplate and into the adjacent vertebra

Lymphatics are absent in:

- ➥ Epidermis
- ➥ Eye
- ➥ Cornea
- ➥ Lens
- ➥ Articular cartilage
- ➥ Placenta
- ➥ Bone marrow
- ➥ Glottis

▶ Thoracic duct starts as continuation of **cisterna chylii.**

▶ Crosses from right to left at **T 4 level**   PGI 1990

▶ Passes through **aortic opening** of diaphragm.   PGI 1999

▶ **Primary lymphoid organs** are Thymus and Bone marrow.

▶ Lymphatics are **not present** in Brain, Choroid, Internal ear, Cornea   KOL 2008

➲ Skull:

High Yield for AIPGME/AIIMS/PGI 2013

Scaphocephaly	**Boat shaped skull** due to premature union of saggital suture.
Acrocephaly/Oxycephaly	**Pointed skull** due to premature union of coronal suture.
Plagiocephaly	**Twisted skull** due to assymetrical union of sutures.
Trigonocephaly	**Triangular prominence** of forehead. due to premature fusion of metopic suture;

Brachycephaly	**Short and broad skull** Seen in Cleidocranial dysostosis Seen in Downs Syndrome Seen in Achondroplasia
Dolicocephaly	**Long and thin skull** Seen in Marfans syndrome
Anencephaly	Vault of skull not developed resulting in the absence of a major portion of the **brain, skull, and** scalp

➲ Miscellaneous Points

➡ **Arc of Buehler:** Persistent embryological anastomosis between Celiac trunk and Superior Mesentric Artery
➡ **Arc of Riolan:** anastomosis between middle and left colic artery
▶ **Crooks Hyaline change:** change in pituitary basophils caused by elevated cortisol levels
▶ **Zellbalen:** neuroendocrine cells in nests seen in Carotid Body Tumor (Chemodectoma)
▶ **Nervus hesitans:** Deep peroneal nerve
▶ Carcinoma **head** of pancreas produces **obstructive jaundice**
▶ **Tail** of pancreas can be injured in spleenectomy.

➲ Eponym Nerves:

High Yield for AIPGME/AIIMS/PGI 2013

▶ Nerve of Bell	Long thoracic nerve✱
▶ Buffer nerve	Carotid sinus and vagal fibres from aortic arch
▶ Saphenous nerve	Longest/ largest cutaneous branch of femoral nerve ✱
▶ Herrings nerve	Branch of glossopharyngeal nerve to carotid sinus✱

►	Exners nerve	Nerve from pharyngeal plexus to cricothyroid membrane.
►	Nerve of Grassi	"Criminal nerve" branch of right posterior vagus to gastric cardia.
►	Nerve of Laterget	Crows foot formation, parallel to lesser curvature of Stomach, branch of anterior vagus.
►	Vidian nerve	Greater pertrosal +deep pertrosal nerve (N of Pterygoid canal)✳
►	Nerve of Wrisberg: (2 nerves)	Nervus intermedius (branch of Facial nerve)✳✳
		Medial cutaneous nerve of forearm ✳✳

➲ High Yield for 2012

→ **Aldermans nerve:** auricular branch of vagus

→ **Arnolds nerve:** auricular branch of vagus

→ **Jacobsons nerve:** tympanic branch of glossopharyngeal

→ **Nervi erigentes:** parasympathetic nerves S2,S3,S4

→ **Singular nerve:** inferior vestibular nerve supplying posterior semicircular nerve.   AP 2007

→ **Thickest <u>cutaneous</u> nerve:** Greater occipital nerve

→ **Thickest nerve:** sciatic nerve

→ **Dentists nerve:** inferior alveolar nerve

→ **Longest thoracic nerve:** nerve of bell

→ **Nervus spinosus:** meningeal branch of mandibular nerve

→ **Nerve of Kuntz:** 'An inconstant intrathoracic ramus which joins the 2nd intercostal nerve to the ventral ramus of the 1st thoracic nerve, proximal to the point where the latter gave a large branch to the brachial plexus is known as the 'nerve of Kuntz'

→ **Galen's:** nerve (ansa galeni) branch of the superior laryngeal nerve to the recurrent laryngealnerve;

Freys syndrome/ Baillargers syndrome: ✳✳✳

Due to abnormal and inappropriate regeneration Auriculotemporal branch of trigeminal nerve there is rednesss, sweating especially on cheeks while eating, talking. (gustatory sweating)

➲ Petrosal Nerves: High yield for 2011-2012

➢ **Greater petrosal nerve** is a branch of facial nerve and is parasympathetic to lacrimal glands, glands of pharynx and nose. (Injury causes absence of lacrimation.   AIIMS 2010

➢ **Lesser petrosal nerve** is a branch of glossophayngeal nerve and is parasympathetic to parotid gland.

➢ **Deep petrosal nerve** is a branch of plexus around internal carotid artery and joins greater petrosal nerve to form nerve of pterygoid canal (Vidian Nerve)

➢ **External petrosal nerve** is a branch of sympathetic plexus around middle meningeal artery.

Greater petrosal nerve+Deep petrosal nerve=Nerve of Pterygoid Canal (Vidian Nerve)

Parasympathetic secretomotor fibres to parotid traverse through: **Tympanic plexus/Lesser petrosal nerve**

➲ Cervical Spinal Nerves

High Yield for AIPGME/AIIMS/PGI 2013

Cervical spinal nerves have cutaneous branches which supply areas of skin in the face and scalp.

The named branches are the great auricular, lesser occipital and greater occipital nerves.

Great auricular nerve

→ And is derived from the anterior primary rami of the second and third cervical spinal nerves.

→ It passes up from the neck, lying on sternocleidomastoid, towards the angle of the jaw, and supplies much of the lower part of the auricle of the ear, and skin overlying the parotid gland.

Lesser occipital nerve

→ The lesser occipital nerve is a branch of the cervical plexus

→ It ascends along the posterior border of sternocleidomastoid to supply the scalp above and behind the ear and a small area on the cranial surface of the auricle.

Greater occipital nerve

→ The greater occipital nerve represents the posterior primary ramus of the second cervical spinal nerve.

→ It pierces trapezius close to its attachment to the superior nuchal line and ascends to supply the skin of the back of the scalp up to the vertex of the skull.

➲ Important Points About Veins:

High Yield for AIPGME/AIIMS/PGI 2013

▶ **Great cerebral vein of Galen** is formed by **union of internal cerebral veins.** PGI 1998

▶ Great cerebral vein of Galen drains into **straight sinus.** MAH 2006

▶ Facial vein communicates to cavernous sinus via:

    Superior opthalmic vein,

    Inferior opthalmic vein,

    Deep facial vein.

▶ **Long saphenous vein** is the **largest and longest** superficial vein of lower limb formed on medial side of dorsal venous arch.

▶ **Injury to great saphenous vein corresponds to area of femoral nerve distribution** AI 2008

▶ Portal vein is formed behind the neck of pancreas by union of **superior mesentric and spleenic vein.** DNB 2000

    MAH 2000

▶ **Normal pressure is 5-10 mm Hg**

▶ Portal venous system is **valveless.**

▶ **Left suprarenal** drains into left renal vein.

▶ **Left testicular vein** drains into left renal vein.

▶ **Left ovarian vein** drains into left renal vein.

▶ **Batesons vertebral venous plexus is valveless.**

1

ANATOMY

⊃ Excepts in Anatomy✱✱✱

High Yield for AIPGME/AIIMS/PGI 2013

- ▶ All muscles are mesodermal in origin **except** muscles of Iris (Sphincter pupillae and dilator pupillae) which are ectodermal➤➤

- ▶ All Pharyngeal arches persist **except** fifth which disappears.➤➤

- ▶ All intrinsic muscles of Larynx are supplied by recurrent laryngeal nerve **except** cricothyroid which is supplied by external laryngeal nerve.➤➤   **MAH 2005**

- ▶ All major salivary gland are supplied by facial nerve **except** Parotid gland (Although passes through the substance of parotid)➤➤

- ▶ All divisions of Trigeminal nerve **except** Mandibular division lie in lateral wall of Cavernous sinus➤➤

- ▶ All muscles of pharynx are supplied by pharyngeal plexus **except** stylopharyngeus which is supplied by Glossopharyngeal nerve.➤➤

- ▶ All muscles of soft palate are supplied by pharyngeal **plexus** except tensor palati which is supplied by Nerve to medial pterygoid.➤➤

- ▶ All muscles of tongue are supplied by hypoglossal nerve **except** palatoglossus which is supplied by pharyngeal plexus➤➤   **TN 2008**

⊃ Joints

High Yield for AIPGME/AIIMS/PGI 2013

⇨ Fibrous joints:

➡ Sutures:	Skull	**PGI 1998**
➡ Syndesmosis:	Inf. Tibiofibular joint	
➡ Gomphosis:	Tooth in socket	

⇨ Cartilaginous joints:

▶ Primary cartilaginous (Synchondrosis):	Joint between epiphysis and diaphysis➤➤	
	First costochondral joint.	**AI 2004**
▶ Secondary cartilaginous (Symphisis):	Symphisis pubis, Manubriosternal joint	**KERALA 1996**
▶ Syndesmosis:	Inferior tibiofibular joint	**AP 1991**
▶ Hinge joint:	Elbow, ankle, **IP joint**	**JK BOPEE 2012**
▶ Pivot Joint: ➤	Sup and inf radioulnar joint	
▶ Condyloid joint	TM joint	**DNB 2007**
▶ Ellipsoid joint:	Wrist joint, MCP	**KERALA 1996**
▶ Saddle/ sellar joint: ➤➤	Ist MCP, sterno clavicular	**APPG 2006, MP 1998**
▶ Ball and Socket variety:	Shoulder, Hip	

TYPES OF EPIPHYSIS DNB 2011

PRESSURE EPIPHYSIS	1. *Articular*
	
	2. *Takes part in transmission of weight*
	
	EXAMPLES :
	
	  ✓ **Head of femur**✱ AIIMS 1986
	
	  ✓ **Lower end of Fibula**✱

TRACTION EPIPHYSIS	1. *Non articular*
	
	2. *Does not take part in transmission of weight*
	
	3. *Provide attachment to one or more tendons which exert traction on epiphysis*
	
	EXAMPLES:
	
	  ✓ **Tubercles of humerus**✱ AI 2003
	
	  ✓ **Trochanters of femur**
	
	  ✓ **Mastoid process**✱ AIIMS 1993

ATAVISTIC EPIPHYSIS	1. *Phylogenetically an independent bone which in man becomes fused to another bone.*
	
	EXAMPLE:
	
	  ✓ **Coracoid process of Scapula**✱ JK BOPEE 2012
	
	  ✓ **Os Trigonum**✱ AMU 1988

ABERRANT EPIPHYSIS	EXAMPLES
	
	  ✓ **Ephysis of head of first metacarpal**✱
	
	  ✓ **Epiphysis at the base of other metacarpal bones**✱

⇨ **Struthers' ligament:**

✱ It is not a constant ligament and can be acquired or congenital.

✱ Its clinical significance arises form the fact that the **median nerve, passes in the space between the ligament and the humerus,** and in this space the nerve may be compressed leading to supracondylar process syndrome.

✱ Coracobrachialis is more important morphologically than functionally. It represent the medial compartment of the arm.

✱ In some animals the **muscle is tricipital**. In man the **upper** two heads have fused, but the musculocutaneous nerve passes between the remnants of these two heads.

✱ <u>The third head (and the lowest) head of the muscle has disappeared in man</u>.Occasional persistence of the lower head is associated with the presence of the so called "ligament of struthers" which is a fibrous band extending

⇨ **Bursitis: High Yield for 2012**

> **Bursitis is inflammation of a bursa**, which is a thin-walled sac lined with synovial tissue.
> The function of the bursa is to facilitate movement of tendons and muscles over bony prominences

- **Subacromial bursitis (subdeltoid bursitis)** is the most common form of bursitis. Trochanteric bursitis involves the bursa around the insertion of the gluteus medius onto the greater trochanter of the femur.

- **Olecranon bursitis** occurs over the posterior elbow, and when the area is acutely inflamed, infection should be excluded by aspirating and culturing fluid from the bursa. Achilles bursitis involves the bursa located above the insertion of the tendon to the calcaneus and results from overuse and wearing tight shoes.

- **Retrocalcaneal bursitis** involves the bursa that is located between the calcaneus and posterior surface of the Achilles tendon.

- **Ischial bursitis (weaver's bottom)** affects the bursa separating the gluteus medius from the ischial tuberosity and develops from prolonged sitting and pivoting on hard surfaces.

- Iliopsoas bursitis affects the bursa that lies between the iliopsoas muscle and hip joint and is lateral to the femoral vessels.

- **Anserine bursitis** is an inflammation of the sartorius bursa located over the medial side of the tibia just below the knee and under the conjoint tendon and is manifested by pain on climbing stairs.

- **Prepatellar bursitis (housemaid's knee)** occurs in the bursa situated between the patella and overlying skin and is caused by kneeling on hard surfaces. Treatment of bursitis consists of prevention of the aggravating situation, rest of the involved part, administration of a nonsteroidal anti-inflammatory drug (NSAID), or local glucocorticoid injection.

⇨ **Bursitis of knee joint:**

- **Housemaid's knee** is the result of inflammation of **Prepatellar bursa**   MP 2009
- **Miners beat knee** is the result of inflammation of **Prepatellar bursa**
- **Clergymans knee** is the result of inflammation of **subcutaneous infra patellar bursa.**

⇨ **Structures Pasing Between/Piercing: High Yield for AIPGME/AIIMS/PGI 2013**

- ✓ Structure **passing between two heads of gastrocnemius:** sural nerve
- ✓ Structure **passing between two heads of lateral pterygoid:** Maxillary artery
- ✓ Structure **passing between pronator teres:** median nerve
- ✓ Structure **passing between two plains of fibres of supinator:** posterior interosseous nerve
- ✓ Structure **passing through tarsal tunnel:** posterior tibial nerve
- ✓ Structure **passing through choroid fissure of eye:** hyaloids artery
- ✓ Structure **passing through foramen of Vesalius:** emissary vein
- ✓ Structure passing **through carotid sheath:** internal carotid/ common carotid artery, internal jugular vein, vagus nerve. **External carotid is External to sheath**   UPSC 2007
- ✓ Structure **piercing corocabrachialis :** Musculocutaneous nerve
- ✓ Structure **piercing clavipectoral fascia (encloses subclavius):**
  lateral pectoral nerve, thoracoacromial vessels Cephalic vein   DNB 2011 & COMED 2009
- ✓ Structure **piercing thyrohyoid membrane:** Internal laryngeal nerve

⊃ Differentiate between: High yield for 2011-2012

☐ **Meckel's band (Meckel's ligament):** Portion of the anterior ligament of the malleus that extends from the base of the anterior process through the petrotympanic fissure.

☐ **Meckel's cartilage:** A cartilaginous bar about which the mandible develops.

☐ **Meckel's cavity** (Meckel's space) the cavity, or cleft, between two layers of dura over the petrous portion of the temporal bone that encloses the roots of the trigeminal nerve and the trigeminal ganglion.

☐ **Meckel's diverticulum** Diverticulum of the ileum derived from the unobliterated yolk stalk.

☐ **Meckel's ganglion** The sphenopalatine ganglion or the second division of the trigeminal nerve.

☐ **Meckel's cave (Meckel's space)** The cavity, or cleft, between two layers of dura over the petrous portion of the temporal bone that encloses the roots of the trigeminal nerve and the trigeminal ganglion.

⊃ Important Structures Accompanying: High Yield for AIPGME/AIIMS/PGI 2013

- **Axillary nerve** accompanies posterior humeral circumflex artery.
- **Radial nerve** accompanies profunda brachii vessels
- **Short saphenous vein** accompanies sural nerve.
- **Great saphenous vein** accompanies saphenous nerve.
- **Superior thyroid vessels** accompany external laryngeal nerve
- **Superior laryngeal vessels** accompany internal laryngeal nerve
- **Inferior laryngeal vessels** accompany recurrent laryngeal nerve

Remember "Rule of 45"

Following structures are 45cms long in human body:

- Spinal cord
- Vas deferens
- Femur
- Thoracic duct

Questions of AIPGME 2011

☐ **Type of joint seen in the growth plate :** Primary Cartilagenous joint.	AIPGME 2011
☐ **Muscle not affected in low radial nerve palsy :** Extensor carpi radialis longus	AIPGME 2011
☐ **Diaphragm develops from :** Septum transversum, Pleuroperitoneal membrane, Cervical myotomes	AIPGME 2011
☐ **Muscular component of dorsal aorta develops from:** Paraxial mesoderm	AIPGME 2011
☐ **pneumatic bones are:** Frontal , Ethmoid, Maxilla	AIPGME 2011
☐ **Seen in injury to common peroneal nerve** Foot drop, Injury to neck of fibula	AIPGME 2011
☐ **Main blood supply of neck of femur:** Medial circumflex femoral	AIPGME 2011

1

ANATOMY

1

Important Revision Questions. One liners asked frequently

☐ <u>VON Bruns nests</u> are seen in urothelium	COMED 2008
☐ Urinary bladder is lined by: transistional epithelium	UP 2007
☐ Trigone of bladder develops from: **Mesonephric duct**	TN 2008
☐ Trapezoid body is present at: **Pons**	TN2008
☐ Lateral rotator of hip: **Piriformis**	TN 2008

▶ "<u>Abductor</u>" of vocal cord is: posterior cricoarytenoid	COMED 2008
▶ "<u>Abductor</u>" of vocal cord is: posterior cricoarytenoid	UP 2007
▶ "<u>External laryngeal nerve</u>" supplies cricothyroid	COMED 2008
▶ "<u>Tensor</u> of vocal cords is cricothyroid	JK 2008
▶ <u>Parasympathetic</u> Preganglionic to parotid travel in lesser petrosal nerve	COMED 2008
▶ "Central artery of Retina" is a branch of <u>Opthalmic artery</u>	UP 2007
▶ Maxillary nerve passes through "<u>Foramen Rotundum</u>"	UP 2007
▶ Platysma is supplied by <u>Facial nerve</u>	PGI 2007

▶ Spleenic artery lies in <u>spleenorenal ligament</u>	UPSC 2007
▶ **Renal Angle** lies between <u>12 th rib and lateral border of sacrospinalis</u>	AIIMS 2007
▶ Nerve supply of pyramidalis <u>is subcostal nerve</u>.	Manipal 2006
▶ Blood supply of <u>lung tissue proper</u> is by Bronchial arteries.	JK 2008
▶ <u>Herrings bodies</u> are present in <u>neuro</u>hypophysis	JK 2008
▶ **Middle meningeal artery** is a branch of internal maxillary artery	AI 2006
▶ Tail of pancreas lies in <u>spleenorenal ligament</u>.	UP 2007
▶ Gall bladder is lined by <u>simple columnar epithelium</u>	AIIMS 2007

▶ Glossopharyneal nerve supplies Stylopharyngeus muscle	JK 2009
▶ Nerve supply of trapezius: <u>Accessory nerve</u>	MAHE 2007
▶ <u>Erbs point</u>: **C5 and C6**	COMED 2007
▶ Erb Duchnee paralysis involves 5th and 6th Cervical nerves.	COMED 2007
▶ <u>Winging of scapula is</u> due to injury to Long thoraxic nerve.	PGMCET 2007
▶ Axillary sheath is derived from <u>prevertebral fascia</u>	PGMCET 2007
▶ Axillary nerve supplies : <u>Deltoid and Teres minor</u>	PGI 2006
▶ Klupkes palsy involves: <u>C7, C8, T1</u>	PGMCET 2007
▶ Nerve passing through spiral groove of humerus is: <u>Radial nerve</u>	TN 2005
▶ Function of median nerve in carpal tunnel is to <u>abduct the thumb</u>.	AIIMS 2005

Questions Likely to be repeated.

- Tendon of Flexor Hallucis longus passes below sustanteculum tali — AI 2010
- **Deltoid ligament** is attached to **medial malleolus, spring ligament, susteteculum tali.** — AIIMS 2009
- <u>Right</u> **gastroepiploic artery** is a branch of **gastroduodenal artery.**
- Nerve supply of vocal cords is by: **Internal laryngeal and recurrent laryngeal nerves** — MP 2005
- One of the commonest area of colonic ischemia is called **Sudeck's point** — MP 2009
- The sinoatrial node is usually supplied by a nodal branch from the:**Right coronary artery** — MP 2008
- The loss of opposition movement of the thumb is due to injury to this Nerve:**Median Nerve** — MP 2007
- **Pelvic splanchnic nerves** supply **rectum, urinary bladder, uterus.** — AIIMS 2009
- **Sphincter of Oddi** consists has <u>three</u> **sphincters** — AIIMS 2009
- **Urothelium** lines **ureters, minor calyx and urinary bladder.** — AIIMS 2009
- **Aortic hiatus** contains **azygous vein, thoracic duct.** — AIIMS 2009
- <u>Enopthalmos</u> is due to **palsy of orbitalis muscle.**
- Cranial nerve VIII affects: **equilibrium.** — AIIMS 2009
- **Vaginal sphincter** is formed by: **external urethral sphincter, pubovaginalis, Bulbospongiosus** — AIIMS 2009
- The embryological first pharyngeal arches remains: **Sphenomandibular ligament** — UP 2007
- Adductor canal lies beneath the: **Sartorius** — UP 2007
- Medial medullary syndrome occurs due to thrombosis of the: **Vertebral arter** — UP 2006
- In testes **"Thermostat"** is : **Dartos and cremater** — UP 2006
- **"Dropped shoulder"** occurs due to paralysis of: **Trapezius** — UP 2006
- Lateral rotator of hip: **Piriformis** — TN 2008
- Drainage of Posterior ethmoidal sinus is at: **Superior meatus** — TN 2008
- Maxillary sinus opens into the: **Middlemeatus of the nose in the lower part of the hiatus semilunaris** — TN 2006
- Extensor of Shoulder join: **Teres majo** — TN 2007
- The characteristics features of Lymph node is: **Germinal centre** — TN 2007
- External laryngeal nerve supplies: **Cricothyroid muscle** — PGI 2000
- Vidian nerve is: **Nerve of Pterygoid cana** — TN 2006
- Position of vagus nerve in relation to carotid sheath is: **Posterior** — TN 2008
- Hypoglossal nerve carries fibres from**Hypoglosal nucleus and 1st cervical spinal nerve** — MP 2009
- **Cells present in cerebellar cortex** are: **granule, golgi, basket, stellate, purkinje.**
- Fascia around nerve bundle of branchial plexus is derived from **Prevertebral fascia** — DNB 2008
- Delphic nodes are **Pretracheal** — DNB 2008

1

ANATOMY

♯ Paramesonephric duct in males remains as: **Prostatic utricle**   MH 2010

♯ **Stapedial artery** is derivative of second branchial arch   MH 2010

♯ Artery supplying blood to trigeminal ganglion **Cavernous part of internal carotid artery**   MH 2010

♯ Carpometacarpal joint of thumb is **Saddle** type of joint

♯ The abductor of vocal cord is: **Posterior cricoarytenoid**   MHPGMCET 2009 & MH 2010

♯ Erb's palsy occurs due to involvement of **Upper trunk** of brachial plexus: MHPGMCET 2001

♯ Lymphatics of suprarenal gland drain into **Para-aortic** lymph nodes: MH 2010

♯ Portal Acinus in liver is centered on **Hepatic arteriole**

♯ Urogenital diaphragm is made of Deep transverse perinea, Perineal membrane,

   Sphincter urethrae   MH 2010

■ **Fascia around brachial plexus** is derived from **prevertebral fascia.**   AIIMS 2008

■ **Tredlenburgs test** is positive in **injury to <u>superior</u> gluteal nerve**   AIIMS 2008

■ **Gluteus medius is supplied by superior gluteal nerve.**   AI 2010

■ **Permanent mucosal folds** are: **spiral valve of Heister, plicae semilunaris, transverse**

   rectal fold   AIIMS 2008

■ **Terminal** lymph nodes for colon are **preaortic**   AIIMS 2008

■ The fate of the notochord is that it **Persists as nucleus pulposus of the**

   intervertebral disc   MAH 2012

■ Sequestration of lung is supplied by **Systemic arteries**   UP 2008

■ Lines of Gennari are seen in: **Visual cortex**   TN 2005

■ Radial nerve supplies : **brachioradialis**   TN 2004

■ Great vein of Galen in formed by: **Internal cerebral veins & straight sinu**   TN 2004

■ The 'oral diaphragm' is formed by the **Mylohyoid** muscle: TN 2004

■ Ascending pharyngeal artery is the branch of: **External carotid artery**   TN 2004

■ Gartner's duct is remnant of **Wolffian duct**

■ Kerckring's centre for ossification is associated with: **Occipital bone**   DNB 2006

NOTES

NOTES

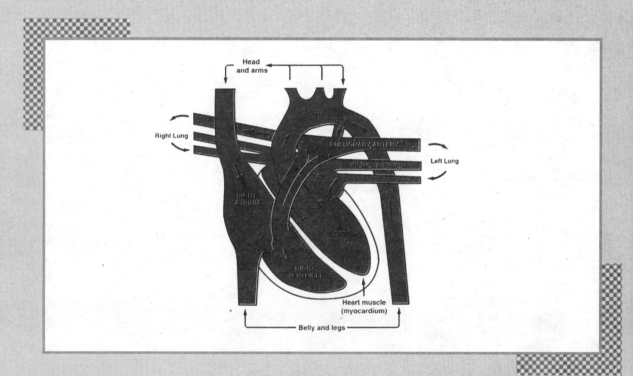

PHYSIOLOGY

Na K ATPASE PUMP

➲ High Yield for 2012

➡ Na K ATPase Pump is an active, electrogenic pump moving three sodium ions outside and in place two potassium ions inside utilizing ATP. It helps in **intrusion** of K^+.   **AIIMS 92**

➡ It accounts for 20% of energy utilized by cells.

➡ Thus its coupling ratio is 3:2. ☛☛   **MAH 2012, ASSAM 2004**

➡ Extracellular binding site is **OUBAIN**.   **JIPMER 2006**

➡ Its activity is inhibited by **oubain and related cardiac glycosides.** ☛☛

➡ It is a **P type ATP ase** (super family of cation transporters) ☛☛

➡ Also called **E1 /E2 Type ATPase** responsible for carrying ions across cell membranes ☛☛☛

➡ Type: **heterodimer heterogeneous**   **UP 2005**

➡ **Is an example of active transport**   **AIIMS 2006**

➡ Resting membrane potential of a **skeletal muscle** is -90mV. ☛

➡ Resting membrane potential of a **smooth muscle** is -50 to -75mV. ☛

➡ Resting membrane potential of a **cardiac muscle** is -85 to -95mV. ☛☛

➡ The resting membrane potential in the **nerve fiber is -70mV.** ☛   **JK BOPEE**

➡ The resting membrane potential in the **rods** is -40mV.

➡ The resting membrane potential of **inner ear cell** is -60mV.

CELLS IN WHICH ACTIN POTENTIAL IS GENERATED:

Nerve cells not neuroglia

Muscles   **PGI 2011**

Contractile tissues

Glands   **PGI 2011**

➡ Resting Membrane Potential is <u>due to</u> : K^+✱   **(PGI 03)**

➡ Resting Membrane Potential is <u>close to</u> isoelectric potential of : Cl^-✱   **(AI 93)**

➡ IPSP is due to <u>Cl^- influx</u>✱   **(NIMHANS 01)**

➡ EPSP is due to <u>K^+influx</u>✱   **(NIMHANS 01)**

✓ For action potential; threshold stimulus is required.

✓ Nerve conduction follows <u>**All or None phenomenon**</u>.

✓ <u>**Axon**</u> has the lowest threshold potential in a nerve fibre.

✓ Nerve impulse travels <u>**in one direction only**</u> at synapse.   **AI 1996**

☐	RMP is close to	Isoelectric potential of chloride	
☐	RMP is due to	Pottasium	PGI 2003
☐	IPSP is due to	Chloride	
☐	Amplitude is due to	Chloride	

⮌ Presynaptic Inhibition   AIIMS 2009

➡ Occurs where the "terminal of one neuron makes synaptic contact with the presynaptic ending of a second neuron which in turn excites a third neuron."

➡ The first neuron controls the "amount of excitatory transmitter released from the second neuron and hence the level of stimulation of the third neuron."

➡ Control is exerted by the release of an inhibitory neurotransmitter. (Mostly the inhibitory transmitter substance is **GABA** (Gamma amino butyric acid).

➡ The inhibitory neurotransmitter →increases the Cl- conductance of the presynaptic nerve ending. The increase in Cl- conductance →causes a partial depolarization of the presynaptic nerve ending and→ a **decrease in the magnitude of the action potential** in the presynaptic nerve ending. →This in turn **reduces Ca++ entry** which consequently reduces the amount of excitatory neurotransmitter released by the nerve terminal into the synaptic cleft (the amount of neurotransmitter released from the presynaptic neuron is directly proportional to the magnitude of calcium influx). →Thus the magnitude of the postsynaptic potential is reduced. Reducing the magnitude of the postsynaptic potential decreases the probability that an action potential will be generated by the postsynaptic cell.

⮌ Chemical Classification of Neurotransmitters:

High Yield for AIPGME/AIIMS/PGI 2013

Biogenic Amines

➡ Catecholamines: Dopamine, norepinephrine (NE), and epinephrine

➡ Indolamines

➡ Serotonin and histamine (5-Hydroxytryptamine or 5-HT)

Amino Acids

➡ GABA—Gamma ()-aminobutyric acid

➡ Glycine

➡ Aspartate

➡ Glutamate

Neuropeptides

➡ Substance P

➡ Endorphins and Enkephalins

➡ Somatostatin, gastrin, cholecystokinin, oxytocin, vasopressin, Leutinizing hormone releasing hormone (LHRH)

PHYSIOLOGY

2

Purines

- Adenosine
- ATP

Gases and Lipids

- Nitric Oxide (NO)
- Carbonmonooxide (CO)
- Cannabinoids

⇨ **Acetylcholine (Ach)**

Acetylcholine (Ach) was the first neurotransmitter to be identified. It is the most abundant neurotransmitter in the brain

- Released at **neuromuscular junctions** and some ANS neurons
- Synthesized by enzyme **choline acetyltransferase**
- Degraded by the **enzyme acetylcholinesterase (AChE)**

⇨ **Catecholamines**

Catecholamines-Dopamine, norepinephrine (NE), and epinephrine are **synthesized from Tyrosine**

- Is involved in **reward-pleasure and learning**
- Dopamine is the principle neurotransmitter involved in **Addiction pathway**

⇨ **Serotonin**

- Broadly distributed in the brain, derived from **Tryptophan** involved in sleep, dreaming, hunger and arousal
- Play roles in **emotional behaviors and the biological clock**
- Depletion of serotonin in brain leads to **depression**

⊃ **GABA**

- GABA—Gamma ()-aminobutyric acid is the **major inhibitory neurotransmitter** in CNS
- Synthesized from **decarboxylation of Glutamate**
- Involved in **regulating anxiety**
- May be related to **eating or sleep disorders**

⇨ **Endorphins, Enkephalins and Substance P**

- Substance P is the **mediator of pain signals**
- Endorphins and Enkephalins act as **natural opiates**; reduce pain perception
- They also depress physical functions like breathing and may produce physical dependence

⇨ **Purines such as ATP**

- Purines such as ATP:
- Act in both the CNS and PNS
- **Produce fast or slow responses**
- **Induce Ca2+ influx in astrocytes**
- **Provoke pain sensation**

⇨ **Nitric Oxide (NO)**

- Synthesized on **demand**
- Activates the intracellular receptor guanylyl cyclase to cyclic GMP
- Involved in **learning and memory**

⇨ **Endocannabinoids**

- Lipid soluble; synthesized on demand from **membrane lipids**
- Bind with **G protein-coupled receptors** in the brain
- Involved in **learning and memory**

⊃ **Blood Brain Barrier: (High Yield for 2011/2012)**

✓ Membranes are generally **assymetrical.**

✓ Plasma membrane is composed mainly of **proteins.**

✓ Protein content: 55%

✓ Phospholipid: 25%

✓ Function of phospholipid is **transduction of signals and enzyme activation.**

✓ Lipids and proteins in cell membrane interact by **hydrogen bonds.**   PGI 2007

✓ Fluidity of membranres depends on **lipid content.**

✓ **Saturated fatty acids** increase transistion temperature and decrease fluidity.

✓ **Unsaturated fatty acids** decrease transistion temperature and increase fluidity.   AIIMS 2005

— Cerebral blood vessels are unique in that the junctions between vascular endothelial cells are nearly fused. The paucity of pores is responsible for what is termed the blood-brain barrier.

— This lipid barrier allows the passage of lipid soluble substances but restrict movements of those that are ionized or have large molecular weight.

— CO_2, O_2 and lipid soluble substances (such as most anaesthetics) freely enter the brain, where as most ions, proteins and large substances such as mannitol penetrate poorly.

— Water moves freely, across the BBB.

— Mannitol, an osmotically active substance that does not normally cross the BBB, causes a sustained decrease in brain water content and is often used to decrease brain volume

— BBB may be disrupted by severe hypertension, tumors, trauma, stroke, infection, marked hypercapnia, hypoxia and sustained seizure-activity.

► Most of pottasium is intracellular

► Mx pottasium is found in skeletal muscles

► In response to tissue injury intracellular pottasium shifts to extra cellular space.

⮌ The Cell Membrane: (High Yield for 2011/2012)

► Main constituent is the protein.	AIIMS 1994
► Lipids are regular but assymetrically arranged.	
► Membrane lipids are amphiphatic.	
► Are arranged as a bilayer.	
► Signal transduction and enzyme activation are the functions of phospholipid part.	
► The fluidity of cell membrane is increased by Poly unsaturated fatty acids.	AIIMS 2005
► Lipids and proteins intreact by hydrogen bonds.	PGI 2007
► RBC Membrane is specially having spectrin (maintains integrity) and glycophyrin.	AIIMS 2002
► Lipid bilayer is most permeable to urea.	
► Lipid bilayer acts as a gel.	
► Protein: lipid ratio is 2:1.	

⮌ Basement Membrane

► Contains laminin	AIIMS 2007
► Nidogenin	AIIMS 2007
► Enactin	
► Type IV collagen	PGI 2006
► Degeneration mediated by metalloproteineases	AI 2007

⮌ Functions of Organalles Commonly asked: (High Yield for 2011/2012)

► Synthesis of lipids occurs in agranular Endoplasmic Reticulum	AI 2007
► Synthesis of proteins occurs in Rough ER	
► Intracellular sorting and packing is done in Golgi complex	
► Cell shape and motility are a function of Microtubules	AI 1995
► Catabolism of H_2O_2 is a function of Peroxisomes	AI 1994
► Site of ATP synthesis is Mitochondria.	PGI 2002

2

⇨ **Microfilaments**

Microfilaments are the **"thinnest"** cytoskeleton components (5-7 nm wide). They are usually composed of one of several types of actin protein. Microfilaments are contractile, but to contract they usually must interact with myosin

- **Intermediate filaments** Intermediate filaments are intermediate in thickness (10-12 nm) between microtubules and microfilaments. Examples:
- **Cytokeratins** in epithelial cells,
- **Vimentin** in, fibroblasts

⊃ **Marker of: High Yield for AIPGME/AIIMS/PGI 2013**

▶ Plasma membrane: adenyl cyclase, 5 nucleotidase		PGI 2006
▶ Golgi bodies: galactosyl transferase		AI 1995
▶ Mitochondria: Glutamic dehydrogenase		PGI 2005

⊃ **Fluids: High Yield for AIPGME/AIIMS/PGI 2013**

- ☐ Water constitutes between 50% and 70% of total body weight.
- ☐ The water of the body is divided into three functional compartments.
- ☐ The intracellular water, represents between 30% and 40% of body weight.
- ☐ **The extracellular water** represents approximately 20% of body weight and is divided between intravascular fluid, or plasma (5% of body weight), and interstitial, or extravascular, extracellular fluid (15% of body weight).
- ☐ Intracellular Fluid. Measurement of intracellular fluid (ICF) is determined indirectly by subtraction of the measured extracellular fluid (ECF) from the measured total body water. The intracellular water is **between 30% and 40% of body weight**, with the largest proportion in the skeletal muscle mass. Because of the smaller muscle mass in the female, the percentage of intracellular water is lower than in the male. The chemical composition of ICF **with potassium and magnesium** the principal cations, and **phosphates and proteins the principal** anions.
- ☐ **Extracellular Fluid.** The total ECF volume represents approximately 20% of body weight. The ECF compartment has two major subdivisions. **The plasma volume** is approximately 5% of body weight in the normal adult. **The interstitial, or extravascular, ECF volume**, obtained by subtracting the plasma volume from the measured total ECF volume, accounts for approximately 15% of body weight.
- ☐ The interstitial fluid is further complicated by having a rapidly equilibrating or functional component as well as several more slowly equilibrating, or relatively nonfunctioning, components. The nonfunctioning components include connective tissue water as well as transcellular water, which includes cerebrospinal and joint fluids. This nonfunctional component normally represents only 10% of interstitial fluid volume (1% to 2% of body weight) and is not to be confused with the relatively nonfunctional ECF, often called a third space, found in burns and soft tissue injuries.
- ☐ The normal constituents of ECF are with **sodium the principal cation and chloride and bicarbonate the principal anions**

Electrolyte	Function	Distribution
Sodium (Na$^+$)	➡ Essential role in fluid and electrolyte balance- accounts for half the osmolarity of ECF. ➡ Role in generation of action potentials.	Represents about 90% of extracellular cations. Level in blood controlled by aldosterone, ANP, and ADH.
Potassium (K$^+$)	➡ Establishes resting membrane potential and essential in the repolarisation phase of action potentials in nervous and muscle tissue. ➡ Aids maintenance of fluid volume in cells. ➡ Helps regulate pH.	Most abundant intracellular cation. Blood serum level controlled by aldosterone.
Calcium (Ca^{2+})	➡ Roles in blood clotting, neurotransmitter release, maintenance of muscle tone, and excitability of nervous and muscle tissue.	Most abundant mineral in the body due to bone content. Principally extracellular. Blood level controlled chiefly by Parathyroid hormone (PTH).
Chloride (Cl$^-$)	➡ Helps balance anions in different fluid compartments.	Most prevalent extracellular anion. Diffuses easily between interstitial space and ICF. Level controlled indirectly by aldosterone – due to relationship with sodium.
Bicarbonate (HCO$_3^-$)	➡ Major buffer of H$^+$ in plasma. ➡ Helps maintain correct balance of anions and cations in ECF and ICF.	Second most prevalent anions in extracellular fluid. A small amount found in intracellular fluid. Blood level controlled by kidneys which can both form and excrete bicarbonate.

Remember:

➜ **If an isotonic salt solution is added to or lost from the body fluids,** only the volume of the ECF is changed. The acute loss of an isotonic extracellular solution, such as intestinal juice, is followed by a significant decrease in ECF volume and little, if any, change in ICF volume. Fluid is not transferred from the intracellular space to refill the depleted extracellular space as long as the osmolality remains the same in the two compartments.

➜ **If water alone is added to or lost from the ECF,** the concentration of osmotically active particles changes. Sodium ions account for most of the osmotically active particles in ECF and generally reflect the tonicity of other body fluid compartments. If ECF is depleted of sodium, water passes into the intracellular space until

→ Osmolality is again equal in the two compartments.

→ The concentration of most other ions within the ECF compartment can be altered without significant change in the total number of osmotically active particles, thus producing only a compositional change. For instance, a rise of the serum potassium concentration from 4 to 8 mEq. per liter would have a significant effect on the myocardium, but it would not significantly change the effective osmotic pressure of the ECF compartment. Normally functioning kidneys minimize these changes considerably, particularly if the addition or loss of solute or water is gradual.

→ An internal loss of ECF into a nonfunctional space, such as the sequestration of isotonic fluid in a burn, peritonitis, ascites, or muscle trauma, is termed a distributional change. This transfer or functional loss of ECF internally may be extracellular (e.g., as in peritonitis) or intracellular (e.g., as in hemorrhagic shock). In any event, all distributional shifts or losses cause a contraction of the functional ECF space.

⇨ **Regulation of Fluid Transfer among Compartments**

The transfer of fluid between vascular and interstitial compartments occurs at the capillary level and is governed by the balance between hydrostatic pressure gradients and plasma oncotic pressure gradients.

This relation is stated by the <u>Starling equation</u>:

$$Jv = Kf (DP - Dp)$$

Where:

- Jv is rate of fluid transfer between vascular and interstitial compartments, Kf is the water permeability of the capillary bed,
- DP is the hydrostatic pressure difference between capillary and interstitium, and
- Dp is the oncotic pressure difference between capillary and interstitial fluids

Under normal circumstances, interstitial tissue pressure is low, and the DP term in the Starling equation represents the integrated hydrostatic pressure gradient from arteriolar to venular ends of a capillary. Since interstitial fluid is protein poor, the Dp term in the Starling equation represents the oncotic pressure of plasma proteins, principally albumin; 5 grams of albumin per deciliter of plasma exerts an oncotic pressure of about 15 mm Hg.

⇨ **Diffusion**

For the diffusion of small water-soluble molecules (e.g. sodium, chloride and glucose) across capillary endothelium, the size and number of the pores (which vary depending upon the site) is not rate limiting and movement is dictated by blood supply, i.e. is 'flow limited'. These movements are dictated by the Fick equation (diffusion rate = blood flow/arteriovenous concentration difference) and Fick's law of diffusion which relates the diffusion rate:

- Directly to the diffusion coefficient of the solute (related to molecular size and therefore weight);
- Directly to the area of the capillary membrane;
- Directly to the concentration gradient;
- Inversely to the thickness (and hence permeability) of the membrane

The filtration of fluid is a passive process proceeding at a rate dictated by:

➡ The filtration coefficient of the membrane (influenced by its surface area and permeability);

➡ The hydrostatic pressure gradient (greater within the arterial end of the capillary but consistent across a glomerulus);

➡ The colloid osmotic pressure gradient, in a relationship described by Starling's law of ultrafiltration. The net filtration is out of the capillary at the arterial end and into the capillary at the venous end.

➲ Channelopathies with (Channels): High Yield for AIPGME/AIIMS/PGI 2013

➡ Epilepsy Benign neonatal familial convulsions (K)

➡ Generalized epilepsy with febrile convulsions plus (Na)

➡ Periodic Hyperkalemic periodic paralysis (Na)

➡ Hypokalemic periodic paralysis (Ca)

➡ Myotonia Myotonia Congenita (Cl)

➡ Paramyotonia congenita (Na)

➡ Deafness Jorvell and Lange-Nielsen syndrome (K)

➡ Autosomal dominant progressive deafness (K)

MOLARITY

Molarity is defined as the gram molecules (moles) of solute per liter of solution.

Molality

Molality is defined as the gram molecules (moles) of solute per kilogram of solvent.

At all body temperatures 1 kg of water is regarded as occupying 1 liter.

The terms molarity and molality should not be confused. For dilute aqueous solutions they are approximately equal, but in the body the distinction is marked.

OSMOLARITY

One liter of solution containing 1 mole of undissociated solute represents an osmolarity of 1 osmol/L or 1000 mosmol/L. An aqueous solution of such concentration will exert an osmotic pressure of 22.4 atmospheres under ideal conditions and with an ideal membrane.

OSMOLALITY

Osmolality is applicable when the concentration of solute is molal. This term, unlike osmolarity, takes account of the solute volume.

For undissociated non-electrolyte solutions the molarity (molality) and osmolar (osmolal) concentrations are identical. For a substance dissociating fully into ions, however, each ion has the same osmotic effect as an undissociated molecule (i.e. dissociation increases the osmotic effect beyond that expected in terms of the molar content of the undissociated solute).

2

PHYSIOLOGY

►	Water constitutes roughly 60% of body weight.	PGI 2007
►	Na, Cl, HCO₃ are Predominantly in ECF.	PGI 2006
►	K, P, Mg are predominantly in ICF.	

⊃ Measurement of Body Fluids: (High Yield for 2011/2012)

►	Total Body water	about 60% of body weight
►	ICF	40%
►	ECF	20%

►	Total body water:	Tritrated water, Deuterium Oxide, Antipyrine	(AIIMS 87)
►	ECF:	Inulin, Mannitol	(AIIMS 03)
►	Plasma volume:	Evans Blue, radiolabelled albumin,	(AIIMS 05)

►	ECF is rich in:	Na^+	
►	ICF is rich in:	K^+	(PGI 90)
►	Endolymph is rich in:	K^+	(TN 99)

⇨ Anion Gap:

►	Anion gap= **unmeasured** ions in plasma.
►	Normal cations in plasma: Na^+, K^+, Ca^{++}, Mg^{++}
►	Normal anions in plasma: Cl^-, HCO_3^-, albumin, phosphate, lactate.
►	Sum of positive and negative charges is equal
►	Anion gap=: $(Na^+ + K^+) - (Cl^- + HCO_3^-)$
►	Normal AG = **10-12 mmol/l**	SGPGI 2002

⊃ Terms Frequently Asked: High Yield for AIPGME/AIIMS/PGI 2013

►	**Endocytosis:** Substance transported into cell by infoldings of cell membrane around substance and internalizing it.	
►	**Pinocytosis:** Engulfing liquid substances by enfolding of cell membrane.	
►	**Phagocytosis:** Engulfing soild substances by enfolding of cell membrane.	
►	**Exocytosis:** Reverse of endocytosis.	
►	**Emiocytosis:** Excretion of specific hormones and granules by cell is emiocytosis. Requires calcium.	AIIMS 1993
►	**Transcytosis:** Vesicular transport within cell.(epithelial cells of intestine)	PGMEEE 2006

⊃ Proteins in vesicular Transport: (High Yield for 2011/2012)

AP 1 clathirin: Involved in transportation from Golgi bodies to lysosomes
AP 2 clathirin: Involved in transportation to endosomes
CO -PI: Coating proteins in vesicles for transportation between endoplasmic reticulum and Golgi apparataus
CO -PII: Coating proteins in vesicles for transportation between endoplasmic reticulum and Golgi apparataus
Dynamin: Vesicle formation from Golgi complex and cell membrane
Docking protein: V snare protein and T snare proteins present on target cells

⇨ Cutaneous Vascular Responses

► White reaction: appearance of pale stroke line when pointed object is drawn lightly over skin. Due to precapillary sphincter contraction.

► Triple response:

1. Red reaction: red line appearing at site of injury.

Due to dilatation of precapillary sphincter histamine and bradykinin

2. Flare: diffuse irregular outside red reaction due to dilatation of arteriole and precapillary sphincter.

3. Wheal: swelling or localized edema within area of flare.

Due to increased capillary permeability.

► Dermatographia: striking triple response on touching the skin.

⊃ Muscle Contraction (High Yield for 2011/2012)

► The skeletal muscle fibres are cylindrical in shape.

► The length varies from 1 mm to 15 cm. The width varies from 10 microns to 80 microns.

► Each muscle fibre has a thick sarcolemma.

► The cytoplasm is acidophilic and granular and is composed of **Actin, Myosin and Tropomyosin.**

► The Cytoplasm contains longitudinal **Myo fibrils or Sarcostyles** which are striated transversely.

► Each Myofibril or Sarcostyles is formed of smaller filaments called as **Myofilaments**.

► The Myofilaments are of two types:

➥ Thin or Actin Filaments

➥ Thick or Myosin Filaments

► The Transverse striations are due to presence of dark and light bands.

► The **Sarcomere** is the unit of contraction.

► It is formed of Actin and Myosin.

► Actin is present in light **band** and Myosin is present in the **dark band.**

2

PHYSIOLOGY

Remember:

- ■ **A:** anisotropic; broad, dark; **remains constant in width despite degree of contraction**

- ■ **I:** isotropic; broad, light; only thin filaments (no thick); **narrows during contraction**

- ■ **Z:** (Zwischenscheiben) bisects I band; **drawn together during contraction.**

- ■ **H:** (Heller) light band bisects A band; only thick filaments (no thin); **narrows during contraction**

  JIPMER 1981

- ■ **M:** (Mittelscheibe) denser band bisects H band.

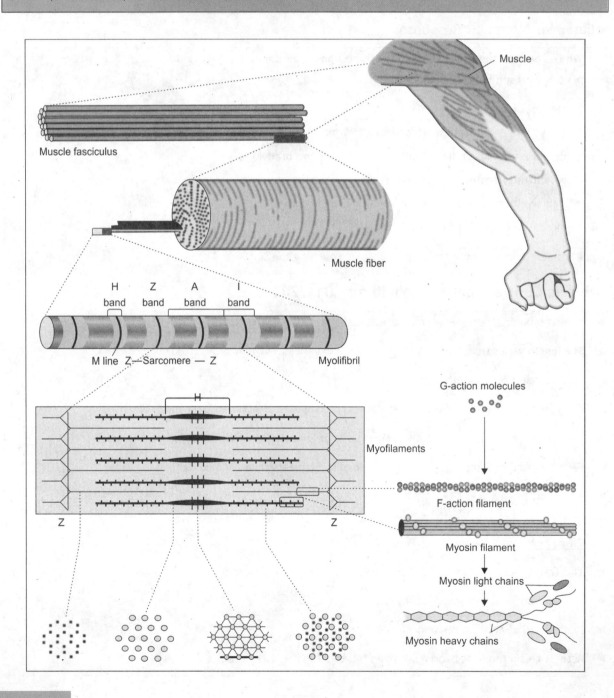

- Heads of Myosin contain actin binding site and possess <u>ATPase</u> activity.
- Tropomyosin is a relaxing protein.
- Troponin I inhibits interaction of myosin with actin.
- Troponin T binds other troponins to tropomyosin.
- Troponin C has binding sites for calcium which initiates contraction.

Tropomyosin covers the **active sites of actin.**   AI 2002

- RMP of skeletal and cardiac muscle is **-90 m V.**
- Repolarization is due to <u>Pottasium Efflux.</u>
- Depolarization is due to <u>sodium influx</u>.
- **Treppe or stair case phenomenon** is due to increased <u>avalibility of Calcium</u> for binding to troponin C.

Muscle Contraction:

- The released calcium binds to troponin on the thin filaments which then act on **tropomyosin** to allow repeated binding of the myosin cross-bridges to actin. Each binding is associated with a conformational change in the cross-bridge that exerts a force on the thin filament toward the center of the sarcomere. The cross-bridge cycle requires **adenosine triphosphate (ATP), which is split by an ATPase** on the cross-bridge.

- If ATP is depleted, the cross-bridges remain attached to the thin filaments and the muscle becomes stiff, as in rigor mortis. When ATP is available, the unloaded fiber shortens, the thin filaments are propelled into the A band, and the Z disks are pulled closer together in every sarcomere. The active state subsides with calcium reuptake by the SR; interaction between actin and the cross-bridges ceases and relaxation sets in.

DNB 2011

⇨ **Remember:**

- ▶ Rheobase is the <u>minimum amount of current</u> to cause excitation.

- ▶ Chronaxie is the <u>shortest duration</u> for a stimulation to excite tissue with a current strength twice the rheobase.   AIPGME 2012

- ✓ Newbornes have <u>longer chronaxies</u>
- ✓ Skeletal muscles have <u>shorter chronaxies</u>
- ✓ <u>Cold</u> lengthens chronaxie
- ✓ <u>Vagal stimulation</u> shortens chronaxie

For smooth muscle contraction presence of cellular calcium is essential to cause contraction.   AIIMS 2002

Force of muscle contraction is independent of amplitude of action potential.   AI 2004

Nerve fibres and anaesthesia:

SUSCEPTIBILITY : Type C > type B> type A   AIIMS 2008

Nerve fibres and pressure

SUSCEPTIBILITY : Type C < type B< type A   AIIMS 2005

⇨ **Golgi Tendon Organ:**

▶ Is an <u>encapsulated</u> sensory receptor	
▶ Detects <u>muscle tension</u>	**AIIMS 2008**
▶ Involved in <u>inverse stretch reflex</u>	
▶ 3-25 muscle fibres on an average are attached to golgi tendon organ.	
▶ Impulses are transmitted by type <u>I b nerve fibres</u>	**ANDHRA 2004**
▶ Is <u>inhibitory and protective</u>.	
▶ Golgi tendon reflex is bisynaptic	**UP 2001**

⇨ **Muscle Spindle: (High Yield for 2011/2012)**

▶ 3-12 mm long structure containing intrafusal muscle fibres enclosed in capsule of connective tissue.	
▶ Is a receptor for <u>myotactic or stretch reflex</u>	**AP 1990**
▶ Central zone has <u>no actin and myosin</u>	
▶ Peripheral zone has actin and myosin.	**JIPMER 2002**

Are of two types:
- ✓ Intrafusal
- ✓ Extrafusal

Intrafusal are of two types:
- ✓ nuclear bag and
- ✓ nuclear chain fibres

Two types of sensory nerve endings are:
- ✓ primary annulospiral endings
- ✓ secondary flower spray endings

▶ Neurapraxia : no anatomic disruption	
▶ Axonometesis: axon and myelin disruption	**PGI 2006**
▶ Neurontemesis: complete division of nerve.	
▶ Degeneration distal to cut end: Wallerian degeneration.	

⇨ **The skeletal muscle fibres are two types: Red Fibres and white fibres**

Red Fibres	White Fibres
ⓞ Have **irregular** striations	ⓞ Have **Regular** striations
ⓞ Have **Central** nuclei	ⓞ Have **peripheral** nuclei
ⓞ Have **rich vascular** supply	ⓞ Have **poorer** blood supply
ⓞ **Non Fatiguable**	ⓞ Are **Fatiguable**

Ⓞ Are poor in mitochondria, Myoglobin , fats	Ⓞ Are rich in Myoglobin, fats
Ⓞ Example :Skeletal muscle	Ⓞ Examples: diaphragm, muscles of eye, mastication.
Ⓞ They react quickly, with brief, forceful contractions, but cannot sustain contraction for long periods.	Ⓞ Their contraction in response to nervous stimulation is slow and steady, resulting in their designation as slow fibers
Ⓞ They are thus termed fast fibers	

⊃ Red Blood Cell

- Mature Red cell is **8 micrometer** in diameter.
- Mature Red cell is **anucleate**.
- Mature Red cell is **discoid** in shape.
- Mature Red cell is **pliable**.
- Normal red cell production results in daily replacement of **0.8-1%** of all circulating red cells.
- Average life of red cell is **100-120** days.
- Haematopoiesis is the process by which formed elements of the blood are produced.
- In the BM (Bone Marrow) first morphologically recognizable precursor is the **PRO**normoblast and "**not normoblast**".
- **Erythropoietin** is produced by the peritubular cells within the kidney.
- There is daily replacement of 0.8-1% of all circulating red cells.

"**Haematopoiesis** "is the process by which formed elements of the blood are produced. Stem cells are capable of producing all classes of cells.

In the BM (Bone Marrow) first morphologically recognizable precursor is the "**PRO**normoblast ". This cell can undergo **4-5 cell divisions** that result in production of 16-32 mature red cells.

Erythropoietin (EPO) is produced by the peritubular cells within the kidney. These cells are **specialized epithelial cells**. A small amount of EPO is also produced by **Hepatocytes**.

⇨ Cardiovascular Physiology:

► Artery/Arteriole	**Resistance vessel** ☛	(JIPMER 04)
► Capillary(Mx Surface area)	**Exchange Vessel** ☛	(AI 05)
► Vein	**Capacitance vessel**☛	UP 2008

► BP= Cardiac output x Peripheral resistance		(PGI 98)
► BP measured by sphygmomanometer is less than arterial BP actually.		
► Small cuff	= High BP	
► Thick walled vessels	= High BP	
► Obesity	= High BP	AIIMS 2001

▶	Pulse Pressure	=	Systolic pressure –Diastolic Pressure➤➤	
▶	Mean Arterial Pressure	=	Diastolic Pressure +1/3 of Pulse Pressure	AIIMS 2011

▶ **Ventricular End Diastolic Volume**: Volume of blood in ventricular cavity at the end of atrial contraction (n)=120 ml. Determines **Preload** (PGI 98)

▶ **Ventricular End Systolic Volume**: Volume of blood in ventricular cavity at the end of ejection (n)= 40 ml

▶ **Stroke volume**: Volume of blood ejected with each heart beat. CO/HR (n)= 70 - 80 ml➤➤

▶ **Ejection Fraction**: Ratio of stroke volume to End Diastolic Volume (SV/EDV) **(n)=50-70%**   DNB 2011

▶ **Cardiac output**: Volume of blood expelled from one side of heart per minute ➤➤

Can be detected by:

✓ Ficks principle

✓ Echocardiography

✓ Thermodilution.

▶ **Cardiac index=CO/Body surface area** ➤➤   (PGI 04)

▶ **Normal cardiac index IS 3.2**   UP 2002

⇨ **Frank – Starling Law**

This principle illustrates the relationship between cardiac output and left ventricular end diastolic volume (or the relationship between stroke volume and right atrial pressure.)

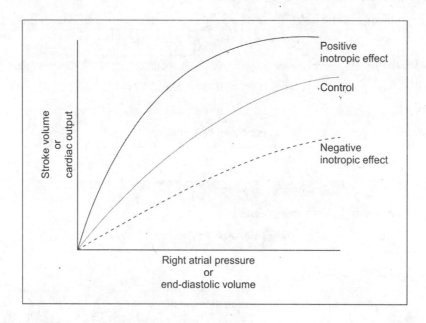

➥ The Frank Starling principle is based on the length-tension relationship within the ventricle. If ventricular end diastolic volume (preload) is increased it follows that the ventricular fiber length is also increased, resulting in an increased 'tension' of the muscle.

- In this way, cardiac output is directly related to venous return, the most important determining factor of preload. When heart rate is constant, cardiac output is directly related to preload (up to a certain point.)

- An increase in preload will increase the cardiac output until very high end diastolic volumes are reached. At this point cardiac output will not increase with any further increase in preload, and may even decrease after a certain preload is reached.

- Also, any increase or decrease in the contractility of the cardiac muscle for a given end diastolic volume will act to shift the curve up or down, respectively. **Regional blood flow:**

✓ Blood flow is controlled mainly by arterioles.

✓ Velocity of blood is maximum in large veins.

✓ Blood flow of liver> kidney >brain>heart.

✓ Carbon dioxide produces <u>vasodilation in brain</u>.

✓ Exercise produces <u>venoconstriction in Splanchnic circulation</u>.

✓ Exercise produces <u>increase in coronary circulation</u>.

✓ Hypoxia produces <u>vasoconstriction in pulmonary circulation</u>.

✓ PGE_1, PGI_2 produce <u>renal vasodilation</u>.

⇨ **Myocardial Action Potential**

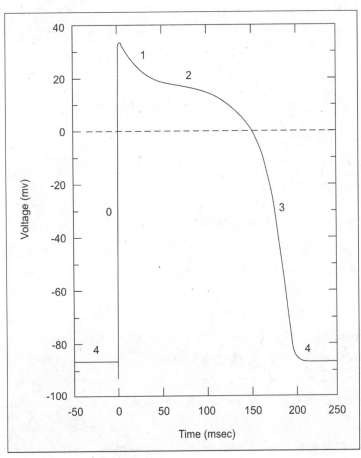

Phase 0 - rapid depolarization

- Rapid **sodium influx**
- These channels automatically deactivate after a few ms

Phase 1 - early repolarisation

- efflux of **potassium**

Phase 2 - plateau

- slow influx of **calcium**

Phase 3 - final repolarisation

- efflux of **potassium**

Phase 4 - restoration of ionic concentrations

- Resting potential is restored by Na^+/K^+ ATPase
- There is **slow entry of Na^+** into the cell decreasing the potential difference until the threshold potential is reached, triggering a new action potential

⇨ **Ventricular Muscle**

▶ Phase 0	▶ Membrane Depolarization	▶ ↑permeability to Na
▶ Phase1	▶ Rapid Repolarization	▶ ↓permeability to Na, ↑permeability to K
▶ Phase2	▶ Slow Repolarization	▶ ↑permeability to Ca
▶ Phase3	▶ Rapid Repolarization	▶ Inactivation of Ca channels, ↑permeability to K

⇨ **Pace Maker Cells:**

- ▶ Slow upstroke Action Potential
- ▶ Smaller magnitude of Action Potential
- ▶ No Fast Sodium channels
- ▶ Spontaneous Depolarization

⇨ **Inotropic State (Myocardial Contractility)**

A number of factors determine the level of ventricular performance at any given ventricular end-diastolic volume

- **Adrenergic Nerve Activity** The quantity of norepinephrine released by adrenergic nerve endings in the heart is determined by the adrenergic nerve impulse traffic. This mechanism is the most important one that acutely modifies myocardial contractility under physiologic conditions.

- **Circulating Catecholamines** When stimulated by adrenergic nerve impulse, the adrenal medulla releases catecholamines, which, when they reach the heart, augment both heart rate and myocardial contractility.

- **The Force-Frequency Relation** The position of the myocardial force-velocity curve is also influenced by the rate and rhythm of cardiac contraction; e.g.: ventricular extrasystoles result in postextrasystolic potentiation, presumably by increasing the quantity of Ca^{2+} that enters the cardiac cell. The contractility of the normal (but not of the failing) heart is augmented by an increase in frequency of contraction.

- Exogenously Administered Inotropic Agents Isoproterenol, dopamine, dobutamine, and other sympathomimetic agents, cardiac glycosides, Ca^{2+}, amrinone, milrinone, and other phosphodiesterase inhibitors all improve the myocardial force-velocity relation and therefore may be used to stimulate ventricular performance.

- Physiologic Depressants Included among these are severe myocardial hypoxia, ischemia, and acidosis. Acting either singly or in combination, these influences depress the myocardial force-velocity curve and left ventricular work at any given ventricular end-diastolic volume.

- Pharmacologic Depressants These include many antiarrhythmic drugs such as procainamide and disopyramide; calcium antagonists such as verapamil; beta blockers; and large doses of barbiturates, alcohol, and general anesthetics as well as many other drugs.

- Loss of Myocytes When a sufficiently large portion of ventricular myocardium becomes nonfunctional or necrotic, as occurs transiently during ischemia and permanently in myocardial infarction total ventricular performance at any given level of end-diastolic volume becomes depressed.

⊃ Exercise: Physiological Change

Blood pressure
- Systolic increases, diastolic decreases
- Leads to increased pulse pressure
- In healthy young people the increase in MABP is only slight

Cardiac output
- Increase in cardiac output may be 3-5 fold
- Results from venous constriction, vasodilation and increased myocardial contractibility, as well as from the maintenance of right atrial pressure by an increase in venous return
- Heart rate up to 3-fold increase

stroke volume
- Up to 1.5-fold increase

⊃ Regional Blood Flow

✓ Blood flow is controlled mainly by arterioles.	AI 2005
✓ Velocity of blood is maximum in large veins.	
✓ Blood flow of liver> kidney > brain > heart	
✓ Carbon dioxide produces vasodilation in brain.	AI 2005
✓ Exercise produces venoconstriction in Splanchnic circulation	
✓ Exercise produces increase in coronary circulation.	
✓ Hypoxia produces vasoconstriction in pulmonary circulation.	AIIMS 2006
✓ PGE1, PGI2 produce renal vasodilation.	

⇨ **Changes in Isotonic Exercise**

- Heart rate rises.
- Respiratory rate rises.
- Stroke volume increases.
- Systolic BP moderate rise.
- Diastolic BP **unchanged** or **falls.**
- Cardiac output rises.

⇨ **Changes in Isometric Exercise:**

- Heart rate rises.
- Systolic BP rises.
- Diastolic Bp rises.
- Respiratory rate rises.
- Stroke volume is unchanged.
- Blood flow to muscles is decreased.

⊃ **Myocardial Action Potential ✳ (High Yield for 2011/2012)**

Phase 0 - rapid depolarization

- Rapid **sodium influx**
- These channels automatically deactivate after a few ms

Phase 1 - early repolarisation

- Efflux of **potassium**

Phase 2 - plateau

- Slow influx of **calcium**

Phase 3 - final repolarisation

- Efflux of **potassium**

Phase 4 - restoration of ionic concentrations

- Resting potential is restored by Na^+/K^+ ATPase
- There is **slow entry of Na^+** into the cell decreasing the potential difference until the threshold potential is reached, triggering a new action potential

⇨ **Ventricular Muscle**

▶ Phase 0	▶ Membrane Depolarization	▶ ↑permeability to Na
▶ Phase1	▶ Rapid Repolarization	▶ ↓permeability to Na, ↑permeability to K
▶ Phase2	▶ Slow Repolarization	▶ ↑permeability to Ca
▶ Phase3	▶ Rapid Repolarization	▶ Inactivation of Ca channels , ↑permeability to K

⇨ **Pace Maker Cells:**

► Slow upstroke Action Potential

► Smaller magnitude of Action Potential

► No Fast Sodium channels

► Spontaneous Depolarization.

⊃ **Inotropic State (Myocardial Contractility)**

A number of factors determine the level of ventricular performance at any given ventricular end-diastolic volume

➡ **Adrenergic Nerve Activity** The quantity of norepinephrine released by adrenergic nerve endings in the heart is determined by the adrenergic nerve impulse traffic. This mechanism is the most important one that acutely modifies myocardial contractility under physiologic conditions.

➡ **Circulating Catecholamines** When stimulated by adrenergic nerve impulse, the adrenal medulla releases catecholamines, which, when they reach the heart, augment both heart rate and myocardial contractility.

➡ **The Force-Frequency Relation** The position of the myocardial force-velocity curve is also influenced by the rate and rhythm of cardiac contraction; e.g., ventricular extrasystoles result in postextrasystolic potentiation, presumably by increasing the quantity of Ca^{2+} that enters the cardiac cell. The contractility of the normal (but not of the failing) heart is augmented by an increase in frequency of contraction.

➡ **Exogenously Administered Inotropic Agents** Isoproterenol, dopamine, dobutamine, and other sympathomimetic agents, cardiac glycosides, Ca^{2+}, amrinone, milrinone, and other phosphodiesterase inhibitors all improve the myocardial force-velocity relation and therefore may be used to stimulate ventricular performance.

➡ **Physiologic Depressants** Included among these are **severe myocardial hypoxia, ischemia, and acidosis.** Acting either singly or in combination, these influences depress the myocardial force-velocity curve and left ventricular work at any given ventricular end-diastolic volume.

➡ **Pharmacologic Depressants** These include many antiarrhythmic drugs such as **procainamide and disopyramide; calcium antagonists such as verapamil; beta blockers; and large doses of barbiturates, alcohol, and general anesthetics** as well as many other drugs.

➡ **Loss of Myocytes** When a sufficiently large portion of ventricular myocardium becomes nonfunctional or necrotic, as occurs transiently during **ischemia and permanently in myocardial infarction** total ventricular performance at any given level of end-diastolic volume becomes depressed.

⇨ **Exercise: Physiological Change**

Blood pressure

➡ Systolic increases, diastolic decreases

➡ Leads to increased pulse pressure

➡ In healthy young people the increase in MABP is only slight

2

PHYSIOLOGY

Cardiac output

- Increase in cardiac output may be 3-5 fold
- Results from venous constriction, vasodilation and increased myocardial contractibility, as well as from the maintenance of right atrial pressure by an increase in venous return
- Heart rate up to 3-fold increase

Stroke volume

- Up to 1.5-fold increase

⇨ **Central Venous Pressure:**

- Normal Pressure: -2 cm H_2O to 12 cm H_2O
- Causes of ↓CVP: Non cardiogenic shock
- Causes of ↑CVP: Heart Failure, Expansion of Blood volume, PEEP

⇨ **Isometric Contraction:**

Mitral and tricuspid valve close (c-c)	AI 2000
Aortic and pulmonary valve open	

⇨ **Isometric Relaxation:**

Mitral and tricuspid valve open

Aortic and pulmonary valve close

- Normal coronary blood flow is 250 ml at rest.
- It is 5% of cardiac output.
- Blood flow to left ventricle is twice that of right ventricle.
- Atrial blood flow is half of ventricular flow.
- Most of coronary blood flow occurs in diastole.

► Chrontropic effect:	Effect on heart rate.
► Ionotropic effect:	Effect on force of contraction.
► Dromotropic effect:	Effect on conduction of impulses through heart.
► Bathmotropic effect:	Effect on excitability of heart.

➲ **Electrophysiology**

- SA node discharges <u>most rapidly</u>
- SA node is located <u>sub epicardially</u>.
- <u>Pace maker cells</u> are present in SA node.   JKBOPEE 2012
- AP of SA and AV node are due to <u>calcium.</u>
- RMP of myocardial fibres is -<u>90 m V</u>

► Depolarization is from <u>endocardium to epicardium.</u> AIIMS 1995

► Repolarization is also from <u>endocardium to epicardium.</u>

► Speed of conduction is <u>fastest in Purkinje fibres.</u> PGI 2005

► Speed of conduction is <u>least in AV node.</u>

⇨ **Waves of Normal ECG:**

Wave/ segment	From - To	Cause	Duration (second)
P wave		Atrial depolarization	0.1
QRS complex		Ventricular **Depolarization** (UP 07)	0.08 – 0.10 (AI 96)
T wave		Ventricular **Repolarzation**	0.2
P - R interval	Onset of P wave to onset of Q wave		0.18 <u>(0.12 to 0.2)</u>
Q - T interval	Onset of Q wave & end of T wave		0.4 - 0.42

The 12 conventional <u>ECG</u> leads record the difference in potential between electrodes placed on the surface of the body.

These leads are divided into two groups:

Six extremity (limb) leads and six chest (precordial) leads. The extremity leads record potentials transmitted onto the frontal plane and the chest leads record potentials transmitted onto the horizontal plane

The six extremity leads are further subdivided into three bipolar leads (I, II, and III) and three unipolar leads (aVR, aVL, and aVF).

Each bipolar lead measures the difference in potential between electrodes at two extremities:

► **lead I left arm-right arm voltages,**

► **lead II left leg-right arm, and**

► **lead III left leg-left arm.**

The six chest leads are unipolar recordings obtained by electrodes in the following positions:

► lead V_1, fourth intercostal space, just to the right of the sternum;

► lead V_2, fourth intercostal space, just to the left of the sternum;

► lead V_3, midway between V_2 and V_4;

► lead V_4, midclavicular line, fifth intercostal space;

► lead V_5, anterior axillary line, same level as V_4; and

► lead V_6, midaxillary line, same level as V_4 and V_5.

2

⊃ The Cardiac Vector

▶ The frontal plane vector, or axis, is the **sum of the electrical potentials of the cardiac cycle as reflected in the frontal plane of the body.**   **PGI 2011**

▶ By combining frontal plane bipolar leads I, II, and III with frontal plane unipolar leads aVR, aVL, and aVF, a hexaxial reference system that illustrates all six leads of the frontal plane can be constructed and the mean QRS, P, and T wave vectors in the frontal plane can be approximated by determining their net magnitudes and direction in any two of the three standard leads.

▶ The normal QRS axis lies between **0 and +110 degrees;**

▶ **Superior axis deviation** (between -45 and -90 degrees) and **right axis deviation** (between +110 and ±180 degrees) are considered **abnormal.**

▶ Leftward deviation of the mean frontal plane QRS axis can occur with advancing age in the absence of clinically overt heart disease.

▶ Both the normal frontal plane P wave and T wave axes usually correspond to the normal QRS axis and point in the same general direction.

Remember:

➥ **First-degree AV block**, more properly termed **prolonged AV conduction**, is classically characterized by a PR interval >0.20 s, ☞

➥ **Second-degree heart block** (intermittent AV block) is present when some atrial impulses fail to conduct to the ventricles. ☞

➥ **Mobitz type I second-degree AV block**

✓ (AV Wenckebach block)

✓ Is characterized by progressive PR interval prolongation prior to block of an atrial impulse.

✓ This type of block is almost always localized to the AV node and associated with a normal QRS duration, although bundle branch block may be present. ☞☞

➥ In **Mobitz type II second-degree AV block,**

✓ Conduction fails suddenly and unexpectedly without a preceding change in PR intervals.

✓ It is generally due to disease of the His-Purkinje system and

✓ Is most often associated with a prolonged QRS duration. ☞☞

➥ **Third-degree AV block**

✓ Is present when no atrial impulse propagates to the ventricles.

✓ If the QRS complex of the escape rhythm is of normal duration, occurs at a rate of 40 to 55 beats per minute, and increases with atropine or exercise, AV nodal block is probable.

✓ Congenital complete AV block is usually localized to the AV node.

▶ **Refractoriness** is a property of cardiac cells that defines the period of recovery that cells require after being discharged before they can be reexcited by a stimulus.

▶ **The absolute refractory period** is defined by that portion of the **action potential** during which no stimulus, regardless of its strength, can evoke another response.

► The **effective refractory period** is that part of the **action potential** during which a stimulus can evoke only a local, nonpropagated response.

► The **relative refractory period** extends from the end of the effective refractory period to the time that the tissue is fully recovered. During this time, a stimulus of greater than threshold strength is required to evoke a response, which is propagated more slowly than normal.

⮕ Heart Sounds (High Yield for 2011/2012)

Heart sounds	Occurs during	Cause	Characteristics
First	Isometric contraction & ejection period☞	Closure of AV valves(Mitral Tricuspid)✸✸	Long, soft, & low pitched. Resembles the word '**LUBB**'
Second	Protodiastole & part of isometric relaxation☞	Closure of semilunar valves(Aortic, Pulmonary)✸✸	Short, sharp, & high pitched. Resembles the word '**DUBB**'

Third Heart Sound is due to **Rapid Ventricular filling**✸✸

Fourth Heart sound is due to **ventricular distension caused by forceful atrial contraction.**✸✸

Heard during ventricular filling phase.	AI 2007
Correlates with second filling phase	KOL 2008

⇨ Waves in JVP

➡ '**a**' wave - 1st positive wave & it's due to <u>atrial systole.</u> ✸✸	DNB 2011

➡ '**x**' wave - fall of pressure in atrium, coincides with **atrial diastole**✸

➡ '**c**' wave - its due to rise in atrial pressure during **isometric contraction** during which the <u>AV valves bulges into atrium. ✸</u>

➡ '**x₁**' wave - occurs during ejection period, when AV ring is pulled towards ventricles causing distension of atria.

➡ '**v**' wave - occurs during **isometric relaxation** period or during atrial diastole.

➡ '**y**' wave - due to <u>opening of AV valve</u> & emptying of blood into ventricle. ✸	UP 2006

<u>The Bainbridge reflex, also called the atrial reflex,</u>

➡ Is an increase in heart rate due to an increase in central venous pressure.

➡ Increased blood volume is detected by stretch receptors located in both atria at the venoatrial junctions

➡ The **Bainbridge reflex** and the **Baroreceptor reflex** act antagonistically to control heart rate.

➡ The baroreceptor reflex acts to decrease heart rate when blood pressure rises.

► When blood volume is increased, the Bainbridge reflex is dominant;

► When blood volume is decreased, the baroreceptor reflex is dominant

The oculocardiac reflex,

- Also known as Aschner phenomenon,
- Is a **decrease in pulse rate associated with traction applied to extraocular muscles** and/or compression of the eyeball.
- The reflex is mediated by nerve connections between the **trigeminal cranial nerve and the vagus nerve of** the **parasympathetic nervous system.**

⇨ **Respiratory Physiology:**

▶ Number of alveoli in man: 300 million.		
▶ Carbon dioxide is primarily transported in arterial blood as bicarbonate		AI 2005
▶ Oxygen delivery to tissues depends on		
✓ **Cardiac output**		
✓ **Hb**		
✓ **Affinity of Hb for oxygen**		
▶ Normal value of Po2 is: **80 mm Hg**		AIIMS 1999
▶ Arterial Co 2 Level is: **40 mm Hg**		PGI 2004

⇨ **Physiology of Respiration:**

▶ During inspiration intrapleural pressure becomes <u>more negative</u>.	PGI 2006
▶ Respiration stops in late expiration because of <u>dynamic compression of airways</u>.	
▶ Total lung capacity depends on <u>compliance</u>.	
▶ Nitrogen wash out method detects <u>functional residual capacity</u>.	
▶ FRC is <u>not estimated by spirometry</u>.	PGI 2004
▶ <u>Slow and deep</u> breathing are the most economical way of breathing.	

⇨ **The all important Respiratory Volumes:**

Measurement	Value (Male/Female)	Calculation	Description
Total lung capacity (TLC)☛☛	= 6.0 / 4.7 <u>L</u>✱	= IRV + Vt + ERV + RV	The volume of air **contained in the lung** at the end of <u>maximal inspiration</u>.✱ CUPGEE 2002 **Depends on lung compliance** UP 2000
<u>**Vital capacity**</u> **(VC)**☛☛	= 4.8 / 3.6 L✱	= IRV + Vt + ERV	The amount of air that can be **forced out of the lungs** after a <u>maximal inspiration</u>.✱ Rohtak 97
Forced vital capacity (FVC)	= 4.8 / 3.7 L		The amount of air that can be **maximally forced out of the lungs after a maximal inspiration.** Emphasis on speed. ✱

Measurement	Value (Male/Female)	Calculation	Description
Tidal volume (Vt)	= 500 / 390 mL✷	IC- IRV	The amount of <u>air</u> breathed in or out during normal <u>respiration</u>. The volume of air an individual is normally breathing in and out.✷ AI 2001
Residual volume (RV)☞☞	= 1.2 / 0.93 L✷		The amount of **air left in the lungs after a maximal** <u>exhalation</u>. The amount of air that is always in the lungs and can never be expired (i.e.: the amount of air that stays in the lungs after maximum expiration).✷
Expiratory reserve volume (ERV)	= 1.2 / 0.93 L		The amount of **additional air** that can be pushed out after the end expiratory level of normal breathing. (At the end of a normal breath, the lungs contain the residual volume plus the expiratory reserve volume, or around 2.4 litres. If one then goes on and exhales as much as possible, only the residual volume of 1.2 litres remains).✷
Inspiratory reserve volume (IRV)	= 3.3 / 2.3 L✷	measured IRV=VC-(TV+ERV)	The **additional air** that can be inhaled after a normal tidal breath in. The maximum volume of air that can be inspired in addition to the tidal volume.
<u>Functional residual capacity</u> (FRC)	= 2.4 / 1.9 L (PGI 80)(AI 93)	= ERV + RV	The **amount of air left in the lungs after normal expiration.** AIIMS 1993
Inspiratory capacity (IC)	= 3.8 / 2.7 L	= TV + IRV	The **maximal volume that can be inspired following a normal expiration.**✷
Anatomical <u>dead space</u>✷	= 150 / 120 mL		The **volume of the conducting airways.** Measured with <u>Fowler method</u>.
Physiologic dead volume✷	= 155 / 120 mL		The anatomic dead space +alveolar dead space. Under normal conditions equal to anatomic dead space.✷✷ DNB 2011

VENTILATION PERFUSION RATIO

- ➡ Ideally Ventilation = Perfusion ie V/Q =1
- ➡ Apex of Lung   V>Q   **Wasted Ventilation**   (AI 98)
- ➡ Base of Lung   V<Q   **Wasted Perfusion**
- ➡ With exercise   V/Q approaches zero

2

PHYSIOLOGY

⇨ **Important Points asked in Examinations**

➥ The volume of lung after quite expiration is **ERV**	**(Bihar 2004)**
➥ Minute alveolar ventilation is: **3.5 - 4.5L**	**(Bihar 2004)**
➥ Physiological dead space in normal adult: **100 ml**	**(Bihar 2004)**
➥ V/P ratio is ideal in: **Apex of lung**	**(DPG 2004)**
➥ In a normal adult, ratio of physiological and anatomical dead space is:	**(DPG 2005)**
➥ FRC comprises of: **Amount of air remaining in lungs at end of normal expiration**	**(DPG 2005)**
➥ Vital capacity is: **Maximum volume expired after complete inspiration**	**(DPG 2006)**

⇨ **Pulmonary Circulation**

- ➥ Is a **Low Resistance,**
- ➥ **High Compliance** Bed.
- ➥ Hypoxia produces **pulmonary vasoconstriction.**(unique feature)

Response to high altitude

➥ ↑Ventilation (EARLIEST CHANGE)	**KERALA 2001**
➥ ↑Sensitivity of central receptors	
➥ ↑response of carotid bodies.	**AI 2004**
➥ ↑Erythropoietin	
➥ ↑2 3 DPG	
➥ ↑Mitochondria	
➥ ↑Renal excretion of Bicarbonate	
➥ Respiratory alkalosis	**PGI 2004**
➥ Pulmonary edema when occurs is due to increased pulmonary capillary pressure.	**PGI 1999**

- ➥ **Type I cells** or **type I pneumocytes,**
- ✓ These are squamous epithelial cells that make up **97%** of the alveolar surfaces.
- ✓ They are specialized to serve as **very thin** (often only 25 nm in width) gas-permeable components of the blood-air barrier

- ➥ **Type II cells.**
- ✓ Are also **called type II alveolar cells, type II pneumocytes, great alveolar cells, and alveolar septal cells,** cover the remaining **3%** of the alveolar surface.
- ✓ They are interspersed among the type I cells, to which they attach by desmosomes and occluding junctions. Type II cells are **roughly cuboidal with round nuclei;**
- ✓ Type II cells are **secretory cells** secreting pulmonary **surfactant.** **PSC 2004**

➡ **Alveolar macrophages.**

✓ Known also as **dust cells**, these large monocyte-derived representatives of the mononuclear phagocyte system are found both on the surface of alveolar septa and in the interstitium.

✓ They also **phagocytose blood cells** that enter the alveoli as a result of heart failure.

✓ These alveolar macrophages, which stain positively for iron pigment **(hemosiderin),** are thus designated **heart failure cells.**   COMED 2006

➡ **Clara cells**

✓ Are non-mucous and non-ciliated <u>secretory</u> <u>cells</u> found in the <u>primary bronchioles</u> of the <u>lungs</u>.

✓ Main functions of Clara cells are to **protect the bronchiolar <u>epithelium</u>.** By secreting a small variety of products, **including <u>Clara cell secretory protein</u>** (CCSP) and a component of the lung <u>surfactant</u>.

✓ They are also responsible for **detoxifying harmful substances** inhaled into the lungs.

SURFACTANT

▶ **Is (Dipalmitoyl Lecithin)**☜☞   Kerala 94

▶ It is secreted by **Type II** Pneumocyte☞   AI 2005

▶ Synthesis begins at <u>16-18 weeks</u> of gestation.

▶ Maintains alveolar integrity.

▶ Breaks structure of water in alveoli.   AIIMS 2007

▶ Deficiency causes **Hyaline Membrane Disease**☜☞

▶ **Smoking** ↓ surfactant production.

▶ **Surfactant :**

✓ ↓ **Surface Tension**☜☞

✓ ↑ **Compliance** ☞

▶ **Prevents pulmonary edema**☜☞

▶ **Glucocorticoids accelerate surfactant production.**   UP 2007

▶ **It is used therapeutically nowadays.**

▶ **Deficiency Causes**

✓ **IRDS,**   COMED 2007

✓ **HMD,**

✓ **Patchy atelectasis,**

✓ **Pulmonary alveolar proteinosis.**☜☜☞

Nernest Equation /Chloride shift:

Bicarbonate diffuses into plasma and same quantity of chloride diffuses into RBC in venous circulation. ☞☞☞

JIPMER 92

✓ In place of bicarbonate chloride moves into RBC from plasma.☞

✓ Occurs in one second.

▶ **Bohr Effect:**

✓ **Affinity of Oxygen for Hb decreases with fall in pH.** JIPMER 95

▶ **Haldane effect**

✓ Is reverse of Bohr effect. ☞

✓ **Binding of Oxygen with hemoglobin displaces carbon dioxide from blood.**☞

✓ **Deoxygenated Hb binds more H+ than oxy hemoglobin.** ☞

▶ **Hering Bruer reflex:**☞☞ Overinflation of lung causes stretch receptors in bronchi and bronchioles to send inhibitory signals to inspiratory centre through vagus. **(Distension of lung causes slowing of respiratory rate.) It helps in maintainence of tidal volume.** AIIMS 2011

▶ **Heads Reflex.Inflation of lungs induces more inflation.** AIIMS 2003

▶ **Heads Reflex is due to irritant receptors in lungs.**

▶ **J receptor reflex:** ☞☞ J receptors are present in close association with pulmonary capillaries.✶✶

On stimulation of j receptors, **apnea followed by hyperapnea**, bradycardia and hypotension occurs. ✶✶Bronchospasm also occurs.

▶ **Daven port diagram is used to determine type and severity of Acidosis/Alkalosis.**☞☞

▶ **Siggard Anderson Nomogram is used for calculating abnormalities of acid base balance.**✶✶ **(Plasma Bicarbonate)**

⇨ **Control of Respiration:**

▶ Inspiratory centre✶	▶ **Dorsal Medulla**
▶ Expiratory centre✶	▶ **Ventral** Medulla
▶ Pneumotaxic centre ✶	▶ Pons(DORSAL) UP 2005
▶ Apneustic centre ✶	▶ Pons

Rhythmic respiration is initiated by a small group of synaptically coupled pacemaker cells in the **Pre-Botzinger complex** on **either side of the medulla between the nucleus ambiguus and the lateral reticular nucleus.** These neurons discharge rhythmically, and they produce rhythmic discharges in phrenic motor neurons.

- ☐ **Dorsal respiratory group** of Neurons: Inspiration. ☞☞ (DIVE)

- ☐ **Ventral respiratory group** of Neurons: Expiration☞

- ☐ **Peripheral chemoreceptors** are located in Carotid and Aortic bodies.☞

- ☐ **Transection of brain stem** produces <u>irregular and gasping respiration</u>.(less smooth respiration)

- ☐ **Damage to pneumotaxic centre** causes <u>slow and deep respiration</u>.

- ☐ **Damage to vagi nerves** <u>causes increase in depth of inspiration</u>.

- ☐ Only <u>hypercapnia</u> not Hypocapnia stimulates receptors.   **AI 1995**

- ☐ **Respiratory centre** is inhibited during swallowing and vomiting.

⇨ **Oxygen Hb Dissociation Curve:**

Oxygen Hb dissociation curve is 'S' shape or sigmoid shape. AIIMS , PGI, JK BOPEE, UPSC, KAR, DNB

To Left (←)	To Right (→)
☐ ↑CO	☐ ↑$[H^+]$☞ , ↓pH
☐ HbF	☐ ↑Temp
☐ ↓pCO_2	☐ ↑pCO_2
☐ ↓2, 3-DPG	☐ ↑2, 3-DPG
☐ ↓Temp	

⇨ **Additional:**

Shift to left		Shift to right	
➡ Increase Ph		➡ Decrease pH☞☞	
➡ Decrease in temp	**AIIMS 1999**	➡ Increase in temp	
➡ Foetal blood		➡ Excess of 2, 3 DPG	
➡ Oxygen affinity of Hb.	**AI 2003**		
		➡ Increase PCO_2 (Bohr effect)	**UP 2005**
		➡ Sickle cell Hb.	**PGI 2001**
		➡ Shock	
		➡ RDS	**JIPMER 1995**
		➡ CHF	

Important Points about Hb-O_2 Dissociation Curve Are

- ➡ At PO_2 of 100mm Hg, Hb is 100% saturated. O_2 is bound **to all four heme groups**

- ➡ At PO_2 of 40mm Hg, Hb is 75% saturated. O_2 is bound to 3 of the 4 heme groups

- ➡ At PO_2 of 25mm Hg, Hb is only 50% saturated, O_2 is bound to 2 of the 4 heme groups

- ➡ The curve is **sigmoid shaped** showing **positive cooperativety**

2   PHYSIOLOGY

▶ In anemia 2, 3 DPG concentration increases.   TN 1999

▶ 2, 3 DPG <u>unloads</u> oxygen to tissues

➲ **Questions Asked in (AIIMS 87, AI 86, AI 90)**

▶ In a healthy adult, 24 hour production of CO_2 is about **330 liters.** ☞☞

▶ Diffusion capacity for carbon dioxide as compared to that of O_2 is **20 times.** ☞

▶ Average area of the alveolar walls in contact with capillaries in both lungs is about <u>70 sq.m.</u>

▶ Diffusion capacity of lungs for CO_2 is **10-30 ml/min/mm Hg.**

▶ Normal composition of **venous blood** is PO_2 - **40 mm Hg, PCO_2 -46 mm Hg and Hb saturation 75%.**

▶ **Peak expiratory flow** rate is <u>400-500 L/mt.</u> ☞☞

▶ The presence of Hb increases the O_2 carrying capacity of the blood by **70 fold.**

▶ Intra-pleural pressure (recoil pressure) required to prevent collapse of the lung — **4 mm Hg** in presence of surfactant.

▶ Intrapleural pressure at the end of deep inspiration is - **4 mm Hg.**

▶ Intrapleural pressure during expiration is - **2 mm Hg.**

▶ **Hypoxia** causes "pulmonary vasoconstriction" but "cerebral vasodilation." ☞☞

▶ In lungs <u>Angiotensin I is converted into Angiotensin II.</u> ☞☞

▶ **Transport of CO_2 is maximum in the form of** <u>bicarbonate.</u> ☞✳

➡ **Type I cells** or **type I pneumocytes,** and **squamous alveolar cells,** these are squamous epithelial cells that make up **97%** of the alveolar surfaces.

➡ **Type II cells.** Are also **called type II alveolar cells, type II pneumocytes, great alveolar cells,** and **alveolar septal cells,** cover the remaining **3%** of the alveolar surface. They are interspersed among the type I cells, to which they attach by desmosomes and occluding junctions. Type II cells are **secretory cells** secreting pulmonary **surfactant.**

➡ **Alveolar macrophages.** Known also as **dust cells,** these large monocyte-derived representatives of the mononuclear phagocyte system are found both on the surface of alveolar septa and in the interstitium. Macrophages are important in removing any debris that escapes the mucus and cilia in the conducting portion of the system. They also **phagocytose blood cells** that enter the alveoli as a result of heart failure. These alveolar macrophages, which stain positively for iron pigment **(hemosiderin),** are thus designated **heart failure cells.**

➡ **Clara cells** are non-mucous and non-ciliated <u>secretory cells</u> found in the <u>primary bronchioles</u> of the <u>lungs.</u> Clara cells are dome-shaped and have short <u>microvilli.</u> One of the main functions of Clara cells is to **protect the bronchiolar** <u>epithelium.</u> They do this by secreting a small variety of products, **including <u>Clara cell secretory protein</u>** (CCSP) and a component of the lung <u>surfactant.</u> They are also responsible for **detoxifying harmful substances** inhaled into the lungs .Clara cells were originally described by their namesake, <u>Max Clara</u> in 1937. Clara cells are **mitotically active** cells. They divide and differentiate to form both ciliated and non-ciliated epithelial cells.

2

➥ Pulmonary neuroendocrine cells (PNEC) are specialized airway <u>epithelial cells</u> that occur as solitary cells or as clusters called <u>neuroepithelial bodies</u> (NEB) in the <u>lung</u>.

➥ Brush cells, also termed **tuft, caveolated**, multivesicular, and fibrillovesicular cells, are part of the epithelial layer in the gastrointestinal and respiratory tracts.

⊃ High Yields Points in Respiratory Physiology Never Forget

✓ Dead space air in respiratory system is **not exchanging gas with capillary blood.**

✓ First 150 ml of inspiration fills **Anatomic dead space**. This contributes only to total ventilation but not alveolar ventilation. **DNB 2011**

✓ Intrapleural pressure is usually **negative** during restful breathing. It becomes more negative during inspiration.

✓ **Compliant lungs** are easy to inflate and posses low recoil.

✓ **Non compliant** lungs are difficult to inflate.

✓ An **obstructive pattern** is associated with large lung volumes but small volume is expired slowly.

✓ A **restrictive pattern** is associated with reduced lung volumes but small volumes are often expired rapidly.

⊃ Never to be Forgotten

	CO_2	pH	HCO_3
Respiratory Acidosis✱✱	↑	↓	↑
Respiratory Alkalosis✱✱	↓	↑	↓
Metabolic Acidosis✱✱	No change	↓	↓
Metabolic Alkalosis✱✱	No change	↑	↑

➤ $P\,CO_2$ is the most important variable in regulation of Ventilation.

➤ Central Chemoreceptors respond to changes in [H^+]

➤ Peripheral Chemoreceptors respond to changes in PO_2, PCO_2, H^+ conc. of arterial blood.

▶ <u>Cheyne-Stokes breathing</u> is characterized by **irregular pattern** of respiratory dysfunction (**apnea and hyperapnea**) suggests that central respiratory mechanism are no longer functioning adequately.

▶ Opium poisoning, uremia, CCF, Hypoxia☛

▶ <u>Apneustic breathing</u> is seen after head trauma and is characterized by inspiratory breath holding that lasts many seconds, followed by brief exhalations.

▶ <u>Biot's breathing</u> is seen in some patients with CNS disease (e.g, **meningitis**). It consists of periods of **normal** breathing interrupted suddenly by periods of apnea.☛

▶ <u>Hysterical breathing</u> may produce **hyperventilation** i.e.: rapid, intense breathing that causes the $PaCO_2$ to decrease.☛☛

▶ <u>Kussmaul breathing</u> occurs in diabetic coma and consists of **continuous, rapid, deep breathing**. seen in Diabetic ketoacidosis, uremia☛☛

► <u>Ondines curse:</u> loss of automatic respiratory control☛☛

► <u>Apnea:</u> cessation of respiration.☛

⇨ **Cyanosis**

► Reduced Hb>4 gm/dl.☛☛

► Oxygen saturation <85%.☛

► Methhemoblobin>1.5 gm/dl.☛   PGI 2007

► Sulfhemoglobin >0.5 gm/dl☛

⇨ **Nitrogen Narcosis**

➥ Is an **effect on the brain** of gaseous nitrogen that **occurs to divers who go below 100 feet depth of sea.**

➥ At great depths below the sea level, the pressure is quite high

➥ At such high pressures **to prevent the lungs from collapsing, air is supplied at very high pressure.** This exposes the blood in the lungs to extremely high alveolar gas pressure, a condition known as **Hyperbarism.**

➥ Nitrogen is an inert gas which at sea-level pressure has no significant effect on the body. At pressures of 4-5 atmospheres, approx 30 to 40 m (100 feet- 140) below sea level nitrogen produces varying degrees of narcosis.

➥ The symptoms resemble **Alcohol intoxication** thus it is known as **"Raptures of the Depths".**

➥ Manual dexterity is maintained, but intellectual function is impaired.

➥ The mechanism of the narcotic effect of the nitrogen is similar to most other gas anesthetics i.e. **it dissolves in the fatty substances in neuronal membranes.**

➥ Because of its physical effect on **altering ionic conductance** through the membrane reduces neuronal excitability.

The Diffusing Capacity for CO (DLCO)

➥ Is measured as an index of diffusing capacity because its uptake is diffusion-limited. DLCO is proportionate to the amount of CO entering the blood (VCO) divided by the partial pressure of CO in the alveoli minus the partial pressure of CO in the blood entering the pulmonary capillaries.

➥ The normal value of DLCO at rest is about 25 mL/min/mm Hg. It increases up to three-fold during exercise because of capillary dilation and an increase in the number of active capillaries.

Difference between Obstructive Lung Disease and Restrictive Lung Disease✳✳✳✳

Obstructive lung disease	Restrictive lung disease
❏ TLC ↑	❏ TLC ↓
❏ RV↑	❏ RV↓
❏ TV↓	❏ TV↓

2

❑ VC↓	❑ VC↓
❑ FEV1↓	❑ FEV1↓
❑ FVC↓	❑ FVC↓
❑ FEV1/FVC↓	❑ FEV1/FVC↑
❑ PaCO2↑	❑ $PaCO_2$ (N)or ↓

⇨ **Carbon Monoxide Poisoning Causes:**☜☜☜☜

- — "Normal" PO_2☜☜
- — ↓Oxygen saturation.☜☜
- — Metabolic Acidosis☜
- — Cherry red skin discoloration☜
- — CO has 210 times more affinity for Oxygen than Hemoglobin.☜☜
- — Form of Hypoxia produced is anemic hypoxia.☜
- — Oxygen dissociation curve shifts to left.✱✱

- ▶ Hypoxic hypoxia : ☜☜ High altitude, Respiratory diseases Test by: PaO_2✱
- ▶ Anemic hypoxia: ☜ Anemia, CO Poisoning. Test by Oxygen content (HB%)✱
- ▶ Stagnant hypoxia:☜ Cardiogenic shock Test by A-V difference of O_2✱
- ▶ Histotoxic Hypoxia: ☜ Cyanide poisoning. Test by A-V Difference/ PO_2 of Venous blood✱

⮑ **HYPOXIA:**

✓ Low arterial PO_2	AIIMS 1984
✓ Oxygen affinity also decreases.	
✓ Response to oxygen is good.	
✓ Hypoxic hypoxia is the mc type.	AIIMS 1986
✓ Causes rise in pulmonary arterial pressure.	

- ✓ Carbon dioxide is the most potent stimulus for respiration.
- ✓ Carbon dioxide affects respiratory centre by influence on H+ concentration in CSF
- ✓ ↑CO_2 causes:

- ▶ CNS Depression
- ▶ ↓ventilation
- ▶ ↓Sensory acuity
- ▶ Confusion, coma, death

⇨ **Oxygen Toxicity Causes**

CNS Effects (Bert Effect)✳✳

- Hyperirritability
- ↑Muscular twitching
- Convulsions
- Dizziness, Irritability, disorientation

Pulmonary Effects (Smith Effect)

- Tracheobronchial irritation✳
- Pulmonary edema✳
- Congestion and atelectasis✳

Retinal Effects:

- Retrolental fibroplasia✳
- Retinal damage✳

Burnt out Tissue

- Due to ↑metabolic rates and excess heat production with tissue damage

---

Mountain Sickness: adverse effects of Hypoxia at High Altitude.

Develops 8-24 hours after arrival and lasts 4-8 days.

Low PO_2 stimulation is the main cause leading to ↑ ventilation blowing of CO_2 which inhibits respiratory centre causing respiratory distress.

- ► Expansion of gases in GIT occurs → Nausea , Vomiting
- ► Pulmonary edema(↑Permeability) → Breathlessness
- ► Cerebral edema (Cerebral vasodilation) → Headache, irritability, Insomnias, Weakness

⇨ **Carbon Monoxide Poisoning**

- **Carbon monoxide poisoning** is often listed as **a form of anemic hypoxia** because
- There is a deficiency of hemoglobin that can carry oxygen, although the hemoglobin concentration is normal.
- Carbon monoxide is also toxic to **cytochromes in the tissues** ,but the amount of carbon monoxide required to poison cytochromes is 1000 times the lethal dose;
- Tissue Toxicity thus plays no role in clinical carbon monoxide poisonoing.

⇨ **Other Important Facts**

- **Commonest form of hypoxia is hypoxic hypoxia**
- **Stagnant hypoxia** is due to slow circulation in organs like the kidneys and the heart during shock
- **Histotoxic hypoxia** is due to inhibition of tissue oxidative processes commonly due to **cyanide poisning**
- **Hyperbaric oxygen is most useful in the treatment of anemic hypoxia** followed by histotoxic hypoxia.

Acclimatization is by:☛☛	
✓ Hyperventilation	
✓ ↑Hb	
✓ Polycythemia	
✓ ↑Mitochondria	
✓ ↑Cardiac Output	
✓ ↑2,3 DPG	
✓ ↑Diffusion capacity	
✓ Reticulocytosis	
✓ ↑erythropoetin	JIPMER 1990

➲ Physiology

⇨ Renin - Angiotensin - Aldosterone System
Adrenal Cortex

▶ **Zona Glomerulosa** (on outside) **Mineralocorticoids** mainly aldosterone ✹✹
▶ **Zona Fasciculata** (middle) **Glucocorticoids** mainly cortisol
▶ **Zona Reticularis** (on inside) **Androgens** mainly dehydroepiandrosterone (DHEA)

➲ Kidneys:

▶ Each kidney contains about one million nephrons.	
▶ Juxtra medullary nephrons constitute only 15% of nephrons.	
▶ Filtration barrier of kidneys is formed by:	AI 1995
✓ Podocytes	
✓ Endothelial cells	
✓ Basement membrane	

Renin	(AIIMS 07)

— It is released by **JG cells** in kidney in response to **reduced renal perfusion, low Na$^+$**	
— Converts angiotensinogen to angiotensin I.	
— Factors stimulating renin secretion✹✹	UP 2001
➡ low BP☛☛	UP 2001
➡ hyponatraemia ☛	
➡ sympathetic nerve stimulation☛	
➡ catecholamines☛	
➡ erect posture☛	

⇨ **Juxta Glomerular Apparatus**

It is composed of **three parts**

- **The JG Cells:** They are basically **myoepithelial granular cells** present in the wall of <u>afferent arteriole</u>. These cells are in close contact with the blood of the afferent arteriole.

- **Macula Densa:** These are <u>simple cubical cells</u> of the distal convoluted tubule.

They are tall cells with granular cytoplasm. They have no basement membrane.

- **The Polar Cushion:** They are small cells present in between the afferent and the efferent arteriole.

Angiotensin

- ACE in lung converts angiotensin I --> angiotensin II
- **Produced in liver**   UP 2004
- Vasoconstriction leads to raised BP
- Stimulates thirst ✳
- Stimulates aldosterone and ADH release✳✳

⇨ **Thirst:**

— Osmoreceptors are located in **anterior hypothalamus.**

— Thirst is under hypothalmic control.

— Increased thirst is produced by stimulation of thirst centre in **preoptic nucleus of hypothalmus.**

— **Vasopressin secretion is regulated by osmoreceptors located in organum vascolusum and supraoptic crest.**

⮑ **Vasopressin Receptors: High Yield Topic**

- There are at least three kinds of vasopressin receptors: V1A, V1B, and V2.

- All are G protein-coupled.

- **The V1A and V1B receptors** act through phosphatidylinositol hydrolysis to increase the intracellular Ca2+ concentration.

- **The V2 receptors** act through Gs to increase cAMP levels.The mechanism by which vasopressin exerts its antidiuretic effect is activated by V2 receptors and involves insertion of protein water channels in the luminal membranes of the principal cells of the collecting ducts.

- **V1Areceptors mediate the vasoconstrictor effect of vasopressin.**

- **V1A receptors are also found in the liver and the brain. The V1B receptors (also called V3 receptors) appear to be unique to the anterior pituitary, where they mediate increased ACTH secretion from the corticotropes.**

Aldosterone

- Released by **zona glomerulosa**

- Causes retention of Na^+ in exchange for $K^+/H+$ in distal tubule.

- Aldosterone is produced in **zona glomerulosa** of adrenal glands. ✳

- It binds to MR (Mineralocorticoid receptors) in renal tubular cells.

⇨ **It Causes**

▶ Increased Na reabsorption☛

▶ Increased potassium excretion.☛

▶ Increased hydrogen secretion.☛

▶ Increased ammonia excretion☛

▶ Increased magnesium excretion.☛

↑ Renin ↑Aldosterone✳✳✳

- Renovascular Hypertension

- Fibromuscular Dysplasia

- Diuretic use

- Malignant Hypertension

- Reninoma

Sites of Action of Hormones:

- Aldosterone: Cortical ducts and distal tubules✳

- Angiotensin II: Afferent arteriole constriction, reduces GFR.✳

- ADH: Medullary collecting duct✳✳

- ANP: Collecting duct✳

⇨ **Commonly Asked and Repeated Questions in Renal Physiology**

☐ Major part of glomerular filtrate is absorbed in PCT.		AI 1992
☐ Substances **completely** reabsorbed in PCT —		
☐ Glucose,		AP1998
☐ Proteins, amino acids, vitamins, acetoacetate.		
☐ Bicarbonate.		AI 2005

☐ Water		AI 2001
☐ In presence of vasopressin mx reabsorption of water occurs in PCT.		AI 2003
▶ Substances **partially** absorbed in PCT—Na. K, Cl (7/8 reabsorbed in PCT).		(UPSC 02)
▶ Maximum water absorption occurs at PCT. ☛☛		
▶ Glucose transport occurs with sodium.		(PGI 2000)
☐ Substances **secreted** in PCT: H+, PAH (para amino hippurate). creatinine. ☛		
☐ H+ are **actively secreted** in proximal tubules, distal tubules, collecting ducts. ☛		
☐ **Hyperosmolality in the interstitum** is the prerequisite for excretion of concentrated urine.		
☐ Urea is reabsorbed from inner medullary **collecting ducts** only in presence of **ADH.** ☛		
▶ K+ is **actively secreted** in Late Distal tubules and Collecting ducts. ☛		
▶ Macula densa is the <u>epithelial cells of the **distal tubule**</u> that comes to contact with the arterioles.		UPSC 1997
▶ Tubuloglomerular feed back is mediated by sensing NaCl in macula densa.		AI 2006
▶ **Juxtaglomerular cells** produce **renin.** ☛☛		
▶ Are smooth muscle cells of <u>afferent arteriole.</u>		
▶ Lies in relation to glomerulus		
▶ Consists of macula densa		
▶ **Renin** acts on <u>angiotensinogen</u> & convert it into angiotensin I. ☛☛		

▶ Loop of henle does not handle urea.		PGI 1997
▶ Urea has no T m value		

Remember:

➲ Hydrostatic and Osmotic Pressure

☐ Colloid osmotic pressure: is a major determinant of intravascular volume. Albumin is the main osmotically active protein in plasma.

☐ The balance between colloid osmotic pressure and capillary hydrostatic pressure determines the balance between intravascular and extracellular fluid spaces.

☐ A significant degree of hypovolemia and hemoconcentration may take place either because of excessive capillary hydrostatic pressure from an increase in the ratio of post- to precapillary resistance or because of a reduction in plasma protein and consequent reduction of plasma oncotic pressure. Fewer plasma proteins may circulate as a result of increased capillary permeability and loss of plasma proteins from the intravascular to the extracellular space.

□ The transfer of fluid between vascular and interstitial compartments occurs at the capillary level and is governed by the balance between hydrostatic pressure gradients and plasma oncotic pressure gradients. This relation may be stated by the f Starling equation: Jv = Kf (DP - Dp) where Jv is rate of fluid transfer between vascular and interstitial compartments, Kf is the water permeability of the capillary bed, DP is the hydrostatic pressure difference between capillary and interstitium, and Dp is the oncotic pressure difference between capillary and interstitial fluids. Under normal circumstances, interstitial tissue pressure is low, and the DP term in the Starling equation represents the integrated hydrostatic pressure gradient from arteriolar to venular ends of a capillary.

Since interstitial fluid is protein poor, the Dp term in the Starling equation represents the oncotic pressure of plasma proteins, principally albumin; 5 grams of albumin per deciliter of plasma exerts an oncotic pressure of about 15 mm Hg.

Four groups include most edematous states characterized by abnormal Starling forces

► First, the systemic venous pressure may be increased because of primary cardiac disorders, such as **right-sided heart failure or constrictive pericarditis.**

► Second, local elevations in pulmonary or systemic venous pressure may occur, as in **left-sided heart failure, vena caval obstruction, or portal vein obstruction.**

► Third, a reduction in plasma oncotic pressure, and consequently a net increase in the tendency for fluid to transudate from capillaries to interstitium, accounts plausibly for edema formation in the **nephrotic syndrome**. Circulatory albumin concentrations of <3.2 grams per deciliter are usually insufficient to prevent transudation of fluid across capillary beds.

► Finally, **a combination of these factors may be responsible for edema**. For example, both hypoalbuminemia and portal hypertension are major contributory factors to developing ascites in hepatic cirrhosis.

Dehydration or acute volume depletion secondary to blood loss leads to a fall in RBF and GFR secondary to a decrease in cardiac output, activation of the renin-angiotensin-aldosterone system, and an increase in renal sympathetic nerve activity. As the filtered load of sodium decreases, the proximal tubule increases sodium reabsorption. Because the vasoconstrictive effect of angiotensin II affects the efferent glomerular arteriole to a greater degree than the afferent arteriole, the filtration fraction is increased, thereby increasing the oncotic pressure in the peritubular capillaries.

A number of factors modulate glomerulotubular balance .The hemodynamic regulation of oncotic pressure in peritubular capillaries seems to have a dominant role. At relatively low concentrations, angiotensin II has a vasoconstricting effect on efferent, but not afferent, glomerular arterioles. Therefore, this agent, by increasing the glomerular filtration fraction, can increase peritubular capillary oncotic pressure and thereby enhance proximal tubular rates of sodium absorption. At high concentrations, angiotensin II, like norepinephrine, produces afferent glomerular arteriolar constriction, resulting in reductions in GFR and in renal ischemia. AIIMS 2011

2

PHYSIOLOGY

➲ **Site of Action of Diuretics: High Yield for AIPGME/AIIMS/PGI 2013**

Thiazides	
➥ Chlorthiazide	Distal tubule
➥ Hydrochlorthiazide	Distal tubule
➥ Chlorthalidone	Distal tubule
➥ Indapamide	Distal tubule
➥ Metolazone	Proximal and distal tubules
Loop diuretics	
➥ Frusemide	Loop of Henle
➥ Bumatenide	Loop of Henle
➥ Ethacrynic acid	Loop of Henle
Carbonic anhydrase inhibitors	
➥ Acetazolamide	Proximal tubule✲
Potassium sparing diuretics	
➥ Spironolactone	Distal tubule and collecting duct
➥ Triamterene	Distal tubule and collecting duct
➥ Amiloride	Distal tubule and collecting duct

▶ Filtration fraction= GFR/RPF=20%✲✲		(PGI 84)
▶ Clearance=Urine concentration x flow rate/Plasma Concentration✲		
✓ If Clearance < GFR, there is net tubular reabsorption.✲		
✓ If Clearance > GFR, there is net tubular secretion ✲		
✓ If Clearance = GFR, there is no net secretion/reabsorption✲		
▶ GFR=inulin clearance "NOT" Insulin=125ml/min☞		JKBOPEE 2012
▶ RPF=PAH Clearance=500-800☞		(AIIMS 84,85) (TN 02)
▶ Normal creatinine levels: 0.6-1.2mg%.		AI 1993
▶ Urea clearance: 88ml/minute.		AIIMS 1988

⇨ **Important Enzyme Deficencies**

❑ 21α Hydroxylase deficiency:	Hypotension, Hyponatremia, Hyperkalemia☞☞	
❑ 17 Hydroxylase deficiency:	Hypertension, Ambigious genitalia☞☞	
❑ 5 α Reductase deficiency:	↓Testosterone → Feminization.☞	

Substance	Site of absorption
▶ Iron:	Duodeneum (Delhi 85) (AI 91) (AIIMS 07)
▶ Calcium	Jejunum
▶ Folate	Jejunum
▶ Vit B 12	Terminal ileum
▶ Bile salts	Terminal ileum

- ❑ Oxyntic cells of gastric gland contain receptors for PGE_2, "M_3", H_2, Somatostatin.
- ❑ SOMATOSTATIN anatagonizes insulin secretion. DNB 2011
- ❑ Chief cells/Zymogen cells secrete Pepsinogen
- ❑ Oxyntic/Parietal Cells secrete Intrinsic Factor and HCl. (Kerala 94)

➲ Gastric Intrinsic Factor: High Yield for 2011-2012

— A glycoprotein secreted into the lumen of the stomach, is necessary for vitamin B12 absorption from the ileum. DNB 2011

— Absence of this factor results in deficiency of vitamin B12 with consequent development of pernicious anemia.

— Because the liver stores high quantities of vitamin B12, a deficiency of this vitamin may take several months to develop after production of gastric intrinsic factor ceases.

Remember: After intrinsic factor binds cobalamin, the intrinsic factor-cobalamin complex passes down the small intestine until it reaches the distal 60 cm of the ileum, where it binds to a specific receptor of the brush border. In the absence of the terminal ileum, intrinsic factor-mediated cobalamin absorption ceases, although large doses of cobalamin (milligram in contrast to microgram amounts) may lead to adequate absorption by passive diffusion throughout the gastrointestinal tract. DNB 2011

⇨ Somatostatin

- ❑ (Is a peptide) DNB 2011
- ❑ Has GH inhibitory properties
- ❑ Somatostatin also inhibits basal and stimulated TSH secretion.
- ❑ Somatostatin is also present in the D cells of the pancreatic islets and the gut mucosa as well as the myenteric neural plexus. Via paracrine and endocrine actions it suppresses the secretion of insulin, glucagon, cholecystokinin, gastrin, secretin, vasoactive intestinal polypeptide (VIP), and other gastrointestinal hormones, as well as such functions as gastric acid secretion, gastric emptying, gallbladder contraction, and splanchnic blood flow.
- ❑ Recently, analogues of somatostatin have been found to be effective in the treatment of acromegaly, carcinoid tumors, VIP-secreting tumors, TSH-secreting pituitary tumors, islet-cell tumors, and diarrhea of a number of causes.

Remember: Other important Cells of GIT, Hormones and their Function

Hormone	Source of secretion	Actions
Gastrin	G cells of stomach; duodenum, jejunum, Ant. Pitutary, Pancreas and Brain (JIPMER 90)	Stimulates the secretion of gastric juice. Increase the gastric motility (DNB 2001) Stimulates the release of pancreatic hormones.
Secretin	S cells of **duodenum**, jejunum and ileum	Stimulates secretion of watery, alkaline and pancreatic secretions. (AI 88)(PGI 99)
		Inhibits gastric secretion AI 2008 **Causes contraction of pyloric sphincter.** AI 2008 Most potent stimulus is <u>acidic chyme</u>. UP 1996
Cholecytokinin	I cells in **duodenum**, jejunum and ileum	Stimulates **contraction of gall bladder** (PGI 2000) Activates secretin; **Inhibits** gastric motility; Increases secretion of enterokinase and intestinal motility. <u>Protein</u> stimulates CCK secetion. AMU 1999
Gastric inhibitory peptide (GIP)	K cells in **duodenum and jejunum**	Inhibits secretion of gastric juice, gastric motility and increase insulin secretion.

⇨ **Gastric Secretion**

Stimulated by:	
▶ Stomach distension	
▶ Acetylcholine	
▶ Gastrin	PGI 2001
▶ Histamine	PGI 2001
Decreased by:	
▶ H2 blockers	
▶ Secretin	
Gastric emptying:	
▶ Stimulated by gastrin and distension of stomach	
▶ Decreased by cholecystokinin.	

Motilin is a **polypeptide** secreted **by enterochromaffin cells.**

➥ It acts on **G protein** coupled receptors. Motilin is a 22 amino acid polypeptide hormone which in humans is encoded by the MLN gene.

➡ Motilin secreted by endocrine M cells (these are not the same M cells that are in Peyer's patches) that are numerous in crypts of the small intestine, especially in the duodenum and jejunum.

➡ Based on amino acid sequence, motilin is unrelated to other hormones. Because of its **ability to stimulate gastric activity**, it was named "Motilin." ☛☛

➡ Its circulating level increases at approximately **100 minutes** in interdigestive state and is the **major regulator of MMC s** that control GIT motility in between meals.   **UP 2005, JK BOPEE 2007**

➡ **Erythromycin** binds to these motilin receptors and is used for treating "gastric hypomotility." ☛

➡ Pacemaker of small intestine is in second part of duodenum   **UP 2004**

☐ **Cephalic phase** of gastric secretion is mediated by: **parasympathetics**

☐ **Gastric phase** of gastric secretions is mediated by **hormones.**   **AI 1993**

☐ Intestinal motility is stimulated by:

✓ **Distension**   **AI 2007**

✓ **Ach**   **AI 2007**

✓ **Cholecystokinin**

☐ Gastrocolic reflex is a **mass reflex.**

☐ **Enterogastric reflex**: chyme entering intestines inhibits gastric motilty.

☐ Stimulated by:

— **Duodenal distension.**

— **Acidity of duodenal chyme**   **PGI 1998**

— **Osmolarity of chyme**

— **Protein/ fat breakdown products**

Enterogastric reflex is a neurally mediated decrease in gastric motility caused by

— **Products of protein digestion.**

— **H+ ions in duodenum and**

— **Distention of duodenum.**

Factors decreasing gastric motility are

— **GIP**

— **CCK**

— **Vagotomy**

— **Fear**

2

➲ Sites of Absorption

- ► Iron is actively absorbed in **duodenum.**
- ► Fat is maximally absorbed in **jejunum.**   AMU 1995
- ► Vitamin B 12 is absorbed in **ileum.**
- ► Calcium is maximally absorbed in ileum   UP 2004
- ► Maximum absorption of bile is seen in **ileum.**
- ► Electrolytes are absorbed in **colon.**   AI 2006

➪ Dietary Fibre

- ► Increases bulk of stools   PGI 2007
- ► ↑metabolism of sugar in GIT   PGI 2007
- ► Decreases stool transit time
- ► Prevent against colonic cancer
- ► Examples:
  - ☐ Pectin   AI 1999
  - ☐ Cellulose
  - ☐ Hemicellulose

➪ D-xylose Absorption Test

Is used to determine proximal small intestinal absorption of D-xylose (a pentose).

- ➡ Various duodenal and jejunal mucosal disorders (not disorders of pancreatic secretion) are associated with decreased D-xylose absorption.
- ➡ After a 25 g oral dose of this simple sugar, urine is collected for 5 hours and the levels of D-xylose are estimated. Excretion of less than 4.5 grams indicates malabsorption.

➪ Fat

- ☐ Fat is the **largest reserve** of energy in body.   PGI 2007
- ☐ Fat is maximally absorbed in **jejunum.**   AMU 1995
- ☐ **Short chain Fatty acids** are maximally absorbed in **Colon.**
- ☐ Digestion of fats occurs by:
  - ✓ Gastric lipase   PGI 2002
  - ✓ Collipase
  - ✓ bile salts
  - ✓ Pancreatic lipase
- ☐ Fat in stool **>6 gms/day** is indicative of malabsorption   PGI 2K
- ☐ Bile absorption is maximum in **ileum.**

⇨ **Leptin**

— Associated with puberty	KOL 2008
— Secreted from adipose tissue	
— Decreased hunger	

⇨ **Bile**

- ❑ Secreted by hepatocytes.
- ❑ Most potent stimulant for bile secretion is **bile salts**.   AIIMS 1997
- ❑ Composed of water, Bile salts, Cholesterol.
- ❑ Bile salts are **amphiphatic.**
- ❑ Primary Bile Acids: **Cholic acid, Chenodeoxycholic acid**
- ❑ Secondary Bile Acids: **Deoxycholic acid, Lithocholic acid**
- ❑ <u>Cholagouges</u> are substances causing gall bladder contraction.
  - ✓ CCK
  - ✓ Fatty acids
  - ✓ Amino acids
- ❑ <u>Cholerectics</u> are substances increasing secretion of bile
  - ✓ secretin
  - ✓ bile salts
  - ✓ vagal stimulation

➲ **Enterohepatic Circulation: High Yield for 2011-2012**

- ➥ Bile acids are **efficiently conserved** under normal conditions.
- ➥ Unconjugated, and to a lesser degree also conjugated, bile acids are absorbed by passive diffusion along the entire gut.
- ➥ Quantitatively much more important for bile salt recirculation, however, is the **active transport mechanism for conjugated bile acids in the distal ileum**
- ➥ The reabsorbed bile acids enter the portal bloodstream and are taken up rapidly by **hepatocytes, reconjugated, and resecreted into bile (enterohepatic circulation).**
- ➥ The **normal bile acid pool size is approximately 2 to 4 g.**
- ➥ During digestion of a meal, the bile acid pool undergoes at least one or more enterohepatic cycles, depending on the size and composition of the meal.
- ➥ Normally, the bile acid pool circulates approximately 5 to 10 times daily.
- ➥ Intestinal absorption of the pool is about 95% efficient, so fecal loss of bile acids is in the range of 0.3 to 0.6 g/d.

➡ This fecal loss is compensated by an equal daily synthesis of bile acids by the liver, and thus the size of the bile acid pool is maintained.

➡ Bile acids returning to the liver suppress de novo hepatic synthesis of primary bile acids from cholesterol by inhibiting the rate-limiting enzyme cholesterol 7□-hydroxylase.

➡ While the loss of bile salts in stool is usually matched by increased hepatic synthesis, the maximum rate of synthesis is approximately 5 g/d, which may be insufficient to replete the bile acid pool size when there is pronounced impairment of intestinal bile salt reabsorption.

⇨ **Gallbladder and Sphincteric Functions**

In the fasting state, the sphincter of Oddi offers a high-pressure zone of resistance to bile flow from the common bile duct into the duodenum.

This tonic contraction serves to

(1) prevent reflux of duodenal contents into the pancreatic and bile ducts and

(2) promote bile filling of the gallbladder

The major factor controlling the evacuation of the gallbladder is the peptide hormone cholecystokinin (CCK), which is released from the duodenal mucosa in response to the ingestion of fats and amino acids.

⇨ **CCK Produces**

(1) powerful contraction of the gallbladder,

(2) decreased resistance of the sphincter of Oddi,

(3) increased hepatic secretion of bile,

(4) enhanced flow of biliary contents into the duodenum.

Hepatic bile is "concentrated" within the gallbladder by energy-dependent transmucosal absorption of water and electrolytes.

Almost the entire bile acid pool may be sequestered in the gallbladder following an overnight fast for delivery into the duodenum with the first meal of the day. The normal capacity of the gallbladder is **30 to 50 mL of bile.**

⊃ **Insulin: High Yield for AIPGME/AIIMS/PGI 2013**

➡ Insulin acts through activation of **"receptor tyrosine kinase activity"**. ☞☞

➡ Insulin receptor has **two subunits:** ☞

➡ **Alpha subunit:** which is extracellular and binds to insulin ☞

➡ **Beta subunit:** which is transmembranous and has tyrosine kinase activity functioning in signal transduction ☞

Insulin **Increases**

➡ Glucose uptake ☞

➡ Glycogen synthesis ☞   **JIPMER 1992**

➡ Protein synthesis ☞

➡ Fat synthesis ☞   **JIPMER 1992**

Insulin **decreases:**

- Gluconeogenesis
- Glycogenolysis
- Lipolysis

▶ Insulin is a "**polypeptide**" Hormone	
▶ **Sanger was awarded Nobel prize for sequencing Insulin structure.**	**AIIMS 2011**
▶ Insulin is an "**anabolic**" hormone.	
▶ Is a **hypoglycemic** hormone.	**PGI 2002**
▶ Insulin is secreted by **Beta cells** of Pancreas	**KERALA 1991**
▶ **Secreted along with Cpeptide in 1: 1 ratio.**	**PGI 2006**
▶ **In fetus secretion begins by 3 month.**	**AIIMS 2005**
▶ Insulin Secretion is stimulated by **increased blood glucose.**	
▶ Insulin Secretion is **inhibited by epinephrine.**	**(PGI 03)**
▶ Insulin is prepared on a large scale by **recombinant DNA technology** from m RNA.	
▶ Pork insulin differs from human insulin by one amino acid only.	
▶ **Insulin DOES NOT** cross placenta.	**MAHE 2001**

- ▶ Alpha cell – Glucagon
- ▶ **Beta cells – Insulin, Amylin** **AIIMS 2011**

Amylin is secreted by Beta Cells of Pancreas. Amylin is a peptide of 37 amino acids, which is also secreted by the beta cells of the pancreas in addition to Insulin.

Some of its actions are:

- Inhibits the secretion of glucagon;
- Slows the emptying of the stomach;
- Sends satiety signal to the brain.

All of its actions tend to supplement those of insulin, reducing the level of glucose in the blood.

A synthetic, modified, form of amylin (pramlintide) is used in the treatment of Type 2 diabetes.

- ▶ Delta cells – Somatostatin **(AI 89)**
- ▶ F or PP cells – Pancreatic polypeptide

⇨ **Effects of Insulin on Various Tissues**

Liver
- ✓ Increased glycogen synthesis
- ✓ Increased protein synthesis
- ✓ Increased lipid synthesis
- ✓ Decreased ketogenesis
- ✓ Decreased glucose output due to decreased gluconeogenesis, increased glycogen synthesis, and increased glycolysis.

Muscle

- ✓ Increased protein synthesis
- ✓ Increased glucose entry
- ✓ Increased glycogen synthesis
- ✓ Increased amino acid uptake
- ✓ Decreased protein catabolism
- ✓ Decreased release of gluconeogenic amino acids
- ✓ Increased ketone uptake
- ✓ Increased K+ uptake

Adipose tissue

- ✓ Increased glucose entry
- ✓ Increased glycerol phosphate synthesis
- ✓ Increased triglyceride deposition
- ✓ Activation of lipoprotein lipase
- ✓ Inhibition of hormone- sensitive lipase
- ✓ Increased K+ uptake

⮞ **Hormones**

⇨ **Hormones can be divided into five major classes:**

(1) amino acid derivatives such as ✷✷

- ✓ dopamine,
- ✓ catecholamines, and
- ✓ thyroid hormone;

(2) small neuropeptides such as ✷✷

- ✓ gonadotropin-releasing hormone (GnRH),
- ✓ thyrotropin-releasing hormone (TRH),
- ✓ somatostatin, and
- ✓ vasopressin;

(3) large proteins such as ✷✷

- ✓ insulin
- ✓ luteinizing hormone (LH), and
- ✓ PTH produced by classic endocrine glands;   (AIIMS 05)

(4) steroid hormones such as ✷✷

- ✓ cortisol and
- ✓ estrogen that are synthesized from cholesterol-based precursors; and

(5) vitamin derivatives such as ✱✱

✓ retinoids (vitamin A) and

✓ vitamin D

➡ A variety of peptide growth factors, most of which act locally, share actions with hormones. ☞☞

➡ As a rule, amino acid derivatives and peptide hormone interact with cell-surface membrane receptors.

➡ Steroids, thyroid hormones, vitamin D, and retinoids are lipid-soluble and interact with intracellular nuclear receptors.☞☞   (PGMCET 07)

➲ Secondary Messengers

▶ cAMP	PGI 2005
▶ DAG	PGI 2005
▶ IP 3	
▶ Ca^{++}	AIIMS 2006
▶ Protein kinase	
▶ NO acts as cellular signalling molecule.	AI 2005

C AMP mediates action of

✓ PTH,	
✓ LH,	
✓ FSH, HCG	
✓ ADH	AIIMS 1995
✓ Calcitonin	
✓ Glucagons	

C GMP mediates action of

✓ ANF,	
✓ NO,	AIIMS 1994
✓ Insulin acts through <u>tyrosine kinase.</u>	PGI 2001

Ca^{++}, Phosphatidyl inophosphate mediates action of

✓ Ach,

✓ angiotensin II,

✓ Oxytocin

▶ Thyroid hormones act on intracellular receptors	
▶ Retinoic acid, act on intracellular receptors	PGI 2011
▶ (Steroids) act on intracellular receptors	
▶ Androgens, estrogen, progesterone, glococorticoids, mineralocorticoids act on intracellular receptors	PGI 2006
▶ Vitamin D3 and thyroid belong to steroid receptor family.	UP 2004

⇨ **Calcium Metabolism**

Parathormone:

- **Stimulates osteoclastic activity,** thereby increasing bone resorption by mobilizing calcium and phosphate; ☛☛

- **Increases the reabsorption of calcium** by the renal tubules, thus reducing the urinary excretion of calcium; ☛

- **Ugments the absorption of calcium from the gut;** ☛   PGI 01

- **Calcium reabsorption takes place from <u>proximal</u> small intestine.**   PGI 1999

- **Reduces the renal tubular reabsorption of phosphate,** thus promoting phosphaturia. ☛

Calcitonin:

- Is secreted by the **"Parafollicular cells"** of the **"Thyroid"** (thyrocalcitonin).☛☛

- It lowers the serum calcium and affects calcium storage in bones; quite the opposite action of parathormone.   (AI 06)

- **Acts by decreasing bone absorption.**   PGI 1999

- **That means inhibits osteoclastic activity.**   AI 2005

Parathyroid hormone-related protein (PTH-rP):

- Is a **hypercalcaemic factor** with similar bioactivity to that of parathyroid hormone.☛☛

- Low calcium levels stimulate its secretion   AIIMS 2007

- Since its isolation from cancer cell lines and carcinoma of the breast, strong evidence has emerged that it is an **important hormonal mediator of cancer-associated hypercalcaemia** in patients with solid tumours.☛

                                                                                   AI 2005

⇨ **Calcium**

- Calcium is absorbed in **proximal small intestine.**

- Absorption is increased by acidic pH, proteins

- Absorption is decreased by **phosphates and oxalates**.

- Ionized form is the active form of calcium   AI 2008

- Organs having role in calcium metabolism are:

Liver, Kidney and skin   DNB 2011

A decrease in the concentration of free calcium ions in plasma results in

- ✓ **Increased neuromuscular irritability** and tetany.   AI 2001
- ✓ peripheral and perioral paresthesia,
- ✓ carpal spasm,
- ✓ pedal spasm, anxiety, seizures,
- ✓ bronchospasm, laryngospasm,

- ⊙ **Chvostek's sign,**

- ⊙ **Trousseau's sign,** and

- ⊙ **Erb's sign,** and

- ⊙ <u>Lengthening</u> of the QT interval of the electrocardiogram.   AIIMS 2003

Substance	Serum calcium	Serum phosphate
Vitamin D	↑	↑
PTH	↑	↓
Calcitonin	↓	↓

2

⊃ Pituitary Gland: High Yield for AIPGME/AIIMS/PGI 2013

The anterior pituitary is often referred to as the **"master gland"** Called **Hypophysis cerebri.**

Remember <u>Epiphysis cerebri is Pineal Gland</u>

The anterior pituitary gland produces six major hormones:

(1) prolactin (PRL),

(2) growth hormone (GH),

(3) adrenocorticotropin hormone (ACTH),   PGI 2003

(4) luteinizing hormone (LH),

(5) follicle-stimulating hormone (FSH), and

(6) thyroid-stimulating hormone (TSH)   PGI 2003

▶ Pituitary hormones are secreted in a **pulsatile manner,**

▶ The pituitary gland weighs ~600 mg

▶ Is located within the **sella turcica** ventral to the diaphragma sella.

▶ The **hypothalamic-pituitary portal plexus** provides the major blood source for the anterior pituitary

▶ The posterior pituitary is supplied by the inferior hypophyseal arteries.

The Posterior Lobe is directly innervated by hypothalamic neurons (supraopticohypophyseal and tuberohypophyseal) nerve tracts) via the pituitary stalk." **Pitucytes" are cells of posterior Pitutary along with Herring Bodies.**

DNB 2011

Thus, posterior pituitary production of **vasopressin (antidiuretic hormone; ADH) and oxytocin.**   PGI 2001

Is particularly sensitive to neuronal damage by lesions that affect the pituitary stalk or hypothalamus.

✓ Vasopressin and oxytocin are typical **Neural** Hormones. They are secreted into the circulation by nerve cells.

✓ The term **neurosecretion** is classic for these two hormones.

✓ Both are synthesized in Para ventricular and Supraoptic nuclei and transported via hypothalmoneurohypophyseal tracts to posterior pituitary.

✓ **Posterior lobe of pituitary** is important in their formation and they are synthesized as a part of large precursor molecule.

✓ Both vasopressin and oxytocin have a **characteristic neurophysin** attached with them. In the granules of the neurons that secrete them.

✓ **Neurophysin I in case of oxytocin** and **Neurophysin II** in case of Vasopressin.

✓ These neurophysins were initially thought to be binding molecules but now they are thought to be parts of precursor molecule.

✓ The vasopressin and Neurophysin II after being secreted forms secretory granules called **Herrings bodies.**

- The **neurohypophysis**, or posterior pituitary gland, is formed by axons that project from large cell bodies in the supraoptic and paraventricular nuclei of the hypothalamus to the posterior portion of the sella turcica.

- The **neurohypophysis** produces two hormones: **(1) arginine vasopressin (AVP), also known as antidiuretic hormone (ADH); and (2) oxytocin.**   DNB 2011

- AVP acts on the renal tubules to induce water retention, leading to concentration of the urine. Oxytocin stimulates postpartum milk letdown in response to suckling.

- Like other peptide hormones destined for secretion, newly synthesized AVP-neurophysin II precursor is translocated from the cytosol to the endoplasmic reticulum, where the signal peptide is removed and the prohormone folds and oligomerizes before moving through the Golgi apparatus to the **neurosecretory vesicles;** there it is **transported down the axons and further cleaved to AVP, neurophysin II, and copeptin.** Stimulation of the neurons results in an influx of calcium, fusion of the **neurosecretory vesicle** with the cell membrane, and extrusion of its contents into the systemic circulation.

- The <u>posterior pituitary peptide "oxytocin"</u> also has an antidiuretic action, although oxytocin is a much less potent antidiuretic agent than is vasopressin.   DNB 2011

⇨ **Somatomedins:**

- Are polypeptide growth factors secreted by liver, and other tissues, which mediate the growth-promoting effects of GH.
- Somatomedins exhibit sequence homology with insulin and proinsulin, they belong to the insulin family.
- Because of their resemblance to insulin, they can bind to insulin receptors and elict insulin-like effects.
- At least four somatomedins have isolated, but by far the most important of these is **somatomedin C** (also called IGF-I)

The somatomedins, have characteristics:

↦ **Regulation of their concentration in serum by growth hormone,**

↦ **Stimulation of sulfate incorporation into the cartilage proteoglycan chondroitin sulfate,**

↦ **Insulin- like effects on both adipose and muscle tissue, and**

↦ **Mitogenicity for fibroblasts.**

⊃ **Growth Hormone**

Is a protein hormone that is synthesized and secreted by cells called somatotrophs in the anterior pituitary.

⇨ **Physiologic Effects of Growth Hormone**

Direct effects are the result of growth hormone binding its receptor on target cells.

Indirect effects are mediated primarily by a insulin-like growth factor-I (IGF-I), a hormone that is secreted from the liver and other tissues in response to growth hormone. A majority of the growth promoting effects of growth hormone is actually due to IGF-I acting on its target cells.

⇨ **Effects on Growth**

- The major role of growth hormone in stimulating body growth is to stimulate the liver and other tissues to secrete IGF-I. IGF-I stimulates proliferation of chondrocytes (cartilage cells), resulting in bone growth.

▶ Growth hormone does seem to have a direct effect on bone growth in stimulating differentiation of chondrocytes.

▶ IGF-I also appears to be the key player in muscle growth. It stimulates both the differentiation and proliferation of myoblasts. It also stimulates amino acid uptake and protein synthesis in muscle and other tissues.

⇨ **Metabolic Effects**

▶ Growth hormone has important effects on protein, lipid and carbohydrate metabolism. In some cases, a direct effect of growth hormone has been clearly demonstrated, in others, IGF-I is thought to be the critical mediator, and some cases it appears that both direct and indirect effects are at play.

▶ **Protein metabolism:** In general, growth hormone **stimulates protein anabolism** in many tissues. This effect reflects increased amino acid uptake, increased protein synthesis and decreased oxidation of proteins.

▶ **Fat metabolism:** Growth hormone enhances the utilization of fat by stimulating triglyceride breakdown and oxidation in adipocytes.

▶ **Carbohydrate metabolism:** Growth hormone is one of a battery of hormones that serves to maintain blood glucose within a normal range. Growth hormone is often said to have **anti-insulin activity, because it supresses the abilities of insulin to stimulate uptake of glucose in peripheral tissues and enhance glucose synthesis in the liver.** Somewhat paradoxically, administration of growth hormone stimulates insulin secretion, leading to hyperinsulinemia.

⇨ **Reproductive Physiology**

➡ Potency: **Dihydrotestosterone>Testosterone>Androstenendione**

➡ **Testosterone is converted to DHT** by enzyme **"5 α reductase".**

➡ Testosterone is converted into **estrogen and estrodial** by "aromatase".

➡ FSH stimulates formation of **Secondary follicle to Graffian Follicle**

➡ **Estrogen** is responsible for **"Proliferative"** phase

➡ **LH surge stimulates ovulation.**   AIIMS 2007 DNB 2011

Female reproductive cycles result from coordinated signaling by hypothalamic, pituitary, and ovarian hormones. Pulsatile secretion of gonadotropin-releasing hormone stimulates pituitary production of LH and FSH. During the follicular phase of the menstrual cycle these peptide hormones regulate ovarian secretion of estrogen and direct maturation of follicles, one of which increases 1000-fold in diameter and becomes dominant for ovulation. FSH induces LH receptors in ovarian granulosa cells, and both LH and FSH induce aromatase as part of the mechanism that enhances estrogen production. LH and FSH increase during the follicular phase and, with follicle development, estrogen secretion rises. <u>Positive feedback effects of estrogen result in the mid-cycle surge of LH and FSH, which induces ovulation</u>

➡ LH **maintains corpus luteum.**   AI 1997

➡ **FSH receptors** are present on **granulosa cells.**   AIIMS 2006

➡ **Progesterone** is responsible for **"Secretory"** phase

- Male **sex hormones** are called the androgens (secreted by leydig cells); testosterone, dihydro testosterone & androstenedione.
- **Mullerian** ducts gives rise to female accessory sex organs such as **vagina, uterus & fallopian tube.**
- **Wolffian** duct gives rise to **male accessory sex organs such as epididymis,** vas deferens & seminal vesicles. ☞☞
- **Fetal testes** begin to secrete the testosterone at about 2nd **to** 4th **month of** embryonic life.
- The **secretion from seminal vesicles** contains <u>fructose,</u> phophorylcholine, fibrinogen, ascorbic acid, citric acid, pepsinogen, acid phosphatase & prostaglandin.
- Fructose & citrate acts as **fuel** for the spermatozoa.
- **Prostatic secretion** is rich in enzymes, <u>zinc</u> & citrate. ☞☞☞   COMED 2007
- Androgen appears to be essential for spermatogenesis. Whereas FSH is required for spermatic maturation.

⮑ Menopause Causes HAVOC

- <u>H</u>ot flushes
- <u>A</u>trophy <u>v</u>agina
- <u>O</u>steoporosis
- <u>C</u>oronary artery disease
- Features
- — ↓Estrogen   DNB 2003
- — ↑FSH↑LH
- — ↑ GnRH

- **Prolactin** increases Dopamine Synthesis   AI 1994
- **Dopamine** inhibits Prolactin Synthesis
- **Dopamine agonists** (Bromocriptine) inhibit Prolactin synthesis.

⮑ Important Points in Reproductive Physiology

- ► Spermatogenesis occurs at **lower temperatures** at about 32^0C. ☞☞
- ► Spermatozoa **acquire motility** in epididymis.☞☞   UP 2008
- ► **Capacitation** (Fertilization capabilities)occurs in **female genital tract**☞   AIIMS 2009
- ► Sperms move at a speed of **1- 3 mm/min.**☞   AI 1988
- ► Semen contains **high concentration of prostaglandins.**☞
- ► Sperms reach uterine tubes in **30-60 minutes** after copulation.☞
- ► In female genital tract don't survive for more than **48 hours.**   ORISSA 1991
- ► **Estrogen** content of fluid in **Rete Testis** is high. ☞

► Spermatozoa contain a special enzyme **Germinal Angiotensin II Converting enzyme**.

► Testosterone is produced from pregnanalone.   AI 1990

► **Testosterone is produced by Leyding cells.**   AI 2006

Sertoli Cells:

Play an important role in the **development of germ cells and regulation of spermatogenesis.**

They maintain the structural integrity and compartmentalization of seminiferous tubules, deliver nutrients and produce proteins that support spermatogenesis, and regulate the movement and release of maturing sperm within the tubule. Sertoli cells also produce **müllerian inhibiting substance** and **inhibin**, a glycoprotein that inhibits follicle-stimulating hormone secretion from the pituitary gland.

► **CART WHEEL** appearance of nucleus is seen in <u>sertoli cells</u>

► Blood testis barrier is formed by <u>sertoli cells</u>.   **MP 2K**

► Receptors for FSH are present in <u>sertoli cells</u>.   **AIIMS 2007**

► Inhibin is secreted by <u>sertoli cells</u>.   AI 2004

► Androgen binding protein is secreted by sertoli cells 2011

⊃ Newer Concepts

➡ The negative feedback effects of <u>inhibin,</u> a peptide produced by <u>testicular Sertoli cells and ovarian granulosa cells,</u> are predominantly on FSH at the pituitary. Inhibin causes a dose-related decrease in the sensitivity of gonadotrophs to GnRH, but there may also be a hypothalamic site of action.   PGI 2011

➡ The related ovarian protein, <u>activin,</u> stimulates FSH synthesis and release from the pituitary.

➡ Another gonadal peptide, <u>follistatin,</u> also inhibits the oophorectomy- and GnRH-induced rises in FSH selectively, primarily by binding to activin.

➡ These ovarian peptides are also found in the pituitary and therefore may have additional local effects on gonadotropin secretion.

⇨ The Corpus Luteum

➡ Is formed <u>from the granulosa and theca cells</u> of the former preovulatory follicle following ovulation.

➡ It secretes <u>progesterone and Estradiol</u> for approximately 14 days.   **PGI 2011**

➡ It then degenerates unless fertilization occurs.

➡ The lifespan of the corpus luteum may depend in part upon prostaglandins and prolactin as well as upon progestin. If fertilization occurs, hCG, which is similar to LH, is secreted by the developing blastocyst and helps to support the corpus luteum until the fetoplacental unit can support itself.

⊃ "Naturally" Occurring Estrogens

✓ **Estradiol**   **PGI 2011**

✓ **Estrone**   **PGI 2011**

✓ **Estriol**

⊃ Thyroid Hormones: High Yield for AIPGME/AIIMS/PGI 2013

▶ The thyroid gland produces two related hormones, **thyroxine (T_4) and triiodothyronine (T_3)** Thyroid hormones act through **nuclear hormone receptors** to modulate gene expression.   **AIIMS 2011**

▶ TSH, secreted by the **thyrotrope cells of the anterior pituitary** serves as the **most useful physiologic marker of thyroid hormone action.**   **UPC 2007**

▶ Thyroid hormones **feed back negatively to inhibit TRH and TSH production**

▶ Thyroid hormones are **derived from a large iodinated glycoprotein.**

▶ **Iodide uptake** is a **critical first step** in thyroid hormone synthesis.

▶ Iodide uptake is mediated by **the Na^+/I^- symporter (NIS),** which is expressed at the basolateral membrane of thyroid follicular cells, followed by **Organification, Coupling, Storage, Release**

▶ **TSH is the dominant hormonal regulator** of thyroid gland growth and function.

▶ Excess iodide transiently inhibits thyroid iodide organification, a phenomenon known as the **Wolff-Chaikoff effect**

▶ T_4 is secreted from the thyroid gland in at least 20-fold excess over T_3.

▶ Both hormones circulate bound to plasma proteins, including **thyroxine-binding globulin (TBG), transthyretin (TTR, formerly known as thyroxine-binding prealbumin, or TBPA), and albumin.**

                                                                                                                          PGI 2001

▶ Thyroid hormones act by binding to nuclear receptors, termed **thyroid hormone receptors (TRs) a and b.**

⇨ Effects

➥ Brain Maturation

➥ <u>Bone Growth (Mediate Epiphyseal closure)</u>   **DNB 2011**

➥ BMR ↑

➥ Beta adrenergic effects

Wolf Chaikoff effect is Iodine itself inhibits organic binding. **Iodine excess also can lead to goitrous hypothyroidism through iodine-induced inhibition of thyroid hormone formation (Wolff-Chaikoff effect).** This occurs especially in patients with underlying thyroid disease. The thyroid is unable to reduce iodide uptake in spite of increased iodide stores, and the inability to escape from the Wolff-Chaikoff effect leads to goitrous hypothyroidism.

                                                                                                                          DNB 2011

▶ Hypertrophy of Zona Glomerulosa✳	**Conns Syndrome**☞	
▶ Hypertrophy of Zona Fasiculata✳	**Cushings Syndrome**☞	
▶ Adrenal Cortical Atrophy✳	**Addisons Disease**☞	
▶ Hypertrophic Adrenal Medulla✳	**Phaeochromocytoma**☞	
▶ Hypertrophic Adrenal Medulla✳✳	**Neuroblastoma**☞	

⇨ **Hormones ↑in Stress**

▶ Adrenaline	
▶ Vasopressin	**PGI 2004**
▶ Cortisol	
▶ Glucagon	
▶ Epinephrine	
▶ Insulin is not increased	**UP 2008**

⇨ **Melatonin**

▶ Is a pineal hormone	**AI 1996**
▶ Is serotegenic	
▶ Is secreted **predominantly at night** in both day - and night-active species,	
▶ **Exogenous melatonin increases sleepiness** and may potentiate sleep when administered to good sleepers attempting to sleep during daylight hours at a time when endogenous **melatonin** levels are low.	
▶ Increased <u>serotonin N acetyl transferase activity</u> occurs in darkness.	**AIIMS 2003**

⇨ **Serotonin**

Seratonin:

- Is produced by **argentaffin cells** of the gastrointestinal tract and is necessary for GIT motility. These cells may grow into locally malignant **argentaffinomas,** otherwise known as **carcinoid tumors.** These tumors develop in small intestine or in the appendix.

- The patient complains of flushing, sweating, intermittent diarrhea and often has fluctuating hypertension.

- Normally, about 1% tryptophan molecules are channelled to serotonin synthesis. But in carcinoid syndrome, up to 60% is diverted to serotonin. Therefore, **niacin deficiency** (pellagra) may also be seen in carcinoid syndrome.

HIAA (5-Hydroxy indole acetic acid) in Urine:

- It is increased in carcinoid tumors in the gut or bronchus, tropical sprue, Whipple's disease, oat cell carcinoma of the bronchus. If urine 5 HIAA exceeds 25 mg/day, diagnosis of carcinoid syndrome can be made. Metastatic carcinoid tumor (functioning) shows higher values. Since 5 HIAA secretion may be intermittent, repeated testing is required.

- It is decreased in depression, small intestinal resection, phenylketonuria and Hartnup's disease.

⇨ **Sleep**

▶ **EEG waves are called Berger rhythm.**
▶ **Normal EEG is bilaterally symmetrical.**
▶ **Alpha waves: 8-13 Hz. seen in awake patient with eyes closed.**
▶ **Beta waves: ≥14 Hz. seen in awake with eyes open.**

▶	Theta waves: 4-7 Hz. Seen in hippocampus.	ASSAM 2003
▶	Delta waves: 3-5 Hz. Seen in deep sleep.	AI 2007
▶	DTAB is order of increasing frequency. (Digest TAB)	

⇨ **REM Sleep**

✓	Light phase with difficult arrousal.	
✓	Called <u>paradoxical</u> sleep.	

Disorders of REM Sleep:

✓	Night mares (remembered)	AI 2000
✓	Narcolepsy	
✓	Nocturnal penile tumescene.	

⇨ **NREM Sleep**

✓	↓ BP
✓	↓ HR

Disorders of NREM sleep:

✓	Sleep walking
✓	Sleep talking
✓	Night terror
✓	Bruxism
✓	Nocturnal enuresis

➲ **Iron Metabolism**

▶	The major role of **iron** is to carry O_2 as part of the heme	
▶	O_2 also is bound by a heme protein in muscle, **myoglobin**.	
▶	**Iron** also is a critical element in **iron**-containing enzymes, including the **cytochrome system** in mitochondria.	
▶	**Iron** absorbed from the diet or released from stores circulates in the **plasma bound to transferrin**, the **iron** transport protein.	JKBOPEE 2012
▶	In a normal individual, the average red cell life span is **120 days.**	
▶	The balance of **iron metabolism** in the organism is tightly controlled and designed to conserve **iron** for reutilization.	
▶	There is no excretory pathway for **iron**, and the only mechanisms by which **iron** is lost from the body are blood loss (via gastrointestinal bleeding, menses, or other forms of bleeding) and the loss of epidermal cells from the skin and gut.	
▶	**Iron** absorption takes place largely in the proximal small intestine.	

⇨ **Haemoglobin**

▶ Hb A	▶ Alpha 2, Beta 2
▶ Hb F	▶ Alpha 2, Gamma 2
▶ Hb A 2	▶ Alpha 2, Delta 2
▶ Hb H	▶ Beta 4 **
▶ Hb S	▶ Beta 6 val- glu
▶ Hb Barts	▶ Gamma 4**

⊃ **Fetal Hemoglobin: High Yield for AIPGME/AIIMS/PGI 2013**

- ➥ The feature of fetal hemoglobin is that it has higher affinity for oxygen than adult hemoglobin.

- ➥ O2 saturation of the maternal blood in the placenta is so low that the fetus might suffer hypoxic damage if fetal red cells did not have a greater O_2 affinity than adult red cells.

- ➥ This difference in O_2 affinity between the two is because, fetal hemoglobin binds to 2, 3 DPG less effectively than adult hemoglobin.

- ➥ Binding of **2-3, DPG** to the hemoglobin decreases its affinity for oxygen i.e., it shifts the O_2 dissociation curve to right.

- ➥ HBF reacts less with 2, 3-DPG and so is able to bind O_2 more tenaciously, accounting for the left shifted O_2 dissociation curve at birth.

- ➥ Concentration of fetal hemoglobin at birth. **HbF- 70-80%** of total hemoglobin.

⇨ **Blood Coagulation Factors**

▶ 1, 2, 5, 7, 9, 10	▶ Produced in liver*
▶ 2, 7, 8, 9, 10	▶ Levels increased with oral contraceptives*
▶ 2, 7, 9, 10	▶ Vitamin K required*
▶ 5, 8	▶ Unstable in stored blood*
▶ 5, 10	▶ Good for growth of hemophilus organisms*

⊃ **Physiology of Eye**

- ▶ **Rods** are responsible for dim light or night vision or **scotopic vision.** (Electric Rods are used at night)

- ▶ **Cones** are responsible for **colour vision**, sensitive to day light and acuity of vision.

- ▶ **Rhodopsin** is the photosensitive pigment of rods cells.

- ▶ **Hem holtz Theory** states that there are 3 kinds of cones in retina corresponding to three colours.

DNB 1991

► Most sensitive in Green light and least sensitive in Red light   (PGI 80)

► Photosensitive pigment in cones are

  ➥ **Porpyropsin - Red**

  ➥ **Iodopsin - Green**

  ➥ **Cyanopsin - Blue**

► Test for **visual acuity** - **Snell's chart** (distant vision) and **Jaeger's chart** (near vision).

► Test for color blindness - **Ishihara's colour chart.**

► Mapping of visual field - **Perimetry.**

► **Nearest point** at which the object is seen clearly is about 7 to 40 cm.

► **Farthest point** is infinite.

➥ <u>**Protanomoly**</u> refers to defect in **red cones**👈👈   AMU 1992

➥ <u>**Deutranomoly**</u> refers to defect in **green** cones.👈👈

➥ <u>**Trianamoly**</u> refers to defect in **blue** cones.👈👈

➲ Occular Physiology: High Yield for AIPGME/AIIMS/PGI 2013

➥ Fovea centralis **or macula lutea** is a thinned out rod free portion of the retina

➥ Cones are densely packed here

➥ There are very few cells and no blood vessels overlying the receptors

➥ It is the point where **visual acuity is greatest**

➥ The <u>Fovea</u> is a small shallow depression in the central region of the eye located such that

➥ Most of the incident light collected by the cornea and lens is focused onto this region.

➥ Most of the inner layers of the retina are markedly reduced or absent and what dominates is a layer of photoreceptors

➥ **Composed entirely of cone cells** for very **fine discrimination of colors and details.**

➥ Retinal vessels are also absent in the region of the fovea. Is most sensitive part of eye.

➥ **Visible range of electromagnetic spectrum of human eye : 370-740 nm**   PGI 2004

➥ **Relative color and luminosity of photoreceptive input under changing light are regulated and maintained by: Amacrine cells.**   AIIMS 2004

➥ **Parvocellular pathway from lateral geniculate nucleus to visual cortex is most sensitive for stimulus of color contrast.**   AI 2005

➥ **Blobs of visual cortex are associated with color processing.**   AI 2006

Cell Adhesion Molecules

Cells are attached to Basal Lamina and each other by cell adhesion molecules (CAMs)

They are:

Integrins☜

Adhesion molecules of IgG Superfamily☜

Cadherins☜

Selectins☜

Nitric oxide ✱

➲ High Yield for AIPGME/AIIMS/PGI 2013

✓ Nitric oxide is **NO**☜☜

✓ It is also called as **EDRF (Endothelial derived relaxing factor).**☜☜   AIIMS 2007

✓ It is produced from **arginine** by enzyme NO synthetase.☜☜   AIIMS 2007

✓ NO has a short t ½ **(4 seconds).**

✓ It acts via **c GMP** pathway.   (AIPGME 05) (AIIMS 93)

➥ It **relaxes smooth muscles** specifically☜

➥ It **prevents platelet aggregation.**☜

➥ It functions as a **neurotransmitter.**☜

➥ It mediates **bactericidal actions of macrophages**☜☜

Acts as:

➥ **Free radical**   PGI 2001

➥ **Vasodilator**   PGI 2001

➥ **Oxidizing agent**   PGI 2001

➥ **Catalyst**

▶ NO, ANP,BNP act through **c GMP**

▶ Remember:

▶ Calmodulin is **Ca Dependent**   (PGI 02)

▶ Calmodulin acts through **Protein Kinase**

➲ Inflammatory Mediators

▶ **Histamine** is present in mast cells, basophils, enterochromaffin cells

▶ Has three types of receptors H1, H2, H3.

▶ Formed by **decarboxylation of histdine**   AI 2008

▶ Alter venular permeability

▶ **Mediates triple response**   AI 2008

⊃ Natriuretic Peptides: High Yield for AIPGME/AIIMS/PGI 2013

Atrial distention and/or a sodium load cause release into the circulation of atrial natriuretic peptide (ANP), a polypeptide; a high-molecular-weight precursor of ANP is stored in secretory granules within atrial myocytes.

Release of ANP causes:

- Excretion of sodium and water by augmenting glomerular filtration rate,   UP 2006

- Inhibiting sodium reabsorption in the proximal tubule, and   MAHE 2003

- Inhibiting release of renin and aldosterone; and

- Arteriolar and venous dilatation by antagonizing the vasoconstrictors   UP 2006

Thus, ANP has the capacity to oppose sodium retention and arterial pressure elevation in hypervolemic states.

The closely related brain natriuretic peptide (BNP) is stored primarily in cardiac ventricular myocardium and is released when ventricular diastolic pressure rises.

Its actions are similar to those of ANP.

Circulating levels of ANP and BNP are **elevated in congestive heart failure** but not sufficient to prevent edema formation.

In addition, in edematous states (particularly heart failure), there is **abnormal resistance to the actions of natriuretic peptide**

Increase the concentrations of cyclic GMP in the kidney, adrenal glomerulose, vascular smooth muscle, and platelets. Elevated circulating concentrations of ANP and particularly BNP correlate with a poor prognosis in heart failure

- **Natriuretric substance**
- **Promotes sodium excretion.**
- **Decreases blood pressure**
- **Acts by c GMP Pathway.**   MAH 2K

⇨ Mechanoreceptors

The "**Encapsulated**" mechanoreceptors include:

- **Pacinian corpuscles** in skin and connective tissues that sense (rapidly adapting touch) **pressure and vibration**. They look like onion bulbs.   NIMHANS 2006

- **Meissner's corpuscles** in dermal papillae of non-hair bearing skin of hands, feet, genitalia, nipples, and mouth that provide tactile discrimination. They look like nutmegs.

- **Ruffini's corpuscles** in skin and joints that respond to **stretch and pressure**

- **Golgi tendon organs** located where muscle inserts into tendon sense stretch for proprioception

- **Muscle spindles** in skeletal muscles are composed of nerve endings in association with specialized intrafusal muscle fibers that function to **detect stretch** for reflexes

The "**Nonencapsulated**" endings include:

- **Peritricial nerve endings** around hair follicles that detect touch through movement of hair

- **Merkel's discs** on non-hair bearing skin such as the hands that perceive touch. It is present in epidermis.   ICS 2005

⇨ Important Regions of CNS

► The **Locus Ceruleus** ☞ is a dense collection of neuromelanin-containing cells in the rostral pons. It appears blue-black in unstained brain tissue .These cells contain <u>norepinephrine.</u>

► The **Basal nucleus of Meynert**☞ is one of the structures that degenerates in <u>Alzheimer's disease</u>.

► The **Caudate nucleus**☞ degenerate in <u>Huntington's disease(GABA ergeic) neurons</u>   AIIMS 2004

► The **Substantia nigra**☞ contains the nigrostriatal neurons that are the source of striatal dopamine. This cell group **degenerates in** <u>Parkinson's disease.</u>

► The **Ventral Tegmental area** ☞is located in the midbrain and is an important source of dopamine for the limbic and cortical areas. Over activity of this cell group is a popular theory of the etiology of <u>Schizophrenia</u>

⊃ Normal Cerebral Physiologic Values: High Yield for AIPGME/AIIMS/PGI 2013

- Cerebral Metabolic Rate (CMR) : 3-3.8 ml/100 g/min (50 ml/min)
- Cerebral blood flow (CBF) : 50 ml/100 gm/min (750 ml/min)
- Cerebral perfusion pressure (CPP) : 80-100 mm Hg
- Intracranial pressure (ICP) : <10 mm Hg
- CPP = MAP (Mean Arterial Pressure) - ICP (or central venous pressure
- which even in greater)
- Cerebral autoregulation range. MAP 60-160 mm Hg.
- Normal total CSF production: 21 ml/Hr (500 ml/day)
- Total CSF volume: 150 ml.

⇨ Limbic System

- Limbic ⟶ Marginal.
- A group or a system of structures lying between cerebral cortex and Hypothalamus.
- Anatomically:
- Subcallosal Gyri.
- Cingulate Gyri. (Jharkhand 2005)
- Parahippocampal Gyri.
- Hippocampal formation Hippocampus Gyrus, Dentate Gyrus,Parahippocampal Gyrus
- Amygdaloid Nucleus. (Jharkhand 2005)
- Mammillary bodies.
- Anterior thalamic nucleus.

⊃ Aphasia: High Yield for AIPGME/AIIMS/PGI 2013

► **Aphasia** should be diagnosed only when there are deficits in the formal aspects of language such as naming, word choice, comprehension, spelling, and syntax.

► Dysarthria and mutism do not, by themselves, lead to a diagnosis of **aphasia**.

▶ In approximately 90% of right handers and 60% of left handers, **aphasia** occurs only after lesions of the left hemisphere.

▶ A language disturbance occurring after a right hemisphere lesion in a right hander is called crossed **aphasia**.

⇨ **Wernicke's Aphasia**

✓ Damage: **Comprehension is impaired for spoken and written language.**   APPG 2006

✓ Language output is **fluent**

✓ The tendency for paraphasic errors may be so pronounced that it leads to strings of neologisms, which form the basis of what is known as "jargon **aphasia**."

⇨ **Broca's Aphasia**

✓ Brocas area is present in **inferior frontal gyrus.**   UP 2003

✓ **Concerned with word formation.**   AI 2007

✓ Damage: **Speech is nonfluent**, labored, interrupted by many word-finding pauses, and usually dysarthric.

✓ **Brocas:** <u>Broken</u> **Speech**

⇨ **Global Aphasia**

✓ Speech output is nonfluent, and comprehension of spoken language is severely impaired. Naming, repetition, reading, and writing are also impaired.

✓ This syndrome represents the **combined dysfunction of Broca's and Wernicke's areas** and usually results from **strokes that involve the entire middle cerebral artery** distribution in the left hemisphere.

⇨ **Conduction Aphasia**

✓ Speech output is fluent but paraphasic, comprehension of spoken language is intact, and repetition is severely impaired. Naming and writing are also impaired.

⇨ **Anomic Aphasia**

✓ This form of **aphasia** may be considered the "minimal dysfunction" syndrome of the language network. Articulation, comprehension, and repetition are intact, but confrontation naming, word finding, and spelling are impaired.

⇨ **Main Hypothalamic Nuclei and Their Functions:** ⟶

ⓞ	Thirst and water balance➛	Supraoptic nucleus	AIIMS 2004
		Supraoptic nucleus controls <u>ADH secretion</u>.	COMED 2008
ⓞ	Hunger➛	Lateral nucleus	
ⓞ	Satiety	Ventromedial nucleus	DNB 2011
ⓞ	Regulation of Autonomic Nervous system	Anterior Hypothalamus	

⓪ Circadian Rhythm	Suprachiasmatic nucleus
	The suprachiasmatic nuclei, located just above the optic chiasm, are important in regulating circadian rhythms of the body. The pituitary has an intrinsic rhythm of small amplitude with a frequency of every 2 to 10 minutes. Superimposed upon this intrinsic rhythm is that from the pulsatile release of hypophysiotropic releasing factors, with or without the withdrawal of a corresponding inhibitory factor. Rhythms that are shorter than a day are referred to as ultradian rhythms. The next layer of rhythmicity is the circadian rhythm, i.e., rhythms with approximately 24-hour periodicity. These rhythms are usually synchronized with the 24-hour period by a periodic environmental cue, such as the dark-light cycle. The suprachiasmatic nucleus functions as a circadian pacemaker and receives light-induced electrical impulses from the retina via the retinohypothalamic tract, finally transmitting those impulses to the pineal, where they are converted to hormonal signals. DNB 2011
⓪ Heat production	Posterior hypothalamus
⓪ Cooling	Anterior hypothalamus
⓪ Sexual functions	Septate nucleus
⓪ Control of anterior pituitary	By releasing factors
⓪ Control of posterior pituitary	By hormones produced in hypothalamic nuclei

⇨ Functions of Hypothalamus

► Food intake		AIIMS 1995
► Temperature control		
► Hypophyseal control		AI 1997
► Non shivering thermogenesis is because of noradrenaline.		AI 2002
► Non shivering thermogens are secreted by heart, liver small intestine		
► Non shivering thermogenesis is mediated byß 3 receptors.		PGI 2003
► Heat loss depends mostly on environmental temperature.		

⊃ Temperature Regulation: High Yield for AIPGME/AIIMS/PGI 2013

➧ Heat loss from body depends on outside temperature	
➧ Temperature regulation is under hypothalmic control.	
➧ Sweating as a result of exertion is mediated through sympathetic cholinergic fibres.	
➧ Vasodilation is seen as the first response to high temperature.	
➧ Non shivering thermogenesis in adults is due to **norepinephrine** and not brown fat.	AI 2002
➧ Non shivering thermogenesis is mediated through **ß3 receptors.**	PGI 2003

- Piloerection is not significant physiological response to low temperature in humans.thyroxine is important for cold adaptation.   AI 2006
- Shivering is regulated by **Posterolateral hypothalamus**   DPG 2005

⇨ **Ascending tracts of Spinal Cord:**

Situation	Tract	Function
Anterior white funiculus	Anterior spinothalamic tract	"Crude" touch sensation
Lateral white funiculus	Lateral spinothalamic tract	Pain and temperature sensation
	Ventral spino cerebellar tract	Subconscious kinesthetic sensations
	Dorsal spino cerebellar tract	Subconscious kinesthetic sensations
	Spinotectal tract	Concerned with spinovisual reflex
	Fasiculus dorsolateralis	Pain and temperature sensations
	Spinoreticular tract	Conciousness and awareness
	Spinoolivary tract	Proprioception
	Spinovestibular tract	Proprioception
Posterior white funiculus	Fasiculus gracilis Fasciculus cuneatus	✓ Tactile sensation ✓ Tactile localization ✓ Tactile discrimination ✓ "Vibratory" sensation ✓ "Conscious kinesthetic sensation" ✓ "Stereognosis"

⇨ **Descending Tracts of Spinal Cord**

Situation	Tract	Function
Pyramidal tracts	Anterior corticospinal tract Lateral corticospinal tract	▶ Control voluntary, skilled movements✱ ▶ Forms upper motor neurons✱ ▶ Forms pyramids UP 2007
Extra Pyramidal Tracts	Medial longitudinal fasciculus	▶ Coordination of reflex ocular movement ✱ ▶ Integration of movements of eyes and neck
	Anterior vestibulospinal tract	▶ Maintenance of muscle tone and posture✱
	Lateral vestibulospinal tract	▶ Maintenance of position of head and body during acceleration✱
	Reticulospinal tract	▶ Coordination of voluntary and reflex movements.✱ ▶ Control of musicle tone. ▶ Control of respiration and blood vessels.
	Tectospinal tract	▶ Control of movement of head in response to visual and auditory impulses. ✱
	Rubrospinal tract	▶ Facilitatory influence on flexor muscle tone. ✱
	Olivospinal tract	▶ Control of movements due to proprioception. ✱

2

⇨ **The Main Somatosensory Pathways to Consciousness**

Sensation	Receptor	Pathways
Pain and Temperature	Free nerve endings	<u>Lateral</u> spinothalamic, spinal lemniscus
Light touch and pressure	Free nerve endings	<u>Anterior</u> spinothalamic, spinal lemniscus
Discriminative touch, vibratory sense, conscious muscle joint sense	Meissner's corpuscles, pacinian corpuscles, muscle spindles, tendon organs	Fasciculus gracilis and cuneatus Dorsal column medial medial lemniscal pathway

⇨ **Muscle Joint Sense pathways to the Cerebellum**

Sensation	Receptor	Pathways
Unconscious muscle joint sense	muscle spindles, tendon organs, joint receptors	Anterior and posterior spinocerebellar

▶ Main **excitatory neurotransmitter** in CNS is: Glutamate	AIIMS 2004
▶ Main inhibitory neurotransmitter in CNS is GABA	

⇨ **Action of Sympathetic & Parasympathetic Divisions of ANS:**

Effector Organ		Sympathetic Division	Parasympathetic Division
Eye	Ciliary muscle	Relaxation ☛	Contraction
	Pupil	**Dilatation** ☛	Constriction
Lacrimal secretion		Decrease	Increase
Salivary secretion		Decrease in secretion and vasoconstriction	Increase in secretion and vasoconstriction
GIT	Motility	**Inhibition** ☛☛	Acceleration
	Secretion	**Decrease** ☛	Increase
	Sphincters	constriction	Relaxation ☛
Gall bladder		Relaxation	Contraction
Urinary bladder	Detrusor muscle	Relaxation	Contraction
	Internal sphincter	**Constriction**	Relaxation ☛☛
Sweat glands		Increase in secretion ☛	-
Heart rate and force		Increase	Decrease ☛
Blood vessels		Constriction of all blood vessels except those in heart and skeletal muscle	Dilatation
Bronchioles		Dilatation ☛☛	Constriction ☛

PHYSIOLOGY

2

Flight or Fright response is seen in Sympathetic stimulation. Example of seeing a lion and subsequent body respone.

➡ ↑BMR: To run away	
➡ Vasodilation of vessels of heart and skeletal muscle	
➡ Dilatation of Pupils: To increase field of vision to escape Not to Frighten the lion	
➡ Urinary and fecal spincters need to close. No need of micturating/defecating at this stage	
➡ Increase heart rate	UP 2000
➡ Increase blood pressure	UP 2000
➡ Increase total peripheral resistance	UP 2000

➲ Cerebellum High Yield for AIPGME/AIIMS/PGI 2013

➡ Purkinje cells are the **largest neurons** in the body.	
➡ The axons of Purkinje cells are the **only output** from cerebellar cortex and these pass to deep nuclei. **AI 1994**	
➡ From the cerebellar nuclei they project to other parts (Thalamus, Brainstem).	
Layers of Cerebellum	
➡ Molecular layer	
➡ Purkinje Layer	
➡ Granular Layer	
Nuclei of Cerebellum	
➡ Dentate	DELHI 1998
➡ Emboliform	
➡ Globoose	
➡ Fastigial	
Types of Neurons in Cerebellum	
➡ Golgi cells	PGI 2000
➡ Basket cells	
➡ Granule cells	
➡ Stellate cells	
➡ Purkinje cells <u>(end in cerebellar nuclei)</u>	JIPMER 1992

Remember:

➡ The Cerebellum is **not a Sensory Organ**	
➡ Removal of cerebellum does not result in loss of any sensation	
➡ The Cerebellum Is **not a motor Organ**	
➡ Stimulation of cerebellum does not produce movement	
➡ **The function of cerebellum is:**	
➡ It coordinates and smoothens the action of different muscle groups	AIIMS 2004
➡ It times their contraction properly	
➡ In this way it produces smooth and accurate movements	PGI 2004

➲ Diseases of the Cerebellum: High Yield for AIPGME/AIIMS/PGI 2013

➥ Diseases of the cerebellum result in inability to do movements smoothly and accurately. This condition is called **cerebellar ataxia or cerebellar asynergia.**

➥ **Disturbance of Gait:** Gait is similar to that of as drunken person; Lesion in one cerebellar hemisphere results in a tendency to fall towards that side. {Right Side of Body is under control of Right Cerebellar hemisphere}. Lesions of cerebellar ataxia are not corrected by vision.

➥ **Decomposiotion of movements:** A movement is broken into components i.e.: the Shoulder, elbow and the wrists move separately and not in a synchronized way.

➥ **Dysmetria:** Inability to stop a movement at a desired point. ie overshooting, past pointing, etc.

➥ **Dysadiadochokinesia:** Inability to stop one movement and immediately to follow it up with other movement of opposite nature i.e. rapid pronation and supination.

➥ **Scanning speech:** Due to lack of synergy of muscles used in speaking, the spacing of sounds is irregular with pauses at wrong places.

➥ **Hypotonia**

➥ **Decreased tendon reflexes**

➥ **Intention tremor**   JK BOPEE 2011

➥ **Sometimes Nystagmus**

➲ Basal Nuclei or Basal Ganglia

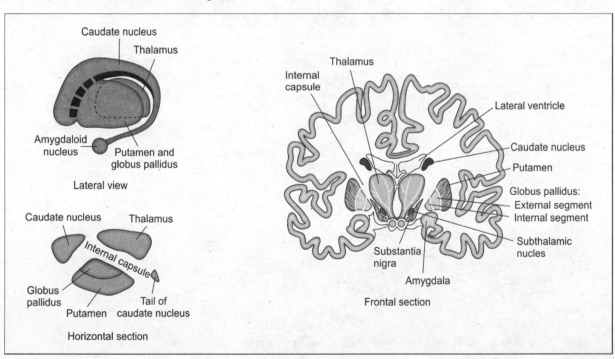

2

- ➡ "sub cortical"
- ➡ "intra cerebral"
- ➡ "grey matter masses"
- ➡ They are concerned with <u>planning and programming of movements</u>.   PGI 2005

They Include:

1. Caudate nucleus + Lentiform nuclei (**Corpus Straitum**)   PGI 2004
2. Amygdaloidal nucleus
3. Claustrum

Functions:

The basal ganglia are concerned with the control of **skilled movements, coordinated movements as well as involuntary movements and regulation of reflex and muscular activity.**   PGI 2002

As a result disease processes effecting basal ganglia can lead to diseases which can be:

More Movements (Hyper kinetic), Less Movement (Hypo kinetic)

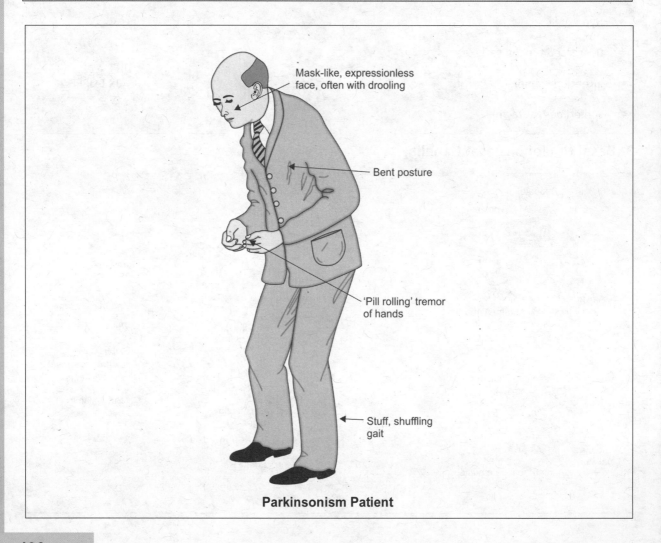

Mask-like, expressionless face, often with drooling

Bent posture

'Pill rolling' tremor of hands

Stuff, shuffling gait

Parkinsonism Patient

(1) **Acalculia:** A selective impairment of mathematical ability

(2) **Achalasia:** Condition in which food accumulates in the esophagus and the organ becomes highly diluted. It is due to increased resting lower oesophageal sphincter tension and incomplete relaxation of this sphincter on swallowing.

(3) **Ageusia:** Absence of the sense of taste

(4) **Agnosia:** Inability to recognize objects by a particular sensory modality even though the sensory modality itself is intact. Lesions producing these defects are generally in the parietal lobe.

(5) **Akinesia:** Difficulty in initiating movements and decreased spontaneous movement.

(6) **Ataxia:** In coordination due to errors in the rate, range, force and direction of movement.

⮑ Superficial Reflexes - Mucus Membrane Reflexes

REFLEX	STIMULUS	RESPONSE	AFFERENT NERVE	CENTER	EFFERENT NERVE
Corneal reflex	Irritation of cornea	Blinking of eye (closure of eyelids)	V Cranial nerve	Pons	VII Cranial nerve
Conjunctival reflex	Irritation of conjunctiva	Blinking of eye	V Cranial nerve	Pons	VII Cranial nerve
Nasal reflex (sneezing reflex)	Irritation of nasal mucus membrane	Sneezing	V Cranial nerve	Motor nucleus of V Cranial nerve	X Cranial nerve and upper cervical nerves
Pharyngeal reflex mucus membrane	Irritation of pharyngeal gagging opening	Retching or of mouth	IX Cranial nerve X Cranial	Nuclei of nerve	X Cranial nerve
Uvular reflex (while talking)	Irritation of uvula	Raising of uvula	IX Cranial nerve X Cranial	Nuclei of nerve	X Cranial nerve

⮑ Superficial Reflexes- Cutaneous Reflexes

REFLEXES	STIMULUS	RESPONSE	CENTER-SEGMENTS of spinal cord involved
Scapular reflex	Irritation of skin at the interscapular space	Contraction of scapular muscles and drawing in of scapula	C_5 to T_1
Upper abdominal reflex	Stroking the abdominal wall below the costal margin	Ipsilateral contraction of abdominal muscle and movement of umbilicus towards the site of stroke	$T_{6,7,8,9}$
Lower abdominal reflex	Stroking the abdominal wall at umbilical and iliac level	Ipsilateral contraction of abdominal muscle and movement of umbilicus towards the site of stroke	$T_{10,11,12}$

REFLEXES	STIMULUS	RESPONSE	CENTER-SEGMENTS of spinal cord involved
Cremasteric reflex	Stroking the skin at upper and inner aspect of thigh	Elevation of testicles	$L_{1,2}$
Gluteal reflex	Stroking the skin over glutei	Contraction of glutei	$L_{4,5} S_{1,2}$
Bulbocavernous reflex	Stroking the dorsum of glans penis	Contraction of bulbocavernous	$S_{3,4}$
Anal reflex	Stroking the perianal region	Contraction of anal sphincter	$S_{4,5}$

➲ Deep Reflexes

REFLEX	STIMULUS	RESPONSE	CENTER-SPINAL SEGMENTS INVOLVED
(1) Jaw Jerk	Tapping the middle of the chin with slightly opened mouth	Closure of mouth	Pons - V Cranial nerve
(2) Biceps Jerk	Percussion of biceps tendon	Flexion of forearm	$C_{5,6}$
(3) Triceps Jerk	Percussion of triceps tendon	Extension of forearm	$C_{6,7,8}$
(4) Supinator Jerk or radial periosteal reflex	Percussion of tendons over distal end (styloid process) of radius	Supination and flexion of forearm	$C_{7,8}$
(5) Wrist tendon or finger flexion reflex	Percussion of wrist tendons	Flexion of corresponding finger	$C_{8,T1}$
(6) Knee Jerk or patellar tendon reflex	Percussion of patellar ligament	Extension of leg	$L_{2,3,4}$
(7) Ankle Jerk or Achilles tendon reflex	Percussion of Achille's tendon	Planter flexion of foot	$L_5 S_1 S_2$

⇨ **Difference between Upper Motor Neuron Lesion and Lower Motor Neuron Lesion:**

POINTS	UMNL	LMNL
* Paralysis.	* Spastic type.	* Flaccid type.
* Tone of muscles.	* Hypertonic ($\uparrow\uparrow$)	* Hypotonic ($\downarrow\downarrow$)
* Muscle wasting.	* Slight.	* Pronounced. **JK BOPEE 2011**
* Reflexes (Deep).	* Hyper-reflexia.	* Hypo-reflexia.
* Superficial reflexes.	* Change.	* no change

➲ Susceptibility of Nerve Fibers: High Yield for AIPGME/AIIMS/PGI 2013

► Pressure	➥ type A
► Hypoxia	➥ type B
► Anesthesia	➥ type C

- Type A α have **largest diameter, Highest conduction velocity, function in Proprioception**
- Type A and B are **Myelinated.**
- Type C has **least diameter, least conduction velocity, unmyelinated.**
- Nerve conduction velocity is more in **upper limbs than in lower limbs.**

⇨ **Blood Brain Barrier: It is formed by**

- Capillary Endothelium.
- Basement Membrane.
- Foot Processes of Astrocytes.

⟳ **Features**

- It is a **selective barrier,** only certain substances can pass across the barrier.
- The permeability of the barrier is **inversely related to the size of the molecules.**
- The permeability of the barrier is **directly related to the lipid solubility** of the substance.
- The barrier is **more permeable to certain substances in the newborn** than in the adults. It is because of the fact that it is under developed in the new born and especially in the preterm fetuses.
- The barrier **undergoes breakdown** in case of direct injury to brain or secondary to toxin/chemical induced damage.
- The **Tight Junction** between the endothelial cells is responsible for the Blood Brain Barrier.
- The Blood Brain Barrier is **deficient at some regions** in the CNS e.g.: in next table

⇨ **Areas Lacking Blood Brain Barrier**

- Area Postrema.
- Organum Vasculosum of the lamina terminalis.
- Subfornical organ.
- The posterior pituitary.

These areas are called as Circum Ventricular Organs

⟳ **Important Molecules: (High Yield for 2011/2012)**

— P53:	▶ Tumor suppressor gene
— bcl$_2$:	▶ Negative regulator of Apoptosis
— fas:	▶ Activator of apoptosis
— c myc:	▶ Transcription factor which commits cells to mitosis
— ras:	▶ G protein. Most commonly mutated gene in Solid Tumors
— Caspaces:	▶ Activates Apoptosis

➲ Changes in Exercise: (High Yield for 2011/2012)

▶ Oxygen uptake	
▶ <u>Right shift</u> of oxygen Hb Dissociation curve	
▶ Ventilation	
▶ CO_2 Excretion	
▶ HR↑	
▶ CO ↑	AIIMS 2007
▶ RR ↑	AI 1998
▶ BP↑	
▶ Blood flow To brain unaltered	AI 2008
▶ Insulin sensitivity	
▶ Causes Hyperkalemia	
▶ Endorphin levels ↑(Relieves depression)	AIIMS 2005

⇨ Changes in Aging

▶ Vital capacity **decreases**	PGI 2001
▶ Glucose tolerance **decreases**	
▶ GFR **decreases**	
▶ Colonic motility **decreases**	
▶ Bone mass **decreases**	
▶ BP **increases**	
▶ Prostate size usually **increases**	
▶ Brain **atrophies**	
▶ Vaginal mucosa **atrophies**	
▶ Haematocrit remains same	AIIMS 1993

➲ Some Laws of Physiology High Yield for AIPGME/AIIMS/PGI 2013

1) **Laplace's Law** For a globular structure, P= 2T/r Where P: transmural force T: wall tension r : radius of the globular structure	PGMCET 2007
2) **Frank- Starling's Law :** The force of contraction is directly proportional to the initial length of muscle fibre.	
3) **All or None Law:** The action potential fails to occur if the stimulus is sub threshold in magnitude, and it occurs with constant amplitude and from regardless of the strength of the stimulus, if the stimulus is at or above threshold intensity.	
4) **Bell- Magendie Law:** In the spinal cord, the **dorsal roots are sensory and the ventral roots are motor.**	

5) **Landsteiner' s Law:**

a) Where an **agglutinogen is present on the membrane of RBC, the corresponding agglutinin must be absent in the plasma of that person.**

b) Where in an individual, the **RBCs are devoid of an agglutinogen, plasma shall contain the corresponding agglutinin.**

6) **Fick's Law**

This law states: $V_g = A/T \times D (P_1 - P_2)$

Where V_g = volume of the gas diffusing through the membrane per min

A = total surface area of alveolo-capillary membrane of the two lungs taken together

T = thickness of alveolo-capillary membrane

D = diffusion constant of the gas

$P_1 - P_2$ = pressure of the gas in the alveoli and within the capillary blood

7) **Dermatomal Rule:** When pain is referred, it is usually to a structure that developed from the same embryonic segment or dermatome as the structure in which the pain originates.

8) **Monro - Kellie Doctrine:** Brain tissue and spinal fluid are essentially incompressible, hence the volume of blood, spinal fluid and brain in the cranium at any time must be relatively constant.

9) **Weber Fechner Law**

It states that the **magnitude of the sensation felt is proportionate to the log of the intensity of the stimulus.**

AI 1997

In other words: $R = KS^A$

Where R = sensation felt

S = intensity of the stimulus and for any specific sensory modality

K and ^{A} = are constants

10) **Law of Projection:** No matter where a particular sensory pathway is stimulated along its course to the cortex, the conscious sensation produced is referred to the location of the receptor. This principle is called Law of Projection

JK BOPEE 2011

Involved in **phantom limb** sensation

AIIMS 2005

11) **Size principle:** In general, **slow muscle units are innervated by small, slowly conducting motor neurons** and fast units by large, rapidly conducting motor neurons.

⇨ **Sites of Important Receptors:**

► Hearing:	✓ Hair cells of <u>organ of Corti</u>.	UP 2008
► <u>Rotational</u> acceleration:	✓ Hair cells of <u>semicircular canals</u>	
► <u>Linear acceleration</u>:	✓ Hair cells of <u>utricle and saccule</u>	UP 2005
► Arterial BP:	✓ <u>Stretch receptors</u> in Carotid sinus/ Aortic arch	
► Arterial PO_2 and PCO_2:	✓ <u>Glomus cells</u> of Aortic and Carotid Bodies	

⇨ **Important Substances**

▶ Bradykinin: stimulation of visceral smooth muscle.		UP 2007
▶ Nitric oxide: vasodilator.		AIIMS 2007
▶ Clathirin: receptor mediated endocytosis.		MAHE 2005

➲ Bradykinin

▶ Are cleaved from plasma precursors by enzymes known as kallikreins;
▶ Bradykinin is potentially significant because of its **potency and the release of kinin-forming enzymes from mast cells**. Septic shock often follows a trimodal pattern of hemodynamic presentation: "warm" shock, "cold" shock, and MOSF.
▶ **Early sepsis** is often associated with a decrease in systemic vascular resistance, due most likely to the release of vasodilatory mediators such as bradykinin and histamine and an increase in cardiac output ("warm" shock). Endotoxin can result in the release of bradykinin via the activation of Factor XII (Hageman factor), kallikrein, and kininogen. Bradykinin is a **potent vasodilator and hypotensive agent**s well as mediator of pain **(algesic agent)**   PGI 2011
▶ It is **cardioprotective**
▶ Vasodilation is mediated by **B2 RECEPTORS**
▶ ACE plays an important role in the degradation of bradykinin and the neuropeptide substance P, and these mediators may be important in forming angioedema.

Chaperones and enzymes involved in folding of proteins at rough ER:

✓ **Bip (immunoglobulin heavy chain binding protein)**
✓ **GRP 94 (Glucose regulated protein)**
✓ **Calnexin**
✓ **PDI (Protein disulfide isomerase)**
✓ **PPI (Peptidyl-proly cis-tras isomerase)**

➲ Chaperones: (High Yield for 2011/2012)

➡ Present in wide range from bacteria to human.
➡ So called **heat shock proteins.**
➡ Facilitate and favour the interactions in the polypeptide chain to finally give the specific conformation of a protein.
➡ Cause **proper folding of proteins.**
➡ They are **inducible.**
➡ Bind to hydrophobic regions of unfolded protein and aggregates protein.
➡ Most of them are associated with ATPase activity.
➡ Found in **cytosol, mitochondria and ER.**

➲ Neuropeptide Y. (High Yield for 2011/2012)

- It is a **polypeptide containing 36 amino acid residues** that is closely related to pancreatic polypeptide.
- It is present in many parts of the brain and the autonomic nervous system. In the autonomic nervous system, although not in the brain, much of it is locatedin noradrenergic neurons, from which it is released by high-frequency stimulation.
- It augments the vasoconstrictor effects of norepinephrine.
- Circulating neuropeptide Y from sympathetic nerves increases with severe exercise in humans. In the hypothalamus, **it mediates increased appetite and increases in food intake.**
- Y1, Y2, Y4, Y5, and Y6 receptors for this polypeptide have been cloned.

⇨ Ubiquitin

- Ubiquitin is "itself a protein" that "degrades other proteins". i.e "unfriendly" for proteins. ☛☛
- It is a "highly conserved "protein.☛☛
- Degradation by Ubiquitin occurs in "Proteosomes" by a process which is "ATP dependent".☛☛
- Before degradation proteins are bound to binding proteins.
- Ubiquitin tags proteins for degradation.☛

⇨ Sirtuins

Are proteins that keep cells alive and healthy in the face of stress by coordinating avariety of hormonal networks, regulatory proteins and other genes. Sirtuins bring about the effects of calorie restriction on a brain system, known as the somatotropic signaling axis, that controls growth and influences. The sirtuins are a highly conserved family of NAD+-dependent enzymes that regulate lifespan in lower organisms. Recently, the mammalian sirtuins have been connected to an everwidening circle of activities that encompass cellular stress resistance, genomic stability, tumorigenesis and energy metabolism.   MAH 2012

➲ Important Questions Lately Asked

Non respiratory function of lung is SODIUM EXCHANGE.	AI 2010
BMR is closely dependent on lean body mass	AI 2010
BMR is low in obesity	AI 2010
Maximum absorption of water in gut occurs in jejunum	AI 2010
Hot water bag use in colic of intestines works by inhibiting adrenergic receptors	AI 2010
Epinephrine decreases insulin secretion	AI 2010
Nitric oxide acts on GIT primarily by smooth muscle relaxant action	AI 2010
In standing position venous return is effected by deep fascia and calf muscles	AI 2010
Cortical representation of body in cerebrum is "vertical"	AIIMS 2009
Capacitation of sperms occurs in "uterus".	
Muscle spindle detects muscle "length".	AIIMS 2009

PHYSIOLOGY

2

- ❑ Function of **spino cerebellar tract** is "smoothening and coordinating movements".   AIIMS 2009
- ❑ Maximum "**potassium**" **ion secretion** occurs in which body fluid: saliva   AIIMS 2009
- ❑ "**Circadian rhythm**" is controlled by "Suprachiasmatic nucleus".   AIIMS 2008
- ❑ **Mean circulatory pressure** is arterial pressure taken at a point when heart stops beating.   AIIMS 2008
- ❑ **Mineralocorticoids receptors** are present at: hippocampus, colon, kidney   AIIMS 2008
- ❑ **Weber Feschner law** is magnitude of stimulus strength perceived is α log of intensity of stimulus strength.   AIIMS 2008
- ❑ **Maximum post prandial motility** is seen in "descending colon"   AIIMS 2008

NOTES

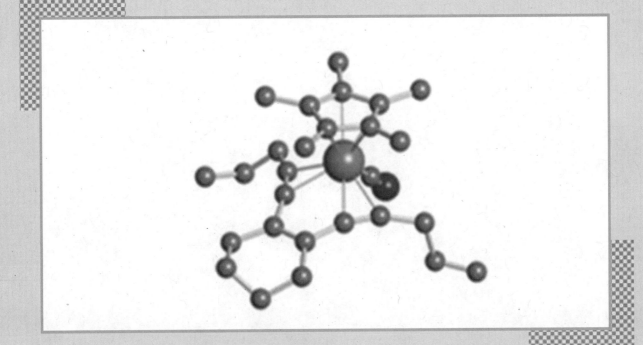

BIOCHEMISTRY

⟳ Important Points about DNA (Repeated in AIPGME, PGI)

Deoxyribonucleic acid (DNA) is the "hereditary material" of the cell.

▶ DNA consists of two strands of nucleotides wrapped around each other to form a complex **double helix** ☞☞

▶ The building blocks of each strand are deoxyribonucleotides, which consist of one of four bases—

▶ Adenine **(A)**, guanine **(G)**, cytosine **(C)**, and thymine **(T)**—a sugar-deoxyribose, and a covalently joined phosphate group☞☞.   **PGI 2004**

▶ The deoxyribose molecules are linked by phosphates to form the backbone of DNA.

▶ The **double helix** is held together by the <u>hydrogen bonds</u> that form between the bases on the two complementary strands oriented in antiparallel directions. ☞☞   **AIIMS 1992**

▶ RNA is similar to DNA except that the **deoxyribose sugar of DNA is replaced by a ribose moiety** in RNA, and **instead of Thymine T**, RNA **uracil (U) is present.**☞☞

▶ Bases are <u>perpendicular</u> to DNA.   **PGI 2006**

▶ **"Transcription"** results in the production of a **precursor messenger RNA (pre-mRNA)** that contains both intron and exon sequences. ✳

▶ The **"introns" are excised.**✳✳   **AI 2004**

▶ Exons are ligated together in a two-stage splicing process that results in a mature mRNA that can be exported from the nucleus and translated to produce the desired protein. ☞

▶ While still in the nucleus, the spliced mRNA undergoes further processing.

▶ <u>The 5' end</u> of the RNA is capped by a **guanosine** derivative✳,

▶ A string of adenylic acid residues **(polyA) is added to its** <u>3' end</u> to stabilize the transcript for transit within the cellular environment.☞☞

▶ **Watson and Crick theory** pertains to **DNA.**   **PGI 2005**

▶ **Human genome contains** <u>3×10^9 base pairs</u>.   **UP 2007**

▶ <u>Histones</u> are proteins present in DNA.   **UP 2007**

▶ New DNA synthesis occurs in <u>interphase</u>   **SGPI 2005**

▶ <u>B DNA</u> is the predominant form seen.

▶ DNA is negatively charged at physiological pH.

<u>"CIRCULAR" DNA:</u>

Found in:

- ❏ Virus   **PGI 2011**
- ❏ Bacteria
- ❏ Chloroplast   **PGI 2011**
- ❏ Mitochondria   **PGI 2011**

Histones:

— Nucleosomes are separated by spacer DNA to which histone, H1 is attached.

— Histones "are highly conserved and can be grouped into five major classes: H1/H5, H2A, H2B, H3, and H4". These are organized into two super-classes as follows:

— core histones – H2A, H2B, H3 and H4

— linker histones – H1 and H5

The linker histone H1 binds the nucleosome and the entry and exit sites of the DNA, thus locking the DNA into place and allowing the formation of higher order structure.

⇨ **Enhancers** PGI 2011

▶ Tissue and developmental activation of individual globin genes depends in part upon short DNA sequences called enhancers. These are located in the 5′ and 3′ flanking sequences and possibly in the introns of the genes. An important enhancer activating the entire non-a gene complex (called the locus control region [LCR]) has been tentatively identified several thousand bases upstream of the e gene.

▶ These regulatory DNA sequences are called cis acting elements. They achieve their biologic effects via their interaction with trans acting factors, i.e., nuclear DNA binding proteins that specifically bind to these sequences, thereby promoting or inhibiting transcription.

▶ Several "transcription factors" have been found to bind the globin gene promoters and enhancers. Many of these protein factors appear to be nonspecific in that they can activate a number of genes in many tissues if they gain access to their binding sites.

⊃ **Bases in DNA**

➥ Purines contain "two rings" in their structure☛☛

➥ Pyrimidines contain "only one ring".☛

▶ Between A and T: 2 double bonds

▶ Between G and C: 3 double bonds

▶ Thermostability depends on GC bonds

▶ Purines = Pyrimidines (Chargaffs rule)

⊃ **Remember: Important Points Likely to be asked**

High Yield for AIPGME/AIIMS/PGI 2013

— Most DNA occurs as "Right Handed" Double Helical called "B DNA."☛☛

— "Rare" "Left Handed" Double Helical called "Z DNA".☛☛

— "Negative" super coiling occurs if DNA is wound loosely.☛☛

— "Positive" super coiling occurs if DNA is wound tightly.☛☛

— Topoisomerases are enzymes that change amount of supercoiling in DNA molecules.

— DNA Topoisomerase II can induce negative supercoiling or Remove Positive super coils ☛✳

— DNA Topoisomerase I can relax supercoiling.☛

Heterochromatin	Euochromatin
✓ Highly condensed	✓ Loosely condensed
✓ Inactive	✓ Active

▶ **Prokaryotes** have **single origin** of Replication.

▶ **Eukaryotes** have **multiple origin** of Replication.

— New synthesized strand is <u>made</u> in 5'→3' direction.☞☞   PGI 2003

— Template is <u>scanned</u> in 3'→5'direction.☞☞

— New synthesized strand is **complimentary and antiparallel.**☞

— **Daunorubicin** and **Doxorubicin** exert their effect by intercalating between bases of DNA and thereby interfering with activity of **Topoisomerase II**☞

— **Cisplatin** on the other hand binds tightly to DNA causing **structural Distortion.**☞

➲ Important Points about DNA and RNA (Memorize Keenly)

DNA Repair: Single strand✱	▶ Single strand, excision-repair-specific glycosylase <u>recognizes and removes damaged base.</u> ▶ Endonuclease <u>makes a break several bases to the 5' side.</u> ▶ Exonuclease <u>removes short stretch of nucleotides</u>. DNA polymerase <u>fills gap</u>. ▶ DNA ligase <u>seals.</u>
DNA/RNA/protein synthesis direction	▶ DNA and RNA are **both synthesized in 5'→3'** direction. ▶ Protein synthesis also proceeds in the **5'→ 3'** direction.
Types of RNA✱	▶ mRNA is **largest** type of RNA. ▶ rRNA is the **most abundant** type of RNA. ▶ tRNA is the **smallest** type of RNA.

Polymerases: RNA✱	**Eukaryotes:** ▶ **RNA polymerase I** make **rRNA.** ▶ **RNA polymerase II** makes **mNA.** ▶ **RNA polymerase III** makes **t RNA.** ▶ No proofreading function. RNA polymerase II opens DNA at promoter site (A-T-rich upstream sequence-TATA and CAAT). ▶ α-amanitin inhibits RNA polymerase II. **Prokaryotes:** ▶ RNA polymerase makes all three kinds of RNA.
Start and Stop codons✱ AIIMS 1982	▶ AUG (or rarely GUG) is the **initiation codon.** JK BOPEE 2012 ▶ AUG codes for methionine, which may be removed before translation is completed. In prokaryotes the initial AUG codes for a formyl-methionine (f-met).

cont...

cont...

	► Stop codons:
	   ✓ UGA,
	   ✓ UAA,
	   ✓ UAG.

"Promoter" ✱ "Enhancer "✱	► <u>Site</u> where RNA polymerase and multiple other transcription factors bind to DNA upstream from gene locus. ► <u>Stretch of DNA</u> that alters gene expression by binding transcription factors. ► May be close to, far from, or even within (in an intron) the gene whose expression it regulates.

Remember:

Methionine having anticodon UAC is the first amino acid required in binding to the initiation codon AUG on m-RNA. In bacteria and in mitochondria the initiator t-RNA carried an N-formylated methionine but in eukaryotes the methionine is not formylated.

➲ (t RNA Special Features)

►	Anticodon is present in <u>t RNA</u>.	
►	Abnormal purines can be present on <u>t RNA</u>.	AI 2001
►	Thymidilated RNA is present on <u>t RNA.</u>	
►	Modified bases are present on <u>t RNA</u>.	AI 2006
►	Clover leaf pattern is seen in <u>t RNA</u>.	

►	<u>CISTRON</u> is the smallest fundamental unit coding for DNA synthesis.	PGI 2006
►	<u>Leucine zipper complex</u> is a DNA binding protein.	
►	<u>Zinc</u> regulates binding of proteins to DNA.	
►	<u>ZINC finger</u> is a nuclear receptor and steroids bind to it.	AIIMS 2006

➲ DNA Replication: (High Yield for 2011/2012)

►	Okazaki fragments are <u>DNA fragments with RNA head</u>.	APPG 2006
►	Okazaki fragments are <u>formed during replication</u>.	PGMCET 2007
►	Okazaki fragments are <u>involved in DNA replication</u>.	AI 1996
►	DNA replication proceeds in one direction.	PGI 2011
►	Microsatellite sequence is <u>short sequence repeat DNA</u>.	AI 2006
►	Proteins binding to DNA contain zinc.	AI 1997
►	Protein synthesis occurs mainly in <u>ribosomes.</u>	CUPGEE 1996

⇨ **Functions of Different Types of DNA Polymerases in Eukaryotes**

In Eukaryotes	
➡ DNA Polymerase δ synthesizes **leading** strand CONTINUOUSLY	PGI 2011
➡ DNA Polymerase α synthesizes **lagging** strand ☞	
➡ DNA Polymerase γ replicates **mitochondrial DNA** ☞	
➡ DNA Polymerase β	
➡ DNA polymerase ε participate in **DNA Repair.** ☞	

Functions of Different Enzymes. Kindly don't take any examination without remembering this table

➲ **High Yield for AIPGME/AIIMS/PGI 2013**

Site	Prokaryotic	Eukaryotic
Recognition of origin of replication	DNA A Protein	
Unwinding of DNA Helix	Helicase AIIMS 1997	▶ Helicase DNB 2011
Stabilization of unwound Template strand	Single stranded binding protein(SSB)	▶ Single stranded binding protein(SSB)
Synthesis of RNA Primers	Primase	▶ Primase
Synthesis of DNA		
Leading strand+ Proof reading.	DNA Polymerase III	▶ DNA Polymerase δ
Lagging strand	DNA Polymerase III	▶ DNA Polymerase α
Removal of RNA Primers	DNA Polymerase I	
Joining of Okazaki Fragments	DNA ligase	▶ DNA ligase MAH 2012
Removal of <u>Positive super coils</u>	DNA Topoisomerase II (DNA gyrase)	▶ DNA Topoisomerase II

Remember important points in Protein synthesis:

➲ **Steps of Protein Synthesis (High Yield for 2011/2012)**

➡ **Activation of amino acids.**
➡ **Initiation**
➡ **Elongation**
➡ **Termination**

▶ RNA contains **Ribose** instead of Deoxyribose and **uracil** instead of thymine. ☞☞
▶ Most RNAS exist as **single stranded** structures. ☞
▶ rRNA is the **"most common"**/Abundant type. It is a structural component of Ribosomes ☞
▶ tRNA is the **"smallest"**type. It functions to <u>transport amino acids to ribosomes</u> ☞
▶ mRNA is the most **"heterogeneous"** type. <u>Carries information specifying amino acid sequence of protein to ribosomes</u> ☞
▶ Prokaryotic RNA is 70 S(30S and 50S) ☞

BIOCHEMISTRY

3

► 5O S is further subdivided into: 23S and 5S.	PGI 2011
► Eukaryotic RNA is **80S** (40S AND 60S)	
► "Ribozymes" <u>not ribosomes</u> are RNA molecules with enzymatic activity.✱✱	
► <u>Fidelty enzyme</u> in protein synthesis is amino acyl t RNA synthetase.	AI 1998
► <u>Sn RNP</u> processes RNA.	ICS 1998
► <u>AMBER codon</u> is termination codon.	AIIMS 2001
► <u>Chaperones</u> function in protein folding	AI 2003

⇨ **Important Difference in Prokaryotes and Eukaryotes Regarding Protein Synthesis are**

✱ Prokaryotic mRNAs are **polycistronic** i.e. with several coding regions with its own initiation codon. It can produce separate species of polypeptide while eukaryotic mRNA is **monocistronic** i.e. codes for only one polypeptide chain.

✱ The **releasing factors** utilized in termination are 3 in prokaryotes RF-1, RF-2 & RF-3 while in eukaryotes it is only one- eRF.

✱ In prokaryotes three **initiation factors** are known (IF-1, IF-2 & IF-3) whereas in eukaryotes there are at least 10.

⊃ **RNA: High Yield for AIPGME/AIIMS/PGI 2013**

► RNA contains **Ribose** instead of Deoxyribose and **uracil** instead of thymine.	
► Most RNAS exist as **single strand**ed structures.	
► rRNA is the "**most common**"/Abundant type. **It is a structural component of Ribosomes**	
► tRNA is the "**smallest**"type. It functions to transport amino acids to ribosomes	
► tRNA has abnormal purine bases	AI 2001
► tRNA has the highest percentage of modified base	AI 2002
► mRNA is the most "**heterogeneous**" type. Carries information specifying amino acid sequence of protein to ribosomes	
► Prokaryotic RNA is **70 S**(30S and 50S)	UPSC 2003
► Eukaryotic RNA is **80S**(40S AND 60S)	
► Normal role of Micro RNA is: **Gene Regulation**	AI 2009
► Splicing Activity is a function of: **sn RNA**	AI 2009
► The sigma (σ) subunit of prokaryotic RNA polymerase: **Specifically recognizes the promoter site.**	AI 2003

⇨ **RNA Polymerase**

► In bacteria <u>RNA polymerase</u> synthesizes almost all of the RNA.
► RNA polymerase is a <u>multi subunit enzyme.</u>
► One component of RNA polymerase is <u>the sigma subunit</u> "which enables RNA Polymerase to recognize **promoter regions** on the DNA".
► Other component is "<u>the rho factor or termination factor</u>" which enables RNA Polymerase to recognize **termination regions** on the DNA.

3

➲ **Mitochondrial DNA**

⇨ **AIIMS/PGI Favourite**

▶ Thirteen out of 100 polypeptides required for oxidative phosphorylation are coded by mitochondrial DNA.

▶ Defects in **oxidative phosphorylation** are most likely as a result of alterations in mt DNA as it has a **mutation rate about ten times greater** than nuclear DNA."☞   **PGI 2011**

▶ MATERNALLY inherited   **PGI 2011**

▶ This is because there are no introns and a mutation invariably strikes a coding sequence (axon)."☞☞

▶ Tissues with **greatest ATP requirement** (CNS, Skeletal muscle, Heart muscle, Kidney, Liver) are most affected.

▶ Mitochondrial DNA is **maternally inherited** because mitochondria from sperms do not enter the fertilized egg.

▶ Mitochondrial DNA is Closed and **circular** and 16.5 kb in length.   **AI 2006**

▶ **MELAS** (Mitochondrial Encephalopathy, Lactic Acidosis and Stroke like episodes) are attributed to Mitochondrial mutations.

Other diseases associated with mt DNA are:

— Lebers Hereditary Optic Neuropathy ☞☞☞

— MELAS (mitochondrial encephalopathy with lactic acidosis and stroke like episodes)   **DNB 2001**

— Myopathy✳

— MERRF Syndrome: (myoclonic epilepsy and ragged red fibres)   **PGI 2006**

— Cardiomyopathy

— Strokes

— Lactic acidosis

— External Opthalmoplegia☞☞

— Optic atrophy☞☞

— NARP (Neuropathy, ataxia and retinitis pigmentosa)

— Pearsons syndrome

— Sensorineural deafness

— Diabetes mellitus

❑ **A DNA:**
  ✓ right handed helix.
  ✓ has 4 base pairs per turn.

❑ **B DNA:**
  ✓ 10 base pairs per turn.
  ✓ most common type, right handed

❑ **Z DNA:**
  ✓ left handed helix.
  ✓ has 12 bases per turn. z refers to zigma fashion of its poly nucleotide.

▶ <u>GENOME</u>: total genetic information in a cell.

▶ <u>HUMAN GENOME</u>: genetic information present in a single set of 23 chromosomes.

▶ <u>HUMAN GENOME PROJECT</u>: identification of all genes in human DNA ,determine base sequences that make DNA

⇨ **Transposons**   **JK BOPEE 2004/2003**

▶ Are **pieces of DNA** that move readily from the one site to another either within or between the DNA's of bacteria, plasmids and bacteriophages.

▶ They are also known as **"jumping Genes"**.   **COMED 2005**

▶ They can **code for:**

— drug resistance,

— enzyme,

— toxin or a variety of metabolic enzymes

▶ They can either cause mutation in the gene into which they insert or alter the expression of nearby genes.

▶ In contrast to plasmids or bacterial viruses, transposons **are not capable of independent replication.**

▶ They **replicate as a part of recipient DNA.**

⮑ **Bacteriophages: High Yield for AIPGME/AIIMS/PGI 2013**

➡ Bacteriphages are **viruses that infect bacteria.**

➡ Bacteriophages resemble most viruses in having a **protein coat called a capsid** that surrounds a molecule of DNA or RNA.

➡ Typical phages have **hollow heads**. The fibres have the ability to bind to specific molecules on the bacterial cell surface.

➡ When a phage binds to bacterial cell surface it is called **adsorption**. The phage then undergoes penetration, in which the viral DNA is injected through the tail into the host.

There are two types of phages

✳ **Lytic or virulent phages**

✳ **Temperate/Prophages**

Lytic or virulent phages

✳ Lytic phages **multiply inside the cell and release a burst of phages through the membrane, lysing the cell.**

Prophages or temperate phages

✓ Prophages or temperate phages on the other hand **do not immediately lyse the bacteria they infect. Instead, they integrate their DNA into host DNA creating a phage.**

Transduction:

➾ Transduction occurs when bacteriophage carries a piece of bacterial DNA from one bacterium to another.

➾ Transduction is not only confined to transfer of chromosomal DNA, episomes and plasmid may also be transduced. Just as there are two types of phages, there are two types of transduction.

➾ Lytic phages cause **generalized transduction.**

➾ Temperate phages cause **specialized transduction.**

➲ Medically Important Enzymes Frequently Asked ☞

Reverse Transcriptase:👈👈👈   PGI 2003

➡ Is an <u>RNA dependent DNA Polymerase</u>   PGI 2011

➡ <u>Requires an RNA Template</u> to direct the synthesis of new DNA.✶✶

➡ AZT, ddC, ddI **(Antiretrovirals)** act on reverse transcriptase.

▶ **HIV-1 is** a single-stranded plus-sense RNA virus. The RNA-dependent DNA polymerase, or reverse transcriptase, is packaged within the virion core and is responsible for replicating the single-stranded RNA genome through a double-stranded DNA intermediate, which in turn serves as the precursor molecule for proviral integration within the host cell genome. The reverse transcriptase of HIV-1 is a magnesium-requiring RNA-dependent DNA polymerase responsible for replicating the RNA viral genome. Agents that block such steps (including reverse transcriptase inhibitors) can prevent cells from being newly infected.

▶ **The hepatitis B virus core** consists of a nucleocapsid formed of aggregated hepatitis B core protein (HBcAg) dimers, containing incompletely double-stranded circular DNA, and the DNA polymerase/reverse transcriptase.

▶ **The initial step in the life cycle of HTLV is** attachment of the virus envelope glycoprotein to an unknown cell surface receptor, which results in preferential infection of CD4, T-helper cells, for HTLV-I, and CD8 cells for HTLV-II. Following uptake and uncoating, viral RNA is transcribed by reverse transcriptase, an RNA-dependent DNA polymerase complexed to the RNA in the core of the virus particle, into double-stranded DNA. This double-stranded viral DNA is integrated into the host cell nucleus by the virally encoded integrase, resulting in cell infection that may be lifelong.

Restriction endonucleases 👈👈   AIPGME 2012

➡ Are <u>Bacterial enzymes that cleave double stranded DNA</u> into smaller fragments.✶✶

➡ Each enzyme cleaves DNA at a specific 4-6 base long nucleotide sequence producing DNA segments called **"restriction fragments".**

➡ These enzymes form either **sticky ends or blunt ends** on the DNA.

➡ The DNA sequence recognized by a restriction enzyme is called a **restriction site.**

Telomerase

Is an enzyme that completes replication of Telomers. 👈👈👈

☐ **Telomeres** are <u>repetitive sequences at ends</u> of DNA✶

☐ <u>Telomerase</u> is present in **embryonic cells, stem cells and cancer cells.**✶

❏ DNA polymerase is **unable to replicate the end of a DNA chain** completely, resulting in loss of DNA with each replication. This problem has been solved by a mechanism that replicates **tandem repeats of a six-nucleotide sequence (GGGTTA) to the ends of each chromosome.** These repeated sequences are called **telomeres** and are replicated through an <u>RNA-dependent DNA polymerase called telomerase.</u> ✱

❏ **Normal somatic cells do not express telomerase**, and the replicative lifetime of such cells is limited to approximately 30 cell divisions due to the progressive loss of telomere repeats; the limit imposed on somatic cell division is called the <u>Hayflick limit</u>✱✱✱, at which time replicative senescence occurs.

◉ **Germ cells express telomerase** and have a long (possibly unlimited) replicative lifetime.   PGI

◉ **Cancer cells express telomerase** and in cancer cells is thought to be a component of the neoplastic process, assuring that the cell will be able to undergo many divisions without inducing senescence or genetic catastrophe. Inhibition of **telomerase** activity in cancer cells could have antitumor effects.   PGI

◉ **Human pluripotential stem cells** express high levels of **telomerase**, an enzyme that is essential for allowing repeated replication of the ends of eukaryotic chromosomes.   PGI

❏ **The capacity to divide indefinitely** is provided by activation of **telomerase,**✱✱ which allows continued replication of chromosomes by addressing the unique need of chromosome ends to be continually renewed to a proper length to allow normal mitosis.

❏ **The capacity to invade and metastasize** is conveyed by elaboration of **matrix metalloproteases and plasminogen activators**✱✱ and the capacity to recruit host stromal cells at the site of invasion through tumor-induced angiogenesis.

➲ Prions: High Yield for AIPGME/AIIMS/PGI 2013

Prions are proteins which are normally found in the body. Prions become infectious or pathogenic due to misfolding of the proteins.

❏ Prions are **normally present in human.** The prion protein, endogenous to the human is PrP (which is a glycoprotein rich in β sheets).

❏ **PrPsc is the infectious form of the Prion.** (It is formed due to mutation in PrP)

❏ The key to becoming infectious lies in changes in **three dimensional conformation of PrP** i.e. there is abnormality in protein folding (the α helical secondary structure of PrP changes to β sheets in PrPsc).

❏ So, **PrPsc is a misfolded PrP** and this conformational difference cause PrPsc to resist proteolytic degradation.

❏ **Misfolded proteins are quite dangerous for the body because they possess a remarkable property that they can cause other normally folded prions to distort into the same misfolded state.** Thus misfolded proteins i.e. prions are able to replicate and spread throughout tissue without using either DNA or RNA.

❏ The infective agent is thus an **altered version of a normal protein which acts as a template** for converting more normal protein to the pathogenic conformation.

⇨ **Carbonic Anhydrase**

Is the fastest acting enzyme.
Inhibitors Include:
* Acetazolamide
* Dichlorphenamide
* Methazolamide
CA inhibitors are used as
➡ Antiglaucoma agent
➡ Altitude sickness.
➡ Antiparalytic (familial periodic paralysis.)
➡ Diuretic, urinary alkalinizing
➡ Antiurolithic (uric acid calculi; cystine calculi

⊃ **Defects in DNA Repair: High Yield for AIPGME/AIIMS/PGI 2013**

Xeroderma Pigmentosa✶✶	
❏ Extreme <u>UV</u> sensitivity☞☞	
❏ DNA <u>polymerase I</u> defective.	**AI 2004**
❏ Exposure of cell to UV light can result in the covalent joining of two adjacent **pyrimidines (Usually Thymines) producing a dimer.**	**AI 2000**
❏ **Nucleotide excision repair defect is a feature.**	**AIIMS 2005**
❏ These Thymine dimmers prevent DNA polymerase from replicating the DNA strands.	
❏ Pyrimidine dimmers can be formed in the skin cells of humans exposed to **"unfiltered sunlight"**.	
❏ In Xeroderma Pigmentosa, **"the cells can't repair the damaged DNA"**, resulting in accumulation of mutations and skin cancers.	
❏ The disease is produced by absence of enzyme **UV specific Exinuclease/Endonuclease"**.	
⓪ **Excessive freckling** ✶✶	
⓪ **Multiple skin cancers**✶	
⓪ **Corneal ulcers**☞☞	

Hereditary Non Polyposis Colorectal Cancer(Lynch Syndrome)✶✶
It results from mutations in genes **(hMlh2/hMsh2)** encoding enzymes that carry out DNA mismatch repair.

⊃ **Genetic Code**

➡ Each codon has **three bases.**✶✶	
➡ There are **64 codons** written in 5'→3' direction.✶	
➡ Code is "unambiguous" (<u>Each codon specifies no more than one amino acid</u>).✶	**TN 1995**
➡ Code is "degenerate". (<u>More than one codon can specify a single amino acid</u>).✶	**AIIMS 2006**
➡ Code is "universal"(Same in all organisms)✶	
➡ Code is **comma less.**✶	

⇨ **Mutations**

➡ Transistion: A point mutation that replaces <u>purine-pyrimidine base pair with different purine-pyrimidine</u> base pair.➤➤

➡ Transversion: A point mutation that replaces <u>purine-pyrimidine base pair with different pyrimidine-purine</u> base pair.➤➤

⇨ **Kindly Understand this Table**

Mutation		Effect on Protein
▶ Silent:	New codon specifies "**same**" amino acid	None
▶ Missense:	New codon specifies "**new**" amino acid	Decrease in function
▶ Non sense:	New codon is "**Stop**" codon	usually non functional ICS 1998
▶ Frameshift:	Deletion/addition of base	usually non functional

⇨ **Disorders of Collagen Synthesis**

▶ Scurvy	▶ Deficent hydroxylation secondary to **Ascorbate deficency**
▶ Osteogenesis imperfecta	▶ Mutations in collagen genes
▶ Ehler Danhlos syndrome	▶ Mutations in **collagen genes, Lysine and Hydroxylase** genes
▶ Menkes disease	▶ Deficent cross linking secondary to **Cu deficency**

⇨ **The Collagens: High Yield for AIPGME/AIIMS/PGI 2013**

✓ Are a large group of <u>triple-helix</u> structural matrix proteins.	PGI 2011
✓ <u>Have glycine residues</u> at every third position.	PGI 2011
✓ <u>Vitamin c</u> is needed for post translational modification.	PGI 2011
✓ <u>Type I collagen</u> is the major structural component of bones, skin, and tendons.	
✓ <u>Type II</u> is found predominantly in cartilage.	
✓ Type III is found in association with Type I, although the ratio varies in different tissues.	
✓ Type IV collagen is found in basement membranes in association with mucopolysaccharides and laminin, whereas.	
✓ Type V is found in the cornea in association with Type III and is important in maintaining transparency.	

⇨ **Scurvy (Biochemical Basis) (High Yield for 2011-2012)**

➡ Hydroxylation of proline residues requires the presence of vitamin C.

➡ In individuals who suffer from a deficiency of this vitamin, **the a-chains of the tropocollagen molecules are unable to form stable helices, and the tropocollagen molecules are incapable of aggregating into fibrils.**

➡ This condition, known as scurvy, first affects **connective tissues with high turnover of collagen, such as** periodontal ligament and gingival.

- Because these two structures are responsible for maintaining teeth in their sockets, the symptoms of scurvy include bleeding gums and loose teeth. If the vitamin C deficiency is prolonged, other sites are also affected.

- These symptoms may be alleviated by eating foods rich in vitamin C.

- **Hunters glossitis or Moellers glossitis** is due to deficiency of: Vitamn B12
- **Median rhomboid glossitis:** absence of filliform pappliae
- **Raw beefy tongue** is due to niacin deficiency
- **Woody legs** are due to viamin c deficiency
- **Cork screw hair pattern** is due to vitamin c deficiency
- **Leutic glossitis:** feature of syphilis
- **Encephalomalacia** can occur due to vitamin E deficiency

⇨ **Mutation is Detected by**

▶ Single strand confirmational polymorphism.   AI 2002
▶ PCR
▶ DNA sequencing.

⊃ **Elastin: High Yield for AIPGME/AIIMS/PGI 2013**

- Elastin is a **connective tissue protein** with elastic or rubber like properties.
- Elastic fibres are found in **lungs, walls of large arteries and elastic ligaments.**
- Elastin is synthesized from **tropoelastins** which is rich in "**proline and lysine**".
- In the **extra cellular matrix** tropoelastins is converted to elastin.
- In elastin **three allysyl side chains** plus **one lysyl side chain** form the Desmosine cross links unique to Elastin in extracellular matrix.   JK BOPEE
- Alpha 1 antitrypsin **prevents** elastin degradation.
- **Deficiency** of Alpha 1 antitrypsin can cause **emphysema.**   AIIMS 2000

- ✳✳✳Desmosine, the intermolecular and intramolecular cross link between the chains of elastin polypeptide, may be useful as a **marker of a lung injury in adult respiratory distress syndrome (ARDS). Higher urine desmosine levels are associated with mortality in patients with acute lung injury.**Desmosine is not metabolically absorbed, reused, or catabolized by the body, but rather **eliminated unchanged in the urine** as low molecular weight peptides. The lung is relatively rich in elastin, a timed collection could be used as an index of elastin degradation in vivo. Ref: Am. J. Physiol. Lung Cell. Mol. Physiol. October 1, 2006 291:L566-L571

⇨ **Diagnostic Techniques (Updated)**

Blot type	Material Analyzed
▶ Southern blot	— DNA
▶ ASO titer	— DNA
▶ Northern blot	— RNA AI 2007

▶ Microarray	— RNA or c DNA	
	— Detects genetic transfer of disease	AI 2010
▶ Western blot	— Protein	
▶ ELISA	— Protein/ antibodies	
▶ Proteomics	— Proteins	
▶ Dot Blot✷✷	— DNA, RNA or Protein	
▶ FISH	— Rapid method of chromosome identification.	AIIMS 2007, AI 2010
▶ RFLP	Detects	
	— Mutation	
	— Repeat trinucleotide patterns	
	— Deletions	
	— Chromosome structure	
	— Measuring long DNA molecules	
Linkage analysis	— Detects DNA polymorphisms in a family	
RT PCR	— Detects haemophilia	

❑ Genomics: study of structure of genes and their products.	PGI 2005
❑ Proteomics: Study of all proteins expressed in a genome, including their abundance, distribution, post translational modification, function and interaction with other molecules.	AI 2007
❑ DNA library: Collection of "cloned restriction fragments" of DNA of an organism	
❑ Genomic library: is a collection of "fragments of double stranded" DNA obtained by digestion of total DNA of an organism with restriction endonucleases and subsequent ligation to appropriate vector.	
❑ Probe: is a single stranded piece of DNA usually labeled with radio isotope that has nucleotide sequence complimentary to DNA molecule of interest.	
❑ Nucteotide sequence of a probe is complimentary to DNA of interest called Target DNA	
❑ Vector is a molecule of DNA to which fragment of DNA to be joined is attached.	

➲ Polymerase Chain Reaction (High Yield for 2011/2012)

▶ Is enzymatic DNA amplification.	AI 1999
▶ The polymerase chain reaction (PCR) is now the most frequently used technique in molecular biology. Used to study a specific area of DNA using short complementary sequences of DNA (oligonucleotides) from both the 3' and the 5' ends of the DNA to be studied.	
▶ These oligonucleotides build copies of the DNA (amplifies) using a heat stable polymerase (Taq 1).	AIIMS 1997
▶ It is then possible to heat the mixture and the DNA strands will separate.	
▶ Substances Required:	
✓ Primers,	
✓ DNA Polymerase,	PGI 2011
✓ Mg.	AIIMS 2007
▶ On cooling, the DNA can once more be duplicated and the process repeated again and again leading to an exponential increase in the copies of the two fragments.	

▶ The main advantages of this technique are that

  ⓞ It is very quick,

  ⓞ Highly sensitive and very robust and it

  ⓞ Can be used to study mRNA as well as DNA. **PGI 2003**

▶ It can also be used to study very small amounts of almost any tissue, e.g. the **blood spots** on a Guthrie card or the cells found in a mouth wash sample.

▶ The technique is widely used in **molecular diagnosis of genetic disease**

▶ It is also being used in **infectious disease** to confirm the presence of infectious agents and in immunology to identify the human leukocyte antigen (HLA) haplotype.

⇨ **Amino Acids**

➤ Phenylalanine and Tyrosine are precursors of **Cathecolamines**☞☞

Phenylalanine is an essential amino acid for growth whose anabolic products include

  ▶ Tyrosine, **PGI 2011**

  ▶ Thyroid hormone,

  ▶ Adrenergic neurotransmitter (Adrenaline) **PGI 2011**

  ▶ Melanin

"Chymotrypsin" is involved in cleaving <u>carbonyl groups</u> **of aromatic amino acids like**

  ➤ Tryptophan **PGI 2011**

  ➤ Tyrosine

  ➤ Phenylalanine **PGI 2011**

➤ **Tryptophan** is precursor for **Serotonin, Niacin**☞☞ **DNB 2011**

➤ **Valine and isoleucine** are **branched chain amino acids** whose metabolism is abnormal in MSUD. (**Maple Syrup Urine Disease**)☞☞ **AI 2010**

➤ Proline has an **imino group.**☞☞

➤ **Essential AA:** **JK BOPEE 2011, AIIMS 2007**

  Arginine,Histidine,Isoleucine,Leucine,Lysine,

  Methionine,Phenylalanine,Threonine,Tryptophan, Valine☞☞

  Naturally occurig amino acids are L isomers. **JK BOPEE 2011**

— **Histidine is a buffer at normal pH.**

— It can protonate or deprotonate.

— Dissociation constant closest to physiological p H is histidine.

➤ Leucine is present in **transmembrane region of proteins.**

➤ **Most non polar amino acid** is leucine. **AI 1998**

— Glycine is the smallest and simplest AA.☞☞

— Glycine is responsible for **flexibility of proteins.**☞☞

— Glycine is optically inactive.

— Glycine does not have anomeric carbon atom. **AIIMS 2002**

— Glycine lacks chilarity. **AI 1996**

⇨ **Arginine Functions**

- ✓ As a vasodilator
- ✓ regulates blood flow
- ✓ Neurotransnmitter
- ✓ Bactericidal
- ✓ Medates penile erection
- ✓ Inhibits platelet aggregation

- ➡ Most of the amino acids do not absorb visible light and hence are **colourless.**
- ➡ Aromatic amino acids are the only amino acids that absorb light. **They are:**
- ⓪ **Tryptophan (contains indole ring)**   DELHI 1987
- ⓪ **Tyrosine**
- ⓪ **Phenylalanine and**
- ⓪ **Histidine**
- ⓪ **Tryptophan** is the **major** amino acid contributing to ability to absorb light in the range of **250-290 nm.**

⇨ **Amino Acids**

▶ Melatonin is synthesized from **tryptophan.**	MAH 2012
▶ **Thyroxine is synthesized from tyrosine**	DNB 2011
▶ Norepinephrine is synthesized from **tyrosine**	
▶ Dopamine is synthesized from **tyrosine**	
▶ Tryptophan can be **converted into vitamin.**	
▶ Ammonia is produced in kidney from **glutamine.**	JIPMER 1999
▶ Ammonia is detoxified in brain to **glutamine**	JK 2003
▶ Phenyl alanine is a **precursor of tyrosine**	AI 2002
▶ **Creatinine is synthesized from glycine, arginine, methionine**	KAR 1994
⓪ Risk of MI is increased with **homocysteine.**	
⓪ **Cysteine** is the reducing agent in glutathione	
⓪ Buffering action of blood is due to **histidine.**	PGI 2006

⇨ **Remember**

"Glucogenic" amino acids are:

- — Alanine, Arginine, Asparagine, Aspartate
- — Cysteine
- — Glutamate, Glutamine, Glycine
- — Methionine, Theronine, Valine

"Ketogenic" Amino acids are:

- — Leucine, Lysine

⇨ **Classification of Amino Acids**

Amino acids are usually classified into 5 types based on the properties of their side chains (R groups), in particular, their polarity, or tendency to interact with water at biological pH (near pH 7.0). The polarity of the R groups varies widely, from nonpolar and hydrophobic (water-insoluble) to highly polar and hydrophilic (water-soluble).

* **Nonpolar, Aliphatic R Groups:** Glycine, Alanine, Proline, Valine, Leucine, Isoleucine and Methionine.
* **Nonpolar, Aromatic R Groups:** Phenylalanine, tyrosine, and tryptophan.
* **Polar, Uncharged R Groups:** Serine, Threonine, Cysteine, Asparagine, Glutamine.
* **Polar, positively Charged (Basic) R Groups:** Lysine, Arginine and Histidine.
* **Polar, Negatively charged (Acidic) R Groups:** Aspartate and Glutamate.

- Hydroxylation of **proline** in fibroblasts generates the modified amino acid hydroxyproline. This is an example of post-translational modification. Hydroxyproline is involved in stabilizing the three-dimensional triple helix structure of collagen.
- **Cysteine** is unique in its ability to form a covalent disulfide bond with another cysteine residue elsewhere in the protein molecule, thereby forming a cystine residue. Such strong disulfide bonds stabilize the three-dimensional structure of the protein.
- **Glycine** is abundant in fibroblasts since it constitutes every third amino acid in the primary sequence of collagen. However, glycine is not hydroxylated.
- **Serine, tyrosine and threonine** can all be phosphorylated post-translationally to form phosphoserine, phosphotyrosine, and phosphothreonine, respectively. These phosphorylated amino acids are believed to play a role in signal transduction.

⊃ **Mechanism Pathway of Important Enzymes: High Yield for AIPGME/AIIMS/PGI 2013**

Pathway	G protein	Protein Kinase	Examples
▶ c AMP	Adenyl cyclase	Protein Kinase A	✓ Glucagon ✓ Epinephrine
▶ PIP2	Phospholipase	Protein Kinase B	✓ Vasopressin
▶ C GMP	Guanyl cyclase	Protein Kinase C	✓ ANF ✓ NO

⊃ **Proteins: High Yield for AIPGME/AIIMS/PGI 2013**

▶ 1° Structure	Specific order of Amino Acids in peptide chain	
▶ 2° Structure	Spatial relationship of <u>neighboring</u> Amino Acid residues. eg α Helix	
▶ 3° Structure	Spatial relationship of <u>distant</u> Amino Acid residues by arrangement of	
▶ 4° Structure	Spatial relationship <u>between individual Polypeptide chains.</u>	

KERALA 1994

3

⇨ **Alpha Helix, Beta Sheet and Beta Bends are Secondary Structures**

▶ **Alpha helix** can be composed of more than one polypeptide chains. It is a spiral structure with polypeptide backbone and side chains of amino acids.☞

▶ It is stabilized by **hydrogen bonds.**☞☞   AI 1991

▶ Each turn of the helix has **3.6 amino acids**☞

▶ Proline disrupts alpha helix because of geometric incompatibility of **imino group of proline.**

▶ Beta <u>sheets</u> are **secondary structures** in which all peptide bonds are involved in hydrogen bonding.☞   AI 2004

▶ Beat sheets are both parallel and anti parallel.

▶ Secondary structure of **prion proteins** is beta sheet.   AI 2008

▶ Beta <u>bends</u> are also called **reverse turns.**

▶ Beta bends often **contain glycine.**☞☞

▶ Proline can also be present.☞

▶ **Motifs** are <u>super secondary structures</u>.✳

▶ **Domains** are a type of <u>tertiary structure</u>✳

✓ **Primary structure:** Peptide bonds

✓ **Secondary structure:** hydrogen bonds

✓ **Tertiary structure:** disulfide bonds

✓ **Quarternery structure:** homodimers/ heterodimers.   AI 2006

⇨ **Detection of Protein Structure**

▶ **Primary structure** of proteins is detected by <u>Edmans degradation</u>.

▶ **Secondary, tertiary and quaternary structure** is detected by **x ray diffraction/ crystallography**

▶ **SDS PAGE** is used for **separation and purification of individual proteins** on <u>basis of size</u>.   PGI 2003

▶ **SDS PAGE** is used for **determining** <u>molecular weight of a protein</u>.   AIIMS 2004

▶ **Affinity chromography** separates proteins by <u>their binding affinity</u>

▶ **Gel filtration chromatography** separates proteins **on basis of** <u>size</u>.

▶ **Ion exchange chromatography** separates proteins **on basis of their** <u>charge</u>.
Exchange of ions in solution form with that of surface occurs here   AI 2010

▶ **Iso electric focusing** separates proteins **on basis of their** <u>isoelectric pH.</u>

▶ **Hb electrophoresis** is done on basis of <u>charge</u>.   AIIMS 2007

3

⊃ Denaturation of Proteins

▶ Amino acid sequence is <u>conserved.</u>	AIIMS 2008
▶ Unfolding is seen.	AIIMS 2008
▶ <u>Disruption</u> of secondary structure occurs.	
▶ Biological function is <u>not conserved</u>.	AIIMS 2008
▶ <u>Re covery is not possible</u> after denaturation.	
▶ <u>Gaunidine</u> is a denaturing substance.	
— Folding of proteins is due to disulfide bonds.	
— Chaperones assist in protein folding.	

⊃ Important Elements

⇨ Components of Enzymes

▶ Magnesium:	<u>Kinases, Phosphatases</u>, Ribonuclease, Adenyl cyclase, Transketolase☜☜☜
▶ Copper:	Cytochrome Oxidase, Tyrosinase, Superoxide dismutase☜☜
▶ Zinc:	Carboxy peptidase
▶ Molybedenum:	Xanthine Oxidase, Sulfite oxidase DNB 2011
▶ Manganese:	Pyruvate Carboxylase☜

⊃ Effects of Mineral Deficiencies: High Yield for AIPGME/AIIMS/PGI 2013

▶ arsenic	(impaired growth, infertility),
▶ boron	(impaired energy metabolism, impaired brain function),
▶ nickel	(impaired-growth and reproduction),
▶ silicon	(impaired growth) and
▶ vanadium	(impaired skeletal formation).

Zn is a co factor in many enzymes. Some of the important ones are:

— Carbonic anhydrase ☜☜
— Lactate/Alcohol Dehyrogenase ☜☜
— DNA polymerase ☜
— RNA polymerase
— Alkaline phosphatase

⇨ Globulins

▶ Alpha 1 globulins: AFP, α_1AT, Trypsin☜☜
▶ Alpha 2 globulins: Cerruloplasmin, Haptoglobin☜
▶ Beta globulin: Transferrin, CRP, Hemopexin☜

3

⇨ **Enzymology**

- ► Enzymes **don't alter** Energy of <u>Reaction.</u>🖛🖛
- ► Enzymes **lower** Energy of <u>Activation</u>🖛
- ► V_{max}=Maximum velocity with specified amount of enzyme🖛
- ► K_m =concentration of substrate required to produce half V max🖛
- ► **Enzyme activity is measured as micromoles/ min.**   PGI 2006

⇨ **"Competetive" Inhibition**

- ▶ Is reversible🖛🖛🖛
- ▶ Substrate and inhibitor resemble each other.🖛
- ▶ V max is same, Km is increased.🖛✳   PGI 1998
- ▶ Substrate affinity to enzyme is **lowered**🖛

⇨ **"Noncompetetive" Inhibition**

- ▶ Is reversible or irreversible🖛
- ▶ Substrate and inhibitor don't resemble each other.🖛
- ▶ V max is decreased , Km is unaltered🖛✳
- ▶ Substrate affinity to enzyme is not lowered🖛

⇨ **"Allosteric" Inhibition**

- ▶ Here inhibitor binds to enzyme at a site different than active site.🖛🖛
- ▶ **Does not follow Michels menton Kinetics.**
- ▶ Follows **sigmoid kinetics.**
- ▶ Km is raised but V max is unchanged in some allosteric inhibition reactions.

⇨ **Terms Asked**

- ⓪ **Coenzyme: non protein** organic compounds.   PGI 1994
- ⓪ **Abzyme** is **antibody** with catalytic activity   AIIMS 1998
- ⓪ **Ribozymes** are **RNA molecules** with catalytic activity   PGI 2002

Remember:

- ☐ Michels Menton (Km) reflects the **affinity of enzymes** to that substrate.🖛🖛   MP 2002
- ☐ It is equal to the substrate concentration at which reaction velocity is half of V max.🖛
- ☐ **Low Km** reflects **high affinity** of enzyme.🖛🖛
- ☐ **High Km** reflects **low affinity** of enzyme.🖛🖛

➲ Enzyme Designations: High Yield for AIPGME/AIIMS/PGI 2013

▶ Lyase: fumarase	AMU 2003
▶ Ligase: glutamine synthetase	
▶ Oxidase: tyrosinase	UP 2001
▶ Transferase: hexokinase	WB 2001

➲ Metabolic Processes and their Sites: High Yield for AIPGME/AIIMS/PGI 2013

Processes occurring in <u>cytosol</u>:

— Glycolysis☛☛	AIIMS 2007
— Glycogenolysis☛	
— Glycogenesis☛	
— HMP Shunt (Pentose phosphate synthesis)☛	
— Fatty acid <u>synthesis</u>☛	
— Bile acid synthesis☛	
— Cholesterol synthesis☛	

Processes occurring in <u>Mitochondria</u>:

- Fatty acid <u>oxidation</u> (Beta)☛✳
- Electron transport chain☛✳
- Krebs/TCA Cycle☛✳
- Oxidative phosphorylation☛✳

Processes occurring in <u>both mitochondria and cytosol</u>:

- Urea synthesis☛
- Gluconeogenesis ☛

▶ Protein synthesis: RER✳✳
▶ Steroid synthesis: Smooth ER✳✳
▶ Sorting of Proteins: Golgi bodies (Dictyosome)✳✳

➲ Important Tests in Biochemistry (High Yield for 2012)

☐ Zwengers test:	Cholesterol☛☛	
☐ Modified Koopanys test:	Barbiturates	AMU 1984
☐ Fouchets test	Bile pigments ✳✳	
☐ Hays sulfur test	Bile salts ✳✳	
☐ Xanthoproteic test:	Proteins☛☛	
☐ Guaicac test:	Haematuria	KAR 1998
☐ Selivanoffs test:☛	Fructose in urine	
☐ Rotheras test: ☛	Ketone bodies	AI 2010
☐ Gerhardts test:	Ketosis	AIIMS 1985

BIOCHEMISTRY

❑ Molishs test: ☞ Colour test for sugar	JIPMER 2003
❑ Guthries test: ☞ Phenylketonuria	
❑ Millons test: Tyrosinosis	PGI 1983
❑ Exton Rose test: ☞ Glucose Tolerance test	
❑ Cyanide nitroprusside test: ☞ Phenyl ketonuria	
❑ Benedicts test: ☞ Glucose in urine	
❑ Sulkowitz test: Urinary calcium	DNB 1989
❑ Biurate test: Protein	AIIMS 1987

➲ Ketone Bodies: AI-2010: High Yield for AIPGME/AIIMS/PGI 2013

- **Ketone bodies** are intermediary products of fat metabolism and their presence in the blood and then in the urine are indications that the metabolism is disordered or incomplete.
- The three main ketone bodies are **Acetone, Acetoacetic acid and Betahydroxybutyric** acid.
- **Testing for ketone bodies** should be done on fresh urine or the specimen kept at 4°C. **Principle:** Acetone and acetoacetic acid react with sodium nitropruside in the presence of alkali to produce a purple color. **(Rothera test) used for** Ketone bodies.

⇨ Differentiate

❑ Vitamins:	**Organic** Molecules ☞
❑ Coenzyme:	**Non protein** organic molecule ☞
❑ Co factor:	Usually a **metallic ion** eg: Fe in Cytochromes ☞

— Holoenzyme:	enzyme+cofactor
— Apoenzyme:	protein part of holoenzyme
— Prosthetic group:	tightly bound coenzyme that does not dissociate from enzyme

➲ Important Vitamin Deficiencies ✳✳✳ High Yield for AIPGME/AIIMS/PGI 2013

Vitamin	Enzyme	Deficiency State
Thiamine (B1) AI 1985	❑ Pyruvate dehydrogenase ❑ αKetoglutarate dehydrogenase AIIMS 2008 ❑ Transketolase AIIMS 2008 UP 2007	➤ Wernicke Korsakoff Syndrome ☞☞ KERALA 94, AI 88 ➤ Wet Beri Beri ☞ ➤ Dry Beri Beri ☞
Biotin	❑ Pyruvate carboxylase JIPMER 1992 ❑ Acetyl CoA carboxylase ❑ Propionyl CoA carboxylase	➤ Consumption of eggs containing avidin ☞ UP 2007, COMED 2006 ➤ Alopecia, Muscle pains ☞

3

Pyridoxine	☐ Aminotransferases	PGI 1986 JIPMER 1987 KERALA 1988	➤ Isoniazid therapy☞ ➤ Sidderoblastic anemia☞ ➤ Chielosis/stomatitis☞ ➤ Convulsions☞
Riboflavin	☐ Dehydrogenases		➤ Corneal neovascularization☞ ➤ Chielosis/stomatitis☞ ➤ Magenta tongue☞
Niacin	☐ Dehydrogenases		➤ Pellagra☞ ➤ Diarrhoea, Dementia, Dermatitis,☞ Death
Pantothenic AI 1995	☐ Fatty acid Synthase ☐ Fatty acyl CoA synthase		➤ Rare ➤ Burning foot syndrome
Folic-Acid	☐ Thymidylate synthase		➤ Alcholics and pregnancy☞ ➤ Homocystenemia☞ ➤ Macrocytic anemia ➤ Neural tube defects
Vitamin B$_{12}$ Extrinsic factor of castle PGI 1987	☐ Homocysteine methyltransferase ☐ Methyl malonyl CoA mutase		➤ Pernicious anemia☞ ➤ Megaloblastic anemia ➤ Neuropathy ➤ SACD ➤ Methyl malonic aciduria AIIMS 1986,JIPMER 1991
Vitamin C post translation modifier (AI 2005)	☐ Propyl and Lysyl hydroxylase ☐ Dopamine hydroxylase		➤ Diet deficient in citrus ➤ Scurvy☞☞ JK BOPEE 2011

⊃ **Pyridoxine Deficency and Neuropathy: High Yield for AIPGME/AIIMS/PGI 2013**

The pathologic findings are mainly those of axonal degeneration with secondarydemyelination. A specific vitamin deficiency has not been identified in alcoholic neuropathy; similar **polyneuropathies occur with deficiencies of thiamine, niacin, or pyridoxine.** Possibly, alcohol may have a direct toxic effect on peripheral nerves. Treatment consists of a balanceddiet of supplemental B vitamins and abstinence from alcohol. Alcoholics and other nutritionallydeprived persons commonly develop a **mixed axonal-demyelinating polyneuropathy withpain and paresthesias in the feet.** More severe cases develop leg weakness and symptomsinvolving the hands.

MAH 2012

⇨ **Fat Soluble Vitamins**

Vitamin A (acts as hormone)	AIIMS 1999	▶ Night blindness☞☞ ▶ Xeropthalmia☞☞ ▶ Follicular Hyperkeratosis☞

Vitamin D	▶ Rickets ☜
	▶ Osteomalacia
Vitamin E Prevents lipid peroxidation.　　　ORISSA 2005	▶ Hemolysis☜ ▶ Retinitis pigmentosa☜ ▶ Neurological problems
VitaminK ▶ (Gamma carboxylation) 　　　AIIMS 2008, AIIMS 2007, AIIMS 2001 ▶ Post translation modifier.　　　AI 2005	▶ Bleeding tendency with ↑PT normal BT☜

Remember:

⊃ Folate Deficency

Dietary folic acid is conjugated with glutamyl peptides; prior to its absorption, these polyglutamates must be deconjugated to monoglutamates by folic deconjugase, an enzyme found on the microvillus membrane. Folate monoglutamates are absorbed by active transport at low concentrations of folate and by passive diffusion at high concentrations of folate. Folic acid undergoes an enterohepatic circulation. Since its body stores are limited, the major cause of folate deficiency is diet poor in fresh fruits and vegetables. Folic acid deficiency may also occur if there is extensive damage to the proximal small intestine (e.g., nontropical sprue) or secondary to the use of a number of medications (**sulfasalazine, phenytoin, trimethoprim**) that inhibit its absorption.

⇨ Causes

➥ Infections e.g. coxsackie A and B, HIV,(VIRAL)	PGI 2011
➥ Diphtheria, parasitic	
➥ Endocrine e.g. hyperthyroidism	PGI 2011
➥ Infiltrative* e.g. haemochromatosis, sarcoidosis	
➥ Neuromuscular e.g. Duchenne muscular dystrophy, Friedreich's ataxia	
➥ Nutritional e.g. kwashiorkor, pellagra, thiamine/selenium deficiency	
➥ Alcoholics	PGI 2011

Vitamin	Coenzyme	Reaction Type
B_1 (Thiamine)	TPP (thiamine pyrophosphate)	✓ Oxidativedecarboxylation, transketolation.
B_2 (Riboflavin)	FMN, FAD	✓ Oxidation/Reduction
B_3 (Pantothenate	CoA – Coenzyme A	✓ Acyl group transfer
B_6 (Pyridoxine)	PLP (Pyridoxal phosphate)	✓ Transfer of groups to an from amino acids ▶ Transamination,　　　MAH 2012 　➥ Deamination, 　➥ Condensation 　➥ Decarboxylation

B$_{12}$ (Cobalamin)	5-deoxyadenosyl cobalamin,, methylcobalamin	✓ Isomerization of methylmalonyl, synthesis of methionine	
Niacin	NAD$^+$, NADP$^+$	✓ Oxidation/Reduction	
Folic acid	Tetrahydrofolate	✓ One carbon group transfer	
Biotin	Biotin	▶ Carboxylation	MAH 2012
Vitamin K	Vitamin K	✓ Carboxylation of glutamic acid residues	

➲ Hypervitaminosis

Vitamin A:

— Hypercalcemia,

— Hyperostosis,

— Demineralization of bones,

— Pseudotumor cerebri,

— Teratogenic.

Vitamin D:

— Hypercalcemia,

— Hyperphosphatemia.

➲ Vitamin K Dependent Factors

This vitamin is a necessary cofactor for the enzyme that catalyzes the conversion of glutamic acid residues to carboxyglutamic acid residues.

Six of the proteins involved in clotting require conversion of a number of glutamic acid residues to carboxyglutamic acid residues before being released into the circulation, and hence all six are vitamin K-dependent.

These proteins are:

✓ factors II (prothrombin),

✓ VII,

✓ IX,

✓ X,

✓ protein C, and

✓ protein S.   AIPGME 2012

⇨ Haem Proteins

1. Cytochrome
2. Haemoglobin
3. Myoglobin
4. Catalase

⇨ **Haemoglobin**

▶ Haemoglobin is an <u>allosteric</u> protein.

▶ Haem proteins are specialized proteins containing Haem as a <u>prosthetic</u> group. ✱

▶ HAEM in hemoglobin lies in <u>hydrophobic pocket</u>   PGI 2003

▶ HAEM in hemoglobin is bonded to <u>E 7 Histidine</u>.   AIIMS 1983

▶ Iron is present in <u>ferrous</u> state   PGI 1996

▶ Ferrous ions are present in porphyrin rings.

▶ Iron in hemoglobin is held by <u>polar bonds</u>.   AI 91

▶ Haem itself is a complex of Protoporphyrin IX and Ferrous iron. ✱

▶ Hb shows <u>coperative binding</u>.

▶ Haemoglobin binds <u>four</u> molecules of oxygen ✱

▶ Haemoglobin exists in two forms <u>Deoxygenated form or (T)Taut form</u> and ✱

▶ **Oxygenated form or (R) relaxed form.** ✱

▶ Oxygen dissociation curve of Hb is <u>sigmoidal.</u> ✱

▶ Hb is a buffer because of histidine.

▶ **Myoglobin** binds one **molecule of oxygen**

▶ Oxygen dissociation curve of **Myoglobin** is **Hyperbolic**

Gems about Haemoglobin

⊃ **Earliest Haemoglobin**

▶ Hb Gowers	$\alpha_2\varepsilon_2$ ↩	
▶ Hb Fetal	$\alpha_2\gamma_2$ ↩	JK BOPEE 2011
▶ Hb Adult	$\alpha_2\,\delta_2$ ↩	
▶ Hb A$_2$	$\alpha_2\delta_2$ ↩	

⇨ **Revise Configuration of Haemoglobins**

▶ Most common Hb is	HbA ↩
▶ Adult Hb is HbA is:	$\alpha_2\delta\delta_2$ ↩
▶ Fetal Hb is Hb F is:	$\alpha_2\gamma_2$ ↩
▶ Minor Adult Hb is HbA$_2$ is:	$\alpha_2\delta_2$ ↩

➲ **Clinically Important Points About:**

⇨ **Methaemoglobin**

▶ Form of oxidized HB.
▶ (Fe^{2+} replaced by Fe^{3+})
▶ Oxygen carrying capacity ↓
⓪ Phenacetin,
⓪ Primaquine,
⓪ sulfonamides,
⓪ Nitrites,
⓪ Nitrates cause "Methaemaglobinemia."

⇨ **Carboxy Haemoglobin**

▶ Hb combines with CO (**Carbon Monoxide** NOT Dioxide) to form Carboxy Haemoglobin
▶ Affinity of Hb for CO is **200 times** more than that of O_2, hence CO displaces O_2

⇨ **Glycosylated Haemoglobin**

▶ Adult Hb binds with glucose during 120 day life cycle of RBC.
▶ It is an **irreversible reaction.**
▶ **Normally** upto 9% of adult Hb is Glycosylated.
▶ **In diabetes >9 % Hb is glycosylated.**
▶ It is useful for providing picture of "**long term**" state of diabetic control.

➲ **Lysosomal Storage Disease: High Yield for AIPGME/AIIMS/PGI 2013**

Fabry's Disease	Lysosomal Storage Disease	<u>X-Linked Recessive</u>. **Alpha-Galactosidase A** deficiency ------> buildup of **ceramide trihexoside** in body tissues.	**Angiokeratomas** (skin lesions) over lower trunk, fever, severe burning pain in extremities, cardiovascular and cerebrovascular involvement.
Hunter's Syndrome	Lysosomal Storage Disease	<u>X-Linked Recessive</u>. **L-iduronosulfate sulfatase** deficiency ------> buildup of **mucopolysaccharides** (heparan sulfate and dermatan sulfate)	Similar to but **less severe than Hurler Syndrome**. No corneal clouding. Hepatosplenomegaly, micrognathia, retinal degeneration, joint stiffness, mild retardation, cardiac lesions.
Hurler's Syndrome	Lysosomal Storage Disease	<u>Autosomal Recessive</u>. **-L-iduronidase** deficiency ------> accumulation of **mucopolysaccharides** (heparan sulfate, dermatan sulfate) in heart, brain, liver, other organs.	"**Gargoyle-like facies**", progressive mental deterioration, stubby fingers, death by age 10. Similar to Hunter's Syndrome.

➲ Other Mucopolysachroidoses

MPS IIIA, IIIB, IIIC, and IIID

- ☐ **(Sanfilippo Syndromes)**
  - ✓ **Skeletal defects and hepatosplenomegaly are less pronounced** in this group of MPS variants, though progressive behavioral problems, mental retardation, and seizures are present.
  - ✓ Affected patients can survive into the third or fourth decade with progressive CNS disease.

MPS IV

- ☐ **(Morquio Syndrome)**
  - ✓ Characterized by **severe skeletal diseases** that resemble the spondyloepiphyseal dysplasias.
  - ✓ There is extreme shortening of the trunk due to multiple vertebral collapses.
  - ✓ The long bones are relatively spared. Joint laxity can lead to osteoarthritis-like destruction of the joints.
  - ✓ Upper cervical spinal cord compression due to atlantoaxial instability predisposes to subluxation and paralysis. Many patients have mitral valve insufficiency that can be functionally significant.

MPS VI

- ☐ **(Maroteaux-Lamy Disease)**
  - ✓ Mutations in the **arylsulfatase B gene** cause this autosomal recessive disorder.
  - ✓ Intelligence is normal, and the life span can extend beyond three decades.
  - ✓ Cardiac valvular disease and progressive pulmonary hypertension are frequent causes of death.

➲ Carbohydrates

⇨ Glucose ✹✹

- Glucose is a dominant <u>Monosaccharide</u>,
- Glucose is a <u>Hexose</u>
- Glucose is an <u>aldehyde</u> (Aldose)
- **Carbon 1** is the anomeric carbon in aldoses and not carbon 2 which is anomeric in ketoses.
- Glucose is a <u>reducing sugar</u>
- On reaction with **Benedicts reagent** reduces Cu^{++} ions.

Monosaccharides: Are those those carbohydrates that cannot be hydrolysed into simpler forms. They are divided into Aldoses and Ketoses

Aldoses	Ketoses
► Glyceroses	► Dihydroacetone
► Erythroses	► Erythulose
► Ribose✹	► Ribulose
► Glucose✹	► Fructose✹✹

⇨ Disaccharides:

- ✓ Sucrose,
- ✓ Maltose,
- ✓ Lactose

> Lactose: Glucose + Galactose
> Sucrose: Glucose + Fructose
> Maltose: Glucose + Glucose

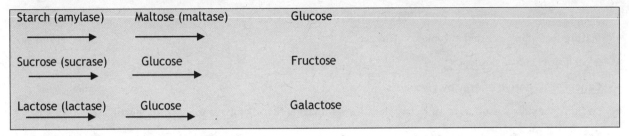

Starch (amylase) →	Maltose (maltase) →	Glucose
Sucrose (sucrase) →	Glucose →	Fructose
Lactose (lactase) →	Glucose →	Galactose

⊃ Oligosaccharides: Maltotriose

Reducing Sugars are:

- Maltose
- Glucose
- Trehalose
- Lactose

- Glucose is the principle substrate of energy metabolism in humans.

- Metabolism of glucose generates ATP via **glycolysis** and mitochondrial oxidative phosphorylation. **A continuous source of glucose** from dietary intake, gluconeogenesis, and degradation of glycogen maintain normal blood glucose levels.

- Sources of glucose in our diet are obtained by ingesting polysaccharides, primarily starch, and disaccharides including lactose, maltose, and sucrose.

- **Galactose and fructose are two other monosaccharides** that provide fuel for cellular metabolism; however, their role as fuel sources is **much less significant than that of glucose.**

- **Galactose is derived from lactose (galactose, glucose),** which is found in milk and milk products. If necessary, galactose can be incorporated into glycogen and thus becomes a source of glucose.

- **Galactose** is also an important component for certain glycolipids, glycoproteins, and glycosaminoglycans.

- **Glycogen,** the storage form of glucose in animal cells, is composed of glucose residues joined in straight chains by α1-4 linkages and branched at intervals of 4 to 10 residues with α1-6 linkages.

- **In skeletal muscle,** stored glycogen is a source of fuel that is used for short-term, high-energy consumption during muscle activity; in the brain, the small amount of stored glycogen is used during brief periods of hypoglycemia or hypoxia as an emergency supply of energy.

- **In contrast, the liver takes up glucose from the bloodstream** after a meal and stores it as glycogen. When blood glucose levels start to fall, the liver converts glycogen back into glucose and releases it into the blood for use by tissues such as brain and erythrocytes that cannot store significant amounts of glycogen.

➲ Glycolysis (High Yield for 2011/2012)

- ➠ Converts glucose to **3 carbon units**.
- ➠ Glycolysis is conversion of glucose to <u>pyruvate</u> under **aerobic** condition. ☞
- ➠ Glycolysis is conversion of glucose to <u>lactate</u> under **anerobic** condition.
- ➠ Mature RBC <u>don't</u> contain enzymes of TCA cycle.   **AIIMS 1994**
- ➠ Glycolysis occurs in <u>cytosol.</u>☞
- ➠ <u>Cancer cells</u> derive energy by glycolysis.   **AIIMS 2001**
- ➠ **Sodium fluoride is used as an anticoagulant for estimating blood glucose to prevent glycolysis**   **DNB 91**
- ➠ Flouride inhibits <u>enolase</u> Al 1995
- ➠ Glycolysis is **regulated at three steps** involving irreversible reactions catalysed by enzymes namely **PGI 98**
- ✓ Hexokinase ☞☞
- ✓ Phosphofructokinase☞☞ (Ist <u>commited</u> step in glycolysis)
- ✓ Pyruvate kinase☞☞
- ▶ Enzymes responsible for complete oxidation of glucose are present in <u>Mitochondria:</u>   **AIIMS 2007**
- ▶ **Sodium flouride and pottasium oxalate** prevent glycolysis(used as anticoagulants)   **AIIMS 2006**
- ▶ <u>Mg</u> is important ion in glycolysis
- ▶ <u>Mallate shuttle</u> is important for glycolysis.
- ▶ Inhibition of glycolysis by oxygen is PASTEUR EFFECT.

⇨ Citric Acid Cycle

Also called "Krebs" cycle.

First substrate of citric acid cycle is pyruvate.   **AIIMS 2007**

ATP is produced in steps catalysed by: **PGI 2006**

- ✓ Isocitrate dehydrogenase
- ✓ Succinate dehydrogenase
- ✓ Succinate thiokinase
- ✓ Malate dehydrogenase

Pyruvate dehydrogenase contains: **AMU 2005**

- ✓ Decarboxylase   **UP 2005, SGPI 2004**
- ✓ Transacetylase
- ✓ Dehydrogenase
- ✓ NAD
- ✓ FAD
- ✓ TPP
- ✓ CoA   **KAR 2001**
- ✓ Lipoic acid.   **JIPMER 2003**

Substrate level phosphorylation occurs in reaction catalysed by: Succinyl Co A **thiokinase**   **PGI 2002**

Thiamine and riboflavin are important for TCA cycle.

➲ Glycogen Synthesis (High Yield for 2011/2012)

- ▶ **Insulin** is produced in the **beta cells of the pancreatic islets.** ☞
- ▶ It is initially synthesized as a single-chain 86-amino-acid **precursor polypeptide, "preproinsulin."**
- ▶ The mature **insulin molecule and C peptide** are stored together and cosecreted from secretory granules in the beta cells.
- ▶ Human **insulin** is now produced by recombinant DNA technology; ☞
- ▶ **Glucose is the key regulator** of **insulin** secretion by the pancreatic beta cell, although amino acids,
- ▶ Ketones, various nutrients, gastrointestinal peptides, and neurotransmitters also influence **insulin** secretion.
- ▶ Glucose stimulates **insulin** secretion through a series of regulatory steps that begin with transport into the beta cell by the GLUT2 glucose transporter
- ▶ Glucose phosphorylation by **glucokinase is the rate-limiting step** that controls glucose-regulated **insulin** secretion.
- ▶ **Insulin** binding to the receptor stimulates **intrinsic tyrosine kinase activity,** leading to receptor autophosphorylation✳✳✳
- ▶ **In the fasting state, low insulin levels promote hepatic gluconeogenesis and glycogenolysis to prevent hypoglycemia. ✳✳✳**
- ▶ Low **insulin** levels decrease glycogen synthesis, reduce glucose uptake in **insulin**-sensitive tissues, and promote mobilization of stored precursors.
- ▶ Reduced **insulin** levels are also permissive in allowing glucagon to stimulate glycogenolysis and gluconeogenesis by the liver and renal medulla. ☞
- ▶ These processes are of critical importance to ensure an **adequate glucose supply for the brain.**

➩ Glycogen Synthesis ✳✳

(Glycogen synthetase) **Activated by**	▶ Insulin ▶ Glucose
Inhibited by	▶ Glucagon ▶ Epinephrine

➩ Glycogen Breakdown✳✳

(Glycogen Phosphorylase) Activated by	▶ Glucagon ▶ Epinephrine
Inhibited by	▶ Insulin ▶ Glucose

➩ Gluconeogenesis

▶ Occurs from **glycerol, alanine, lactate,**	AIIMS 1997, AI 1996
▶ **Major** contributor is <u>alanine</u>	

► Gluconeogenic capabillty is determined by **fructose 1, 6 bi phosphate**	**PGI 2005**
► Enzyme common to "<u>gluconeogenesis and glycolysis</u>" is **phosphofructokinase**	**AI 1997**

⇨ **Enzymes Controlling It☛☛☛**

► Fructose 1,6 Bi phosphate

► Pyruvate carboxylase

► Phosphoenol pyruvate carboxykinase

► Glucose 6 phosphatase

➡ Glycogen cannot be used for energy in muscles	
➡ Muscles cannot make use of glycogen as they lack **G6 Phosphatase**	**AIIMS 1998**
➡ G6 Phosphatase **does not cross cell membrane.**	**AIIMS 2002**

⇨ **Well Fed State:✱✱**

↑Ingestion of glucose. → ↑blood glucose → ↑insulin release → ↑phosphatase activity → ↑fructose 2,6 biphosphatase

⇨ **Fasting State:✱✱**

↓Ingestion of glucose.→ ↓blood glucose→ ↑glucagon release→ ↑cAMP→↑Protein kinase →↓fructose 2,6 biphosphatase DNB 2011

⊃ **Effects of Hormones on Glucose Level in Blood**

High Yield for AIPGME/AIIMS/PGI 2013

1.Effect of Insulin (Hypoglycemic hormone)

1.Lowers blood glucose

2.Favors glycogen synthesis

3.Promotes glycolysis

4.Inhibits gluconeogenesis

2.Glucagon (Hyperglycemic hormone)

1.Increases blood glucose

2.Promotes glycogenolysis

3.Enhances gluconeogenesis

4.Depresesses glycogen synthesis

5.Inhibits glycolysis

3.Cortisol (Hyperglycemic hormone)

1.Increases blood glucose level

2.Increases gluconeogenesis

3.Releases amino acids from the muscle

4.Epinephrine or Adrenaline (Hyperglycemic)

1. Increases blood glucose level

2. Promotes glycogenolysis

3. Increases gluconeogenesis

4. Favors uptake of amino acids

5.Growth Hormone (Hyperglycemic)

1. Increases blood glucose level

2. Decreases glycolysis

3. Mobilizes fatty acids from apidose tissue

➲ Glucose 6 Phosphate Dehydrogenase Deficiency: (High Yield for 2011/2012)

- Is <u>X linked Recessive</u>
- **Most common** enzyme deficiency
- Causes episodic <u>hemolytic anemia</u> because of decreased ability of RBC'S to withstand oxidative stress.☞☞
- G6PD is the <u>first and rate limiting step of HMP shunt</u>.☞☞ responsible for NADPH production.
- NADPH is the co factor for production for glutathione reductase forming reduced glutathione which is a potent antioxidant.
- In its absence H_2O_2 accumulates in RBC causing cell membrane damage leading to hemolysis.
- Pallor,
- Hemoglobinuria,
- Jaundice,
- Heinz bodies,
- Bite Cells are seen.☞
- **Oxidized hemoglobin denatures** and precipitates in the form of Heinz bodies.☞

➲ HMP Shunt: (High Yield for 2011/2012)

Present in cytoplasm and also known as <u>Pentose</u> phosphate <u>pathway</u>.	
Occurs in cytosol	
Important as it produces NADPH.	AIIMS 2003
Occurs in liver, mammary glands, testis, adipose tissue	
No ATP is directly produced or consumed in this cycle.	AI 2008
Generates	
✓ NADPH, ☞	
✓ Ribose 5 P for Nucleotide synthesis, ☞	PUNJAB 2003
✓ Xylulose 5 phosphate,☞	
✓ 6 Phosphogluconolactone,☞	
✓ Glyceraldehydes 3 phosphate, ☞	
✓ Seodoheptulose 7 phosphate.☞	

3

⊃ NADPH is used for

☐ Fatty acid synthesis	AIIMS 1992
☐ Steroid synthesis	
☐ Drug metabolism	
☐ Glutathione reduction	
☐ Generation of superoxide in phagocytes by NADPH oxidase	
☐ Uronic acid pathway.	
☐ **G6PD** is an important enzyme involved in NADPH synthesis	DELHI 2003
☐ Produced in **HMP pathway.**	AIIMS 2003

⊃ ATP Yield

☐ Anaerobic glycolysis: 2 ATP per glucose molecule	
☐ Aerobic glycolysis: 8 ATP per glucose molecule	
☐ Krebs cycle: 12 ATP per acetyl co A	
☐ HMP Shunt: O	
☐ Palitic acid oxidation: 129ATP	
☐ Stearic acid oxidation: 146 ATP	MAHE 2005

⊃ Remember Energy Yield of

☐ Glucose to pyruvate via glycolysis 8 ATP
☐ Glucose to lactate via anerobic oxidation 2 ATP
☐ Pyruvate to acetyl CoA 3 ATP
☐ Acetyl CoA oxidation via TCA cycle 12 ATP

Remember:

► Brain, liver, muscles uses **glucose** as primary fuel.
► Heart uses **fatty acids** as primary fuel.
► In starvation brain and heart use **ketone bodies** as fuel.

⊃ Glycogen Storage Diseases ✱✱✱ (High Yield for 2011/2012)

1. Von Gierke's Disease✱✱ PGI 1985 JK BOPEE 2012	Glucose-6-phosphatase deficiency PGI 2006 MAH 2012	► Protruding abdomen because of marked hepatomegaly, Renomegaly, hypotrophic muscles, truncal obesity, a rounded 'doll face'
		► Severe symptomatic hypoglycemia is frequent, often occurring during the night or after even short periods of reduced caloric intake.
		► Even minor delays or reduction of carbohydrate intake may provoke hypoglycemic attacks that are accompanied by lactic acidosis and hyperuricemia. TN 1995
		► Muscles not involved PGI 1997
		► Hypoglycemia NON responsive to epinephrine AI 2010

2.	Pompe Disease✳✳	Lysosomal alpha-1,4-glucosidase deficiency (Acid maltase deficiency (AMD),	▶ Profound muscle hypotonia, weakness, hyporeflexia, glossomegaly, <u>massive cardiomyopathy</u> without murmurs but no hepatomegaly except with cardiac failure. ▶ The ECG shows a huge QRS complex, left or biventricular hypertrophy and shortened PR interval.
3.	Cori Disease ✳✳	Debranching enzyme	▶ Mild Hypoglycemia, Hepatomegaly
4.	Andersons Disease✳✳ TN 1997	Branching enzyme	▶ Infantile Hypotonia, cirrhosis
5.	Mc Ardle Disease✳ KERALA 1994	Muscle Phosphorylase	▶ Increasing intolerance for strenuous exercise. ▶ Strenuous muscle activity is accompanied by severe cramps and may be followed by myoglobinuria, which can precipitate anuria and renal failure.
6.	Hers Disease✳✳	Liver phosphorylase	▶ Pronounced hepatomegaly, without splenomegaly ▶ Protuberant abdomen due to muscle hypotonia are the most striking features;
7.	Tauris Disease✳✳	Phosphofructokinase Deficency	

⇨ **Von Gierke's Disease**   MAH 2012, JK BOPEE 2012

- A patient present with Hypoglycemia and Hepatomegaly. Hypoglycemia does not respond to epinephrine. Most likely diagnosis is Von Gierke's disease.
- Hepatomegaly, + Fasting hypoglycemia, + Poor growth + Lactic acidosis, Hyperuricemia, Hypertriglyceridemia, and Enlarged kidneys by ultrasound=Von Gierke's Disease M   AH 2012

⊃ **"Mc Ardle Disease" (High Yield for 2011/2012)**

- This disorder is characterized by **increasing intolerance for strenuous exercise.**
- Strenuous muscle activity is accompanied by **severe cramps** and may be followed by **myoglobinuria**, which can precipitate **anuria and renal failure.** In middle life, the fatigue increases and muscle wasting and weakness predominate.
- The **serum CPK** may be permanently or intermittently **elevated.**
- Muscle exercise is normally accompanied by release of lactate and of inosine, hypoxanthine and ammonia through the purine nucleotide cycle. In myophosphorylase deficiency lactic acid production is blocked and release of the purine nucleotide cycle compounds is exaggerated. The ensuing myogenic hyperuricemia is one of the characteristic features of defects of muscle glycogenosis.
- **Phosphorylase activity must be assayed in muscle;**
- **Liver phosphorylase** is presumably **normal**, as is glucose homeostasis.
- DNA mutation analysis is useful in myophosphorylase deficiency as there are common mutations.
- Treatment is symptomatic and consists of the avoidance of strenuous exercise. 'Carbo loading' and a high protein diet are of some help and glucose should always be taken during exercise. Strenuous exercise is always a risk.

BIOCHEMISTRY

⇨ **Galactosemia✳✳ (PGI Favourite)**

▶ Three enzyme deficiencies implicated	
✓ GPUT Deficiency☛☛(Galactose 1 Po_4 uridyl transferase) most common ✳✳	PGI 1995
✓ UDP galactose 4 epimerase deficency	
✓ Galactokinase deficiency	
▶ AR condition	
ⓞ New Borne presents with failure to thrive, vomiting, diarrhoea and jaundice☛	
ⓞ Hepatomegaly,	
ⓞ Cataract (oil drop cataract) ,	
ⓞ Mental retardation,	
ⓞ E.coli sepsis ☛	PGI 2001
▶ Cataract because of accumulation of galactilol.	
▶ Reducing sugar seen in urine. PGI 2001	
▶ Rapid diagnosis and rapid removal of galactose from diet are essential.	

⇨ **Essential Fructosuria (High Yield for 2011/2012)**

▶ Fructokinase deficiency
▶ AR Condition
▶ Benign, asymptomatic
▶ Fructose accumulates in urine
Hereditary Fructose intolerance:
▶ Aldolase B deficiency PGI 1998
▶ Sever hypoglycemia, vomiting, hepatomegaly and hyperuricemia
▶ Hepatic failure and death if not treated.

⇨ **Electron Transport Chain: (High Yield for 2011/2012)**

▶ Electron transport chain is located in inner mitochondrial membrane.	SJ 2002
▶ Internal respiration is exorgenic and catabolic	PGI 2003
▶ Mitochondrial membrane protein contain transporter of NADH, NADPH and ATP	PGI 2003
▶ SGOT is a mitochondrial enzyme	AI 2010
▶ In electron transport chain FADH gives 2 ATP.	PGI 2005
▶ In electron transport chain NADH gives 3 ATP.	PGI 2005
▶ Cyanide inhibits cytochrome oxidase.	KAR 1994
▶ Cyanide inhibits Complex IV.	APPG 2006
▶ Cyanide inhibits electron flow in cytochrome C oxidase.	AIIMS 2006
▶ Cyanide inhibits cellular oxidation.	
▶ Carbon monoxide, cyanide, H_2S and azide inhibit cytochrome oxidase.	COMED 2007
▶ Dinitrophenol is uncoupler of oxidation and phosphorylation.	AI 2007
▶ Uncouplers of oxidative phosphorylation are:	
Snake venom,	
↑ Serum bilirubin,	
↑ T4,	
↑ Free fatty acids	AIIMS 1981

Electron Transport inhibitors✱✱

▶ Rotenone, amobarbital, chlorpromazine　　　(complex I)

▶ Antimycin A, BAL, phenformin　　　(complex II)

▶ Cyanide ,azide,CO, H_2S　　　(complex III)

ATP ase Inhibitors✱✱

▶ Oligomycin, atractyloside, bongregate

Uncoupling agents ✱✱

▶ 2,4 Dinitrophenol

⇨ **ATP Formation is regulated in OXIDATIVE PHOSPHORYLATION by**

▶ NADH Co Q redructase	PGI 2011
▶ Cytochrome C oxidase	
▶ Co Q cytochrome Creductase	PGI 2011

Compounds Affecting Electron Transport Chain and Oxidative Phosphorylation.

⊃ **Nutshell (Inhibitors in Detail): High Yield for AIPGME/AIIMS/PGI 2013**

1.Complex I to Co-Q specific inhibitors

➥ i. Alkylguanides (guanethide), hypotensive drug

➥ II. Rotenone,insecticide and fish poison

➥ iii. Barbiturates (amobarbital),sedative

➥ iv. Chlorpromazine,tranquilizer

➥ v. Piericidin,antibiotic

2.Complex II to Co-Q

➥ i. Carboxin

3.Complex III to cytochrome c inhibitors

➥ i. BAL (british anti lewisite), antidote of war gas

➥ ii. Naphthoquinone

➥ iii. Antimycin

4. Complex IV inhibitors

➥ Carbon monoxide, inhibits cellular respiration

➥ Cyanide CN^-

➥ Azide $N3^-$

➥ Hydrogen sulphide (H_2S)

5. Site between succinate dehydrogenase and Co-Q

➥ Carboxin, inhibits transfer of ions from $FADH_2$

➥ Malonate, competitive inhibitor of succinate DH

6.Inhibitor of oxidative phosphorylation

➥ Atractyloside, inhibits translocase

➥ Oligomycin, inhibits flow of protons through Fo Ionophores, e.g. Valinomycin

3

7. **Uncouplers**
- 2,4-dinitrophinol (2,4-DNP)
- 2,4-dinitrocresol (2,4-DNC)
- CCCP(chlorocarbonylcyanidephenyl hydrazone)

8.**Physiological uncouplers**
- Thyroxine,in high doses
- Thermogenin in brown adipose tissue.

⇨ **Fatty Acids ✳✳✳ (Repeated in 2009, 2010, 2011)**

"Saturated "fatty acids:☛☛
- Butyric acid,
- Palmitic acid,
- Stearic acid.

"Monounsaturated "fatty acids:☛☛   PGI 1983
- Oleic acid,
- Elaidic acid.

"Polyunsaturated" fatty acids PUFA:☛☛
- Linoleic Acid ,
- Linolenic Acid,
- Arachdonic Acid.

⇨ **Significance of PUFA**

- PUFAs are seen in vegetable oils.
- They are nutritionally essential; & are called **Essential Fatty Acids.**
- **Prostaglandins,** thromboxanes & leukotrienes are produced from arachidonic acid.
- PUFAs from integral part of mitochondrial membranes. In deficiency of PUFA, the efficiency of **biological oxidation** is reduced.
- They are the components of **membranes.** Arachidonic acid is 10-15% of the fatty acids of membranes.
- As double bonds are in cis configuration; the PUFA molecule cannot be closely packed. So PUFAs will **increase the fluidity** of the membrane.
- As PUFAs are easily liable to undergo peroxidation, the membranes containing PUFAs are more prone for damage by free radicals.
- The production of DHA (docosa hexa enoic acid) from alpha linolenic acid is limited. DHA is present in high concentrations in fish oils. DHA is present in high concentrations in retina, cerebral cortex and sperms.

⊃ **Essential Fatty Acids are: High Yield for AIPGME/AIIMS/PGI 2013**

— Linoleic acid   JK 2001
— Linolenic acid   PGI 1986, AIIMS 1986
— Ecosopantanoic acid
— Docosa Hexanoic acid
— Arachidonic acid.   PGI 1986

- Most essential is linoleic acid.
- Sunflower oil is a rich source of linoleic acid.
- Breast milk is a rich source of Docosa Hexanoic acid

Lipotrophic factors:

▶ Choline

▶ Betaine

▶ Methionine

⇨ **Cholesterol**

▶ Cholesterol is a **steroid**.

▶ HMG CoA <u>reductase</u> is the rate limiting enzyme.   JK BOPEE 2011

▶ HMG Co A is used both for Cholestrol and ketone synthesis.   AIPGME 2012

▶ Derivatives of cholesterol are:

✓ Palmitic acid

✓ Stearic acid

✓ Bile acids   AIIMS 2007

✓ Squalene

⇨ **Fatty Acid Synthesis (Frequently Repeated)**

Fatty Acid Synthesis

- **Most** fatty acids are synthesized in the "**liver.**"
- Fatty acids to a **lesser extent** are also synthesized in **Lactating breast, adipose tissue and kidney.**
- Fatty acids are synthesized in "**cytosol.**"   AI 1994
- **Carbon atoms** needed for fatty acid synthesis are provided by acetyl co A
- **Energy** for fatty acid synthesis is provided by ATP.
- **Reducing equivalents** for fatty acid synthesis are provided by **NADPH.**   AI 1998
- **Energy is supplied by NADPH.**   AIIMS 2002
- The **regulated step** in fatty acid synthesis is catalyzed by **acetyl CO A carboxylase** which requires Biotin.
- Citrate is the **allosteric activator of enzyme acetyl CO A carboxylase** and
- **Long chain fatty acyl COA is the inhibitor.**
- **Insulin** also activates the enzyme.
- **Epinephrine and glucagon** inactivate the enzyme.
- "Acetyl co A carboxylase" containing Biotin is the rate limiting step.   JIPMER 1991
- It is activated by **insulin** (Promotes fatty acid synthesis)
- **Fatty acid synthetase** is a large multi **enzyme complex** containing Acyl carrier protein, Pantothenic acid)   PGI 1996
- **Carnitine is essential for transport of fatty acids across mitochondrial membrane.**

▶ Beta oxidation of fatty acids produces propionyl Co A.   AI 2003

▶ Beta oxidation of <u>steraic acid</u> produces 147 ATP molecules.

▶ Beta oxidation of <u>palmitic acid</u> produces 129 ATP molecules.   PGI 2005

3

⊃ Brown Fat (Special Characters): High Yield for AIPGME/AIIMS/PGI 2013

- Is abundant in infants.
- Contains abundant mitochondria.
- Thermogenic effect has been linked to that of an electric blanket.
- Uncoupling of metabolism and generation of ATP occurs by **UCP** (uncoupling proteins) But ATP and not high energy ATP is produced.
- There are two pathways:
    - ✓ Inward proton conductance generating ATP.
    - ✓ Second proton conductance not generating ATP.
- The specialized mammalian tissue in which fuel oxidation serves not to produce ATP but to generate heat is: **Brown Fat**   AI 2006

⇨ Ketosis

- ▶ Ketosis results from
- ▶ A marked increase in free fatty acid release from adipocytes, with a resulting shift toward **ketone** body synthesis in the liver.
- ▶ Reduced insulin levels, in combination with elevations in catecholamines and growth hormone, lead to an increase in lipolysis and release of free fatty acids
- ▶ HMGCo A is the precursor of acetoacetate.
- ▶ **Acetoacetate is the first ketone body to be formed.**
- ▶ **Over production of acetyl Co A** Occurs.
- ▶ **In Diabetic Keto Acidiosis**, the **ketone** body, **b-hydroxybutyrate**, is synthesized at a threefold greater rate than acetoacetate
- ▶ Ketone body formation occurs in **Liver**.   **Kerala 1991**
- ▶ **LIVER and MUSCLE don't utilize ketone bodies.**
- ▶ Ketone bodies are by products of **fatty metabolism.**   **AIIMS, UPSC**
- ▶ Ketone bodies are normally produced from **Acetyl Co A.**   **AP 1988**
- ▶ Normal excretion of ketone bodies daily is **1 mg.**   **PGI 1981**
- ▶ Ketone bodies are utilized by conversion of **acetoactetate to acetoacetyl co A.**   **NIMHANS 2001**
- ▶ Ketone body formation without glycosuria is a feature of **starvation.**   **PGI 1997**
- ▶ **Insulin is antiketogenic**
- ▶ **Glucagon is ketogenic**

⊃ Ketoacidosis: (High Yield for 2011/2012)

- Occurs In **type I IDDM.**
- Urinary Acetoacetate, βHydroxy butyrate ↑
- Urinary **Nitroprusside test** Positive

► The hyperglycemia of DKA results from **increased hepatic glucose production** (gluconeogenesis and glycogenolysis) and **impaired peripheral glucose utilization.**

► The decreased ratio of insulin to glucagon **promotes gluconeogenesis, glycogenolysis, and ketone body formation in the liver,** as well as increasing substrate delivery from fat and muscle (free fatty acids, amino acids) to the liver.

► Insulin deficiency also **reduces levels of the GLUT4 glucose transporter,** which impairs glucose uptake into skeletal muscle and fat and reduces intracellular glucose metabolism.

⇨ **Bile**

Major components of bile by weight include water (82%), bile acids (12%), lecithin and other phospholipids (4%), and unesterified cholesterol (0.7)

► The "primary bile acids", <u>cholic acid and chenodeoxycholic acid</u> (CDCA), are synthesized from cholesterol in the <u>liver</u>   JKBOPEE 2012

► Are **conjugated with glycine or taurine,**

► Are excreted into the bile.

► "Secondary bile acids", including **deoxycholate and lithocholate,** are formed in the <u>colon </u>as bacterial metabolites of the primary bile acids.

► In normal bile, the "ratio of glycine to taurine" conjugates is about 3:1.

► Bile acids are detergents that in aqueous solutions and above a critical concentration of about 2 mM form molecular aggregates called **micelles.**

► Cholesterol alone is poorly soluble in aqueous environments, and its solubility in bile depends on both the total lipid concentration and the relative molar percentages of bile acids and lecithin.

► **Normal ratios of these constituents favor the formation of solubilizing mixed micelles, while abnormal ratios promote the precipitation of cholesterol crystals in bile.**

⊃ **Lipoproteins and their Clinical Significance**

⇨ **Frequently Asked**

Lipoproteins are spherical particles made up of lipid and protein molecules.

The major lipids of the lipoproteins are cholesterol, triglycerides, and phospholipids

► **Triglycerides and the esterified form of cholesterol** (cholesteryl esters) are nonpolar lipids that are insoluble in aqueous environments (hydrophobic) and comprise the core of the lipoproteins.

► **Phospholipids** and a small quantity of free (unesterified) cholesterol, which are soluble in both lipid and aqueous environments (amphipathic), cover the surface of the particles, where they act as the interface between the plasma and core components.

► **Apolipoproteins,** also occupies the surface of the lipoproteins; the apolipoproteins play crucial roles in the regulation of lipid transport and lipoprotein metabolism.

Lipoproteins have been classified on the basis of their **densities** into five major classes:

✓ Chylomicrons,

✓ Very low density lipoproteins (VLDL),

✓ Intermediate-density lipoproteins (IDL)

✓ LDL,

✓ High-density lipoproteins (HDL).

► Chylomicron	— Transports dietary cholesterol/ TG from <u>intestine to tissues</u>✱✱(Apo B)	► <u>apoB 48</u>✱ ► apo C II ► apoE
► VLDL Is <u>pre beta lipoprotein</u> JK BOPEE 2012	— Transports TG from <u>Liver to Tissues</u>✱	► <u>apoB 100</u>✱ ► apo C II ► apoE
► LDL	— Delivers cholesterol to cells✱	► apoB 100
► IDL		► ApoE
► HDL	— Picks up cholesterol from blood vessels✱ — Highest electrophoretic mobility — Least lipid content — Good cholesterol	► Apo A1✱ AI 1998

► Apo A activates	LCATAI 2008, MAH 2012
► Apo CI activates lipoprotein lipase.	
► Apo CII activates lipoprotein lipase.	AI 2008

APOLIPOPROTEINS The apolipoproteins (apos) provide structural stability to the lipoproteins and determine the metabolic fate of the particles upon which they reside

➲ Important Points to be remembered

► LDL has only one apoprotein B100.	MANIPAL 2004
► LDL has the **highest Cholesterol content** and is **most atherogenic.**	UP 1997
► Chylomicrons have highest **triglyceride content.**	AIIMS 2007
► Chylomicrons contain Apo A, Apo B, Apo C, Apo E	JHARKHAND 2003
► Chylomicrons transport dietary triglycerides.	
► LDL delivers **cholesterol to extrahepatic tissues (Cells).**	
► LDL has scavenging action.	PGI 1997
► LDL receptors are widely present on cell membranes, liver and extrahepatic tissues.	
► After binding with receptors LDL is taken in by **endocytosis.**	
► A rise of intracellular cholesterol inhibits the synthesis of new LDL receptors.	

HDL is "good" as it scavenges body cholesterol and transports cholesterol from liver to tissues. (reverse cholesterol transport)

COMED 2007

⇨ **Secondary Hyperlipidemias**

Disease	Serum cholesterol	Serum triglyceride
Diabetes	Increased	Increased
Nephritic syndrome	Increased	Increased
Hypothyroidism	Increased	Increased
Biliary obstruction	Increased	Normal
Pregnancy	Normal	Increased
Alcoholism	Normal	Increased
Oral contraceptives	Normal	Increased

⊃ **Familial Hypercholesterolemia ✳✳✳(High Yield for 2011/2012)**

FH is due to mutations in the gene for the LDL receptor and is genetically transmitted as AD

Plasma levels of **LDL cholesterol are elevated at birth** and remain so throughout life.

▶ In untreated adults, total cholesterol levels range from (275 to 500 mg/dL).

▶ Plasma triglyceride levels are typically normal, and ☞☞

▶ HDL cholesterol levels are normal or reduced. ☞

▶ As would be expected of a disorder with decreased numbers of LDL receptors, **the fractional clearance of LDL apo B is reduced.** ☞

▶ **LDL production is increased** because the liver secretes more VLDL and IDL and more IDL particles are converted to LDL rather than taken up by the hepatic LDL receptors.

▶ FH heterozygotes usually develop **severe atherosclerosis in early or middle age.** ☞

— **Tendon xanthomas**, which are due to both intracellular and extracellular deposits of cholesterol, most commonly involve the Achilles tendons and the extensor tendons of the knuckles☞

— **Tuberous xanthomas,**☞ which are softer, painless nodules on the elbows and buttocks, a

— **Xanthelasmas**, which are barely elevated deposits of cholesterol on the eyelids, are common ☞

▶ **Type II Familial Hyper cholestrolemia** is due to **defective LDL receptors** with high LDL and cholesterol levels.✳✳

▶ **Type I Familial Hyperlipoproteinemia** is due to **deficiency of lipoprotein lipase or Apo C II** with increased chylomicrons and triglycerides.✳✳✳

⊃ **Familial Lipoprotein Lipase Deficiency ✳✳✳(High Yield for 2011/2012)**

▶ **Autosomal recessive** disorder

▶ Is due to the **severe impairment or absence of LPL,**(Lipoprotein lipase)

▶ Leading to massive accumulation of **chylomicrons** in plasma. ☞

AIIMS 2000

3

► Manifestations begin in infancy and include

➥ Pancreatitis,

➥ Eruptive xanthomas,

➥ Hepatomegaly, splenomegaly,

➥ Foam cell infiltration of the bone marrow, ➤ and, when the level of triglycerides is (1000 mg/dL), lipemia retinalis. Atherosclerosis is not accelerated.

► The diagnosis is suspected by finding a creamy layer (**chylomicrons**) at the top of plasma that has ➤incubated overnight;

⟴ Abetalipoproteinemia: (High Yield for 2011/2012)

► It is **AR** disease

► **Defective synthesis or secretion of Apo B** with:

► **Low levels of chylomicrons, VLDL and LDL**   PGI 2002

► **Low levels of Cholesterol and Triglycerides.**

Clinical features include

✓ **Fat Malabsorption,**

✓ **failure to thrive,**

✓ **Neuropathy,**

✓ **Spinocerebellar degeneration,**

✓ **Retinitis pigmentosa,**

✓ **Acantholysis.**

Treatment is with low fat, High calorie diet.

► Chylomicrons are Lipoproteins **lowest in density**➤➤

► Chylomicrons are Lipoproteins **largest in size.**➤➤

► Chylomicrons are Lipoproteins with **highest percentage of lipid**➤

► Chylomicrons are Lipoproteins **lowest percentage of protein** ➤

► **Chylomicrons have least electrophoretic mobility**   AI 2010

⇨ Phospholipids Include

► **Plasmalogens**

► **Cardiolipin**

► **Lecithin**   DNB 1990

► **Sphingomyelin**   AIIMS 1984

► **Cephalin**

⇨ **Essential Fatty Acids are**

— Linoleic acid
— Linolenic acid
— Ecosopantanoic acid
— Docosa Hexanoic acid
— Arachidonic acid.

➥ Most essential is <u>linoleic acid.</u>
➥ <u>Safflower oil, Sunflower oil</u> is a rich source of linoleic acid.
➥ Breast milk is a rich source of <u>Docosa Hexanoic acid</u>
➥ Vegetable oils have high concentration of <u>unsaturated</u> fatty acids.
➥ Mustard oil, ground nut oil, fish oil are sources of <u>omega 3 PUFA acids</u>.
➥ Soya bean has high concentration of <u>PUFA.</u>

⇨ **Iodine Number**

— Is the number of grams of iodine absorbed by 100 grams of fat.
— It is a measure of degree of unsaturation of fat.
— Higher the iodine number more is the degree of unsaturation present.
— It is used to assess purity & nutritive value of fat.

⇨ **Saponification Number**

— Is the number of milligrams of KOH needed to saponify completely gram of fat.
— It is inversely proportional to average chain length of fatty acid consitituting the fats.
— It is higher for comprising short chain fatty acids and vice versa.
— **Iodine number** is the number of grams of Iodine absorbed by 100 grams of fat.
— It is a measure of degree of unsaturation of fat.
— Higher the iodine number, more I the degree of unsaturation present.
— It is used assess purity and nutritive value of fat.

Lipid Metabolism Disease	Deficiency
▶ Fabry's	➥ Alpha galactoside- A(Ceramide trihexoside accumulates)
▶ Niemann- Pick's	➥ Sphingomyelinase (RBC appear as foam cells)
▶ Tay- Sach's	➥ Hexosaminidase A
▶ Sandhoff disease	➥ Hexosaminidase A and B
▶ Krabbe Leukodystrophy	➥ Galacto Cerebrosidase
▶ Metachromatic Leukodystrophy	➥ Arylsulfatase A
▶ Gaucher disease	➥ Gluco Cerebrosidase
▶ Tangier Disease	➥ Lipid Metabolism Disturbed (Low Alpha lipoprotein)

⊃ Niemann-Pick Disease: AI-2010

- Deficiency of sphingomyelinase occurs in: Niemann-Pick Disease

- The lipid accumulates in **Reticuloendothelial cells** in the liver and spleen and other cell types throughout the body including the nerve ganglion cells of the central nervous system.

- The **Neurological features** of Niemann-Pickdisease include mental retardation, spasticity, seizures, jerks, eye paralysis (ophthalmoplegia) and ataxia Physical growth is retarded.

- The **Gastrointestinal features** includehepatosplenomegaly, jaundice, hepatic (liver) failure, and ascites (fluid in the abdomen).

- **Eye features** of Niemann-Pick disease include the **"cherry red spot"** in the macula in the center of the retina, **opacity of the cornea.**

- **Respiratory problems** include pulmonary infiltration. Coronary artery disease occurs early. There is easy bruising.

- The sphingomyelin accumulation is due to **deficiency of the enzyme sphingomyelinase.**

- Typical cells (**Niemann-Pick cells**) that have a **characteristic foamy appearance** due to their storage of sphingomyelin.

⊃ Tangiers Disease ☞☞☞(High Yield for 2011/2012)

- ❑ Alpha lipoprotein (HDL)deficiency☞☞
- ❑ ↓HDL,   KCET 2012
- ❑ ↓LDL,
- ❑ ↓apo A because of high catabolic rates.; abnormal cholesterol uptake into and/or efflux from macrophages; increased apo AI clearance
- Large orange tonsils, ✱✱
- Corneal opacities,
- Relapsing polyneuropathy.
- ❑ No premature atherosclerosis

⇨ Lecithin: Cholesterol Acyltransferase (LCAT) Deficiency (Fish-eye Disease)✱✱✱

- ✓ **Decreased LCAT activity** in plasma leads to accumulation of excess unesterified cholesterol in plasma and body tissues☞☞
- ✓ Total plasma cholesterol level variable with
- ✓ **decrease in esterified cholesterol and** ☞
- ✓ **increase in unesterified cholesterol;** ☞
- ✓ **elevated VLDL** level; structure of **all lipoproteins is abnormal**✱
- ⊚ Corneal opacities,
- ⊚ Hemolytic anemia,
- ⊚ Renal insufficiency,
- ⊚ premature atherosclerosis✱✱

⇨ **Wolmans Disease: (AIIMS PAEDIATRICS 2009)**

► AR disorder ☛☛

► Lipid storage disease.☛

► **Lysosomal acid lipase deficiency**✱ causes accumulation of triglycerides, cholestryl esters and other fats within the cells of affected individuals.☛

► **Lipids accumulate** in various organs.☛

► **Calcification of adrenals**✱✱

► Hepatospleenomegaly, poor weight gain, anemia, jaundice, and features of severe malnutrition occur.☛☛

⇨ **Lipid Mobilization**

► **Adipose Tissue breakdown yields Fatty acids plus Glycerol**

► **Hormone** sensitive lipase is responsible

► Hormone **sensitive lipase is activated by:**✱✱

➥ ↑Epinephrine☛☛

➥ ↓ Insulin☛

➥ ↑Cortisol☛

⇨ **Sphingolipids**

➥ **Sphingomyelin:** Phosphorylcholine

➥ **Cerebrosides:** Galactose or glucose

➥ **Gangliosides:** N acetyl neuraminic acid

Disease	Enzyme Deficency	Substance Accumlated	Symptoms
Tay sachs	Hexosaminidase☛☛	Ganglioside✱✱	► **Cherry red spot** in macula ► Psychomotor retardation
Gauchers	Glucocerebrosidase☛	Glucocerebroside✱	► Erosion of bones ► Hepatospleenomegaly ► **Crumpled paper inclusions** in macrophages
Niemann Picks	Sphingomyelinase☛☛	Sphingomyelin✱✱	► Cherry red spot in macula ► Mental ► Retardation ► Zebra body inclusions. ► **Foamy Macrophages**

⇨ **Amino Acid Metabolic Defects**

Phenylketonuria:✳✳ Mousy odour of urine PGI 1997	**Phenylalanine Hydroxylase☞** UP 2007, UP 2006 JKBOPEE 2012	▶ Mental retardation, seizures,, hyperactivity, ▶ Tremor, ▶ Microcephaly, Hypopigmentation, ▶ Failure to grow are features ▶ Musty urine
Alkaptonuria:✳✳	**Homogentisate oxidase☞** JK BOPEE 2011	▶ **Urine darkens on standing** ▶ Pigmentation of the sclerae and ears. ▶ Generalized darkening of the concha, anthelix, and helix of the ear are typical. ▶ Arthritis **KERALA 1997** ▶ Pigmentation of heart valves, larynx, tympanic **membranes, and skin.** ▶ **Arthritis**
Maple syrup urine disease MSUD✳✳	**Branched chain α Ketoacid dehydrogenase.☞**	▶ **Valine, Leucine, Isoleucine defect** ▶ Maple syrup urine ▶ Lethargic baby, Loses weight, Ketosis, Coma
Homocystinuria✳✳ Abnormal methionine metabolism.	**Cystathionine synthetase.☞☞☞**	▶ Mental retardation, MI, Osteeoporosis, ▶ Dislocation of lens. ▶ It is inherited as **AR** triat. ▶ Patients can be responsive to **Vitamin B6** (Pyridoxine)
Albinism✳✳	**Tyrosinase ☞**	▶ White hair ▶ Photosensitivity ▶ Strabismus ▶ Nystagmus ▶ Photophobia

⇨ **Maple Syrup Urine Disease AI-2010**

➥ **Defective metabolism of branched keto acids seen in: Maple syrup urine disease**

➥ Maple syrup urine disease (MSUD), also called branched-chain ketoaciduria, is an autosomal recessive metabolic disorder affecting branched-chain amino acids.

➥ The condition gets its name from the distinctive sweet odor of affected infants' urine.

➥ MSUD is caused by a deficiency of the branched-chain alpha-keto acid dehydrogenase complex (BCKDH), leading to a build-up of the **branched-chain amino acids (leucine, isoleucine, and valine)** and their toxic by-products in the blood and urine.

- The disease is characterized in an infant by the presence of sweet-smelling urine, with an odor similar to that of maple syrup. Infants with this disease seem healthy at birth but if left untreated suffer severe brain damage, and eventually die.

- From early infancy, symptoms of the condition include poor feeding, vomiting, dehydration, lethargy, hypotonia, seizures, ketoacidosis, opisthotonus, pancreatitis, coma and neurological decline.

⊃ Albinism: (High Yield for 2011/2012)

— The most common form of albinism is caused by a deficiency of **copper-dependent tyrosinase (tyrosine hydroxylase),** blocking the production of **melanin** from the aromatic amino acid tyrosine. Affected individuals lack melanin pigment in skin, hair, and eyes, and are prone to develop sun-induced skin cancers, including both **squamous cell carcinomas and melanomas.**

⊃ Amino Acid Transport Defects

⇨ Cystinuria:➤➤➤

- **Defective transport of Basic amino acids (COAL: Cystine, Ornithine, Arginine, Lysine)**
- Cystine calculi and cystine crystals in urine
- Cyanide Nitrosoprusside Test positive

⇨ Hartnups Disease:➤➤

- Defective renal and intestinal transport of **Tryptophan**
- Malabsorption, Ataxia, Pellagrous rash

⇨ Fanconis Syndrome

- Generalized Tubular damage
* Aminoaciduria,
* Glycosuria,
* Phosphaturia (AGP)
- Renal Tubular disorders, Progressive Renal Failure

⊃ Some Important Organic Acidurias: High Yield for AIPGME/AIIMS/PGI 2013

Disorders	Deficient Enzyme	Clinical Features
Methyl malonic aciduria	Methyl malonyl CoA mutase or B12 co-enzyme	Ketoacidosis, hypotonia, hypoglycemia, hyperammonemia, hyperuricemia
Propionic acidemia	Propionyl CoA carboxylase	Ketoacidosis, hypotonia, vomiting, lethargy
MCADH deficiency	Medium chain acyl CoA dehydrogenase	Acidosis, hyperammonemia; Hypoglycemia, fatty liver.

➡ LCADH deficiency	Long chain acyl CoA dehydrogenase	➡ Nonketotic hypoglycemia, ➡ low carnitine,increased acyl carnitine
➡ Glutaric aciduria	Glutaryl CoA dehydrogenase	➡ Ketoacidosis, convulsions progressive neurological defects, cerebral palsy.

⇨ **Defects in the Intestinal Amino Acid Transport**

- ➡ Hartnup's disease
- ➡ Iminoglycinuria
- ➡ Cystinuria
- ➡ Lysinuric protein intolerance
- ➡ Oasthouse syndrome.

⊃ **Urea Cycle (High Yield for 2011/2012)**

- ▶ Takes place in liver and brain.➡➡
- ▶ Ist two reactions occur in mitochondria.➡➡   PGI 2005
- ▶ Ist two reactions are rate controlling reactions.➡➡
- ▶ Combination of "**Hyperammonemia+ ↑Blood Glutamine+↓Blood urea**" suggests defect in Urea Cycle. Lethargy, vomiting, coma are associated.➡➡
- ▶ Source of ammonia in urine is glutamine.   AIIMS 2007

Exopeptidases:
- ☐ Carboxypeptidases
- ☐ Aminopeptidase
- ☐ Prolidase

Endopeptidases:
- ☐ Elastase
- ☐ Trypsin
- ☐ Chymotrypsin
- ☐ Collagenase

⊃ **Important Facts about Urea Cycle**

- ➡ Urea is major disposal form of amino groups derived from amino acids.
- ➡ One nitrogen atom is supplied by **free ammonia and other by aspartate**
- ➡ Carbon and oxygen of urea is derived from carbon dioxide
- ➡ Urea is produced in LIVER & excreted by the KIDNEYS in urine.
- ➡ **First 2 reactions of urea synthesis occur in mitochondria**
- ➡ **Remaining 3 reactions of synthesis occur in cytosol**
- ➡ Ist step in synthesis is formation of carbamoyl phosphate, this is the rate limiting step in urea synthesis.
- ➡ Final step in urea synthesis is cleavage of arginine by arginase enzymes, present only in liver.

⇨ **Genetic Defects in Urea Synthesis**

▶ Carbomyl Phosphate Synthetase	▶ Ornithine Transcarbomylase
▶ ↑Ammonia +↑Blood Glutamine+↓Blood urea	▶ ↑Ammonia +↑Blood Glutamine +↓Blood urea
▶ No increase in Uracil or orotic acid	▶ Increase in Uracil or orotic acid✱✱

⊃ **Urea Cycle Disorders: High Yield for AIPGME/AIIMS/PGI 2013**

Diseases	Enzyme Deficit	Features
Hyperammonemia type 1	CPS-I	Very high NH3 level levels in blood. Autosomal recessive. Mental retardation.
Hyperammonemia type 2	(OTC) Ornithine transcarbamoylase	✓ Ammonia level high in blood. ✓ Increased glutamine in blood, CSF & urine. ✓ Orotic aciduria due to the channelling of carbamoyl phosphate into Pyrimidine synthesis. ✓ X - linked.
Hyperornithinemia	Defective ornithine transporter protein	✓ Failure to import ornithine from cytoplasm to mitochondria. ✓ Defect in ORNT1 gene. ✓ Hyperornithinemia, hyperammonemia & homocitrullinuria is seen (HHH syndrome) ✓ Decreased urea in blood. ✓ Autosomal recessive condition.
Citrullinemia	Argininosuccinate synthethase	✓ Autosomal recessive inheritance. High blood levels of ammonia and citrulline. Citrullinuria (1-2 g/day).
Argininosuccinic aciduria	Argininosuccinate lyase	✓ Argininosuccinate in blood and urine. Friable brittle tufted hair (Trichorrhexis nodosa).
Hyperargininemia	Arginase	✓ Arginine increased in blood and CSF. Instead of arginine, cysteine and lysine are lost in urine.

⇨ **Ammonia is Generated**

- ▶ From amino acids: by Aminotransferase and Glutamate dehydrogenase
- ▶ From urea by urease
- ▶ From amines by amine oxidase
- ▶ From glutamine by glutaminase

⊃ **Defects of Purine and Pyrimidine Metabolism: (High Yield for 2011/2012)**

▶ Orotic Aciduria	Orotic acid phosphoribosyl transferase/OMP decarboxylase	Autosomal recessive Lack of pyrimidine synthesis needed for haematopoesis	A new borne with Megaloblastic anemia with orotic acid crystals in urine

▶ Lesch Nyhan Syndrome☞	Deficiency of HGPRT MAH 2012 JKBOPEE 2012	X linked recessive	A child with cerebral palsy, repeated **self biting** and **needle** shaped crystals in urine with hyperuricemia
▶ Severe combined immunodeficiency ▶ SCID☞	Adenosine deaminase deficency	Autosomal recessive	A boy with severe immunodeficiency with ↓B and↓ T cells

Remember:

— HPRT catalyzes the reaction that combines PRPP and the purine bases hypoxanthine and guanine to form the respective nucleoside monophosphate IMP or GMP and pyrophosphate.　　　　　　**MAH 2012**

— The enzyme is encoded by a single gene located on the X chromosome in region q26-q27. Consequently, affected males are hemizygous for the trait and inherit the mutant allele from their asymptomatic mother, who is a carrier, or are the result of spontaneous gene mutations.

— The deficiency state is generally the result of point mutations, small deletions or insertions, or endoduplication of exons rather than major gene alterations.

➲ Lesch-Nyhan Syndrome: High Yield for AIPGME/AIIMS/PGI 2013

A baby that was apparently normal at birth begins to show a delay in motor development by 6 months of age. At three year of age, the child begins to develop spasticity and writhing movements. At age four, compulsive biting of fingers and lips and head-banging appear. At puberty, the child develops arthritis, and death from renal failure occurs at age 21.

— The patient has a classical case of Lesch-Nyhan syndrome.

— An X-linked disorder due to severe deficiency of **the purine salvage enzyme hypoxanthine-guanine phosphoribosyltransferase (HPRT).**

— This defect is associated with **excessive de novo purine synthesis.**

— **Hyperuricemia,** and the clinical signs and symptoms described.

— The biochemical basis of the often striking self-mutilatory behavior. Treatment with allopurinol inhibits xanthine oxidase and **reduces gouty arthritis, urate stone formation, and urate nephropathy.**

— A **Partial deficiency of HPRT**, the **Kelley-Seegmiller syndrome**, is associated with hyperuricemia but no central nervous system manifestations✱✱

➲ Kelley-Seegmiller Syndrome: (High Yield for 2011-2012)

— A complete deficiency of HPRT, Lesch-Nyhan syndrome, is characterized by
- ↦ Hyperuricemia,
- ↦ Self-mutilative behavior,
- ↦ Choreoathetosis,
- ↦ Spasticity, and
- ↦ Mental retardation.　　　　　　**JKBOPEE 2012**

— A partial deficiency of HPRT, the **Kelley-Seegmiller syndrome**, is associated with hyperuricemia but no central nervous system manifestations.

— In both disorders, the hyperuricemia results from urate overproduction and can cause **uric acid crystalluria, nephrolithiasis, obstructive uropathy, and gouty arthritis.**

— Early diagnosis and appropriate therapy with allopurinol can prevent or eliminate all the problems attributable to hyperuricemia but have no effect on the behavioral or neurologic abnormalities.

⇨ **Gout**   AI 2010

* **Gout is a disorder of Purine** metabolism.
* Gout is a metabolic disease.
* Most often affecting middle-aged to elderly men and postmenopausal women.
* Due to an increased body pool of urate with hyperuricemia.
* It is characterized by episodic acute and chronic arthritis, due to deposition of **MSU (mono sodium, urate)** crystals in joints and connective tissue tophi.
* The risk for deposition in kidney interstitium or **uric acid nephrolithiasis.**

⇨ **Allopurinol**

▶ Allopurinol and its metabolite, oxipurinol (alloxanthine), decrease the production of uric acid by **inhibiting the action of xanthine oxidase,** the enzyme that converts hypoxanthine to xanthine and xanthine to uric acid. ☞

▶ Allopurinol thereby **decreases uric acid concentrations** in both serum and urine. ☞

▶ Also, allopurinol increases reutilization of hypoxanthine and xanthine for nucleotide and nucleic acid synthesis via an action involving the enzyme hypoxanthine-guanine phosphoribosyltransferase (HGPRTase). ☞

▶ The resultant increase in nucleotide concentration leads to feedback inhibition of de novo purine synthesis.

⤷ **Hyperuricemia: (High Yield for 2011/2012)**

◗ **Increased Purine synthesis:** Lesch Nyhan Syndrome, Type I glycogen storage disease. ☞☞

◗ **Increased Purine Turn over:** High purine diet, Myeloproliferative disorders, Exfoliative diseases(Psoriasis)☞

◗ **Decreased uric acid excretion:** Primary gout, Renal failure, alcohol, starvation☞

◗ **Drugs:**

✓ **Thiazides,**

✓ **Loop diuretics,**

✓ **Pyrimidine,**

✓ **Ethambutol,**

✓ **Salicylates,**

✓ **Cytotoxic agents.** ☞

▶ Gout is due to increased purine metabolism.

▶ Uric acid production ↑

▶ Raised uric acid in synovial fluid is a feature.

3

⇨ **"Important Molecules/Substances Frequently asked In Examinations"**
Glycoproteins: (High Yield for 2011/2012)

▶ Glycoproteins are also called **mucoproteins.**

▶ Glycoproteins are proteins that have oligosaccharide side chains covalently attached to their polypeptide back bones.

Prooteins linked with glycosidic bonds   **PGI 2007**

▶ Most of the plasma proteins in humans **except albumin** are glycoproteins.

▶ Certain hormones (HCG, TSH) are also glycoproteins.

▶ "Glycoproteins contain **N terminal signal sequences** which **direct** the growing polypeptide chain to ER

(Endoplasmic Reticulum and Golgi Complex) **where** Carbohydrates are added and

Proteins are **sorted** to their proper destination."

☐ **Functions of glycoproteins:**

1. **Cell surface recognition**   **PGI 2007**

2. **Cell surface antigenicity**☞

3. **Components of extracellular matrix**☞

4. **Composition of globular proteins in plasma.**☞

⇨ **Glycosaminoglycans: High Yield for AIPGME/AIIMS/PGI 2013**

▶ **(GAG)** Glycosaminoglycans are large complexes of **"negatively charged, unbranched heteropolysacchride chains"** usually composed of **"repeating disaccharide"** units.

▶ They produce **"gel like matrix"** and hold large quantities of water.   **AI 2007**

▶ They are also called as **"mucopolysacchrides"**.

▶ They are synthesized in **Golgi bodies.**

▶ They are degraded by **lysosomal hydrolases.**

▶ Deficency of lysosomal hydrolases results in accumulation of GAG causing **mucopolysacchroidoses.**Examples are:

✓ **Chondritin 4 sulfate**☞☞

✓ **Chondritin 6 sulfate.**☞

✓ **Heparin**☞

✓ **Heparin sulfate** ☞

✓ **Keratin sulfate**☞☞

✓ **Dermatin sulfate**☞

✓ **Hyaluronic acid**☞☞

⊃ **Glutathione: (High Yield for 2011/2012)**

▶ Glutathione is a **tripeptide (Glutamyl-cysteinyl-glycine)** present in most cells. It serves as an important reducing agent along with ascorbate, vitamin E and beta carotene.➛➛   **AIIMS 2008**
▶ It **detoxifies hydrogen peroxide**. This reaction catalyzed by selenium requiring glutathione peroxidase forms oxidized glutathione.➛➛
▶ After this cells regenerate the essential glutathione in a reaction catalysed by glutathione reductase.
▶ Glutathione also helps in transport of certain amino acids in to the cell.
▶ It has **"electron donating properties"** and functions as an intracellular reducing agent.**(anti oxidant effects)**➛➛
▶ Reduced glutathione **detoxifies hydrogen peroxide.**➛➛
▶ It acts as a **carrier of amino acids** in kidney.➛
▶ It helps in **conjugation reactions** and **detoxification of xenobiotics.**➛➛   **AIIMS 2008**
▶ Following an acute ingestion of Acetaminophen, sulfate and glucuronide pathways become saturated, resulting in an increased fraction and amount of acetaminophen metabolized to NAPQI and **eventual glutathione depletion.**➛ When this occurs, free NAPQI binds covalently to hepatocytes and causes their lysis (centrilobular necrosis). Less often, hepatotoxicity develops following the chronic ingestion of therapeutic or slightly greater amounts in conditions associated with <u>**decreased glutathione reserves**</u> ➛(e.g., alcoholism, childhood, acute starvation, chronic malnutrition).

⇨ **Other Antioxidants**

❑ **Vitamin A**
❑ **Dimethyl thio urea**
❑ **Dimethyl sulfoxide**
❑ **Allopurinol**
❑ **Vitamin E**
❑ **Vitamin C**
❑ **Catalase**   **JKBOPEE 2012**
❑ **Superoxide dismutase**   **JKBOPEE 2012**
❑ **NADPH**

⊃ **Anti-oxidants: High Yield for AIPGME/AIIMS/PGI 2013**

➥ **Vitamin E** is the lipid phase antioxidant.
➥ **Vitamin C** is the aqueous phase antioxidant.
➥ **Ceruloplasmin** can act as an antioxidant in extracellular fluid.
➥ **Caffeine** is another effective antioxidant.
➥ **Cysteine, glutathione and Vitamin A** are minor antioxidants.
➥ **Beta carotene** can act as a chain breaking antioxidant

⇨ PAF

- PAF is a potent "**Glycerophospholipid** "and a phospholipid activator and mediator of leucocyte functions such as inflammation, platelet aggregation, anaphylaxis
- **Neutrophils, basophils, platelets and endothelial cells** produce PAF.
- PAF Mediates "**bronchoconstriction**".
- PAF Causes "**platelet aggregation**".

⇨ Prostaglandins

LTA$_4$:

✓ Produced in leucocytes, platelets, mast cells, vascular tissue.

LTC$_4$, LTD$_4$, LTE$_4$:

✓ contraction of smooth muscle

✓ Bronchoconstriction

✓ Vasoconstriction

✓ ↑vascular permeability

✓ Components of SRSA.

LTB$_4$:

✓ ↑Chemotaxis

✓ Adhesion of WBC

✓ Release of lysosomal enzymes

Thromboxanes:

✓ Produced mainly in platelets

✓ **Promotes** platelet aggregation

✓ Vasoconstriction

✓ Smooth muscle contraction.

Prostacyclins:

✓ Produced by endothelium of vessels

✓ Vasodilation

✓ **Inhibits** platelet aggregation.

▶ **Cortisol inhibits**	Phospholipase A$_2$
▶ Aspirin, Indomethacin, Phenylbutazone inhibit Both	COX 1 and COX 2.
▶ **Coxibs are selective**	COX 2 inhibitors(Celecoxib)

⇨ Ionophores

- ▶ Ionophores are" **organic molecules**" synthesized by **microbes** to "**facilitate movement of ions across membranes**".☛☚
- ▶ Their properties are because of "**lipophilic nature**" and penetrate lipid membranes.☛☚
- ▶ They have **hydrophilic core and hydrophobic periphery.**☛☚
- ▶ Valinomycin is an ionophore.☛

► Representative ionophores <u>(with the ion(s) they act upon):</u> ☞

1. 2,4-Dinitrophenol **(H+)**
2. Beauvericin (Ca2+, Ba2+)
3. Gramicidin A (H+, Na+, K+)
4. Ionomycin (Ca2+)
5. Monensin (Na+, H+)
6. Nigericin (K+, H+, Pb2+)
7. Salinomycin (K+)
8. Valinomycin **(K+)**

⊃ Lysosomes: (High Yield for 2011/2012)

— Lysosomes function as a form of digestive system for a cell.

— They are membrane bound irregular structures with acidophilic character.

Lysosomes contain many enzymes such as:

✓ Ribonucleases
✓ Deoxyribonucleases
✓ Phosphatases
✓ Glycosidases
✓ Arylsulfatases
✓ Collagenases
✓ cathepsins

Peroxisomes are concerned with catabolism of very long chain fatty acids and are implicated in two
diseases: DNB 2011

➠ X linked Adrenoleukodystrophy
➠ Zellweger syndrome.

⇨ Zellwegers Syndrome

Peroxisomes are **single membrane organalles** that are **responsible for β oxidation of fatty chains.**   DNB 2011

Deficency of Peroxisomes causes **Zellwegers syndrome** with accumulation of long chain fatty acids.

"Substance" Accumulation in Different Diseases

► Accumulation of <u>galactocerebrocide</u> occurs in **Krabbe disease**, which is due to galactocerebrocide deficiency. ✱✱

► Accumulation of **glucocerebroside** occurs in **Gaucher disease**, which is due to defects in β-glucocerebrosidase. The reticuloendothelial cells and CNS are affected.✱

► Accumulation of **GM₂ ganglioside** occurs in **Tay-Sachs disease** because of hexosaminidase a deficiency. The swollen ganglion cells of the retina contribute to a classic sign of Tay-Sachs---the macular cherry-red spot. ✱

► Accumulation of **sphingomyelin** in a variety of organs occurs in **Niemann-Pick disease**, which is due to a defect in sphingomyelinase.✱

► Accumulation of **sulfatide** occurs in **Metachromatic leukodystrophy,** caused by arylsulfatase A deficiency.✱

⇨ I Cell Disease (Very Important)✱✱

► Lysosomal enzymes are glycosylated and modified.
► **In the Golgi complex** specific mannose residues are phosphorylated. ☞

3

▶ This phosphorylation directs them towards lysosomes. In absence of Phosphorylation of their mannose residues, these enzymes are (**not directed to lysosomes**) but to extracellular space and inclusions accumulate in cell.☞☞

Features:

▶ Coarse facial features, Macroglossia, Gingival hyperplasia, Club foot, club hand, Cardio respiratory failure.☞☞☞

Rate limiting steps asked in previous examinations given below

⊃ **(High Yield for 2011/2012)**

▶ Cholesterol synthesis	HMG CoA reductase☞☞	JK BOPEE 2011
▶ Ketone body synthesis	HMG CoA Synthetase☞☞	
▶ Fatty acid synthesis	Acteyl Co A Carboxylase☞	
▶ Bile acid synthesis	7 α hydroxylase☞☞	
▶ Gluconeogenesis	Pyruvate carboxylase☞	
▶ Glycogenesis	Glycogen synthetase☞	
▶ Glycolysis	Phosphofructokinase☞☞	
▶ Cathecholamine synthesis	Tyrosine Hydroxylase☞	
▶ Glycogenolysis	Phosphorylase☞☞☞	
▶ Krebs/TCA Cycle	G6PD☞	
▶ Uric acid synthesis	Xanthine Oxidase☞☞	

⊃ **Important Inhibitors of Medically Important Enzymes:**

High Yield for AIPGME/AIIMS/PGI 2013

❑ Xanthine oxidase: Allopurinol☞☞	
❑ Folate reductase: Methotrexate☞	
❑ Lactate Dehyrogenase: Oxamates	
❑ Dihydrofolate reductase: Amethroptin☞	
❑ Vitamin K synthesis: Dicumarol☞	
❑ Aconitase flouroaceteate	AP 2001
❑ Citrate flouroacetate.	TN 2002
❑ α ketoglutarate dehydrogenase arsenate	
❑ Succinate <u>dehydrogenase</u> malonate	ROHTAK 2004
❑ Enolase fluoride	PGI 1993
❑ Glyceraldehydes 3 phosphate iodoacetate	

⊃ Ion-Exchange

Process in which exchange of ions in solution form with that on to surface form occurs in is Ion exchange

✳ **Ion-exchange chromatography** is a process that allows the separation of ions and polar molecules based on their charge.

✳ It can be used for almost any kind of charged molecule including large proteins, small nucleotides and amino acids. The solution to be injected is usually called a sample, and the individually separated components are called analytes.

✳ It is often used in protein purification, wateranalysis, and quality control. Ion exchange chromatography retains analyte molecules on the column based on coulombic (ionic) interactions.

✳ The stationary phase surface displays ionic functional groups (R-X) that interact with analyte ions of opposite charge. This type of chromatography is further subdivided into cation exchange chromatography and anion exchange chromatography.

✳ The ionic compound consisting of the cationic species $M+$ and the anionic species $B-$ can be retained by the stationary phase. Cation exchange chromatography retains positively charged cations because the stationary phase displays a negatively charged functional group.

⊃ Chromatography: AI -2010

⇨ Salting Out

➡ Proteins are purified using **differences in protein solubility** in varying salt concentrations.

➡ The solubility of proteins varies according to the **ionic strength of the solution**, and hence according to the salt concentration.

➡ Two distinct effects are observed;

➡ **At low salt concentrations**, the solubility of the protein increases with increasing salt concentration (increasing **ionic strength**), and effect termed **salting in.**

➡ As the salt concentration (ionic strength) is increased further, the solubility of the protein begins to decrease.

➡ **At high ionic strength**, the protein will be almost completely precipitated from the solution (**salting out**).

➡ Since proteins differ markedly in their solubilities at high ionic strength, salting-out is a very useful procedure to assist in the purification of a given protein. The **commonly used salt is Ammonium sulfate, as it is very water soluble**.   **AIIMS 2009**

➡ The ammonium sulfate concentration is increased stepwise, and the precipitated protein is recovered at each stage.

➡ The precipitated protein is then removed by centrifugation and then the ammonium sulfate concentration is increased to a value that will precipitate most of the protein of interest whilst leaving the maximum amount of protein contaminants still in solution.

➡ This technique is useful to quickly remove large amounts of contaminant proteins, as a first step in many purification schemes. It is also often employed during the later stages of purification to concentrate protein from dilute solution following procedures such as gel filtration.

➲ Restriction Fragment Length Polymorphism (RFLP) (High Yield for 2011/2012)

* Is a <u>difference in homologous DNA sequences</u> that can be detected by the presence of fragments of different lengths after digestion of the DNA samples in question <u>with specific restriction endonucleases</u>

  PGI 2011

* Is a <u>DNA Variation sequence</u>   **PGI 2011**

* RELP, as a molecular marker, is specific to a single clone /restriction enzyme combination.

* An **RFLP** probe is a labeled **DNA sequence that hybridizes with one or more fragments of the digested DNA sample after they were separated by gel electrophoresis,** thus revealing a unique blotting pattern characteristic to a specific genotype at a specific locus. Short, single-or-low-copy genomic DNA or cDNA clones are typically used as RFLP probes.

* RFLPs are **visualized by digesting DNA from different individuals with restriction enzyme, followed by gel electrophoresis** to separate fragments according to size, then blotting and hybridization to a labeled probe that identifies the locus under investigation. An RFLP is demonstrated when ever the Southern blot pattern obtained with one individual is different from the one obtained with another individual.

* RFLP is an **important tool in**

✓ **Genome mapping,**

✓ **Localization of genes from genetic disorders**   **PGI 2011**

✓ **Determination of risk for diseases, and paternity testing.**

* Test which uses oligomer with single base pair substitution: RFLP   **AIIMS 2009**

➲ Paper Chromatography (High Yield for 2011/2012)

* Technique for **identification and determination of amino acids.**

* **The Principle:** A small amount of solvent is put at the bottom of a jar. A strip of absorptive paper, with a concentrated spot of the mixed amino acids near the bottom, is suspended in the jar so that its end dips into the solvent. The solvent moves slowly up the strip of paper, carrying the amino acids with it. As the amino acids travel at different speeds, they separate from one another. The paper is then treated with a reagent which strains the amino acids so they can be detected and identified. The location reagent used for amino acids is **ninhydrin.**

* **Chromatography paper contains about 15-20% water, held to the paper fibres. This water acts as the stationary phase in paper chromatography. Amino acids are separated according to their solubility in the water and in an organic solvent (the mobile phase) moving up the paper. The most non-polar amino acids migrate the furthest, due to their greater solubility in the organic solvent.**

* **Paper also acts as an adsorbent, having an affinity for polar groups.**

➲ Other Important Biochemical Tests (High Yield for 2011/2012)

➡ Barfoed's test	Differentiates monosaccharides disaccharides
➡ Mucic acid test	Detects galactose
➡ Biuret test	Detects proteins

➡ Xanthopretic test	Detects phenylalanine, tyrosine, tryptophan
➡ Million's test	Detects tyrosine
➡ Sullivan reaction	Detects cysteine
➡ Acrolein test	Detects triglycerides
➡ Leiberman Burchard reaction	Detects cholesterol
➡ Salkowsky's reaction	
➡ Rothera test	
➡ Legal's test	Detects ketone bodies
➡ Gerhardt's test	

⇨ **Urate Crystals**

— Are **negatively bireferingent** when viewed under polarizing microscope
— Appear **yellow** when their axis is parallel to light
— Appear **blue** when their axis is perpendicular to light

⇨ **Crystal Types**

➡ **Glucose**	**Needle shaped crystals**
➡ **Fructose**	**Needle shaped Crystals**
➡ **Maltose**	**Sunflower crystals**
➡ **Lactose**	**Cotton ball crystals**

➲ **Important in Biochemistry: (High Yield for 2011/2012)**

Liver Transaminases

Increased liver transaminase levels in liver disease reflect leakage from injured liver cells. The degree of elevation of the transaminases generally reflects the severity of hepatic necrosis, except in the important setting of alcoholic hepatitis, when levels seldom exceed 200 to 300 I.U. per liter.

Alkaline Phosphatase Activity

Activity of ALP is detected in many tissues, including the liver, bile ducts, intestines, bone, kidneys, placenta, or white blood cells. The serum ALP level is also elevated in a number of conditions not associated with hepatobiliary disease, such as pregnancy, normal growth, bone tumors, and liver tumors (the Regan isoenzyme).

Albumin. Albumin is a useful clinical marker of synthetic function in chronic hepatic insufficiency. It is synthesized only in the liver

Transferrin. Also synthesized in the liver, transferrin has a much shorter half-life than albumin. Changes in transferrin levels reflect more acute changes in liver function than do changes in albumin levels.

Bromsulphalein and Indocyanine Green. These dyes are removed from the circulation by the liver. Such intravenous tests have been used to assess liver dysfunction in the absence of jaundice. Each is a measure of biliary excretion and is a more specific quantitative test than any of the routine tests of liver function or cholestasis.

Galactose Elimination Capacity. This test reflects hepatocellular function but requires multiple determinations over a 2-hour period. Galactose is safe and injected intravenously at a dose that saturates the enzyme system responsible for its elimination. The preliminary step is the initial phosphorylation by galactokinase.

Aminopyrine Breath Test. Aminopyrine as well as caffeine have been used as breath test substances that measure the efficiency of the cytochrome P-450 (microsomal) system where they are metabolized. Aminopyrine is labeled with carbon-14 and given by mouth. Carbon dioxide samples labeled with carbon-14 are collected at intervals over 2 hours. This test reflects the residual functional microsomal mass and, thus, viable hepatic tissue. It has more value in assessing prognosis than for screening. Serial salivary caffeine clearance is a similar measure. Antipyrine clearance can also be measured, but the test requires over 30 hours.

⇨ **Important Enzymes**

* **Lipoprotein lipase** degrades triacylglycerol in circulating plasma lipoprotein particles.

* **Gastric lipase** in the stomach hydrolyses triacylglycerol containing short and medium chain - length fatty acids. This enzyme may be of importance only in the degradation of dietary lipids in infants.

* **Pancreatic lipase**, synthesized by the pancreas and present in pancreatic juice, hydrolyses dietary triacylglycerol in the small intestine.

* **Phospholipase A2** is also synthesized by the pancreas and hydrolyses dietary Phospholipids in the small intestine.

* **Muscle glycogen** is degraded to glucose 1- phosphate, which is converted to glucose 6- phosphate by phosphoglyceromutase.

* **Maximum amount of glycogen in health adults is stored in hepatocytes of liver.**   **JK BOPEE 2012**

* **Glucose 6-phosphate** cannot be converted to glucose because muscle lacks the enzyme glucose 6 phosphatase.

* **Glucokinase** is a liver enzyme that converts glucose into glucose 6-phosphate.

* **Glycogen phosphorylase** is the major degradative enzyme in glycogenolysis, producing glucose 1-phosphate, which, in muscle, cannot lead to the release of free glucose.

⇨ **Aspartate Amino Transferase (AST): AI -2010**

➥ AST catalyse transamination **reaction.**

➥ AST exist two different isoenzyme forms which are genetically distinct, **the mitochondrial and cytoplasmic form.** AST is found in highest concentration in **heart** compared with other tissues of the body such as liver, skeletal muscle and kidney.

➥ **Elevated mitochondrial AST** is seen in extensive tissue necrosis during myocardial infarction and in chronic liver diseases like liver tissue degeneration and necrosis.

➥ The ratio of mitochondrial AST to total AST activity has diagnostic importance in identifying the liver cell necrotic type condition and **alcoholic hepatitis.**

⇨ **Classification of Enzymes**

Class 1.	**Oxidoreductases**: Transfer of hydrogen or addition of oxygen; e.g. Lactate dehydrogenase (NAD); Glucose-6-phosphate dehydrogenase (NADP); Succinate dehydrogenase (FAD); dioxygenases.
Class 2.	**Transferases**: Transfer of groups other than hydrogen. Example, Aminotransferase. (Subclass: Kinase, transfer of phosphoryl group from ATP; e.g. Hexokinase)
Class 3.	**Hydrolases**: Cleave bond and add water; e.g. Acetyl choline esterase; Trypsin.
Class 4.	**Lyases**: Cleave without adding water, e.g. Aldolase; HMG CoA lyase; ATP Citrate lyase. (Subclass: Hydratase; add water to a double bond)
Class 5.	**Isomerases**: Intramolecular transfers. They include racemases and epimerases. Examples, Triose phosphate isomerase.
Class 6.	**Ligases**: ATP dependent condensation of two molecules, e.g. Acetyl CoA carboxylase; Glutamine synthetase; PRPP synthetase.

⇨ **Biochemically useful Competitive Inhibitors**

Drug	Enzyme inhibited
☐ Allopurinol	✓ Xanthine oxidase
☐ 6-mercapto-purine	✓ Adenylosuccinate synthetase
☐ 5-fluorouracil	✓ Thymidylate synthase
☐ Azaserine	✓ Phosphoribosyl-amidotransferase
☐ Cytosine arabinoside	✓ DNA polymerase
☐ Acyclovir	✓ DNAP of virus
☐ Neostigmine	✓ ACh-esterase
☐ Alpha-methyl dopa	✓ Dopa-decarboxylase
☐ Lovastatin	✓ HMGCoA-lowering
☐ Oseltamiver	✓ Neuraminidase
☐ Dicoumarol	✓ Vit.K-epoxide-reductase
☐ Penicillin	✓ Transpeptidase
☐ Sulphonamide	✓ Pteroid synthetase
☐ Trimethoprim	✓ FH2-reductase
☐ Pyrimethamine	✓ FH2-reductase
☐ Methotrexate	✓ FH2-reductase

3

BIOCHEMISTRY

⊃ Enzymes used for Diagnostic Purpose: High Yield for AIPGME/AIIMS/PGI 2013

Enzyme	Used for testing
▪ Urease	▪ Urea
▪ Uricase	▪ Uric acid
▪ Glucose oxidase	▪ Glucose
▪ Peroxidase	▪ Glucose;Cholesterol
▪ Hexokinase	▪ Glucose
▪ Cholesterol oxidase	▪ Cholesterol
▪ Lipase	▪ Triglycerides
▪ Horse radish peroxidase	▪ ELISA
▪ Alkaline phosphatase	▪ ELISA
▪ Restriction endonuclease	▪ Southern blot;RFLP
▪ Reverse transcriptase	▪ Polymerase chain reaction(RT=PCR)

⊃ Non Functional Plasma Enzymes used in Clinical Diagnosis:

High Yield for AIPGME/AIIMS/PGI 2013

Serum Enzymes	Diagnostic use
☐ Amylase and lipase	✓ Acute pancreatitis
☐ Aminotransferases	✓ Myocardial infarction
☐ Aspartate aminotransferase (AST or SGOT)	✓ Viral hepatitis
☐ Alanine aminotransferase (ALT or SGPT)	
☐ Acid Phosphatase	✓ Prostate cancer
☐ Alkaline phosphatase	✓ Obstructive liver diseases, bone diseases and hyperparathyroidism
☐ Creatine kinase	✓ Muscle disorders and Myocardial infarction
☐ Ceruloplasmin	✓ Wilson's disease
☐ Gamma-glutamyl transpeptidase	✓ Liver diseases
☐ Lactate dehydrogenase	✓ Myocardial infarction

Sub cellular Organelle	Marker enzyme
▪ Mitochondria	Inner membrane: ✓ ATP Synthase
▪ Lysosome	✓ Cathepsin
▪ Golgi complex	✓ Galactosyl transferase
▪ Microsomes	✓ Glucose-6-phosphatase
▪ Cytoplasm	✓ Lactate dehydrogenase

➲ Key Enzymes under Well Fed Conditions, Fasting and Starvation

Enzyme	Fed	Fasting	Starvation
Glucokinase	Increase	Decrease	Decrease
Phospho fructokinase1	Increase	Decrease	Decrease
Fructose 1,6 biphosphatase	Decrease	Increase	Increase
Pyruvate carboxylase	Decrease	Increase	Increase
PEPCK	Decrease	Increase	Increase
Glycogen phosphorylase	Decrease	Increase	
Glycogen synthase	Increase	Decrease	Decrease
Carnitine acyl transferase		Increase	Increase
Acetyl CoA carboxylase	Increase	Decrease	Decrease
Hormone sensitive lipase	Decrease	Increase	Increase

PEPCK=phosphor enol pyruvate carboxy kinase; F-6-P=fructose-6-phosphate; F-2, 6-bisP=fructose-2, 6 biphosphate; G-6-P = Glucose-6-Phosphate.

➲ Enzyme Deficiencies in Porphyrias: High Yield for AIPGME/AIIMS/PGI 2013

☐ Erythropoetic porphyria	Ferrochelatase
☐ Heridetary Porphyria	Coproporphynogen Oxidase
☐ Vaiegate Porphyria	Protoporphyrinogen Oxidase
☐ Acute Intermittent porphyria	Porphobilinogen Deaminase
☐ Porphyria cutanea Tarda	URO Decarboxylase
☐ Congenital Erythropoetic porphyria	URO III cosynthetase

➲ Metabolic functions of Subcellular Organelles:

High Yield for AIPGME/AIIMS/PGI 2013

Organelle	Function
Nucleus	➥ DNA replication, transcription
Endoplasmic Reticulum	➥ Biosynthesis of proteins, glycoproteins, lipoproteins, ➥ Drug metabolism ➥ Ethanol oxidation ➥ Synthesis of cholesterol (partial)
Golgi body	➥ Maturation of synthesized protein
Lysosome	➥ Degradation of proteins, carbohydrates, lipids and nucleotides

BIOCHEMISTRY

3

Mitochondria	• Electron transport chain,
	• ATP generation,
	• TCA cycle,
	• Beta oxidation of fatty acids,
	• Ketone body production ,
	• Urea synthesis (part),
	• Heme synthesis (part),
	• Gluconeogenesis (part),
	• Pyrimidine synthesis (part),
Cytosol	• Protein synthesis,
	• Glycolysis,
	• Glycogen metabolism,
	• HMP shunt pathway, transaminations, fatty acid synthesis,
	• cholesterol synthesis, heme synthesis (part), urea synthesis (part),
	• pyrimidine synthesis (part), purine synthesis

⟳ Peroxisomal Deficiency Disease

Adreno leuko dystrophy Defeciency of peroxisomal matrix proteins can lead to **Adreno leuko dystrophy (ALD)** (Brown-Schilder's disease) characterized by progressive degeneration of liver, kidneyand brain. It is a rare autosomal recessive condition. The defect is due to insufficient oxidation of very long chain fatty acids **(VLCFA)** by peroxisomes.

Zellweger syndrome, proteins are not transported into the peroxisomes. This leads to formation of empty peroxisomes or peroxisomal ghosts inside the cells.

Primary hyperoxaluria is due to the defective peroxisomal metabolism of glyoxalate derived from glycine.

⟳ G Proteins: (High Yield for 2010/2011)

— **Guanine nucleotide regulatory proteins (G proteins)** are a **superfamily of guanine triphosphate (GTP) binding** proteins that range from the heterotrimeric forms to monomeric forms, GTPase activating protein (GAP), activated G proteins, and ras-associated nuclear proteins.

— The typical G protein involved in receptor signaling is made up of three subunits: **a, b, and g**. The a subunit binds the nucleotide guanosine diphosphate (GDP) and, when activated via receptor interaction, exchanges GDP for guanosine triphosphate (GTP), which renders the G protein active and able to stimulate an effector molecule. An endogenous guanosine triphosphatase (GTPase) activity then hydrolyzes GTP to GDP, deactivating the G protein. In addition to heterotrimeric G proteins, single polypeptide proteins similar to the a subunit of the heterotrimeric G protein, called the small-G proteins, bind GTP. The prototypes of these small-G proteins are the ras oncogenes: **Ha-ras, Ki-ras, and N-ras.**

— Functionally related GTP proteins are involved in **signal transduction, protein synthesis, microtubule assembly, and oncogene function.** G proteins are also coupled to many pharmacologic receptors that mediate vascular smooth muscle cell contractile responses.

➥ The heterotrimeric G proteins are intrinsic membrane-bound proteins that act as **transmembrane signal transducers in cells and activate intracellular secondary messengers, such as adenylate cyclases and phospholipases**. These heterotrimeric G proteins consist of three distinct subunits: **alpha, beta, and gamma.**

➥ G proteins act as inhibitory and excitatory because of difference in alpha subunit   **AIIMS 2008**

⊃ Questions Asked in   **AIPGME 2011**

☐ **Cardioprotective fatty acid is :** Omega-3 fatty acids   **AIPGME 2011**

☐ **Differential RNA regulation is responsible for deciding whether an antibody will remain membrane bound or gets secreted**   **AIPGME 2011**

☐ **Vitamin K is involved in the posttranslational modification of:** Glutamate   **AIPGME 2011**

☐ **Tests used in the diagnosis of diabetes mellitus are:** FBS , HbA1c , OGTT   **AIPGME 2011**

☐ **Transfer of an amino group from an amino acid to an alpha keto acid is done by:** Transaminases

AIPGME 2011

☐ **Predisposing factors for atherosclerotic plaque formation are:** Apo E deficiency, Oxidised LDL, Increased homocystiene   **AIPGME 2011**

☐ **Urea cycle occurs in:** Liver .   **AIPGME 2011**

☐ **Disorder of protein misfolding are:** Alzheimer's disease , Cystic fibrosis, CJD (Creutzfeld- Jakob disease)

AIPGME 2011

⊃ Important Questions Likely to be Repeated

☐ Northern blot test is used for   **RNA analysis**

☐ Mechanism by which pyruvate from cytosol is transported to mitochondria is: **Proton symport**   **MH 2010**

☐ **Malonate** as a poisons act by causing inhibition of complex IV of respiratory chain except: **MH 2010**

☐ Overdose of vitamin A mainly affects: **Lysosome**   (AIIMS 2007 May) (MH 2010)

☐ Pyridoxal phosphate acts as coenzyme for: Alanine transferase, ALA Synthase, Cystathionine Synthase

MH 2010

☐ Menkes Kinky hair syndrome is characterized by congenital deficiency of: **Copper binding ATPase**

☐ **Histidine** has maximum buffering capacity: **MH 2010**

☐ Von Geirke's disease occurs due to deficiency of **Glucose-6-Phosphatase**   **MH 2012**

☐ Fluoride inhibits: **Enolase**   (MHPGMCET 2008) MH2010

☐ Nicotinamide is derived from: **Tryptophan**   (MHPGMCET 2007) MH 2010

☐ The main enzyme responsible for activation of xenobiotics is: **Cytochrome P-450**

3

BIOCHEMISTRY

- ☐ Vitamin B_{12} and folic acid supplementation in megaloblastic anemia leads to the improvement of anemia due to **Increased DNA synthesis in bone marrow**   **AI 2003**

- ☐ Nitric Oxide Synthase : **Requires NADPH, FAD, FMN and Heme iron**   **AI 2003**

- ☐ **Nitric oxide is synthesized from Arginine.**   **JK BOPEE 2011**

- ☐ Elasticity of the corneal layer of skin is due to the presence of :**Keratin**   **AI 2003**

- ☐ In dividing cells, spindle is formed by : **Tubulin**   **AI 2003**

- ☐ If urine sample darkens on standing: the most likely condition is : **Alkaptonuria**   **AI 2002**

- ☐ A baby presents with refusal to feed, skin lesions, seizures, ketosis organic acids in urine with normal ammonia likely diagnosis is: **Multiple carboxylase deficiency**   **AI 2001**

- ☐ tRNA has abnormal purine bases: **AI 2001**

- ☐ Fatty acids is found exclusively in breast milk **Docosahexanoic acid**   **AI 2001**

- ☐ A crystal has **Molecules are arranged in same orientation and same confirmation**   **AI 2001**

- ☐ Prolonged treatment with INH leads to deficiency of: **Pyridoxine.**   **AIPGEE 2011**

- ☐ **Vitamin B 6 Deficiency symptoms**: Seborrhea, glossitis convulsions, neuropathy, depression, confusion, microcytic anemia   **AIPGEE 2011**

- ☐ Urea cycle occurs in: Liver   **AIPGEE 2011**

- ☐ Vitamin K is involved in the post translational modification of: **Glutamate**   **AIPGEE 2011**

- ☐ **Receptors are present in liver for uptake of LDL:** Apo E and Apo B100

- ☐ **Thiamin requirement increases in excessive intake of:**Carbohydrate

- ☐ **Refsum's disease is due to deficiency of enzyme** Phytanic alpha oxidase   **AIIMS 2008**

- ☐ **In molecular cloning, Blue-white screening is used for:** To identify desired chromosomal DNA insert in plasmid vectors

- ☐ **Nephelometry is based on the principle of** Light attenuated in intensity by scattering   **AIIMS 2007**

- ☐ **Peroxidase enzyme is used in estimating :** Glucose   **AIIMS 2007**

- ☐ Molecular change in Lysosomal storage disorder is: **Mutation of genes encoding lysosomal hydrolases.**   **AIIMS 2007**

- ☐ Intron is not found in:**Mitochondrial DNA**   **AIIMS 2008**

- ☐ Vitamin which is excreted in urine is : Vitamin C   **AIIMS 2008**

- ☐ Cytosolic Cytochrome C mediates **Apoptosis**   **AIIMS 2008**

- ☐ Technique which estimates blood creatinine level most accurately: **Jaffe method**

- ☐ G proteins act as inhibitory and excitatory because of difference in alpha subunit   **AIIMS 2008**

NOTES

3

BIOCHEMISTRY

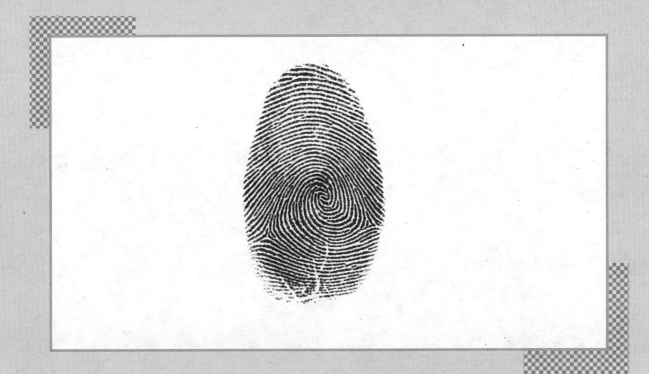

FORENSIC

➲ Basic Terminology Asked in Exams:

✳ **Inquest:** It is the investigation into cause of death conducted in cases of murder, suicide, accidents and Suspicious deaths.☛☛	**TN 1991**
Corners inquest is done in Bombay.	**UPSC 1995**
<u>Police inquest</u> is the commonest type of inquest in india.	**KAR 1994**
In case of death in lock up inquest is conducted by <u>magistrate.</u>	**PGI 1993**
✳ **Subpoena:** is a <u>written document</u> **issued by the court** and served on the witness under a penalty in all cases by the police officer to attend the court for giving evidence on a particular day and time.☛☛ **AMU 2005**	
▶ <u>Criminal cases take priority</u> over civil courts	
▶ <u>Higher courts have priority</u> over lower courts.	
✳ **Conduct money:** It is **fee paid to a witness at the time of serving summons** to cover the expenses for attending the court.☛☛(CIVIL)	**AI 1990**
✳ **Perjury:** It means **telling lies by a witness under oath or failure to tell what he knows or believes to be true.**☛☛	**MAH 1998**

➲ Inquest:

1. **POLICE INQUEST:** Done by officer in charge of a police station, autopsy is done on requisition of senior Head Constable (the person of minimum rank). Police officer visits the scene of crime, prepares a report which includes description of wound, the nature of weapon used and the apparent cause of death. The inquest report (panchnama) is then signed by police officer and two witnesses. If foul play is suspected, the body is sent for autopsy.

2. **CORONER INQUEST:** No longer done in India.

3. **MEDICAL EXAMINER'S INQUEST:** Medical examiner is a forensic pathologist who conducts and supervises inquest. It is considered to be the best form of inquest. Practiced in USA.

4. **MAGISTRATE INQUEST:** Conducted by District magistrate, Sub-divisional magistrate and

   Executive magistrate. It is conducted in following circumstances.

   Executive Exhumation

   Magistrate Death (unnatural) within 7 yrs of **Marriage.**

   Conducted inquest in

   ↪ **Police cases** Death in **P**olicefiring
   ↪ Death in **P**rison
   ↪ Death in **P**olice custody or interrogation
   ↪ Death in **P**sychiatric hospital

Mental ability to make a valid will is: Testamentary capacity.	**AIIMS 1991**
Mc Naughtens rule is for criminal responsibility.	**PGI 2002**

✳ **Dying declaration:** written or oral statement of a person who is dying due to some unlawful act, relating to the cause of his death.☛☛

- **Oath is not necessary** as it is assumed that a dying person will not lie.☛
- **A doctor or any other person** can record the statement in presence of two witnesses.☛
- **Leading questions should not be asked.**☛
- If declarant survives, he is called to **give oral evidence** and dying declaration becomes useless.
- Presence of accused is **not needed.**☛
- **Has lesser legal value.**
- **Medical certificate is a documentary evidence.**   AIIMS 1996

➲ **Dying Deposition:** ☛☛

- **Oath is necessary** ☛
- A **magistrate** records the statement.   AI 1990
- **Leading questions should not be asked.**☛
- Presence of accused /his lawyer is allowed.
- **Has more legal value.**☛☛   TN 1997

➲ **Judicial Magistrate of Second Class** ✳☛

| 1 Year imprisonment | Fine up to Rs 1000 |

➲ **Judicial Magistrate of First Class** ✳☛   **PGI 2006**

| 3 Years imprisonment | Fine up to Rs 5000 |

➲ **Chief Judicial Magistrate** ✳☛

| 7 Years imprisonment | Fine unlimited |

➲ **Assistant Sessions Court**✳ ☛

| 10 Years imprisonment | Fine unlimited |

➲ **Sessions Court**✳☛☛   **KERALA 1999**

| Any sentence authorized by law but death sentence must be confirmed by higher court. |
| **President of india can commute a death sentence.**   JIPMER 1999 |
| **Amnesty for capital punishment vests with president.**   AMU 1998 |

➲ Exhumation ✎✎✎

- Exhumation is the **digging out** of an already buried body from grave.
- Exhumation is done after a written order from <u>First class judicial magistrate</u>.✱   AIIMS 1992
- It should be conducted in **day light.**✱   AIIMS 1992
- Average number of samples of earth taken is: <u>6-7</u>.✱
- Disinfectants **should not be used** on body.✱
- There is **No time limit** for exhumation in India.✱   JK BOPEE 2012
- Exhumation is **not done** for Hindus. ✱

➲ PM (Postmortem)

- PM (Postmortem) should **not be undertaken without permission** from police, Magistrate or Corner.✱✱
- PM is conducted in **day light**✱✱
- PM is conducted by a **practitioner trained** in forensic sciences mostly.✱
- **All body cavities** should be preferably opened and all organs should be examined.
- Doctor should **record all positive and negative findings.**✱
- **Viscera should be preserved** for toxicology analysis✱
- After PM, **opinion should be formed** as to the cause and mode of death and report should be **produced in** <u>triplicate</u>.
- In cases of "<u>Asphyxia</u>", **skull** should be opened first and neck last.✱
- In case of "<u>Newborn</u>", **abdominal cavity** should be opened first.✱

➲ Important Sections

- Sec 118 IPC—Concealing design to commit offence punishable with death or imprisonment for life.
- Sec 176, IPC—Omission to give notice or information to public servant by person legally bound to give it.
- Sec 177 IPC—Furnishing false information.
- Sec 182 IPC—False information with intent to cause public servant to use lawful power to the injury of another person. --Sec 191 IPC—Giving false evidence
- Sec 192 IPC—Fabricating false evidence.✱
- Sec 193 IPC—Punishment for false evidence.✱(Perjury)   AI 2003
- Sec 197 IPC—Issuing or signing false certificates.✱✱
- Sec 201 IPC—Causing disappearance of evidence of offence, or giving false information to screen offenders.
- Sec 203 IPC—Giving false information respecting an offence committed.
- Sec 204 IPC—Destruction of document to prevent its production as evidence.✱
- Sec 284 IPC —Negligent conduct with respect to poisonous substances.

4

FORENSIC

►	Sec 304A IPC—Causing death by negligence. ✱✱	UP 2003
►	Sec 304B IPC- Dowry ✱✱	KERALA 2K
►	Sec 309 IPC—Attempt to commit suicide✱	
►	Sec 313 IPC—Causing miscarriage without woman's consent.	
►	Sec 318 IPC—Concealment of birth by secret disposal of dead body.	
►	Sec 319 IPC—Hurt.	
►	Sec 320 IPC—Grievous hurt. ✱✱	PGI 1992
►	Sec 351 IPC—Assault.	
►	Sec 362 IPC—Abduction.	
►	Sec 375 IPC —Rape. ✱✱	
►	Sec 376 IPC—Punishment for rape.	
►	Sec 377 IPC—Unnatural offences.✱✱	PGMEE 2004
►	Sec 497 IPC—Adultery.	

► Sec 39 Cr. P.C—Every person, aware of the commission of or of the intention of any other person to commit any offence is punishable under I.P.C. shall forthwith give information to the nearest magistrate of police officer of such commission or intention.✱

► Sec 84 IPC—Nothing is an offence which is done by a person who at the time of doing it, by reason of unsoundness of mind, is incapable of knowing the nature of the act or what he is doing is either wrong or contrary to law.✱

➲ Types of Witness

COMMON WITNESS	EXPERT WITNESS	HOSTILE WITNESS
Person who gives evidence about facts observed by himself.	Person who is qualified or experienced in a scientific or technical subject and is capable of giving opinion from the facts observed by him self or others. ✓ Doctor　　　　　　　　　JK BOPEE ✓ Finger print expert ✓ Fire arm expert　　　　　PGMEE 02 　　IMPORTANT POINT IS THAT ANY PROFESSIONAL CAN BE A COMMON WITNESS AS WELL. 　　Say a doctor can be an expert witness as well as a common witness. JK BOPEE 2012	Person who has some motive or interest for concealing part of truth and fact or for giving false evidence

Chain of custody is method to **verify the actual possession** of an object from the time it was identified until it is offered into evidence in the court room.

Cognizable offence: offence for which a **police officer** can arrest a person without warrant from a magistrate eg: rape, murder, robbery.

Privileged communication	Novus Actus Interveniens	Res Ipsa Loquitur
Statement communicated by a doctor to the concerned authorities to protect the interests of community. Eg:issuing statements in case of: • Syphilitic taking bath in a pool. • Driver found to be colour blind • A person with infectious disease working as a cook. UPSC 2001	*Means unrelated action intervening.* A person is responsible for his actions and also for its consequences. Eg a doctor leaving a scissor in the abdomen, doctor becomes negligent AIPGEE 2000	*Means things or facts speak for itself.*

Professional negligence	Criminal Negligence	Contributory negligence
Also called as malpraxis *Is the absence of reasonable care and skill or willful negligence on part of a doctor in treatment of his patient resulting in death/ injury.* AP 1992	*Occurs when doctor shows gross lack of competency, inattention, criminal indifference to patients safety*	*Negligence on the part of patient combined with doctors negligence which contributes to the injury as a direct cause and without which injury could not have occurred.*

Therapeutic misadventure	Vicarious liability
It is a case in which a patient dies due to some unintentional act done by a doctor or hospital. MAHE 1998	*An Employer is responsible not only for his negligence but also for the negligence of his employees.*

Corpus Delicti : (Body of offence, Essence of crime) means elements of any criminal offence   AIIMS 2008

Race is determined by: Cephalic index   PGI 2004, 2003

Cephalic index = $\dfrac{\text{Maximum breadth}}{\text{Maximum length}} \times 100$

◗ Skull Indicies

▶ **Dolicocephalic** skull:	▶ seen in **Aryans**	▶ CI=70 — 75	AI 2004
▶ **Mesati** cephalic skull:	▶ seen in **Europeans/ Chinese**	▶ CI=75 — 80	
▶ **Brachy** cephalic skull:	▶ seen in **Mongols**	▶ CI=80 — 85	

➲ Dentition:

— Dentition study is the best method to study age **up to 14 years.**	**KERALA 1994**
— Hypothyroidism delays dentition.	**PGI 2005**
— Eruption of primary teeth is completed by year: 2—2.5 years	**KERALA 1991**
— **Mixed dentition** is seen in 6—11 years.	**ORISSA 1998**

Temporary teeth	Permanent teeth
▶ Smaller, lighter, narrow	▶ Heavier, stronger , Broader
▶ Crown is <u>china</u> white in color	▶ Crown is <u>ivory</u> white in color
▶ Neck is more constricted	▶ Neck is less constricted
▶ Ridge is present	▶ Ridge is absent
▶ 20 in number	▶ 32 in number
▶ Dental formula is I C M: 2 1 2	▶ Dental formula is I C P M: 2 1 2 3

In case of **Deciduous teeth:**

- **Central lower incisors** appear first at:✳ 6 months
- First molar appears at: ✳ 12 months
- Canine appears at : 18 months
- Second molar appears at : 24 months

In case of **Permanent teeth:**

- **First molar** appears at: ✳ 6 years **JIPMER 2002**
- Canine appears at : ✳ 11 years
- Second molar appears at : 12 years
- **Third molar** appears at: 18 years

➲ Gustafsons Method:

— Age estimation of adult over 21 years depending on **physiological age changes in dental tissue.**

— Remember:

— Gustafsons method is used for age determination in adults by six physiological changes in teeth.

▶ **Attrition**

▶ **Paradentosis**

▶ **Amount of secondary dentin**

▶ **Cementum apposition**

▶ **Degree of root resorption**

▶ **Transparency of root dentine**

AIIMS 2006

Ossification centre for :

▶ Calcaneum appears at:✳   5 th month

▶ Sternum appears at:✳   6 th month

▶ Talus appears at : ✳   7 th month

▶ Lower end of femur appears at :✳   10 th month

▶ Upper tibia appears at :✳   10 th month

▶ Xiphoid process unites with rest of body at about   40 years of age.☞   JK BOPEE

▶ Greater cornu of hyoid bone unites with the body between   40-60 years☞

▶ Any act which is done by a child **under 7 years** of age is not an offence.☞

▶ A child between **7-12 years** is assumed to be capable of committing an offence if he attains sufficient maturity☞.

▶ Sexual intercourse by a man even with his wife under **15 years** or with any other girl **under 16 years** even with her consent is an offence.☞

▶ A child below **14 years** cannot be employed to work in any factory or mine.☞

➲ Dactylography: Frequently Asked

▶ Finger prints can be reliably determined upto depth of **0.6 mm.**☞

▶ **Dalton system or dactylography** is other name for fingerprinting.☞   **PGI 2005**

▶ **Sir William Heschle** used this technique first in India.☞   **AIIMS 2008**

▶ Ridge pattern of finger prints appears as early as **12 weeks of IUL** and is completed by 24 weeks.☞

▶ They are present on **both epidermis as well as dermis.**☞

▶ They remain **constant** throughout life.☞

▶ They are absolutely **individual.**

▶ Even identical twins don't have identical finger prints.☞   **KAR 1996**

▶ **Loops are the commonest** variety followed by whorls, arches and composite.☞   **AI 2005**

▶ Permanent impairment of finger prints occurs in

✓ **Leprosy,**   **AIIMS 2006**

✓ **Electric injury,**

✓ **Radiation exposure,**

✓ **Skin grafting.**☞

▶ One of the best methods of identification.   **RAJ 1997**

⇨ Don't Confuse With:

➥ **DNA finger printing** : This is a technique to **determine paternity/maternity**☞

➥ **Brain fingerprinting** is a technique using electrical brain responses to detect the presence or absence of information stored in brain☞

➥ Electronic sensors measuring EEG activity from different parts of scalp are used.☞

➥ **Dr Lawrence Farewell** invented this technique.

Chelioscopy is study of prints of lips.   AI 2007

4

Signs of Death	Tests For Live Birth
▶ **Diaphnous test** (Finger webs lose lusture)	▶ **Wriedens Test** (air in middle ear)
▶ **Icards Dye Test** (Dye injected IV does not change in color)	▶ **Breslous sign** (air in stomach + Duodenum)
▶ **Magnus Test** (Ligature test)	▶ **Foders Test** (on basis of weight of lungs)
▶ **Winslows Test** (Reflections from mirror over chest move with respiration)	▶ **Pioquets Test** (on basis of ratio of weight of lungs to body)
	▶ **Hydrostatic floatation Test** (lungs float if a child has respired)

Immediate signs of death	Early signs of death	Late signs of death
▶ Insensibility and loss of voluntary power	▶ Pallor	▶ Putrefaction
▶ Cessation of respiration	▶ Primary Flaccidity of muscles	▶ Adipocere formation
▶ Cessation of circulation	▶ Changes in eyes	▶ Mummification
	▶ Cooling of body	
	▶ Post mortem Lividity	
	▶ Rigor mortis	

⊃ Cooling of Body

▶ Is called "**Algor Mortis**" Not Rigor Mortis.

▶ Internal organs take <u>24 hours</u> to cool.

▶ Curve of cooling is <u>sigmoid</u>.

▶ Post mortem caloricity is increase in temperature for first two hours after death by

— **Sun stroke,**

— **Septicemia,**

— **Tetanus,**

— **Strychinine poisoning**

▶ Rate of cooling in **first 6 hours is 2.5°F per hour** and 1.5 -2°F per hour in next 6 hours

▶ **Helps in knowing time since death.**

JIPMER 1998

⊃ Postmortem Hypostasis:

▶ Is bluish purple or purplish red discoloration of skin of dependent part of body after **death due to** <u>capillo venous distension.</u>

▶ Usually develops <u>within 4 hours after death</u> and reaches maximum between 6 and 12 hours.

▶ In cholera it **occurs before death.**

▶ It appears **first in neck** on a body lying on back.

▶ It gets fixed **5-6 hours after death.**

▶ **Starts as blotchy discoloration.**

PGI 1995
PGI 2005

▶ CO poisoning:	**Cherry red color**
▶ HCN poisoning:	**Bright red color**
▶ Potassium chlorate poisoning:	**Choclate colour**
▶ Nitrate, Nitrobenzene:	**Reddish brown**

➲ Muscular Changes:

Primary relaxation	Rigor mortis	Secondary relaxation
▶ In this stage death is somatic.☛☛ ▶ Lasts for **1-2 hours**	▶ Stage of **stiffening of muscles** ☛ ▶ With shortening of fibres. ☛ ▶ **Depletion of ATP** occurs. ▶ **All muscles** (voluntary/involuntary) are affected.☛☛ Muscle stiffens. **KAR 1994** ▶ Appears **first in involuntary** Muscles (Heart) **PGI 2004** ▶ Begins in **eyelids (Upper)** **AIIMS 1992** ▶ Rigor of erector pilae causes cutis anserine. ▶ Also disappears from eyelids first. ▶ In india **begins 1-2 hours after death** ▶ In india **lasts 24-48 hours**(winter)☛☛ 18-36 hours (summer)☛☛	▶ In this stage **muscles become soft and flaccid** due to breakdown of actomyosin. ☛

4

FORENSIC

➲ Putrefaction☛ ☛ ☛

- Putrefaction is a <u>**certain**</u> sign of death.☛
- **Late sign** of death.   **KAR 1994**
- <u>**Clostridium welchi**</u> is the chief agent
- **Externally** greenish discoloration of **flank over cecum** is the first sign.☛   **TN 1991**
- **Internally** greenish discoloration of **flank under surface of liver** is the first sign.☛   **PGI 1998**
- **Larynx and trachea** are the first to putrefy.
- Putrefaction is arrested below 0^0 C and above 48°C.
- **In males** Prostate and testis puterify last ☛   **AIIMS 2003**
- **In females** ovaries and non gravid uterus putrefies last.☛   **AI 2000**
- <u>**Honey combing**</u> in liver is seen.   **KERALA 1991**
- <u>**Foamy liver**</u> is seen.   **AIIMS 1997**
- Putrefaction in <u>**air is twice as in water**</u> and eight times as compared to soil. (Casper dictum) ☛☛

Putrefaction is delayed by:

1. Carbolic acid☛
2. Arsenic☛   **PGI 1992**
3. Strychnine☛
4. Zinc chloride☛

➲ Adipocere Formation: AIIMS 2011

► Also called **saponification**.	PGI 2002
► Occurs in <u>warm humid climate</u>.	KAR 1996
► Because of **hydrolysis and hydrogenation of fat**.	PGI 2002
► **Adipocere is delayed by cold** and formed rapidly by warm humid climate.	
► It is first formed in subcutaneous tissue.	
► Fetuses less than 7 months <u>don't</u> show this change.	

➲ Mummification:

► Modification of putrefaction.	
✓ Dry air condition	PGI 2001
✓ Wind present	PGI 2001
✓ High temperature	
► Dessication, dehydration, shrinkage of cadaver occur but features of body are preserved.	AI 2003
► Time required for complete mummification varies from 3 months to a year or two.	

➲ Mechanical Injuries

Types:

► **Abrasions: Destruction of skin involving superficial layers of epidermis only**

► **Scratches:** caused by sharp object passing across skin.

An **abrasion** is a wound produced by scraping or rubbing, resulting in removal of the superficial layer. Skin abrasions may remove only the epidermal layer.

A **contusion**, or bruise, is a wound usually produced by a blunt object and is characterized by damage to blood vessels and extravasation of blood into tissues.

A **laceration** is a tear or disruptive stretching of tissue caused by the application of force by a blunt object. In contrast to an incision, most lacerations have intact bridging blood vessels and jagged, irregular edges.

An **incised wound** is one inflicted by a sharp instrument. The bridging blood vessels are severed. A **puncture wound** is caused by a long, narrow instrument and is termed penetrating when the instrument pierces the tissue and perforating when it traverses a tissue to also create an exit wound.

Gunshot wounds are special forms of puncture wounds that demonstrate distinctive features important to the forensic pathologist.

► **Graze:** MC type of abrasion. Abrasion caused by violent friction against a broad rough surface as in dragging over the ground is called **brush burn**	AI 1995
► **Pressure abrasion: Ligature mark**	
► **Impact/Imprint/ Patterned abrasion:** Caused by impact of a rough object.	

▶ "Hesitation marks/ tentative cuts": ☞☞	Suicidal attempts	JK BOPEE 2012
▶ "Friction burn/brush burn": ☞	Graze	AI 1995
▶ "Tailing of wound": ☞☞	Incised wound.	
▶ "Patterned abrasion": ☞☞	Pressure injury AIIMS 2005	
▶ "Fracture a la signature": ☞	Depressed fracture AIIMS 2006	
▶ "Crushed hair bulb": ☞	Lacerated wound	

➲ Contusion (Bruises):

▶ Is an effusion of blood into tissues due to rupture of subcutaneous vessel.

▶ It is a superficial **injury**.

Age of bruise

▶ Red: 1-2 hours☞☞

▶ Blue:	few hours-3 days☞ (Deoxyhaemoglobin)	AIIMS 1994
▶ Brown:	4 th day (Haemosiderrin)✴✴	
▶ Green:	5-6 days (Haematodoin)✴	JIPMER 1990
▶ Yellow:	7-12 day (Bilirubin)✴✴✴	
▶ Normal:	2 weeks	

➲ Incised Wounds:

- It is a clean cut through tissues.
- **Length > Depth**☞
- **Tailing of wound** is a feature☞
- **Langerhans lines** determine gaping.   MAHE 1998
- Differentiate from "**incised like wounds**" which are seen on scalp, eyebrows, cheek bones. ☞
- **Hesitation marks, Tentative cuts, Trial wounds** are seen in Suicidal wounds.
- Clean incised wound heals by primary intention.   DELHI 1992
- Lacerated wound appears **incised like in scalp**.   PGI 2001

▶ **Defence** wounds:	result from action of an individual to save himself.☞☞	
▶ **Self inflicted** wounds:	inflicted by a person on his own body☞	
▶ **Fabricated** wounds:	wounds produced by a person on his own body or by another with his consent.☞☞	
▶ **Tentative cuts:**	suicidal attempt.	PGI 2004
▶ **Stab wound:**	depth is maximum.	AI 1991

4

FORENSIC

▶ Contre coup lesion	Head injury✻✻	
▶ Railway spine	Concussion of spine✻	
▶ Blast lung	Pulmonary injury of air blast✻✻	
▶ Pond Fracture	Indented fracture of skull✻ Common in children.	TN 1987 AI 2000
▶ Depressed fracture/ Signature fracture	Outer table of skull driven into diploae✻ From heavy object with small striking surface.	AIIMS 2006 PGI 2000
▶ Gutter fracture	Oblique bullet wound✻	KERALA 2001

Grievous Injury:

- Emasculation☛☛ AI 2004
- Permanent privatation/ loss of sight of either eye.☛☛
- Permanent privatation of hearing of either ear.☛ KAR 2K
- Privatation of any joint☛ PGI 2003
- Destruction /permanent impairing of power of any joint.☛ TN 1990
- Permanent disfigurement of head and face.☛ PGI 2003
- Fracture or dislocation of a bone or a tooth.☛
- Any hurt which endangers life or causes the victim to be in severe bodily pain or is unable to follow his ordinary pursuits for a period of 20 days.☛
- Grievous hurt is punishable under sec: 320 IPC ORISSA

Whip lash injury: due to acute hyper extension of spine. AIIMS 2003

➲ Important Points not to be forgotten in Firearm Injuries

- Choking is a constricting device at the muzzle end of a shot gun.✻✻ TN 1989
- A carbine is a short barreled rifle.✻
- Black gun powder contains: Potassium nitrate, sulfur, charcoal.✻✻ PGI 2006
- Smokeless powder is nitrocellulose.✻ AIIMS 1980
- Incindenary bullets contain phosphorus.
- Gun shot wound is a perforated wound.✻✻
- Tandem bullets: 2 bullets in succession. AIIMS 2007
- Abraded collar, grease collar or dirt collar are present in gun shot entrance wound.✻ AI 1989
- In forensic investigations (X files) bullet is picked up with hands. ROTHAK 1986
- Dermal nitrate test detects gun powder residues. AIIMS 2005

4

⊃ Gun Shot Residues are Detected by:

- Dermal nitrate test   AIIMS 2005
- Neutron activation analysis
- Atomic absorption spectrophotometry
- Scanning electron microscopy with x ray analyzer

Asphyxial Deaths

► Homicidal strangulation with forearm ✳✳	Mugging
► Homicide by hanging a large number of people✳✳	Lynching
► Strangulation with **sticks**✳	Bansidola
► **Manual** strangulation✳	Throttling
► Strangulation by **twisting a lever**✳✳	Garroting
► Mechanical obstruction to airways✳	Suffocation
► Closing the external respiratory opening by **hand**✳✳	Smothering
► Closing mouth and nose **with cloth** and tying it around head ✳	Gagging
► Obstructing within the airways✳	Choking
► Homicidal **smotheringand traumatic asphyxia**✳✳✳	Burking DELHI 1986

Hanging

- ► Is that form of asphyxia which caused by suspension of the body by a **ligature which encircles the neck, the constricting force being the weight of the body.**➤➤   KERALA 1994
- ► **Partial hanging:** Bodies are partially suspended.   TN 1990
- ► The <u>ligature mark</u> in the neck is the most important and specific sign of death from hanging.
- ► <u>Le facies sympathique</u> is seen in hanging.➤➤   AMU 1998
- ► Ligature marks represent printed abrasion.   JIPMER 1998
- ► Saliva may be found dribbling from angle of mouth.➤   AIIMS 1991
- ► Seminal emission is common.
- ► Hyoid bone is fractured in 15-20% cases.➤➤
- ► Cause of death in judicial hanging is fracture dislocation at level of **Second and third or third and fourth cervical vertebrae.**   AMU 1998

4

Strangulation

▶ Is that form of asphyxia caused by **constriction of neck by a ligature without suspending the body.**

▶ Most important sign is **ligature mark.**☞☞

▶ **Intense congestion and deep cyanosis of head and neck** is seen in strangulation.☞

▶ **Petechial haemmorages** are common in eyelids, face, forehead.☞

▶ Fracture of <u>thyroid cartilage</u> is common.☞

▶ **Injury to hyoid is not common.**☞☞

Café Coronary

▶ Café coronary refers to **CAFÉ and CORONARY.**☞☞

▶ Occurs mostly in cafes, restaurants and resembles a coronary attack.

▶ **Mostly overdrunk and deeply intoxicated** people with depressed gag reflex while eating food develop café coronary.☞☞   **PGI 1992**

▶ **Because of Choking, asphyxia or reflex cardiac arrest from stimulation of vagus (Laryngeal nerve).**☞

                                                                                                    JK BOPEE 2012, AIIMS 2002

▶ Mechanism of asphyxia is **choking by a bolus of food** obstructing larynx.☞

Drowning

Signs of drowning are:

▶ Fine copious frothy discharge from mouth and nose.☞☞	AI 2000
▶ Water in stomach or intestines	
▶ Diatoms in Bone marrow ☞	JK 2001
▶ Emphysema aquosum☞	
▶ Cutis anserinus or goose skin☞	AI 1996
▶ Paultafs haemorages☞	AI 1990
▶ Weeds, mud, grass in tightly clutched hands. ☞	

Remember in drowning

• Pupils are usually **dilated**☞☞

• Paultafs hemorrhages are sub pleural hemorrhages as a result of **alveolar wall rupture.**☞

• They are shining, pale bluish red and may be minute to 5 cms in diameter.

• Rarely they may be present on surface.

• **Accidential drowning** is the **most common** type of drowning. ☞ AIIMS 1984

- **Getteler test** is done for drowning and estimates the chloride content of blood in both sides of heart. **AI 1995**
- **Dry drowning** is due to laryngospasm
- **Wet drowning** is secondary to Ventricular fibrillation in fresh water and cardiac arrest in sea water.
- **Emphysema** aquosum is seen in **wet drowning**   **AIIMS 1992**
- **Edema** aquaosum is seen in drowning of **unconscious**.
- **Diatoms** are "**unicellular algae**" suspended in water and their presence in bone marrow and brain signifies drowning.   **AI 1995**
- The extracellular coat of diatoms contains **silica.**

➲ Types of Drowning:

1. Wet drowning

In this the water is inhaled into lungs and the victim has severe chest pain. This is of two types i.e. Fresh water and Salt water drowning.

> * In **fresh water drowning**, large quantities of water cross the alveolar membrane into circulation and produce hypervolaemia. *The red cells swell or burst and haemolysis ensues with liberation of potassium*. The ciculation may suffer 50 percent dilution within 2-3 minutes. The heart is therefore submitted to the insult of **anoxia, hypervolaemia, Potassium excess and sodium deficit.** Anoxia and potassium excess lead to ventricular fibrillation and death in 4-5 minutes.
>
> * In **salt water drowning**, the marked hypertonicity of inhaled water causes loss of fluid from the circulation into the lungs giving rise to fulminating pulmonary edema with progressive **hypovolemia, circulatory shock, and eventually cardiac standstill or asystole**, in about 8-12 minutes.

2. Dry drowning

In dry drowning water does not enter the lungs, but death results from immediate **sustained laryngeal spasm** due to inrush of water into the nasopharynx or larynx.

3. Secondary drowning or near drowning /Post immersion syndrome

Near Drowning is defined as initial survival at least beyond 24 hours of an individual after suffocation due to submersion in fluid. It does not necessarily lead to long term survival and is associated with secondary complications, which require further medical management.

4. Immersion syndrome or Hydrocution

Hydrocution or immersion syndrome refers to sudden death in water **due to vagal inhibition** as a result of
- *Cold water stimulating the nerve endings of the surface of the body,*
- *Horizontal entry into the water with a consequent strike on the epigastrium*
- *Cold water entering ear drums, nasal passage, and the pharynx and larynx which cause mucosal nerve endings stimulation*

⇨ Remember the tests: (AIIMS/AIPGE/PGI Favourites)

► Diatom test	Drowning	AI 1995
► Florence test	Semen	AI 2K
► Getler test	Drowning	AIIMS 2004
► Dermal nitrate test	Gun powder residues	AI 2002

4

FORENSIC

▶ Gustafsons method	Age by dentition	AI 2003
▶ Harrsisons Gilroy test	Detection of heavy metals	AI 2002
▶ Precipitation test	Species identification	AIIMS 2003

➲ Suspended Animation

Condition in which vital functions of body are at such low pitch that they cant be detected by routine methods of clinical examination.

Causes are:

▶ Drowning

▶ Electrocution

▶ Heat stroke

▶ After anaesthesia

▶ Cerebral concussion

▶ Shock

▶ <u>Natural</u> Offences: Rape, Incest

▶ <u>Unnatural offences</u>: Sodomy, Tribadism, Bestality, Buccal coitus

▶ <u>Sexual offences</u>: Incest, Nymphomania, Uranism, Paedophilia

➲ Sexual Perversions Include:

▶ Sadism	Infliction of **pain to partner** is mode of pleasure✴	
▶ Machoism	Infliction of **pain to self** is mode of pleasure✴ Associated with sexual asphyxia (autoerotic hanging)	
▶ Fetichism	Sexual gratification by contact with clothes/parts of opposite sex✴	
▶ Exhibitionism	Exhibition of genitalia✴	
▶ Eonism	Desire to be identified with opposite sex✴	KERALA 1996
▶ Voyeurism	Desire to watch sexual intercourse✴	
▶ Frotteurism	Sexual gratification by rubbing genitals with others✴	
▶ Tribadism	Women-women sex✴	
▶ Lesbianism		
▶ Female homosexuality		
▶ Sodomy	Anal sex✴	
▶ Gerantophilia	Anal sex with **adult**✴	
▶ Paedestry	Anal sex with a **child**. If a boy **(catamite)**✴	AI 1990
▶ Incest	Sexual Intercourse with close relative	
▶ Bestality	Sex with **lower** animal✴	PGI 1987

⊃ Important Terms Commonly Asked:

▶ Tribadism or Lesbianism:	Female homosexuality✳
▶ Sin of Gomorrah:	Buccal Coitus✳
▶ Nymphomania:	Increased sexual desire✳
▶ Enunchs:	Male Prostitutes✳
▶ Castrated enunchs:	Hijrahs✳✳
▶ Lust murder:	Extreme cases of sadism where murder serves as a stimulus for sexual act.
▶ Felatio:	Oral stimulation or manipulation of penis either by male or female.✳
▶ Cunnilingus:	Oral stimulation of female genitalia✳

⊃ Rape

▶ Is a **cognizable offence.**

▶ Medical proof of intercourse is <u>not</u> legal proof of rape.

▶ Statoury rape: <u>rape under 15 years</u>.   **KERALA 1997**

▶ In India there is no age limit under which a boy is considered incapable of committing a rape.   **PGI 1994**

▶ **Slightest penetration of penis within vulva with or without seminal emission or rupture of hymen constitutes a rape.**

▶ Rape is punishable under **Sec 376 IPC.**

⊃ For Examination of a Rape Victim:

▶ Written witnessed consent of patient for examination should be taken.

▶ Collection of specimen should be undertaken.

▶ Photographs, treatment and release of information to police should be under taken.

▶ **Objectives of examination should be:**

▶ To search for physical signs that corroborate with the history given by the victim concerned.

▶ To search for, Collect, Preserve all evidence for laboratory examination.

▶ To treat the victim for any injuries against STD, Pregnancy and prenenting/ lessening of permanent psychological damage.

▶ Shape of nulliparous <u>cervical opening</u> is **circular**   **AI 1998**

▶ Shape of nulliparous <u>cervical canal</u> is **longitudinal.**   **AIIMS 2007**

▶ Ruptured hymen is an important sign of **defloration.**   **AP 1998**

⮑ Indecent Assault:

▶ Offence committed on a female with the intention of outraging her modesty.

▶ Kissing of any body part.

▶ Pressing her breast/ private part

▶ Exposing her genitalia/ breasts

Remember: Tests done for Seminal Stains (AFB Tests)

▶ Acid Phosphatase Test depends on **acid phosphatase** in semen

▶ Florence Test depends on **choline** in semen

▶ Barberios Test depends on **spermin** in semen

▶ Creatine Phosphokinase Test depends on **phospho kinase** in semen

▶ Vagitius: first cry of new born

▶ Vagitus uterinus: cry of a child in uterus

▶ Vagitus vaginalis: cry of a child in vagina.

AIIMS 05

▶ Impotence: inability of a person to perform sexual intercourse

▶ Sterlity: inability of a male to beget children, inability of female to conceive children

▶ Frigidity: inability to start or maintain sexual arousal in female

▶ Impotent quoad: is an individual who is **impotent with a particular woman but not with others**

⮑ Tests done for Blood are:

▶ Benzidine Test	✓ **Preliminary test**
	✓ Hydrogen peroxide and glacial acetic acid are used as reagents
▶ Kastle Meyer Test	✓ Less sensitive, more specific but **NOT** most specific
▶ Takayamas Test	✓ Pink Haemochromogen crystals obtained
▶ Teichmans Test	✓ Brown, Rhombic, Haemic crystals seen
▶ Spectroscopic Test	✓ Confirmatory test
	✓ "Most Specific" test
	✓ Detects **recent as well as past** stains.
▶ Thin Layer Chromatography	
▶ Electrophoresis	

➲ Important Terms:

▶ Knock out:	Chloral hydrate
▶ Run amok:	Cannabis
▶ Magnans symptom:	Cocaine
▶ Flash back:	LSD abuse
▶ Morbid jealousy:	Alcohol

➲ Poisons:

▶ Cerebral
- **Somniferous:** Opium, Barbiturates
- **Ineberient:** Alcohol, Chloroform, ether,
- **Deliriant:** Dhatura, Belladona, Cannabis

▶ **Spinal:** Nux vomica, Gelesium

▶ **Peripheral:** Conium, Curare

▶ **Cardiovascular:** aconite, digitalis, quinine, oleander, tobacco, HCN

▶ **Asphyxiants:** CO, CO_2, H_2S

COMED 2006

➲ Universal Antidote Contains:

• Animal charcoal	2 parts
• Magnesium Oxide	1 part
• Tannic acid.	1 part

AIIMS 1999

➲ Antidotes Used:

▶ OP poisoning✱	— Atropine
▶ Amantia Muscaira✱	
▶ Cyanides✱✱✱	■ Dicobalt edentate
	■ Sodium nitrite
	■ Sodium thiosulfate
	■ Amyl nitrite
▶ Digoxin ✱	— Anti digoxin (Fab)
▶ Paracatemol✱	— N acetyl cysteine
▶ Theophylline✱	— Propranolol
▶ Lead✱	— EDTA
▶ Copper ✱	— Pencillinamine Not Pencillin
▶ Bzd✱	— Flumazenil
▶ Thallium✱	— Prussian blue
▶ Isoniazid✱	— Pyridoxine
▶ Beta Blockers✱	— Glucagon
▶ Methanol✱	— Ethanol

4

FORENSIC

FORENSIC

4

➲ Peculiar Odours (High yield for AIPGME 2012/AIIMS 2011)

■ Fruity odour	► *Ethyl alcohol*
■ Phenolic odour	► *Carbolic acid*
■ Rotten eggs	► *Hydrogen sulfide*
■ Fishy	► *Zinc Phosphide*
■ Bitter almonds	► *Cyanide*
■ Burnt rope	► *Cannabis*
■ Garlic odour	► *Arsenic,* ► *Phosphorus,* ► *Thallium*

► **"Ideal homicide"** poison = Thallium, fluoride compounds.

► **"Commonly used"** homicidal poisons: Arsenic, aconite   **UPSC 2001**

► **"Commonly used "suicidal** poisons: Endrine, Opium, Barbiturates, Organo-phosphorus compounds.

► Poison resembling cholera = Arsenic✱

► Poison resembling tetanus = Strychnine✱

► Poison resembling natural death = Thallium✱

► Poison resembling fading measles = Arsenic

► Poison resembling thyrotoxicosis = Bi-nitro compounds✱✱   **JK BOPEE**

A person comes to you with peculiar odour of breath, pin; point pupils, slow pulse, perspiring skin	► Opium poisoning
A person comes to you with intermittent convulsions, cherry red colour of skin and carboxy haemoglobin in blood.	► Carbon monoxide poisonong
A person comes with clinical and lab findings of respiratory alkalosis, Tinnitus and ketosis	► Salicylate Poisoning

➲ Features of Chronic Mercury Poisoning

► Chronic Mercury poisoning is also called as (<u>Hydragyrism</u>)

► <u>Erethism</u> is mercury   **AIIMS 1998**

► <u>Blue black line</u> on <u>gums</u> with loosening of teeth and necrosis of jaw.

► Brownish mercuric deposits of mercury on lens called <u>Mercuria Lentis.</u> It is an early feature.

► Membranous **colitis** (Diptheria like) with inflammation, ulceration, haemmorage of colon.

- ► Mainly involves Kidneys in **acute poisoning**. (Proximal Convoluted Tubules).☞ AI 1996
- ► Coarse intentional tremors called <u>Danburrys, Hatters,Glass blowers shakes</u>☞☞
- ► **Shaking palsy.** AIIMS 1997
- ► Personality disorders in the form of **Erethesism.**(Neuropsychiatric changes in the form of ☞☞
  - — Shyness
  - — Irritability,
  - — Tremors,
  - — Loss of memory
- ►· **Minimata disease** is due to mercury poisoning by eating fish poisoned by mercury .It occurred along minamata bay.☞

Acrodynia or pinks disease is a pinkish rash starting from tips of fingers and toes with insidious onset.☞
  JK BOPEE 2012

  - ✓ Pink
  - ✓ Painful
  - ✓ Parasthesias
  - ✓ Puffy
  - ✓ Peeling of skin.

- ► When patient becomes unable to dress, write or walk the condition is called as **Concussio mercuralis.**☞
- ► **Dimercaprol (BAL)** is used in treatment of mercury poisoning.

➲ Arsenic Poisoning Features: AIIMS 2011

Cutaneous features:

Aldrich Mee lines on nails✱✱	AI 2003
Hyperkeratosis of palms and soles✱	
Rain drop pigmentation of skin✱	

CNS Features:

- **Polyneuritis✱**
- **Parasthesias✱**
- **Encephalopathy✱**

- ► <u>Red velvety</u> stomach mucosa is seen.☞☞
- ► <u>Rain drop hyperpigmentation</u> is seen.☞ PGI 2006 Retardation of putrefaction occurs.☞
- ► Detected in completely decomposed bodies, ash and charred bones KERALA 1996
- ► Mimicks cholera poisoning AI 1997
- ► Detected by
- ✓ Marshs test, PGI 2003
- ✓ Reinschs test,
- ✓ Gutzeit test.☞☞
- ► <u>Arsenophagists</u> are people who can tolerate high doses of arsenic.☞ AIIMS 1990
- ► <u>Delayed rigor</u> occurs in As poisoning. AI 2003
- ► <u>Golden hair</u> is seen in **As poisoning.** AIIMS 1993

4

⊃ Lead Toxicity

▶ The dangers of **lead** toxicity, the clinical manifestations of which are termed <u>plumbism</u> exposed to **lead** chiefly via paints, cans, plumbing fixtures, and leaded gasoline.

▶ Symptomatic **lead poisoning** is characterized by

— Abdominal pain and irritability followed by

— Lethargy,

— Anorexia,

— Pallor (resulting from anemia), ataxia, and slurred speech.

— Convulsions, coma, and death due to generalized cerebral edema and renal failure occur in the most severe cases.

— Anemia, punctuate basophilia, constipation are seen.   **AI 1992**

▶ <u>Punctuate basophilia</u> is early manifestation of chronic lead poisoning.   **PGI 2003**

▶ A "**lead**" line" appears at the gingiva-tooth border after prolonged high-level exposure. (**Blue line**) **PGI 1995**

▶ <u>Burtonian line</u>.   **AI 2007**

▶ Treatment for **lead** toxicity entails the use of chelating agents, principally **Edetate calcium disodium (CaEDTA)**, dimercaprol, penicillamine, and succimer, which is given orally and has relatively few side effects.

⊃ Phosphorus:

• <u>Garlic</u> like odour☛☛
• <u>Luminscent</u> vomit and faeces☛☛
• **Liver** becomes swollen , yellow (<u>acute yellow atrophy</u>)☛
• Osteomyelitis and necrosis of jaw (<u>Phossy jaw</u>)☛
• Is called **Diwali poison**☛

Arborescent Burns

▶ Arborescent burns are also called as **Filgree, Litchen burgs**   **AIIMS 1998**

▶ Flourescent burns as they resemble the **arborscent/ branching** pattern of tree due to **rupture of small blood vessels** due to lightning.

▶ Joule burns are electricity burns

▶ Flash or spark burns, Crocodile skin appearance skin are high voltage electric burns.   **KERALA 1996**

Antemortem Burn	Postmortem Burn	
▶ Line of Redness **present**	▶ Absent☛☛	**DELHI 1993**
▶ Vesicles contain **Chloride, Albumin**	▶ Contain air☛	**PGI 1996**
▶ Healing **by granulation tissue**	▶ No healing☛☛	
▶ **Soot** in Upper respiratory passage	▶ Absent☛	**JIPMER 1990**
▶ **Carboxy haemoglobin** in blood	▶ Absent☛	**PGI 1999**
▶ ↑Enzymes	▶ No increase☛☛	**PGI 2001**

▶	Pugilistic attitude is due to **protein coagulation.**	AI 2000
▶	Pugilistic attitude is seen in **burns.**	PGI 1999
▶	**Heat haematoma** occurs between *skull and duramater.*	PGI 1997
▶	Elevated levels of **cyanide** can be associated with burns.	AIIMS 2000

⮑ Hemodialysis is done for Poisoning in Blood From:

▶	Barbiturates	AIIMS 1997
▶	Aspirin	AIIMS 1998
▶	Methanol(Alcohol)	AIIMS 1995
▶	Boric acid	
▶	Thiocyanates	
▶	Lithium	
▶	Theophylline	
▶	Atenolol	

⮑ For Dialysis Properties Should be:

- ■ Low molecular weight
- ■ High water solubility
- ■ Low protein binding
- ■ Small volume of distribution
- ■ Long half life
- ■ High dialysis clearance.

Widmark's equation

- Widmark, a Swedish physician did much of the foundational research regarding alcohol pharmacokinetics in the human body.
- In addition, he developed an algebraic equation allowing one to estimate any one of six variables given the other five. Typically, we are interested in determining either the amount of alcohol consumed by an individual or the associated blood alcohol concentration (BAC) given the values of the other variables.

Widmark's equation relates these variables according to:

$$N = W r (Ct + Bt)/0.8z$$

where:

- N = the number of drinks consumed

4

- W = body weight in ounces
- r = volume of distribution (a constant relating the distribution of water in the body in L/Kg)
- Ct = the blood alcohol concentration (BAC) in Kg/L
- ß = the alcohol elimination rate in Kg/L/hr
- t = time since the first drink in hours
- z = the fluid ounces of alcohol per drink
- 0.8 = the density of ethanol (0.8 oz. per fluid ounce)

References:

1. Widmark, E.M.P., Principles and Applications of Medicolegal Alcohol Determination, Davis, CA: Biomedical Publications, 1981, pp. 107-108.

⊃ Causes of Pin Point Pupils:

- ▶ Organophosphorus poisoning
- ▶ Opium/Morphine poisoning
- ▶ Pontine haemmorage
- ▶ Barbiturates
- ▶ Chloral hydrate
- ▶ Carbolic acid poisoning.

⊃ Remember Other Tests:

▶	Arsenic =	Marsh's test, Reinsch's test⬅⬅ asked multiple times
▶	Opium =	Marquis test⬅
▶	Alcohol =	Mc'evan's test⬅
▶	Datura =	Mydriatic test⬅
▶	Phenol =	Green urine test⬅
▶	Imipramine =	Forrest test⬅
▶	Poisonous mushroom=	Meixner test⬅
▶	Salicylic acid=	Trinders test⬅

⇨ Remember:

▶	Stupefying poison⬅⬅	is Datura.
▶	Methaemoglobinaemia ⬅⬅	is caused by poisoning due to **Nitrates.**
▶	**Viperbite** like poison⬅	**Abrus.**
▶	Diwali poisons are ⬅	**Mercury, phosphorous. AI 1988**
▶	Tingling of skin and tongue by⬅	**Aconite poisoning.**
▶	Ochronosis⬅	is seen in Phenol(carbolic acid) poisoning
▶	Chromolachryorrhoea⬅⬅	in organophosphorus poisoning is due to porphyrin
▶	A green line in gums in copper poisoning is	**Clepten line**

➲ Other Important Points in Poisoning:

▶ **Corrigans line** is seen in Copper poisoning

▶ **Aqua Tofana** is a poisonous arsenic solution

➲ Sulfuric Acid

▶ <u>Strongest corrosive</u> poison✳

▶ Stomach mucosa is stained black.   JIPMER 1994

▶ Teeth are <u>chalky white</u>.✳

▶ Perforation of stomach is common.   AMU 1996

▶ Gastric lavage/ emetics are **contraindicated**✳

▶ <u>Vitriolage</u> is common with sulfuric acid.   PGI 1997

▶ Fatal period: <u>12-16 hours</u>.   JK 2003

▶ Throwing of sulfuric acid on other individual is called <u>vitriolage</u>✳

➲ Nitric Acid:

▶ Gives **yellow discoloration** to tissue due to picric acid production **(Xanthoproteic reaction)**✳

▶ Stomach is **greenish in color**

➲ Carbolic Acid:

▶ Characteristic <u>carbolic/ phenolic smell</u>✳

▶ Urine turns green or black on exposure to air **(Carboluria)**✳   PGI 2007

▶ Pigmentation of cornea or cartilages occurs **(Ochronosis)**✳

▶ Stomach looks <u>leathery</u>✳   UP 2004

▶ <u>Retards</u> putrefaction.   AI 1994

➲ Chloral Hydrate

▶ It is used to **increase potency of liquor.**

▶ <u>Dry wine</u>   PGI 2004

▶ Chloral hydrate is also called as **dry wine** is basically a <u>hypnotic</u>. ✳

▶ It has got a rapid action and produces <u>Knock out drops</u>.✳   AMU 1994

▶ It is a **colourless, Crystalline substance with pungent taste.**

▶ In small doses it produces <u>natural sleep</u> but in large doses it causes **CNS Depression** and rapid death.✳

▶ Mixture of alcohol and chloral hydrate is called as <u>Micky Fin</u>.✳

Ricinus communis: ☛☛☛

▶ Derived From castor plant (arandi)

▶ Contains toxalbumen " Ricin"☛

Croton tigilium :➥➥

► Jamalgota

► Seeds contain a toxalbumen "Crotin."➥

Abrus precatorius:➥➥

► Also called Indian liquorice

► Seeds contain active toxalbumen "Abrin" which resembles viperine snake venom.➥   AMU 2007

► They are used for making suis.➥

Capscum annum ➥

► Has pungent odour.

► Active principles are Capsaicin and Capiscin➥

Semecarpus anacardium➥

► Marking nut called builwala

► Contain active principles Semecarpol and Bhilwanol.➥

► Lesion resembles a bruise

Calatropis :➥

Used to: A3

► Produce Artificial bruise.➥➥

► Used as Arrow poison.➥

► Used as Abortion stick for criminal abortion.   COMED 2002

➲ Ophitoxemia: Poisoning by Snake Venom.   AIIMS 1994

Cortilidae ➥➥	Viperiade ➥➥	Elapidae ➥➥	Hydrophidae ➥➥	Colubridae➥➥
Pit viper	Russels viper	Cobra	Sea snake	Bird snakes
Venom of pit viper contains hylauronidase	Venom is hemolytic PGI 2003	Krait Venom is neurotoxic PGI 2004	Venom is myotoxic UPSC 2003	Boom slangs

➲ Important Questions Recently Asked

■ Pest killer in OPD presents with **pain abdomen, garlic odour in breath** and **transverse lines on nails** :
  Arsenic poisoning   AIIMS 2009

■ Less impact causing maximum bruise is seen on **face**.   AIIMS 2009

■ **Destructive power of bullet** is determined by velocity of bullet.   AIIMS 2009

■ **Incised wounds on genitals** are a feature of homicides.   AIIMS 2009

■ **Formication and persecutory delusions** are seen in cocaine poisoning.   AIIMS 2009

■ Pest killer in OPD presents with pain abdomen, garlic odour in breath and transverse lines on nails : Arsenic
  poisoning   AIIMS 2008

■ **Study of death** in all aspects is <u>thanatology</u>   AIIMS 2008

■ **Hydrocution** is **drowning in <u>cold water</u>**   AIIMS 2008

■ **Falanga** is <u>beating on soles</u> with blunt object   AIIMS 2008

■ Constituents of embalming fluid is:

— Formalin,

— Sodium borate,

— Sodium citrate,

— Glycerine,

— Sodium chloride,

— Eosin,

— Water soluble winter green

➲ Garroting High Yield AIPGME 2011/2012

A loop of thin string is thrown around the neck of the victim, who is attacked unawares from his back. This is used to be the official method of judicial execution in Spain, from which also comes the description of the Twisting device. The Spanish Windlass.

"Signature" fracture refers to: Depressed skull fracture **HIGH Yield for 2011-2012**

➲ "Sparrow" Marks High Yield AIPGME 2011/2012

➥ are seen in: <u>Windshield glass injury</u> AIPGMEE 2011
➥ Sparrow's foot marks are <u>bizarre shaped lacerations</u> that result from the face coming in contact with shattered windshield glass.
➥ It is a commonly seen in front seat passengers in road traffic accidents

➲ Dhatura Poisoning :

"Thorn apple" (a spherical fruit with sharp spines)
➥ Atropine, hyoscyamine, scopolamine – active ingredients
➥ Signs and symptoms :
➥ Delirium: Muttering delirium – irrelevant, talking pill rolling movement
➥ S/S

↪ **Drowsiness**
↪ **Dilated pupils**
↪ **Diplopia**
↪ **Drunken gait**
↪ **Dilated blood vessels**
↪ **Dry and hot skin and flushing of the face**
↪ **Death due to respiratory failure**

➥ Fatal dose: 1 gm Fatal period: 1 day
➥ Uses: Road poison/railway platform poison (powdered seeds used by criminals for stupefying,
➥ prior to robbery, rape or kidnapping)
➥ Treatment: **Potassium permanganate + tannic acid, for gastric lavage, Physostigmine is specific anti dote**

4

⊃ Bobbit Syndrome:

Perverted female partner amputes the penis of her male partner.

Gerantophilia:	Sodomy with old patient, serving as passive agent.
Peeping Tom :	Person gets sexual pleasure by observing sexual Activities of other people.
Troilism :	Sexual gratification obtaining by inducing wife for sexual intercourse with other person.
Scopophilia:	Sexual pleasure is obtained by seeing a nude woman in her privacy.
Algolagnia:	Person gets sexual gratification by being bodily tortured.

Primary impact injury—these are produced by the **initial contact with the vehicle**, and may be in the form of abrasion, laceration, or contusions. Most commonly both legs get fractured in the region of impact with bumper of the vehicle **(Bumper fracture)**

Secondary impact injuries - caused by **subsequent contact of body with vehicle after the primary impact.** They usually result from the victim flung into the air after the primary impact and subsequent landing against the hood, windscreen or roof of vehicle. Head injuries are common.

Secondary injuries (Tertiary injuries) - caused by **striking against objects or surfaces other than the vehicle such as road surface or street poles.** Grazed abrasion, flaying injuries, etc. due to being dragged on the road are common.

In Blunt trauma to abdomen most **common organ to be damaged is spleen, liver is the 2nd organ** after spleen. **In Penetrating trauma** to abdomen **small intestine** is the most common organ to be damaged, liver is the 2nd organ after small intestine.

A married woman died in unnatural condition in home within 5 years of marriage. Her parents complained of frequent demand of dowry. Her autopsy will be conducted under section: 176 CrPC

176 CrPC: Magistrate inquiry shall be conducted in dowry death cases. Postmortem will be conducted by 2 doctors where the period of marriage is within 7 years. As in this question death takes place within 5 years of marriage so inquest will be done by magistrate and autopsy will be conducted under Sec 176 CrPC.

⊃ Narcoanalysis

Is a test to **detect truth. In this test subject's imagination is neutralized by making him semiconscious.** In this state it becomes difficult for him to lie. Drugs used for the purpose are
- Scopolamine hydrobromide
- Sodium Amytal or sodium pentothal (TRUTH SERUM)
- Sodium Seconal

⊃ Dhatura: High Yield AIPGME 2011/2012

Thorn apple (a spherical fruit with sharp spines)
Atropine, hyoscyamine, scopolamine – active ingredients
Features:

- ✓ Delirium: Muttering delirium - irrelevant talking pill rolling movement carphologia-picking up imaginary threads from clothes, bed sheets
- ✓ Drowsiness
- ✓ Dilated pupils
- ✓ Diplopia
- ✓ Drunken gait
- ✓ Dilated blood vessels
- ✓ Dry and hot skin and flushing of the face
- ✓ Death due to respiratory failure

Fatal dose: 1 gm (100 seeds)

Fatal period: 1 day

Treatment: Potassium permanganate + tannic acid, for gastric lavage, Physostigmine is specific anti dote

➲ Aconite Poisoning

Signs and symptoms of aconite which is also known as **"Monks Hood", Wolf Bane"**. All the species of the plant is poisonous so the name **"Bish"** or **"Bikh"** meaning the poison is used for them.

Has **sweetish taste which gives it the name Mitha Bish (sweet poison).**

- ▶ Tingling followed by numbness of mouth and throat is characteristic symptom of aconite poisoning.
- ▶ Salivation (not excessive), nausea, vomiting
- ▶ Muscular weakness, convulsion
- ▶ In early stage pupils alternately contract and dilate **(HIPPUS)** but dilated in the later stage.
- ▶ Hypotension, cardiac arrhythmia and AV Block
- ▶ Death may occur from shock or syncope but usually occurs from asphyxia due to paralysis of the respiration.

Treatment – Milk or activated charcoal, stomach is washed with potassium permanganate. Atropine is given to avoid vagal inhibition. Artificial inflation and oxygen inhalation.

➲ High Yield AIPGME 2011/2012

- ➧ **Incendiary Bullets:** A type of army bullet used to cause fire in the target. Usually confined to use in the aircraft.
- ➧ **Tracer Bullet:** This type of bullet leaves a visible mark or 'trace' while in flight so that gunner can observe the strike of the shot.
- ➧ **Dumdum bullet:** Tip is chiselled out, it fragments extensively upon striking.
- ➧ **Express bullet:** Bullet with a hole
- ➧ **Ricochet bullet:** Before striking the object aimed at, it strikes some intervening object first, then after rebounding, it hits the target.
- ➧ **Yawning bullet:** It traverses in an irregular fashion, causes a key hole entry wound.
- ➧ **Tumbling bullet:** It rotates end on end during its motion.

> ➡ **Souvenier bullet:** Left in body for a long time, surrounded by dense fibrous tissue.
>
> ➡ **Frangible bullets:** Designed to fragment on impact.
>
> ➡ **Tandem bullet:** 2 bullets are present in the same cartridge which enter the target object at different points. PIGGYBACK bullet/ TANDEM bullet (tandem = one behind the other): Two bullets are ejected one after the other, first bullet failed to leave the barrel and is ejected by subsequently fired bullet.

➲ Electrical Injuries

- ➡ **Joule burn:** contact electrical and endogenous burn.
- ➡ **Crocodile flash burn:** high voltage burn. Multiple lesions due to **'arc effect'**. Metal particles and the skin at the site of entrance. Death due to ventricular fibrillation.
- ➡ Current pearls and wax drops seen on radiology.
- ➡ **Lightening stroke:** It is an electrical discharge from the cloud to the earth.
- ➡ **Filligree burn/ Litchenburg's flowers:** superficial, irregular, thin resembling <u>the branches of a tree</u> also known as **"arborescent burn"**. Most common site is shoulder flanks. Cause is staining of tissues with Hb due to rupture of smaller blood vessels along the path of current.

Mechanism of injury by lightening:

- ✓ Due to **direct effect of current of very high voltage**, cardiorespiratory failure or sudden cardiac arrest is likely to ensue.
- ✓ **Burning** by the flash of lightening.
- ✓ The atmospheric gases become heated to 20,000 c, and this heating of gases in the path of lightening causes an explosive expansion. **Blast effect of the rapidly expanding air** which may tear the clothing and impart suspicion of foul play.
- ✓ **Compression effect due to air movement** in its return wave produces the changes. So compression effect is <u>after the flash</u>.

➲ Suicidal Injury

- ➡ is on limited accessible areas of the body such as throat, wrist, elbow, or groin **for incised wounds:**
- ➡ left side of the chest over the heart, and abdomen, **for stab wounds;** and

  Right temple, mouth, or pericardium for **gunshot wound.**
- ➡ Suicidal wounds take more or less a **definite direction.**
- ➡ Most persons being right handed, suicidal incised wounds of the neck are usually directed from left to right and tailing off to a superficial incision on the right;
- ➡ Suicidal incised wounds of wrist are directed from above downwards and those on lower limbs form below upwards. Suicidal wounds of chest are on the left side and directed downwards and inwards.

➲ Homicidal Wounds

- ➡ Incised wounds on the **nose, ears and genitals** are usually homicidal and are inflicted on account of jealously.
- ➡ Stab wounds **over the back** are almost always homicidal.
- ➡ Stab wounds over the abdomen, chest and limbs, other than over the heart area are suggestive of homicide.

- Chop wounds of head, face, neck shoulders and extremities are suggestive of homicide or accident.
- Wounds of the head especially over the vertex, if accidents are excluding are presumptive of homicide.
- Defence **injuries**- Presence of defence injuries indicate a homicidal attack. However their absence does not rule out a homicidal attack for it is possible for the victim to be incapable of defence.

⊃ A Bullet's Ability to Produce Tissue Depends on:

1. **Bullet velocity** - A bullet's ability to injure is directly related to its kinetic energy at the moment of impact. Kinetic energy i.e. $E = mc/2$

2. **Tissue density** - The greater the tissue density, the greater is the amount of energy discharged by the bullet passing through it and thus greater the injury. Thus a bullet may cause slight damage to the soft tissue, but extensive damage to hard tissue such as bone.

3. **Hydrostatic force**- Hydrostatic forces increase the impact of injury. When fluid distended hollow organs are hit by the bullet, extensive lacerations are produced due to the explosive displacement of the liquid in all displacements.

⊃ Kerosene Poisoning: High Yield AIPGME 2011/2012

<u>Kerosene exerts its toxic effects on the lungs and CNS</u>

- Clinical features include:
  a) *Cough dyspnea, high feaver, vomiting, drowsiness and coma.*
  b) *Physical signs in lungs are minimal.*
  c) *X-ray film of chest shows ill defined homogenicity or patchy clouding.*
  d) *Picture may resemble milliary mottling.*

- Treatment:
  - Gastric lavage is avoided
  - Patient is kept on O_2
  - **Routine antibiotics are not indicated**
  - Corticosteroids have little beneficial effect.

Poisoning	Features	Postmortem findings
Copper	Nausea, vomiting, diahorrea, liver damage, paralysis, shock, respiratory depression	Bluish tongue/mucosae. Atrophy of internal organs.
Thallium	Gi irritation, vomiting, anorexia, respiratory distress, conjuctivitis, neuritis, ataxia, tremor	Alopecia, fatty liver and fatty change in kidney.
Zinc	Mdetabolic acidosis, hypocalcemia, nausea, vom iting, fever, chills	Degenerative changes in internal organs.

4

⊃ DNA Profiling (also called DNA testing, DNA typing, or genetic fingerprinting)
High Yield AIPGME 2011/2012

* Is a technique employed by forensic scientists to assist in the identification of individuals by their respective DNA profiles.
* **DNA profiles** are encrypted sets of numbers that reflect a person's DNA makeup, which can also be used as the person's identifier.
* DNA profiling should not be confused with full genome sequencing. It is used in, for example, parent testing and criminal investigation.
* DNA profiling uses repetitive ("repeat") sequences that are highly variable, called variable number tandem repeats (VNTR). VNTRs loci are very similar between closely related humans, but so variable that unrelated individuals are extremely unlikely to have the same VNTRs.
- **For highly degraded samples, mitochondrial DNA (mtDNA)** is sometimes typed due to there being many copies of mtDNA in a cell, while there may only be 1-2 copies of the nuclear DNA.
- Forensic scientists amplify the HV1 and HV2 regions of the mtDNA, then sequence each region and compare single-nucleotide differences to a reference.
- Because mtDNA is maternally inherited, directly linked maternal relatives can be used as match references, such as one's maternal grandmother's daughter's son.
- A difference of two or more nucleotides is generally considered to be an exclusion.
- **mtDNA** is useful in determining clear identities, such as those of missing people when a maternally linked relative can be found.
- **mtDNA** can be obtained from such material as hair shafts and old bones/teeth.

Iris Scan High Yield AIPGME 2011/2012

→ It uses both **visible and near-infrared light** to take a clear, high-contrast picture of a person's iris. With near-infrared light, a person's pupil is very black, making it easy for the computer to isolate the pupil and iris
→ Iris scanners are becoming more common in high-security applications because people's eyes are so unique.
→ They also allow **more than 200 points of reference for comparison, as opposed to 60 or 70 points in fingerprints.**
→ The iris is a **visible but protected structure, and it does not usually change over time**, making it **ideal for biometric identification.**
→ Most of the time, people's **eyes also remain unchanged after eye surgery,** and blind people can use iris scanners as long as their eyes have irises.
→ Eyeglasses and contact lenses typically do not interfere or cause inaccurate readings.
→ This technology not only offers **convenience**, but also promises **greater safety and security.** Top airport security officials have recently recognized iris identifiers as an important tool for increasing airport security and for improving upon current immigration practices.
→ The cameras **use harmless infrared light** to record the iris' minute ridges and valleys. They can detect 235 unique details and differentiate between right and left eyes and those of identical twins, whereas a fingerprint has about 70 details. Irises aren't affected by age, eye surgery or disease

➲ AIIMS 2011 QUESTIONS

- **Cardiac polyp** refers to fibrinous clot. AIIMS 2011

- In Civil negligence burden of proof lies with patient. AIIMS 2011

- A Patient with History of garlic odor, pain abdomen, transverse line on nails suffers from **Arsenic poisoning**. Remember: Garlicky odor on breath; Hyperkeratosis, Raindrop Hyperpigmentation, Exfoliative dermatitis, and Mees' lines (transverse white striae of the fingernails); sensory and motor polyneuritis, distal weakness. Radiopaque sign on abdominal x-ray ECG: QRS broadening, QT prolongation, ST depression, T-wave flattening; AIIMS 2011

- Formication & delusions of persecution are seen in **cocaine.** Tactile hallucination is common in cocaine psychosis. This may take the form of small ants crawling over the body so called formication. In cocaine psychosis this type of hallucination occurs together with delusion of persecution and is known as cocaine bug. AIIMS 2011

- Spinal cord autopsy approach used is posterior aspect AIIMS 2011

- Indian medical degree is recognised by- schedule 1 AIIMS 2011

- Adipocere formation requires-humid & optimum temperature AIIMS 2011

FORENSIC

4

NOTES

4

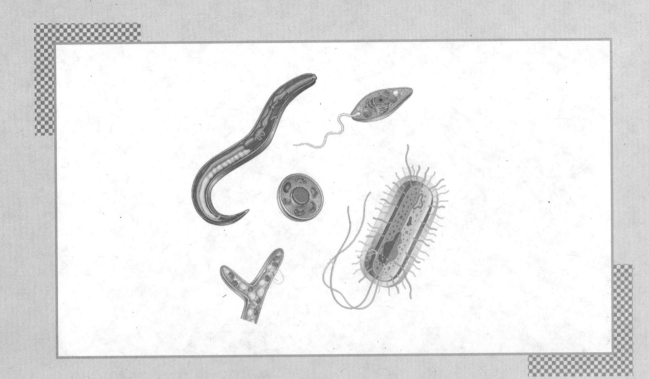

MICROBIOLOGY

⊃ Prokaryotes: (High yield for 2011-2012)

► Absence of <u>nuclear</u> membrane   AI 1999

► Absence of nucleolus

► Absence of <u>organized</u> DNA (no histones)

► Absence of cytoplasmic organalles

► Absence of sterols/ muramic acid

► <u>Bacteria</u> are prokaryotes.

⊃ Eukaryotes: (Repeated in 2008, 2009, 2010)

► Presence of nuclear membrane. **(TWO SEPARATE BILAYERS)**   JK BOPEE 2012

► Presence of nucleolus

► Presence of DNA

► Presence of cytoplasmic organalles

► Presence of sterols/ muramic acid

⇨ Characteristics of different organisms

Characteristics	Viruses	Bacteria	Fungi
► Nucleic Acid	<u>Either</u> DNA/RNA	Both Present	Both present
► Nucleus	Absent	Prokaryotic	Eukaryotic
► Ribosomes	Absent	70S	80S
► Mitochondria	Absent	Absent PGI 2000	Present
► Motility	Nil	Present	Nil
► Reproduction		Binary Fission*	Budding*

⇨ Difference between gram-positive and gram-negative cells

Component	Gram Positive Cells		Gram Negative Cells
Peptidoglycan	Thick	AI 1996	Thin
Teichoic Acid	Present*	PGI 1998	Absent
Lipopolysacchride	Absent*		Present

⇨ **Functions of different components of cell envelop:**

- ► **Capsule:** antiphagocytic and immunogenic ☛

- ► **Capsulated organisms:**

  ✓ Pneumocoocus,   PGI 2003

  ✓ Anthrax bacillus,   PGI 2003

  ✓ Bordetella,

  ✓ Meningococci, (especially complement deficiencies)   KCET 2012

  ✓ Klibesella,

  ✓ Cryptococcus, H. influenza,

  ✓ Bacteroids,

  ✓ V. parahemoltyicus   PGI 2003

- ► **Techoic acid:** attachment to epithelial surfaces and immunogenic ☛

- ► **Cell wall:** rigid support, protection from osmotic damage ☛

- ► **Cytoplasmic membrane:** membranous matrix for respiratory pathways and cell wall synthesis.

- ► **Porin proteins:** passive transport of aqeous materials ☛

- ► **Perplasmic space:** extracellular enzymes, ↓ osmotic pressure ☛

- ► **Inner membrane:** matrix for enzymes of respiratory pathways and cell wall synthesis ☛

⊃ **Lipopolysaccharide (LPS): (High yield for 2011-2012)**

- ➧ Is the major component of the outer membrane of **Gram-negative bacteria.**

- ➧ LPS also **increases the negative charge of the cell membrane** and helps stabilize the overall membrane structure.

- ➧ The LPS molecule is composed of **two biosynthetic entities: the lipid A - core and the O-polysaccharide (O-antigen).**

- ➧ Most **biological effects of LPS are due to the lipid A** part, however, O-antigen (O-ag) plays an important role in effective colonization of host tissues, resistance to complement-mediated killing and in the resistance to cationic antimicrobial peptides that are key elements of the innate immune system.

- ➧ LPS is an endotoxin, and induces a strong response from normal animal immune systems.

It comprises three parts:

1. O antigen (or O polysaccharide)

2. Core oligosaccharide

3. Lipid A

LPS function has been under experimental research for several years due to its role in activating many transcription factors. LPS challenge also produces many types of mediators involved in septic shock.

⇨ **Septic Shock:**

- *Septicemia is defined as the proliferation of bacteria in the bloodstream.*
- *Accompanied by systemic manifestations of sepsis, including rigors, fever or hypothermia (characteristic of gram-negative septicemia with endotoxemia), leukocytosis or leukopenia (characteristic of profound septicemia or viremia), and tachycardia or circulatory collapse.*
- Any organism, including bacteria, fungi, rickettsiae, and viruses, may be involved, but **gram-negative bacteria** that produce endotoxin predominate.
- Septic shock follows a combination of **loss of vasomotor tone, increased capillary permeability, and myocardial depression.**
- Vasoactive substances such as **histamine, serotonin, and prostaglandins,** which increase capillary permeability.
- Complement activation causes white cell aggregates, and factors involved in phagocytosis by leukocytes, such as lysosomal enzymes and oxygen-derived free radicals, may be released, damaging capillary endothelium.
- Clinically, there are two patterns of septic shock:
- **Warm shock** is characterized by tachypnea, rigors, fever spikes, and a hyperdynamic circulation. The periphery is warm to the touch and appears well perfused because of diffuse peripheral dilatation. The veins are dilated, which increases vascular capacitance and causes a reduction in effective blood volume.
- **Cold shock** is characterized by peripheral vasoconstriction and is associated with hypovolemia, occurring most frequently in patients, who have extensive extracellular fluid losses following burns, peritonitis, or intestinal obstruction. A transition from the warm to the cold type may occur if circulating volume diminishes.

Uncontrolled sepsis leads to the development of

- Multiple organ failure, with acute pulmonary failure (ARDS),
- Acute renal failure,
- Hepatic failure,
- Gastrointestinal ulceration and
- Hemorrhage,
- Adrenal failure,
- Cerebral failure as potential additional manifestations,
- DIC precipitated by the release of thromboplastin from damaged tissue into the circulation and consumption of clotting factors and platelets in the microcirculation.

⇨ **Detection techniques:**

- ✓ Flagella are detected by **Dark ground microscopy.**   AI 2001
- ✓ Fimbriae are detected by <u>Haemagluttination</u>
- ✓ Spores are detected by <u>Acid fast (ZN staining)</u>
- ✓ Capsules are detected by **India ink / Quelling reaction.**   KAR 1999

5

MICROBIOLOGY

⊃ Phases of Bacterial Growth Cycle: (High yield for 2011-2012)

Lag Phase↜	Nutrients incorporated	
Log Phase↜	Rapid cell division	UPSC 2000
Stationary Phase↜	Cell Death=Cell formation *(sportulation occurs)*	JK BOPEE 2011
Death Phase↜	Cell death > Cell formation	JK BOPEE 2012

1. **During lag phase,** bacteria adapt themselves to growth conditions. It is the period where the individual bacteria are maturing and not yet able to divide. During the lag phase of the bacterial growth cycle, synthesis of RNA, enzymes and other molecules occurs.

2. **Exponential phase** (log phase or the logarithmic phase) is a period characterized by cell doubling. The number of new bacteria appearing per unit time is proportional to the present population

3. **During stationary phase,** the growth rate slows as a result of nutrient depletion and accumulation of toxic products. This phase is reached as the bacteria begin to exhaust the resources that are available to them. This phase is a constant value as the rate of bacterial growth is equal to the rate of bacterial death. Sportulation occurs here.

4. **At death phase,** bacteria run out of nutrients and die.

⇨ Bacterial conjugation:

► **Bacterial conjugation** is the **transfer of genetic material between bacteria through direct cell-to-cell contact.**↜

► Discovered in 1946 by Joshua **Lederberg** and Edward **Tatum.**↜   UPSC 02

► Conjugation is a mechanism of <u>horizontal gene transfer</u>—

► The prototype for conjugative plasmids is the F-plasmid, also called the **F-factor.** The F-plasmid is an episome (a plasmid that can integrate itself into the bacterial chromosome by genetic recombination) of about 100 kb length. The host bacterium is called F-positive or F-plus **(denoted F+).** Strains that lack F plasmids are called F-negative or **F-minus (F-).**↜

► Bacterial conjugation is often incorrectly regarded as the bacterial equivalent of sexual reproduction or mating.↜

► It is merely the transfer of genetic information from a donor cell to a recipient.↜

► **Multiple drug resistance** is by conjugation.   TN 1986

⇨ Transduction:

Transduction is the process by which DNA is transferred from one bacterium to another by <u>a virus</u>.   AI 2005
It also refers to the process whereby <u>foreign DNA is introduced into another cell via a viral vector</u>.
This is a common tool used by molecular biologists to stably introduce a foreign gene into a host cell's genome.↜
     MAHE 2007

When <u>bacteriophages (viruses that infect bacteria)</u> infect a bacterial cell, their normal mode of reproduction is to harness the replicational, transcriptional, and translation machinery of the host bacterial cell to make numerous virions, or complete viral particles, including the viral DNA or RNA and the protein coat.↜

● Bacterial Transformation: (High yield for 2011-2012)

Bacteria transformation may be referred to as a stable genetic change brought about by <u>taking up **naked DNA**</u> (DNA without associated cells or proteins), and competence refers to the state of being able to take up exogenous DNA from the environment➤ .   JK BOPEE 2011

⇨ Transposons:✱

- **Mobile genetic elements** that can move themselves from one DNA to other. ➤   UP 2007
- Jumping genes. ➤
- Create additional mutations➤
- Have sequences of indirect repeats of bases at each end. ➤

⇨ Sterilization and disinfection:

♯ Critical device

Is a device or item that enters sterile *tissue or the vascular system* and therefore, should be sterile, i.e. IV catheter, surgical instruments, cardiac and urinary catheters, implants, etc.

Critical items confer a high-risk for infection if they are contaminated with any microorganism. Thus, objects that enter sterile tissue or the vascular system must be sterile.

♯ Semi-critical device

Are items that come in contact with *mucous membranes* or *non-intact skin*, i.e. laryngoscope blades, oxygen masks, resuscitation bags, (respiratory therapy and anesthesia equipment), endoscopes, laryngoscope blades, esophageal manometry probes, cystoscopes, etc.

They require high/ intermediate level disinfection between uses.

♯ Noncritical items

Are those that come in contact with intact skin but not mucous membranes

Noncritical items can be divided into noncritical patient care items, such as **stethoscopes, bedpans, crutches, computers and blood pressure cuffs,** and noncritical environmental surfaces like **stretchers, bed rails, patient furniture, shelves and door handles in transport vehicles.**

Virtually, no risk has been documented for transmission of infectious agents to patients through noncritical items when they are used as noncritical items and do not contact non-intact skin and/or mucous membranes.

"A biosafety level is the level of biocontainment precautions required to isolate dangerous biological agents in enclosed facility"*.

There are four levels of biosafety -

- ✱ *Biosafety level - 1*
- ✱ *Biosafety level - 2*
- ✱ *Biosafety level - 3*
- ✱ *Biosafety level - 4*

- *Each level has guidelines for laboratory facilities, safety equipment and laboratory practices and techniques.*

i) Biosafety level - 1 (BSL -1)

- BSL-1 risk group contains biological agents that pose **low risk** to personnel and the environment.

Examples -

→ Agrobacterium radiobacter
→ Aspergillus niger
→ Bacillus thuringiensis
→ E.coli strain K-12
→ Lactobacillus acidophilus
→ Micrococcus leuteus
→ Neurospora crassa
→ Pseudomonas fluorescens
→ Serratia marcescens

⌗ *BSL- 1 is found in water-testing laboratories, in schools, and in colleges teaching introductory microbiology classes.*

⌗ *Work is done on an open bench or in a fume hood.*

⌗ *Standard microbiological practices are used when working in the laboratory.*

⌗ *Decontamination can be achieved by treating with chemical disinfectants or by steam autoclaving.*

⌗ *Lab coats are required and gloves are recommended.*

⌗ *The laboratory work is supervised by an individual with general training in microbiology or a related science.*

ii) Biosafety level-2 (BSL-2)

⌗ BSL-2 risk group contains biological agents that pose moderate risk to personnel and the environment.

⌗ If exposure occurs in a laboratory situation, **the risk of spread is limited and it rarely would cause infection that would lead to serious disease.**

⌗ Effective preventive measures and treatment are available in the event that an infection occurs.

- Agrobacterium radiobacter
- Aspergillus niger
- Bacillus thuringiensis
- E.coli strain K-12
- Lactobacillus acidophilus,
- Micrococcus leuteus
- Neurospora crassa Pseudomonas fluorescens
- Serratia marcescens

Examples -

Bacteria	Viruses	Fungi
• MOTT	• Adeno	• Cryptococcus
• Pneumococci	• Calci	• Candida
• Streptococci	• Corona	• Aspergillus
• Staphylococci	• Herpes	• Dermatophytes
• Enterobacteriaciae	• **Influenza**	
• E.coli		
• Clostridium sp.		
• Bacillus (except anthrax)		

⊞ *Access to the laboratory is restricted.*

⊞ *An autoclave should be readily available for decontaminating waste materials.*

⊞ *Lab coats, gloves and face protection is required.*

⊞ *The laboratory work must be supervised by a competent scientist who understand the risk associated with working the agents involved.*

iii) Biosafety level -3 (BSL-3)

⊞ *BSL-3 risk group contains biological agents that usually produce serious disease.*

⊞ *These agents are usually not transmitted by casual contact.*

⊞ *The laboratory must be a separate building or isolated zone, with double-door entry, directional inward airflow.*

Examples :-

Bacteria	Viruses
- Anthrax	- Lymphocytic choriomeningitis virus
- Brucella	- Hantaan virus
- Coxiella burnetti	- St. Louis encephalitis virus
- Tularemia	- Japanese encephalitis virus
- MAC	- West nile encephalitis virus
- M.tuberculosis	- SARS corona virus
Fungi	
- Coccidioides imitis	
- Blastomyces dermatitides	
- Histoplasma capsulatum	
- Paracoccidioides brazileinsis	

iv) Biosafety level- 4 (BSL-4)

⊞ *BSL-4 risk group contains biological agents that usually produce very **serious** infection that is often untreatable.*

⊞ *These agents are usually easily transmitted from one individual to another, from animal to human or vice-versa, either directly or indirectly, or by casual contact.*

⊞ *Numerous special facilities and precautions are required when working with these agents.*

Example :-

Lassa virus

Marburg virus

Ebola virus

Herpes simiac virus

⇨ **Bacterial Cultures:**

Smith noguchi medium: Spirochetes

Selenite F Broth: Salmonella, shigella

Dorset egg medium: Mycobacterium

Noguchi medium : Borellia

BYCE Medium: Legionella

Lofflers serum slope: Cornyebacterium diphtheria   (AIIMS 2002)

Tellurite Media: Cornyebacterium diphtheria   (AIIMS 2004)

Thayer martin media: N. gonorrhea

Korthof media: Leptospira   (AIIMS2009)

Staurts media: Leptospira

Fletcher media: Leptospira

Choclate agar: H. influenza

Bordet gengou: B. pertusis

Lownstein Johnson: M. tuberculosis

Sabourdars media: Fungi

Skirrows media: *Campylobacter jujeni*   (AIIMS 2004)

EXOTOXIN	ENDOTOXIN	
• Mostly gram-positive bacteria	• Gram-negative bacteria	
• Polypeptides	Lipopolysacchrides	JK BOPEE 2012
• Highly toxic	• Low toxicity	
• Highly antigenic	• Poorly antigenic	
• Toxoids used as vaccines	• No toxoids, no vaccines	
• Heat sensitive	• **Heat stable**	
• Secreted from cell	• Not secreted from cell	

⇨ **Antiphagocytic Structures (C A M P)**

▶ Capsule

▶ Pilli of Nisseria Gonorrhea

▶ M protein of *Streptococcus pyogenes*

▶ A protein of Staph aureus

⇨ **Capsulated Organisms:**

Streptococcus Pneumoniae☞

Klibessela Pneumoniae☞

Haemophilus influenza☞

Pseudomonas Aeruginosa☞

Nisseria meningitides☞

Cryptococcus neoformans☞

⇨ **Understanding toxins commonly asked in Examination. Best in Toxins**

"**P**seudomonas alpha toxin," which is responsible for the tissue damage, **inhibits Protein synthesis** by acting on **EF-2** with a primary target cell in the liver. ☞

The" **diphtheria toxin**" has a similar action, although its target cells are **heart and nerve.** ☞

Anthrax toxin is an "**Adenylate cyclase**" that causes fluid loss from cells. ☞

Botulinum toxin is a "neurotoxin" that **decreases acetylcholine synthesis.** ☞   SGPGI 2001

Cholera toxin acts to increase "adenylate cyclase "activity by **ribosylation of GTP-binding protein.** ☞

Clostridium perfringens **alpha toxin** is a "**lecithinase**" ☞

Escherichia coli labile toxin works in a fashion similar to the cholera toxin. ☞

Pertussis toxin causes fluid loss by "**ribosylating Gi**". ☞

Shiga toxin decreases protein synthesis by inhibiting the "**60S**" ribosomal subunit. ☞

Streptococcal "**erythrogenic**" **toxins** act similarly to the diphtheria toxin, but do so by increasing cytokine production. ☞

Tetanus toxin is a "**neurotoxin**" that "**inhibits the inhibitory neurotransmitters glycine and GABA**". ☞

TSST-1 is a "**superantigen**" that acts by increasing cytokine production and decreasing liver clearance of endotoxin. ☞

⇨ **Remember:**

Clostridium botulinum spores (**found in honey**) in the baby's gastrointestinal tract. Patients improve when honey is removed from the diet. This disorder is most common in children under the age of six months; older children and adults do not appear to be vulnerable to this form of botulism, but are susceptible to botulism caused by ingestion of preformed toxin. ☞

Clostridium difficile causes **pseudomembranous colitis**, especially after antibiotic therapy. ☞   PGI 2004

Clostridium perfringens causes **gas gangrene and gastroenteritis,** and it is not associated with ingestion of honey. ☞   AI 1999

Clostridium tetani causes **tetanus**, and does not cause a food-borne illness in infants. ☞   PGI 2004

5

MICROBIOLOGY

⇨ **Important Bacterial Toxins:**

Coryne Bacterium diptheria	• Diptheria	• Inactivates **EF2**: shuts down protein synthesis • <u>**KCET 2012**</u>
Clostridium tetani	• Tetanus	• Blocks release of **Glycine**
Clostridium boutilinium	• Boutilism	• Blocks release of **Acetyl choline**
Clostridium difficile	• Pseudomembranous colitis	• **Exotoxin <u>B</u>** Cytotoxin disaggregates actin filaments
Clostridium perfringens	• Gas gangrene	• **Alpha Toxin** acting as Lecithinase
Bacillus anthraxus	• Anthrax	• **Edema Factor, Lethal factor**
Staph aureus	• TSS	• Superantigen binding directly to **MHC II**
Stret pyogenes	• Scarlet fever	• **Super antigen**
E. coli	• Watery Diarrhoea	• Stimulates adenylate cyclase **(Gs)**
Vibrio cholera	• Cholera	• Stimulates adenylate cyclase **(Gs)**
Bordetella Pertussis	• Whooping Cough	• Stimulates adenylate cyclase (G_i)

⇨ **Toxins ↑c AMP levels (PACE):**

▶ Pertusis toxin

▶ Anthrax toxin

▶ Cholera toxin

▶ E. coli toxin (labile)

COMED 2003

Site	Important organism
• Skin	• Staph. epidermidis
• Nose	• Staph. aureus
• Mouth	• Strept. viridians
• Dental plaque	• Strept. mutans
• Vagina	• Lactobacillus, E. coli, Group B Strept.
• Colon	• Bacteroids, E.coli
• Throat	• Strept. viridians

Colony Appearance in Culture	Organism	
▶ 1. Draughtsman (Concentric Rings)	Pneumococci	
▶ 2. Medusa Head	B. Anthracis	JIPMER 2004
▶ Frosted Glass		PGI 1985
▶ Inverted Fir Tree in Stab Culture		
▶ String of pearls		
▶ 3. Swimming Growth (Fishy or Seminal Smell)	Proteus	PGI 1982
▶ 4. Swarm of Gnats or Fish in Stream	V. Cholerae	
▶ 5. Stalactite growth	Yersinia Pestis	
▶ 6. Thumb print appearance, Bisected pearls or	B. Pertussis	
▶ mercury drops, Aluminium Paint appearance		
▶ 7. Cigar bundle (globi) appearance	M.Leprae	
▶ 8. Fried egg	Mycoplasma	
▶ 9. Bread crumb	Actinomyces israelii	
▶ 10. Oil Paint	Staphylococci	
▶ 11. School of Red fish	H. ducreyi	
▶ 12. Stately Motility	Clostrida	

⇨ **Gram Positive Bacilli:**

Organism	Characteristics	Disease
▪ Corynebacterium diptheriae	Aerobic Catalase + Non Hemolytic Toxin production	▶ Diptheria
▪ Listeria monocytogenes	Aerobic Hemolytic	▶ Meningoencephalitis in neonates, immunocompromised
▪ Bacillus anthracis ▪ Bacillus cereus ▪ Bacillus anthracis	Aerobic spore forming	▶ Anthrax ▶ Food poisoning (reheated rice) ▶ Most common form: cutaneous (hide porters disease) ▶ Most fatal form: pulmonary (wool sorters disease)

cont...

5

MICROBIOLOGY

cont...

Clostridium welchii Clostridium septicum Clostridium tetani Clostridium Botulinium Clostridium difficile	Anaerobic, spore forming	▶ Food poisoning, gas gangrene ▶ Gas gangrene ▶ Tetanus ▶ Botulism ▶ Pseudomembranous colitis
▶ Mycobacterium tuberculosis	Aerobic, rod shaped	▶ Tuberculosis
▶ M. marinum		▶ Swimming pool granulomas
▶ M. ulcerans		▶ Cutaneous abscesses
▶ M. avium intercellulare		▶ Cervical LAP
▶ M. leprae	First mycobacterium to be discovered. **JK BOPEE 2012** Cannot be cultured, acid fast rods, cooler parts of body Don't follow kochs postulates. **5 % H_2So_4** is used for decolorization.	▶ Leprosy

⇨ **Gram Negative Bacilli:**

Haemophilus influenza Haemophilus para influenza Haemophilus aegipticus Haemophilus ducreyi →	Needs factor X and v, satellite phenomenon Koch weeks bacillus	Acute epiglottitis, meningitis in children, otitis media COPD Exacerbations Conjuctivitis Genital ulcers, chancroid
Bordetella pertusis	Cocco bacillus Bordet Gengou media	Whooping cough
Yersenia pestis Yersenia enterocolitica	Aerobic , bipolar staining	Bubonic plague, pneumonic plague Gastroenteritis, Pseudoappendicitis
Pasturella multicoida	Aerobic	Wound sepsis following dog bites

cont...

cont...

Vibrio cholera / Vibrio para hemolyticus	Aerobic curved motile rod	Cholera / Food poisoning (sea food) shell fish
Campylobacter	Microaerophilic	Acute Diarrhoea (bloody) / Gullian barre syndrome / Reactive arthritis
E. coli / E. coli 0157: H7	Aerobic, lactose fermenter, enterotoxin / Verocytotoxin,shiga like toxin / Non sorbitol fermenting	UTI, Peritonitis, cholecystitis, neonatal meningitis, travelers Diarrhoea JK BOPEE 2012 / HUS, TTP, haemorrhagic colitis
Klibessela pneumoniae	Aerobic, lactose fermenter	Pneumonia (currant jelly)
Proteus mirabilis	✓ Swarming growth on agar / ✓ Aerobic non lactose fermenter / ✓ Peritrichous flagella / ✓ Urease positive	UTI
Shigella	Non lactose fermenters / Non motile	Bacillary dysentry
▶ Bacteroids	▶ Anaerobic, non sporing	▶ Abscesses, septicaemia
▶ Fusobacterium	▶ Anaerobic, non sporing	▶ Vincents angina, gingivitis
Acinetobacter	Anaerobes	Hospital acquired infections

▶ Borrilea vincenti	Aerobic	▶ Vincents angina
▶ Borrilea recurrentis	Anaerobic	▶ Relapsing fever (r-r)
▶ Borrilea duttoni	Anaerobic	▶ Relapsing fever
▶ Borrilea burgdorfei	Anaerobic	▶ Lyme disease
Helicobacter pylori	Spiral, flagellate / Microaerophilic / Urease positive / Invasive / Campys medium, Skirrows agar	Peptic ulcer, gastric cancer, gastric lymphoma / Extra gastric diseases

5

MICROBIOLOGY

► Trepenoma pallidium	Anaerobic, spiral, motile	► Syphilis
► Trepenoma <u>pertenue</u>	Anaerobic	► Yaws
► Trepenoma <u>carateum</u>	Anaerobic	► Pinta
Leptospira icterohaemmorhagica	Anaerobic	Weils disease
Leptospira canicola	Anaerobic	Canicola fever
Rickettsia prowazeki	Obligate intracellular bacteria	<u>Epidemic</u> typhus
Rickettsia mooseri		<u>Endemic</u> typhus
Rickettsia burnetti		Q fever
Ehrilichia chafeensis		Ehrilichiosis
Mycoplasma pneumonia (Eaton agent)	Obligate intracellular <u>bacteria</u>	Primary atypical pneumonia
	<u>smallest</u> free living bacteria	Urethritis, PID
Ureaplasma urealyticum	<u>no</u> cell wall	Pyelonephritis
M. hominis	<u>sterols</u> in membrane	PID

► Actinomyces israelli	<u>Anaerobic</u>, branching filaments, <u>non</u> acid fast, sulfur granules,	► Actinomycosis, lumpy jaw
► Nocardial asteroids	<u>Anaerobic</u> , branching filaments, <u>partially</u> acid fast	► Nocardiosis ,

⇨ **Gems about Staph Aureus:**

► Gram-positive,	AI 1996
► Cluster-forming coccus, <u>non motile, non sporeforming facultative anaerobe</u>.	
► Fermentation of glucose produces mainly lactic acid +	
► Ferments mannitol (distinguishes from S. epidermidis.) +	
► Catalase positive +	
► Coagulase positive +	
► Coagulase is responsible for <u>pathogenecity</u>.	PGI 1998
► Golden yellow colony on agar.	
► Normal flora of humans found on nasal passages, skin and mucous membranes.	
► Food poisoning is due to <u>preformed</u> endotoxin.	
► Occurs <u>within 6 hours of food intake</u>	AIIMS 1996
► <u>Panton valentine leucocidin</u> is seen in staph infections.	KERALA 1997
► Especially diary products involved in poisoning.	AIIMS 2001

CAUSES:

Acute osteomyelitis

Acute mastitis

Botromycosis   PGI 2001

SSSS

Furunculosis, carbuncle   PGI 1989

Acute endocarditis

Sycosis barbae.   PGI 2001

Tropical polymyositis.   UPSC 2007

⇨ **Guidelines for the Control of MRSA:**

- Nasal carriage of S. *aureus* is very common and may be due to hand to nose transmission. A nasal carrier often contaminates his/her own hands by hand to nose contact, then transmits the organism in the course of routine activities. Since, skin to skin contract is the most significant mode of transmission, handwashing is of primary importance in preventing its spread.
- Handwashing, using soap and warm running water, is the single most important measure necessary to control the spread of MRSA.
- Decolonization of patients or staff is not routinely recommended. This has not proved to be an effective control measure, because recolonization usually occurs.
- Fumigation and wearing masks are not major activities for control of spread of MRSA.

TSS is caused by any of several related exoproteins produced by S. aureus.

TSST-1 is the toxin most frequently implicated (causing virtually all menstrual cases), and staphylococcal enterotoxin B is the second most frequent.

Menstruation remains the most common setting for TSS, but the disease can also complicate the use of barrier contraceptives and childbirth. The illness usually begins precipitously, with high fever and a complex of symptoms that may include nausea, vomiting, abdominal pain, diarrhea, muscular pain, sore throat, and headache. Dizziness is common as a manifestation of orthostatic or frank hypotension. The characteristic macular erythroderma develops over the first 2 days of illness. It is usually generalized but is sometimes locally confined; it can be evanescent or persistent. The patient's mental status is often abnormal to a degree that is out of proportion to the degree of hypotension.

⇨ **Gems about Streptococci:**

- C carbohydrate is used for Lancfield classification.   AIIMS 2007
- M protein is mainly responsible for pathogenecity.   AIIMS 1995
- MC organism causing cellulitis: streptococcus pyogenes
- Pikes medium is used.   DNB 2011

5

MICROBIOLOGY

Causes:
- ✓ erysipelas
- ✓ Scarlet fever
- ✓ Purpureal sepsis
- ✓ Non suppurative infections: rheumatic fever, glomerulonephritis

Group A streptococci produce a large number of extracellular products that may be important in local and systemic toxicity and in the spread of infection through tissues. These products include streptolysins S and O, toxins that damage cell membranes and account for the hemolysis produced by the organisms; streptokinase; DNases; protease; and pyrogenic exotoxins A, B, and C. The pyrogenic exotoxins, previously known as erythrogenic toxins, cause the rash of scarlet fever. Since the mid-1980s, pyrogenic exotoxin-producing strains of group A Streptococcus have been linked to unusually severe invasive infections, including necrotizing fasciitis and a systemic syndrome termed the **Streptococcal toxic shock syndrome**

▶ Str. Agalactaciae	▶ Neonatal meningitis, Neonatal sepsis	JK BOPEE 2012
▶ Str. Bovis	▶ Endocarditis	
▶ Str. Pneumonia	▶ Pneumoniae, Otitis media	
▶ Str. Mutans	▶ Dental caries	
▶ Anaerobic streptococci	▶ Purpureal sepsis	
▶ Str. Pyogenes	▶ Erysipelas, Cellulitis,	
	▶ Impetigo, scarlet fever, Rheumatic fever, Acute Glomerulonephritis	
▶ Str. Viridians	▶ Endocarditis	

"Streptococcus agalactaciae":

- ✓ Group b Streptococci., gram positive   AI 2010
- ✓ Beta Hemolytic
- ✓ Bacitracin <u>Resistant.</u>   AI 2010
- ✓ Hydrolyses hippurate
- ✓ C AMP test positive.   AI 2010

⊃ **Acute Meningitis: Commonest Bacterial organisms**✳✳✳

▶ **Neonates:** Group B streptococci, E. coli,	TN 2002
▶ **Infants and children:** H. influenza	
▶ **Adolscents and young adults:** N.meningitidis	
▶ **Elderly:** Strept. Pnemonaie, Listeria Monocytogenes	

Beta hemolysis is shown by:✷✷

- Strep. pyogenes
- Strept agalataciae
- Staph. aureus
- Listeria. monocytogenes
- Bacillus subtilis

Alpha hemolysis is shown by:✷✷

- Strep. pneumonia
- Strep. viridians
- Sterpt, mutans
- Strep. Sanguis
- Enterococcus

⇨ **Gems about S. bovis.**

The main **nonenterococcal group D streptococcal** species that causes human infections is S. bovis. ☛

S. bovis endocarditis is often associated with <u>neoplasms of the gastrointestinal tract</u>. ☛

¾most frequently a colon carcinoma or polyp¾but is also reported in association with other bowel lesions. ☛

S. bovis are reliably killed by penicillin as a single agent, and **penicillin is the treatment of choice for S. bovis infections.** ☛

⇨ **Catalase Positive Organisms Are:✷✷✷**

Staph aureus
Pseudomonas
Aspergillus
Candida
Citrobacter,
Enterobacter,
E.coli,
Klebsiella
Shigella,
Yersinia

5

MICROBIOLOGY

⇨ **Gems about Pneumococcus:**

▶ Gram **positive**	AIIMS 2005
▶ Capsulated	
▶ Most virulent : **type C**	AIIMS 1986
▶ <u>Draughtsman</u> colonies	AMU 1987
▶ <u>Quelling reaction</u> seen	PGI 1986
▶ Vaccine is made from capsule.	PGI 1992
▶ <u>Lanceolate, flame shaped diplococcus</u>	PGI 1982
▶ Bile soluble	
▶ Optochonin **sensitive**	
▶ Virulence is due to <u>capsule</u>	AI 1999

⇨ **Gems about Nisseria Gonococcus:**

▶ Means <u>flow of seeds</u>.	AIIMS 1980
▶ <u>Intracytoplasmi</u>c Gram negative	PGI 1997
▶ Non capsulated	
▶ Don't ferment maltose. Ferments glucose	AI 1996
▶ Kidney shaped	
▶ Causes:	
Urethritis	PGI 2006
Cervicitis	
Salpingitis	
Vaginitis	
Conjunctivitis	
Meningitis, arthritis, endocarditis	JIPMER 1991

⇨ **Nisseria Meningococcus:**

Gram negative diplococcic	
Capsulated	
<u>Carriers</u> are a source of infection	AI 2003
Cause <u>Water house Freiderschein syndrome</u>, Meningitis	

• Nisseria meningitides: ☞	Capsule +	Maltose Fermentation +
• Nisseria gonococcus: ☞	Capsule -	Maltose Fermentation -

⇨ **Gems about Coryne bacterium diptheriae:**

► Gram positive, <u>non motile, non sporing, non capsulated</u>	
► <u>Babes ernest / volutin granules seen/ Metachromatic granules</u> seen	**PGI 1986**
► Lofflers serum slope, Tellurite media used	**KERALA 1991**
► Eleks gel precipitation test used.	
► Incubation period 2-6 days	
► <u>Faucial (tonsillar)</u> not facial diptheria is the commonest type of diphtheria	
► <u>Pseudomembrane</u> formation is a feature.	
► <u>Bulls neck</u> (cervical lymphadenopathy) occurs in diphtheria.	
► Diptheria toxin inhibits protein synthesis.	**JK BOPEE 2012**
► **Toxin is phage mediated**	**KCET 2012**
► Coryne bacterium <u>parvum</u> is used as immunomodulator	**COMED 2005**
► Coryne bacterium <u>pseudotuberculosis</u> is Nocards bacillus.	**AIIMS 1982**
► Coryne bacterium <u>minnusitum</u> causes Erythrassma.	**AI 1988**
<u>Ehrlichs phenomenon</u> is seen in diphtheria.(toxin-antitoxin reaction)	**PGI 2011**

Daisy head colony (C. diptheriae) gravis✱	· **TN 2004**
Frogs egg colony (C. diptheriae) intermedius✱	
Poached egg colony (C. diptheriae) mitis✱	

⇨ **Corynebacterium Minutissiumum:**

— Is a part of normal skin flora.

— It is **lipophilic**, gram positive, aerobic, catalase positive but non spore forming diptheroid.

— It ferments glucose, dextrose, sucrose, maltose and mannitol

- Erythrasma is a <u>**chronic superficial infection of intertriginous areas.**</u>
- Organism causing erythrasma is **Corynebacterium Minutissiumum**.　　　**JK BOPEE 2008**
- Erythrasma produces <u>**coral red flourescene**</u> under wood light secondary to production of porphyrins.

⇨ **Anthrax:**

► Is a Zoonosis	**PGI 2004**
► Gram positive, Non motile, capsulated, sporing	
► <u>Cutaneous</u> anthrax commonest,	
► <u>Painless malignant pustule.</u> (CHARBON)	**(PGI 1985)**
► Hide porters disease is cutaneous anthrax.	
► Wool sorters disease is pulmonary anthrax.	**AIIMS 1986**

5

— Colony woes for a student

— Colony characteristics for the organism

▶ Medusa head   PGI 1981

▶ Inverted fir tree appearance

▶ Frosted glass appearance

▶ String of pearl appearance   PGI 1985

▶ Mc Faydens reaction positive   PGI 1999

▶ PLET medium used.

"Malignant pustule"   PGI 2011

Bacillus anthracis can produce an ulcer (anthrax) with black-based, sharply demarcated edges. The infection generally begins with a small, somewhat pruritic papule at the site of an abrasion, which over the next several days develops into a vesicle containing serosanguineous fluid teeming with organisms. The lesion generally occurs on the upper extremities, especially the arms and hands, or on the face, neck, or other areas that are likely to be exposed to the contaminated animal product or infected soil. As the lesion progresses, ulceration occurs, with formation of a necrotic ulcer base frequently surrounded by smaller vesicles. The characteristic black eschar evolves over several weeks to a size of several centimeters, gradually separating and leaving a scar. This black eschar accounts for the name anthrax, which comes from the Greek word for coal. The edema is frequently nonpitting, gelatinous, and brawny and is very striking. It may be quite extensive, spreading over a wide area in severe cases.

⇨ **Gems about Clostridia:**

Clostridium tetani:

• Gram positive ☛☛	PGI 1984
• **Anaerobic** spore forming bacilli. ☛	
• Motile with swarming tendency.	AI 1995
• Strict anaerobe	

• Spherical and terminal spores☛☛☛	(drum stick)	Cl. tetani	PGI 2003
• Oval and terminal spores: ☛☛☛	(tennis racket)	Cl.difficile	
• Central or sub terminal: ☛☛☛	(spindle)	other species	

Tetanospasmin is the toxin. Blocks release of **inhibitory neurotransmitters glycine/ GABA.**
Generalized tetanus is the mc form.   Most effective way of preventing tetanus is **tetanus toxoid.**

⊃ **Clostridial Myonecrosis (gas gangrene): (AIIMS 09)** ☛☛

▶ 80% of cases are caused by C. perfringens,   AI 1991

▶ <u>Alpha toxin</u> is the most important toxin responsible.

▶ C. novyi, C. septicum, and C. histolyticum cause the other cases.

▶ Typically, **gas gangrene** begins with the **sudden onset of pain in the region of the wound**, which helps to differentiate it from spreading cellulitis.

▶ Once established, the pain increases steadily in severity but remains localized to the infected area and spreads only if the infection spreads.

⇨ **Clostridium botulinium:**

▶ The **CNS is <u>not affected</u>** by the toxin of Cl. botulinium.   AI 2007

▶ **Blocks release of Ach** at synapses and NM junction.

▶ Infant botulism is caused by ingestion of spores.food borne botulism is due to ingestion of preformed toxin.

▶ **Symmetric descending paralysis** is a feature of botulinism   JIPMER 1980

⇨ **Clostridium difficile**

▶ **Causes pseudomembranous colitis**   AI 1991

▶ Is a normal gut commensal   AI 2007

▶ Almost <u>all antibiotics</u> even the ones used in treatment of pseudomembranous colitis can cause the disease

▶ Metronadizole is the DOC

▶ Vancomycin is also effective in treatment

▶ Cytotoxin assay in stools is the best test.

Clostridial gas gangrene or myonecrosis

Occurs in three different settings.

First, and most commonly, traumatic gas gangrene develops after deep, penetrating injury that compromises the blood supply (e.g., knife or gunshot wound, crush injury), creating an anaerobic environment ideal for clostridial proliferation.

C. perfringens accounts for 80% of such infections.   PGI 2011

The remaining cases are caused by

✓ C. septicum,   PGI 2011

✓ C. novyii,   PGI 2011

✓ C. histolyticum,   PGI 2011

✓ C. bifermentans, and

✓ C. fallax.

5

Conditions associated with traumatic gas gangrene are :

- Bowel and biliary tract surgery,
- Criminal abortion, and
- Retained placenta;
- Prolonged rupture of the membranes; or
- Intrauterine fetal demise or missed abortion in postpartum patients.

⇨ **Gems about Enterobacteeraicea:**

- E. coli, klibessela, enterobacter: ☛   Ferments <u>lactose</u>
- Salmonella, shigella, proteus, pseudomonas :☛   Don't Ferment <u>lactose</u> (S2P2)   MAH 2012

Capsular☛☛
Antigen☛☛
Flagellar antigen☛☛
Ferment <u>glucose</u>: E. coli, Proteus, Klibessela☛☛

INCLUDES:

▶ Escherichia,   PGI 2006

▶ Klebsiella,   PGI 2006

▶ Proteus,   PGI 2006

▶ Enterobacter,

▶ Serratia,

▶ Citrobacter,

▶ Morganella,

▶ Providencia, and

▶ Edwardsiella as well as the genus **Actinetobacter** from the family Neisseriaceae

Six distinct "pathotypes" of intestinal pathogenic **E. coli** exist: (1) enterotoxigenic **E. coli** (ETEC); (2) Shiga toxin-producing **E. coli** (STEC)/enterohemorrhagic **E. coli** (EHEC); (3) enteropathogenic **E. coli** (EPEC); (4) enteroinvasive **E. coli** (EIEC); (5) enteroaggregative **E. coli** (EAEC); and (6) diffusely adherent **E. coli** (DAEC). Organisms of these pathotypes are acquired via the fecal-oral rout

ETEC is the most common cause of **traveler's diarrhea**☛☛☛   JK BOPEE 2012

EHEC estimated 50% of all cases of **HUS** are caused by EHEC infection. ☛☛   JIPMER 1988

EPEC is an important cause of **infant diarrhea**☛☛   AIIMS 1995

EIEC shares many features with **Shigella infection**; however, unlike Shigella, EIEC causes disease only at a high inoculum (10^8 to 10^{10} CFU). **Penetrate Hela cells in tissue culture.** ☛☛☛

Sereny test in diagnosis used. **Non motile and Non lactose fermenting.** ☛☛   AIIMS 1999

EAEC: These pathotypes have been described primarily in **developing countries and mostly affect young children.** These strains may also cause some cases of traveler's diarrhea. A high inoculum is required for infection. In vitro, the organisms exhibit a diffuse or **"stacked-brick"** adherence pattern. ☛

⇨ **Gems about PROTEUS**

> ► Causes only 1 to 2% of cases of UTI in healthy women, and *Proteus* species cause **only 5% of cases of hospital-acquired UTI.**
>
> ► **Swarming motility**
>
> ► Fishy / seminal odour   **PGI 1982**
>
> ► **Urease positive**
>
> ► **Dienes phenomenon shown**   **PGI 2002**
>
> *Proteus* is responsible for 10 to 15% of cases of complicated UTI, primarily those associated with catheterization; in the setting of long-term catheterization This high prevalence is due to the ability of *Proteus* to produce **high levels of urease, which hydrolyzes urea to ammonia and results in alkalization of the urine.** ☛   **AI 2001**
>
> This situation, in turn, leads to precipitation of organic and inorganic compounds, with the
>
> ► **Formation of struvite and carbonate-apatite crystals,** ☛
>
> ► **Biofilm formation on catheters, and/or the** ☛
>
> ► **Development of calculi.** ☛
>
> ► *Proteus* becomes associated with the stones and usually can be eradicated only by complete stone removal. Over time, **staghorn calculi** may form and lead to obstruction and renal failure. ☛☛☛

⇨ **Gems about Klibessela**

> ► Causes only a small proportion of cases of community-acquired pneumonia
>
> ► **Friedlandres bacillus.**   **PGI 1997**
>
> ► This infection occurs primarily in hosts with underlying disease, such as **alcoholics, diabetics, and individuals with chronic lung disease.** ☛☛
>
> ► Presentation with earlier, less extensive infection is more common than that with the classic lobar infiltrate with a **bulging fissure.** ☛
>
> ► **Currant jelly sputum** is a feature in lung infections.

⇨ **Gems about SHIGELLA:**

> **Gram negative**
>
> <u>**Non capsulated**</u>
>
> <u>**Non motile**</u>   **AI 1999**
>
> **Lactose non fermenters**
>
> **Ferment mannitol except S. dysentrae**   **MAH 2012**
>
> **Subdivided on basis of <u>Mannitol fermentation</u>**   **AI 1997**
>
> **Most virulent type is S. dysentiae**   **CMC 1986**
>
> **Stool culture is the best test.**   **UPSC 1999**

⇨ **Gems about SALMONELLA:**

▶ Gram negative.

▶ Peritrichate flagella.

▶ Need tryptophan as growth factor.   DNB 1998

▶ Selenite F is used as growth medium.

▶ Affects Payer's patches in intestines.

▶ H antigen is the most immunogenic.   PGI 1996

▶ Vi agglutination detects carriers.   AIIMS 2002

▶ Vi antigen is not seen in normal population.   AIIMS 1991

▶ Blood culture is the gold standard for diagnosis.

▶ Diazo reaction is also used for diagnosis.   AIMS 1985

Widal test:

▶ Test of blood serum that uses an **agglutination reaction** to diagnose typhoid fever.

▶ [After Fernand Widal (1862-1929), French physician.]

▶ The Widal test is a **presumptive serological test** for Enteric fever or Undulant fever.

▶ In case of **Salmonella** infections, it is a demonstration of agglutinating antibodies against antigens

O-somatic and H-flagellar in the blood. ✳

▶ For **brucellosis**, only **O-somatic antigen** is used.

▶ It's not a very accurate method, since patients are often exposed to other bacteria (e.g. Salmonella enteritidis, Salmonella typhimurium) in this species that induce cross-reactivity;

▶ Many people have antibodies against these enteric pathogens, which also react with the antigens in the Widal test, causing a false-positive result.

Test results need to be interpreted carefully in the light of past history of enteric fever, typhoid vaccination, general level of antibodies in the populations in endemic areas of the world.

The highest dilution of the patients serum in which agglutinations occurs is noted, ex. if the dilution is 1 in 160 then the titer is 169.

A single test of O titer of 1:100 or more and of H titer of 1:200 or more is significant.

A rising titer of four fold or higher in an interval of 7 - 10 days is more meaningful than one test.

⇨ **Cautionary factors:**

▶ In endemic areas, low titer of agglutinins is present in the serum of normal persons.

▶ Immunisation with TAB vaccine will show high titres of antibodies to S. typhi, S. paratyphi A and B. (in an infection there will be rise in only one type of antibodies)

► Person who have had past enteric infections or immunisations may develop anamestic reaction during unreleated fever like malaria. There is only a transient rise.

► Bacterial antigens used may contain fimbrial antigens which give false positive results.

► Cases treated early with chloramphenicol show poor antibody response.

► Test may be positive in carriers

⇨ **Gems about Vibrio cholera:**

► Isolated by **Koch**.	**KERALA 1994**
► Most cases are **subclinical**.	**AI 1997**
► Gram negative bacilli ,Aerobic	
► **Non capsulated, comma shaped**	
► <u>**Motile with polar flagellum**</u>	
► Ferments glucose, transported in alkaline medium.	**AI 1994**
► Toxin action is **cAMP mediated**.	**AIIMS 1995**
► **Darting motility**	**TN 1997**
► **Cary Blair medium** used	
► **Venkata Raman** medium used	
► **Humans are the reservoir**	**AI 2010**
► **Survives boiling for 30 seconds**	**AI 2010**
► **Survives in cold temperature (ice for 4-6 weeks)**	**AI 2010**
► causes **rice water stools/ Pea soup Diarrhoea**	
► <u>**Non** halophilic</u>	**AI 2005**

⇨ **Gems about Pseudmonas:**

Pseudomonas aerugenosa is a **gram negative, aerobic, motile bacillus.** ☞☞

Cetrimide agar is the selective media for Pseudomonas aerugenosa ☞☞

EXOTOXIN A inhibits protein synthesis.   **AI 1997**

Pseudomonas aerugenosa produces pigments

✓ **Pyocyanin,**

✓ **Pyoverdin,**   **PSC 2001**

✓ **Pyorubin and**

✓ **Flourescein.** ☞☞

✓ Produces blue green pus☞☞

Virulence factors are:✱

► Pilli, Elastase,Exotoxin,Endotoxin,Alkaline protease,Hemolysin Alginate☞

► Grape like odour

► Slime layer formation

5

Pseudomonas aerugenosa grows at **37-42°C.**

Pseudomonas aerugenosa **hydrolyses arginine** to citrulline and ammonia. ☛☛

Pseudomonas aerugenosa **oxidises indophenols.** ☛☛

Pseudomonas aerugenosa **does not ferment lactose.** ☛☛

Pipercillin Is an anti pseudomonal pencillin. (p-p)   AI 2006

Pseudomonas aerugenosa Causes:

Serious infections in burn patients☛☛☛

Shock with bullous lesions.   JIPMER 1980

Ecthyma gangreonosum☛☛

Shanghai fever☛☛

Hot tub follicultis ☛☛

Multi drug resistance is due to biofilm production in cornea.   AI 2010

Pseudomonas pseudomallei   DNB 2011

Causes "Meliodosis". ☛☛   AI 2005

Also called **Whitmores bacillus.**

Great imitator disease.

Pseudomonas mallei

Causes "glanders". ☛

"Culture sensitivity" of Pseudomonas:

- As a class, the <u>fluoroquinolones</u> are marked by extremely broad activity against gram-negative rods, including Pseudomonas species.

- Monobactams. <u>Aztreonam</u> is the only currently available member of the class of monobactams. It has gram-negative coverage, including most Pseudomonas species.

- The third-generation cephalosporins have greatly expanded activity against gram-negative rods, including many resistant strains, and rival the aminoglycosides in their coverage while having a much more favorable safety profile. In exchange for this gram-negative coverage, most members of this group have significantly less activity against staphylococci and streptococcal species than first- and second-generation cephalosporins. Anaerobic coverage is, generally, rather poor as well. The important distinction in the third-generation cephalosporins is between those with significant activity against Pseudomonas species <u>(cefoperazone and ceftazidime)</u>   PGI 2011

- and those without (cefotaxime, ceftizoxime, and ceftriaxone)

Gems about Yersinia

▶ **Plague** is an **acute, febrile, <u>zoonotic disease</u>** caused by infection with **Yersinia pestis.** ☞

▶ Y. pestis is a **gram-negative coccobacillus** in the family **Enterobacteriaceae.** ☞   **PGI 2006**

▶ It is **microaerophilic, nonmotile, nonsporulating, oxidase** and **urease negative,** and **biochemically unreactive.** ☞
<u>Bipolar staining</u>.
<u>Safety pin appearance</u>.
<u>Waysons staining done for identification</u>
<u>Stalicite growth</u>.   **TN 1995**

▶ The organism is **nonfastidious** and **infective for laboratory rodents.** It grows well, if slowly, on routinely used microbiologic media **(e.g., sheep blood agar, brain-heart infusion broth, and MacConkey agar).** ☞

▶ The colonies are gray-white with irregular surfaces, described as having a "hammered-metal" appearance when viewed microscopically.

▶ When stained with a polychromatic stain (e.g., Wayson or Giemsa), Y. pestis isolated from clinical specimens exhibits a characteristic **bipolar appearance**, often resembling closed safety pins. ☞

▶ **Bubonic plague, the most common form,**   **AIIMS 2004**

▶ Is almost always caused by the bite of an infected flea but occasionally results from direct inoculation of infectious fluids.

▶ Septicemic and pneumonic **plague** can be either primary or secondary to metastatic spread. ☞

▶ Because fleas often bite the legs, femoral and inguinal nodes are most commonly involved; axillary and cervical nodes are next most commonly affected. The **enlarging bubo becomes progressively painful and tender.** ☞

▶ The bubo of **plague** is distinguishable from lymphadenitis of most other causes, however, by its <u>rapid onset, its extreme tenderness, the accompanying signs of toxemia, and the absence of cellulitis or obvious ascending lymphangitis.</u> ☞

▶ Pneumonic plague is most infectious. pneumonic plague develops most rapidly and is most frequently fatal ☞

▶ **Streptomycin is the drug of choice**

▶ Tetracycline is the doc for prophylaxis.   **AIIMS 2002**

⇨ **Gems about Haemophilus:**

▶ **Gram negative cocco bacillus**
▶ Grows on **chocolate agar**
▶ Capsulated
▶ Requires **factor X and V.**   **TN 1999**
▶ **Satellitism** is seen   **PGI 1986**

▶ **Chancroid** is caused by **H. ducreyi.**
▶ Shows **school of fish appearance.**   **AI 1989**

⇨ **Gems about Bordetella:**

▶ Gram negative cocco bacillus

▶ Capsulated

▶ Bordet gengou media used   PGI 1994

▶ Causes whooping cough

▶ Incubation period 1-2 weeks   AIIMS 2005

▶ Thumb printing appearance in culture films.   KAR 1999

▶ Erythromycin prevents spread of disease in children,

Gems about Brucellosis

is a zoonosis.   PGI 2002

Malta fever/ undulant fever/ meditarrean fever.   AIIMS 2008

Gram negative

non capsulated

non motile

non sporing

NO person -person transmission.   AIIMS 2007

⇨ **Causative organisms**

▶ **B.militensis** from goat, sheep, cattle (most common) ☞☞☞

▶ **B.abortus** from cattle☞☞☞

▶ **B .suis** from hogs☞☞

▶ **B. canis** from dogs☞☞

▶ Brucellae are slow-growing, small, aerobic, nonmotile, nonencapsulated, non-spore-forming, gram-negative coccobacilli.

▶ B. abortus, B. suis, B. melitensis, and B. canis are known to infect humans and are typed on the basis of biochemical, metabolic, and immunologic criteria. There are differences in virulence among these four species.

▶ B. melitensis, with a reservoir in sheep, camel and goats, swine, buffaloes, horses may cause severe, acute disease and disabling complications.   PGI 2011

▶ B. canis, spread to humans from infected dogs, causes disease with an insidious onset, frequent relapse, and a chronic course that is indistinguishable from infection related to B. abortus.

➡ Brucella survive in unpasteurized milk for up to 8 weeks.

➡ Brucella is transmitted most commonly through un pasteurized milk/milk products, raw meat and bone marrow. ☞

- It can also be contracted through **inhalation** in farm houses, slaughter houses, labs. Other routes are skin abrasion, inoculation, Conjuctival splashing. 🖙🖙
- The common symptoms are fever, chills, diaphoresis, headache, myalgias, fatigue.
- Patient can look deceptively well with just fever.
- In severe cases Hepatospleenomegaly, Lymphadenopathy, arthritis, meningitis or pneumonia can occur.
- **Rose Bengal Card test** used.   **ROHTAK 1986**
- **Milk Ring test** used.   **JIPMER 1999**
- Diagnosis is by culture, Phage typing, DNA Characteristics, Metabolic profiling(BACTEC)
- Treatment is by combination therapy of **aminoglycoside plus doxycycline for 4 weeks followed by doxycycline plus rifampin for 4-8 weeks.**
- **In pregnancy** TMP-SMZ plus rifampin for 8-12 weeks is given.

⇨ **Bartonella henselae**

- ♯ It is a **slightly curved, small, self-aggregating, gram-negative bacillus** that is capable of twitching motility. B. henselae as an **etiologic agent of cat scratch disease, as well as bacillary angiomatosis.**   **DNB 2011**

- ♯ angiomatosis involves skin and visceral sites with angioproliferative lesions

- ♯ **The lesions of bacillary angiomatosis** assume diverse macroscopic appearances, including an erythematous, polypoid or papular, cutaneous or mucosal pattern; deeply erythematous and indurated dermal plaques; and subcutaneous or visceral nodules. In all of these lesions, a distinctive lobular proliferation of capillaries is seen within a fibrous stroma. Hematoxylin and eosin reveal granular amphophilic material in the interstitium between vessels. This material corresponds to clumps of extracellular bacteria, as viewed with the Warthin-Starry silver stain or with electron microscopy.

- ♯ *Bacillary peliosis is a histologic variant form of bacillary angiomatosis that is characterized by blood-filled cystic spaces, fibromyxoid stroma, and inflammatory cells; it is also associated with B. henselae and occurs most often within the liver and spleen.*

⊃ **Gems About Mycobacterium Tuberculosis**

Mycobacterium tuberculosis complex (consisting of M. tuberculosis, M. bovis, and M. africanum)

⇨ **Mycobacterium tuberculosis:**

- ▶ Discovered by **Robert Koch.**   **TN 2004**
- ▶ **Obligate aerobe**
- ▶ **Acid fast**
- ▶ Acid fastness is due to **mycolic acid and cell wall.**   **AIIMS 1993**
- ▶ Slightly curved rod.
- ▶ LJ Medium **(Lowenstein Jonson Medium)** used.
- ▶ Usually **affects apical and posterior segments of upper lobes.**
- ▶ **Lung** is the mc organ involved.
- ▶ **Tubercular lymphadenitis** is the mc extra pulmonary TB.

5

- ► Rapid diagnosis is by Auramine Rhodamine stain.   ICS 2K
- ► Production of niacin is an important feature.   KERALA 2001
- ► <u>Cord factor</u> promotes virulence.   TN 1998
- ► Mycobacteium <u>Para tuberculosis</u> is <u>Johnes bacillus</u>.   AIIMS 2008

⇨ **Atypical mycobacteria:**

- ► Photochromogen: M. kanasi
- ► Scotochromogen: M.scofulaceum
- ► Non chromagen: MAI
- ► Rapid grower: M. smegmatis

Buruli ulcer is caused by: **M. ulcerans**   COMED 2008

Swimming pool granuloma / Fish tank granuloma is caused by **M. marinum**   AI 1989

⇨ **Gems about M. leprae**

- ► **Gram positive**
- ► Generation time <u>12 days</u>.   MANIPAL 2006
- ► **Acid fast bacilli.** Less acid fast than M. tuberculosis.
- ► <u>Globi and cigar bundle appearance</u> are a feature.
- ► Cultivated in **Armadillo**
- ► Can be grown in **foot pad of mice.**   AIIMS 1994
- ► Spreads by **skin -skin contact.**   KERALA 1995
- ► Lepra cells are <u>histiocytes</u>   DELHI 1993

⇨ **Gems about Treponema palladium:**

Causes **syphilis**

Gram negative spirochete with polar flagellum.

Has **hylauronidase.**

Incubation period **9-90 days**

Primary lesion is a chancre. <u>Painless ulcer</u> with non tender inguinal lymphadenopathy

<u>Condyloma lata</u> is seen in secondary syphilis

Dark ground microscopy is used for diagnosis. 10^4 organisms / ml are needed to be detected.   AIIMS 1981

<u>Leviditti stain</u> is used for staining.   PGI 1986

FTA ABS is a specific test.

VDRL is a slide flocculation test.   TN 1995

VDRL is positive in **secondary syphilis.**   AIIMS 1991

➲ **FALSE POSITIVE VDRL:**

✓ HIV	PGI 2011
✓ Leprosy	PGI 2011
✓ Malaria	
✓ Iv drug abuse	
✓ Pregnancy	
✓ Infectious mononucleosis	
✓ Old age	
✓ CTD	
✓ Relapsing fever	PGI 2011
✓ Hepatitis C	

⇨ **Borellia:**

Borrelia burgdorferi Causes **Lymes disease.**(erythema migrans)

Borrelia recurentis causes **relapsing fever.**   AI 2003

Kellys medium used.

Lymes Disease:

- Causative agent: **B. burgdorferi**

- Vector: **Ixodes tick**

Features:

- **STAGE I:** Localized disease, IP: 3-32 days, **Erythema migrans** at local site.

- **STAGE II:** Disseminated disease, Secondary skin lesions, meningitis, carditis.

- **STAGE III:** Oligoarticular arthritis, Encephalopathy, Polyneuropathy. Acrodermatitis atrophicans.

⇨ **Leptospirosis:**

- ▶ **Spirochetal infection.**

- ▶ Rats, rice and rain associations   AI 2005

- ▶ Transmitted by <u>rat urine</u>.   AI 2002

- ▶ Seen in **sewage workers.**

- ▶ Acute renal failure and jaundice is a feature.

- ▶ Leptospira icteriohaemorrhagica causes Weils disease.   AP 1988

DIAGNOSIS OF LEPTOSPIROSIS

Culture most often become positive after **2-4 weeks.**

Media used for isolation

* Ellinghausen – Mecullough
* Johnson Harris (EMJH) medium
* Fletcher medium
* **Korthof medium**
* **Stuart's medium**

Serological diagnosis

* A fourfold greater rise in antibody titre is diagnostic.
* Antibody reaches detectable level in second week.

Tests used are:

✓ Microscopic agglutination test.
✓ ELISA test
✓ Indirect hemagglutination test
✓ Leptospires grow best under aerobic conditions.
✓ Leptospires remain viable in anticoagulated blood.

Polymerase chain reaction

► **Weil's syndrome**, the most severe form of **leptospirosis**, is characterized by **jaundice, renal dysfunction, hemorrhagic diathesis, and high mortality.** This syndrome is frequently but not exclusively associated with infection due to icterohaemorrhagiae/copenhageni.

⇨ **Gems about Mycoplasma:**

► **Eaton agent.**	**ROHTAK 1986**
► The **smallest free-living organisms** known,	**AIIMS 2005**
► Are **prokaryotes** that are bounded only by a plasma membrane.	**AIIMS 2005**
► Their lack of a cell wall is associated with cellular pleomorphism and **resistance to cell wall-active antimicrobial agents, such as penicillins and cephalosporins.**	**PGI 1999**
► **Fried egg colonies.**	**AIIMS 1986**
► **L forms** seen. (Concept has changed now)	**AIIMS 1986**

— Mycoplasma pneumoniae causes primary **atypical pneumonia**, upper and lower respiratory tract infections.

— M. genitalium and Ureaplasma urealyticum are established causes of urethritis and have been implicated in other genital conditions.

— M. hominis and U. urealyticum are part of the complex microbial flora of bacterial vaginosis.

MYCOPLASMA PNEUMONIAE

► M. pneumoniae causes upper and lower respiratory tract symptoms
► The infection is acquired by **inhalation of aerosols.**

⇨ **Actinomyces**

▶ Gram positive   AIIMS 1995

▶ Non motile

▶ Non sporing

▶ Non acid fast

▶ Non capsulated

▶ Mc form cervico facial

▶ Lumpy jaw is a feature.

Growth of **actinomycetes** usually results in the formation of clumps called **grains or sulfur granules.**   AI 1994

Oral-Cervicofacial Disease

Actinomycosis occurs **most frequently** at an oral, cervical, or facial site, usually as a soft tissue swelling, abscess, or mass lesion that is often mistaken for a neoplasm.

The angle of the jaw is generally involved

⇨ **Nocardia:**

▶ Strict aerobe.

▶ Acid fast.

▶ Causes **Nocardiosis.**

▶ Paraffin bait is used for isolation.

▶ Soil is natural habitat.

▶ Pneumonia is the mc manifestation.

⇨ **Listeria monocytogenes**

Is a **gram-positive cocobacillus** in short chains.   AI 2002

That can be isolated from soil, vegetation, and many animal reservoirs.

Shows **tumbling motility**

also in response to temperature. Motile at 25°c but non motile at temp erature above 37°c.

JK BOPEE 2012

Survives and multiplies in phagocytes.   AIIMS 2005

Human disease due to L. monocytogenes generally occurs in the setting of **pregnancy** or of immunosuppression caused by illness or medication

Antons test used.   AIIMS 1997

• L. monocytogenes grows well in **cold** temperatures.

• L. monocytogenes causes **meningitis and sepsis in neonates.**

• L. monocytogenes causes **meningitis and sepsis in immunocompromised patients.**

• L. monocytogenes during **pregnancy** can cause **abortion, premature delivery or sepsis during postpartum period.**

5

MICROBIOLOGY

⇨ **Campylobacter:**

▶ Are **motile,**

▶ **Non-spore-forming, curved gram-negative rods.**

▶ **Microaerophilic**

▶ The principal diarrheal pathogen **is c. jejuni,** which accounts for 80 to 90% of all cases of recognized illness due to campylobacters.

▶ **Skirrows medium is culture medium**

▶ **Butzlers medium is culture medium**

⇨ **H. pylori :**

▶ is a **gram-negative, spiral, flagellate bacillus**   **PGI 2005**

▶ It is **noninvasive,** living in gastric mucus; a small proportion of the bacterial cells are adherent to the mucosa.

▶ Its spiral shape and flagellae render **H. pylori** motile in the mucous environment,   **PGI 2004**

▶ its efficient **urease** protects it against acid by catalyzing urea hydrolysis to produce buffering ammonia.

▶ In vitro, **H. pylori** is **microaerophilic** and slow-growing and requires complex growth media   **APGEE 2005**

▶ **Complete genomic sequence has been studied**

▶ Causes duodenal ulcers (stronger relation)

▶ Causes gastric ulcers

▶ Prevalence increases with age.

▶ **Transmitted from man-man, fecoorally and orogastric route.**   **PGI 2000**

➥ *Microbiologic culture is most specific but may be insensitive because of difficulty with H. pylori isolation. It Permits determination of antibiotic susceptibility.*

➥ *The test of choice for **documenting eradication is the urea breath test (UBT).***

➥ *Serologic testing is not useful for the purpose of documenting eradication since antibody titers fall slowly and often do not become undetectable.*

⇨ **Urease positive organisms:**

✓ S. aureus

✓ Proteus

✓ H. pylori

✓ Klibessela

✓ Cryptococcus

✓ Nocardia

✓ Diptheroids

✓ Yersenia pseudotuberculosis

✓ Yersenia enterocolitica

Legionellosis

Weakly gram negative bacillus. ☞

Motile, non encapsulated☞

Pleomorhic rods requiring Cysteine and Iron. ☞

Aerosols from natural reservoirs are the most common source of infection

No man to man transmission occurs

No animal reservoir occurs

Disease is limited to humans

Lungs are primarily effected

Legionellosis is an infectious disease caused by bacteria belonging to the genus Legionella

Over 90% of legionellosis cases are caused by Legionella pneumophila, a ubiquitous aquatic organism that thrives in warm environments (25 to 45°C F)

⇨ **Legionellosis takes two distinct forms:**

Legionnaires' disease, also known as "Legion Fever" (archaic), is the more severe form of the infection and produces pneumonia. ☞☞☞

Pontiac fever is caused by the same bacterium, but produces a milder respiratory illness without pneumonia which resembles acute influenza. . ☞☞☞

The time between the patient's exposure to the bacterium and the onset of illness for Legionnaires' disease is 2 to 10 days;

For Pontiac fever, it is shorter, generally a few hours to 2 days.

Grown on BYCE medium (Bufferred Charcoal Yeast Extract)✱   PGI 1999

⇨ **Remember:**

► Meleney's gangrene: Anaerobic bacterial synergistic gangrene is characterized by exquisite pain, redness, and swelling followed by induration. These infections usually involve a combination of Peptostreptococcus spp. and S. aureus; the usual site of infection is an abdominal surgical wound or the area surrounding an ulcer on an extremity☞☞

► Necrotizing fasciitis, a rapidly spreading destructive disease of the fascia, is usually attributed to group A streptococci but can also be caused by anaerobic bacteria, including Peptostreptococcus and Bacteroides spp. Gas may be found in the tissues. ☞☞☞

MICROBIOLOGY

► **Fournier's gangrene** consists of cellulitis involving the scrotum, perineum, and anterior abdominal wall, with mixed anaerobic organisms spreading along deep external fascial planes and causing extensive loss of skin.

► **Neutropenic enterocolitis (typhlitis)** has been associated with **anaerobic infection of the cecum** but ¾ in the setting of **neutropenia** may involve the entire bowel. The primary pathogen is thought by some authorities to be **C. septicum**, but other clostridia and mixed anaerobic infections have also been implicated.

► **Brain abscesses** are frequently associated with anaerobic **bacteria** If optimal bacteriologic techniques are employed, as many as 85% of brain abscesses yield anaerobic **bacteria**¾most often **anaerobic gram-positive cocci (especially peptostreptococci)**, which are followed in frequency by **Fusobacterium and Bacteroides spp**

⊃ Enterococci

► Lancefield **group D** includes the **enterococci,**

► **Enterococci** are distinguished from **nonenterococcal group D streptococci** by their ability to grow in the presence of 6.5% sodium chloride

► Significant pathogens for humans are *E. faecalis* and *E. faecium.*

► These organisms tend to produce infection in patients who are elderly or debilitated or in whom mucosal or epithelial barriers have been disrupted or the balance of the normal flora altered by antibiotic treatment.

► **Urinary tract infections** due to **enterococci** are quite common, particularly among patients who have received antibiotic treatment or undergone instrumentation of the urinary tract.

► **Enterococci** are a frequent cause of **nosocomial bacteremia in patients with intravascular catheters.**

► These organisms account for 10 to 20% of cases of **bacterial endocarditis on both native and prosthetic valves.**

► **Enterococci** are **frequently cultured from** bile and are involved in infectious complications of biliary surgery and in liver abscesses.

► Moreover, **enterococci** are often isolated from **polymicrobial infections arising from the bowel flora (e.g., intraabdominal abscesses)**, from **abdominal surgical wounds**, and from **diabetic foot ulcers.**

⇨ Anaerobic infections:

Non sporing anaerobic bacteria are: **JIPMER 1983**

► Bacteroids fragilis

► Fusobacterium

► Peptostreptococcus

► Actinomyces israelli

⇨ **Microbiology of the colon:**

➡ The human colon is the site of more than 400 bacterial species.

➡ Unlike the stomach and proximal small bowel, both of which have a bacterial count generally considered no greater than 10^5 organisms, the colon has a bacterial concentration that approaches 10^{12} colony-forming units per ml.

➡ The organisms found in the colon vary widely, depending on the clinical situation, but, in general, include large numbers of both aerobic and anaerobic bacteria.

➡ Nearly one third of the fecal dry weight consists of bacteria.

➡ The predominant bacteria are anaerobic and include Bacteroides, Bifidobacterium, and Eubacterium.

⇨ **RICKETTSIAL DISEASES** ✳

- Ricketessia are <u>obligate intracellular</u> parasites.

- Ricketessia divide by <u>binary fission</u>.

- Ricketessial diseases are transmitted by bites of **arthropods**.

- Typical lesion is **vasculitis** and these organisms effect <u>endothelial lining</u> of vessel walls.

- Lab diagnosis is based on **serology** rather than isolation of organisms.

- **Rocky mountain spotted fever**: the most severe of the rickettsial diseases, is caused <u>by Rickettsia rickettsii.</u> ☞

- **Mediterranean spotted fever (boutonnuse fever)** and other spotted fevers: the etiologic agent of mediterranean spotted fever, **R. conorii,** ☞

- **Rickettsial pox** : caused by <u>R. akari.</u> ☞   DNB 2000

- <u>Endemic</u> murine typhus (flea-borne) caused by <u>R. typhi</u>☞

- <u>Epidemic typhus (louse-borne)</u>: due to infection with <u>R. prowazekii</u> is transmitted by the human body louse (pediculus humanus corporis), which lives on clothes and is found in poor hygienic conditions (especially in jails, where the disease it causes is called **jail fever**) and usually in cold areas☞

- **Brill-zinsser disease** is a recrudescent, mild form of epidemic typhus occurring years after the acute disease, probably as a result of immunosuppression or old age. ☞☞☞☞

- **Scrub typhus** caused by <u>R. tsutsugamushi.</u> ☞

- **Ehrlichioses:** ehrlichiae are small, obligately intracellular bacteria with a gram-negative-type cell wall that grow in cytoplasmic vacuoles to form clusters called morulae ☞☞☞

- Two distinct ehrlichia species cause human infections that can be severe and frequent☞☞☞☞

- **E. chaffeensis, the agent of Human monocytotropic ehrlichiosis** infects predominantly mononuclear phagocytic cells in tissues and blood monocytes. ☞☞

- A member of the e. phagocytophila group that infects cells of myeloid lineage is the agent of **Human granulocytotropic Ehrlichiosis.** ☞☞☞

- **Q fever:** results from infection with **C. burnetii.** ☞   COMED 2001

⇨ **Chlamydiae:**

► Are <u>obligate intracellular bacteria</u>	KERALA 1994
► Gram <u>negative</u>	AI 1989
► They possess both <u>DNA and RNA</u>	
► Have a cell wall and ribosomes	
► **Mc Coy and HeLa cells** used for detection	
► Multiply by **binary fission**	
► <u>Elementary body is metabolically inert.(extracellular)</u>	AI 2007
► <u>Reticulate body is active.(intracellular)</u>	
► IDENTIFIED BY Nucleic acid amplification test NAAT	AI 2010
► Inclusion body in conjunctivitis: <u>HP (Halberstaedter prowazeki bodies)</u>	
► Inclusion bodies in LGV : **Miyagawa bodies.**	
► Inclusion bodies in Psittacosis: **Levinthal Colles Lille bodies.**	AIIMS 1985

Pecularities:✳

- Meta chromatic staining: Corynebacterium ✎
- Lancet shaped diplococcic: Pneumococci ✎✎
- Bean shaped diplococcic: Nisseria ✎✎✎
- Bipolar staining: Yersenia ✎✎
- Gulls wing: Campylobacter ✎✎✎

⟳ **Clinical Scenarios: Most Likely Organism:**

► MC cause of lobar pneumoniae in elderly: ✎	Streptococcus pneumonia
► lobar pneumonia with deep red(**Currant jelly**) sputum ✎	Klibessela pneumonia
► Meningitis in **neonate**(Gram **positive** organism):	✓ Strep. Agalactaciae✎
► Meningitis in **neonate**(Gram **negative** organism): ✎	✓ E.coli
► Meningitis in **neonate**(Gram **positive** Rod): ✎✎	✓ Listeria monocytogenes
► Joint pains, skin petechiae , fever, in **young female:** ✎	✓ Gonococcal arthritis
► Patient on **clindamycin** complaining of **Diarrhoea**✎	✓ Clostridium difficile
► Abdominal pain, **bloody** Diarrhoea and **flask shaped ulcers:**	✓ Entameoba histolitica

⇨ **Important culture media:**

Thayer Martin media: ✎	Nisseria Gonorrhea
Choclate agar with Factor X and V: ✎	H. influenza
Bordet Gengou: ✎	Bordetella Pertussis
Lownstein Johnson: ✎	Mycobacterium Tuberculosis
Charcoal Yeast Agar: ✎	Legionella

⇨ **Eponyms:**

Eponyms	
Whitmoores bacillus: ✳	▶ Pseudomonas pseudomallei
Eaton agent: : ✳	▶ Mycoplasma
Johnes bacillus: : ✳✳	▶ Mycobacterium paratuberculosis
Batteys bacillus: ✳	▶ Mycobacterium intercellulare
Freidlanders bacillus✳	▶ Klibsella Pneumoniae
Koch weeks bacillus: ✳	▶ Haemophilus aegipticus
Nocard bacillus: ✳	▶ Cornye bacterium Pseudotuberculosis

⇨ **Tests for Organisms**

1. Ascolis thermoprecipitation test✳	Anthrax, Plague.
2. Xeno Diagnosis✳	Rickettasiae
3. Naegler's reaction (is due to Lecithinase) ✳	Clostrida
4. Green fluroscence on media with neutral red✳	Cl. Tetani
5. Cholera Red reaction indole formation and Nitrates to Nitrites✳	Cholera
6. Strauss reaction✳	Pseudomonas. Mallei
7. Neil Mooser reaction (Tunica reaction) ✳	Rickettsia. mooseri
8. Satellitism✳	H.Influenza
9.	
a) Chinese letter pattern ✳	✓ Diptheria
b) Eleks test ✳	✓ Diptheria
c) Schick test✳	✓ Diptheria
10. Dick test✳	Streptococci/pneumococci
11. Schultz- charlton reaction✳	Streptococci
12. M'Fadyean's reaction✳	B.Anthrax
13. Stormy reaction in Culture✳	Cl. Welchii
14. Milk Ring test (Rose Bengal Card test) ✳	Brucellosis

5

MICROBIOLOGY

15. Von- Pirquet test✱	Tuberculosis
16. Kochs' phenomenon✱	Tuberculosis
17. Francis test (Dick test) ✱	Pneumococci/streptococci
18. String Test✱	V.Cholerae

⇨ **Typical Appearances:** ✱

School of fish:	Haemophilus **ducreyi**←
Satellitism:	Haemophilus **influenza**←
Fried egg colony:	Mycoplasma←
Draughtsman colony:	Pneumococcus←
Swarming growth:	Proteus←
Oil paint appearance:	Staph←

⇨ **Different Motilities:** ✱

Darting motility:	Cholera←
Swarming motility:	Proteus←
Spinning motility:	Fusobacterium←
Tumbling motility:	Listeria←
Motility: *also in response to temperature. Motile at 25°c but non motile at temp erature above 37°c.*	
JK BOPEE 2012	

⇨ **Diagnosis of Urethritis and causative organism:**✱

Gram **negative diplococcic** in PMNs in urethral Exudate: ←← ·	Nisseria gonorrhea
Culture negative specimen with **inclusion bodies**: ←	Chlamydiae trachomatis
Organisms **without cell wall** and **urease positive**: ←←	Ureaplasma Urealyticum
Flagellate protozoa with motility : ←←	Trichomonas vaginalis

⇨ **Vaginal discharge:**✱

Yellow, pH>5, clue cells, amine odour←:	✓ Vaginosis
Cottage cheese discharge, pruritis, Vulvovaginitis:	✓ Candida←
Frothy, **Foamy** discharge and motile trophozites seen:	✓ Trichomonas vaginalis←

⇨ **Virology**

- **Viruses:** Smallest infectious agent containing only one kind of nucleic acid as their genome. ☞☞
- **Virion:** Extracellular infectious particle. ☞   AI 1990
- **Largest virus:** Pox Virus (300 nm). ☞
- **Smallest Virus:** Foot & Mouth Disease Virus (20 nm). ☞
- Capsid is a <u>protein coat</u> surrounding nucleic acids.
- Capsid+nucleic acid is Nucleocapsid.

⇨ **Features of virus:** ☞☞

- ▶ Ribosomes absent☞   AI 1994
- ▶ Mitochondria absent☞
- ▶ Motility absent☞
- ▶ <u>Nucleus absent</u> But Nucleic acid Either DNA or RNA Present. That is why some viruses are DNA Viruses and othes are RNA Viuses. (Common Sense) ☞

- ▶ **Virusoids** are **nucleic acids** that depend on **helper viruses** to package the nucleic acids into virus-like particles.
- ▶ **Viroids** are simply molecules of **naked, cyclical, mostly double-stranded, small RNAs** and appear to be restricted to plants, in which they spread from cell to cell and are replicated by cellular RNA polymerase II.
- ▶ **Prions** are protein molecules that can spread from cell to cell and effect changes in the structure of their normal counterparts (cellular proteins). Prions have been implicated in neurodegenerative conditions such as **Creutzfeldt-Jakob disease, Kuru, and Gerstmann-Straussler disease.** Prions have also been implicated in neurodegeneration associated with human infection with bovine spongiform encephalopathy ("**mad cow** disease").

⇨ **Classification of Viruses**

Nucleic Acid	Capsid Symmetry	Enveloped/Naked	Family	Type of Strand
DNA	Icosahedral	Naked	Parvoviridae	Positive strand
	Icosahedral	Naked	Papovaviridae	
	Icosahedral	Naked	Adenoviridae	
	Icosahedral	Enveloped	Herpes viridae	
	Complex	Complex	Pox	
		Coat	Hepadna	

cont...

5

cont...

	Icosahedral	Naked	**Picorna**	
	Icosahedral	Naked	**Calci**	
	Icosahedral	Naked	**Reo**	Positive strand
	Icosahedral	Enveloped	**Toga**	
	Unknown or Complex	Enveloped	**Flavi**	
		Enveloped	**Areana**	
	Unknown or Complex	Enveloped	**Corona**	
RNA		Enveloped	**Retro**	Positive strand
	Unknown or Complex			
	Unknown or Complex			
	Helical	Enveloped	**Buny**	
		Enveloped	**Orthomyxo**	
		Enveloped	**Paramyxo**	Negative strand
		Enveloped	**Rhabdo**	

▶ Virus with "smallest" genome: ☞	Parvo virus	KERALA 1994
▶ Virus with genome having **double stranded nucleic acid**: ☞	Pox virus, Reo virus	
▶ Virus with "Segmented" RNA : ☞	Influenza virus	AIIMS 1997
▶ Virus with "split" genome: ☞☞	Rota virus	

⇨ **Human slow virus infections**

Virus/agent	Disease
Measles ☞☞☞☞☞☞	▶ Subacute sclerosing panencephalitis.
Papovavarus (JC Virus) ☞☞☞☞☞	▶ Progressive multifocal leucoencephalopathy.
	▶ HIV encephalopathy.
Rubella ☞☞☞☞	▶ Progressive rubella panencephalitis.
Retrovirus ☞☞☞	▶ Acquired Immuno Defeciency syndrome.
Prion disease ☞☞	▶ Kuru
	▶ Creutzfeldt-Jakob disease

⇨ **Pox viruses causing human disease:**

▶ Smallpox	AIIMS 1992
▶ Molluscum contagiosum	AIIMS 1992
▶ Vaccina	
▶ Cow pox	
▶ Monkey pox	
▶ Buffalo pox	
▶ orf	

⇨ **Herpes Virus group includes:**

▶ HSV 1	
▶ HSV2	
▶ Varicella zoster virus	AI 1996
▶ EBV	AI 1995
▶ CMV	PGI 1985
▶ RK Virus	

⇨ **Herpes simplex virus:**

▶ Double stranded DNA virus	AI 1991
▶ Orofacial infection <u>mc</u> caused by HSV 1	
▶ Genital infection <u>mc</u> caused by HSV 2.	

Causes:

Gingivostomatitis

Herpetic whitlow

Corneal infection

Esophagitis

Genital herpes

Herpetic gladiatorum

Meningitis/ encephalitis (HSV 1). MC cause of <u>sporiadiac</u> viral encephalitis.　　　　AI 2010

- Herpes virus 1 causes "Herpes labialis" ☞☞
- Herpes virus 2 causes "Genital herpes". ☞

⇨ **Varicella zoster infection:**

► Caused by VZV,   AI 1999

► Reactivates and can involve eye

► Remains dormant in trigeminal ganglion   AI 2010

► Causes herpes zoster

► Post herpetic neuralgia

► Infectivity lasts 6 days after onset of rash.   AI 2002

⇨ **EBV**

► Belongs to herpes group.

► Binds through CD 21 receptor.

► Diseases caused by EBV:

✓ Oral hairy leukoplakia   AI 2006

✓ Chronic fatigue syndrome

✓ Burkitt's lymphoma   JK BOPEE 2012

✓ Anaplastic nasopharyngeal carcinoma   AIIMS 2004, KERALA 1997

✓ Tonsillar carcinoma,

✓ Angioimmunoblastic lymphadenopathy,

✓ Angiocentric nasal NK/T cell immunoproliferative lesions,

✓ T cell lymphoma,   AI 2004

✓ Thymoma,   PGI 2002

✓ Gastric carcinoma, and

✓ CNS lymphoma from patients with no underlying immunodeficiency.

✓ **Paul bunnel test** is done in infectious mononucleosis.   PGI 1986

⇨ **CMV:**

► MC congenital infections

► Petechiae, hepatospleenomegaly, jaundice are the mc presenting features of congenital CMV infection.

► Cause of <u>heterophile negative</u> mononucleosis. (Kindly remember). Diff from infectious mononucleosis.

► 50% of renal transplant patients with fever 1-4 months after transplant have CMV infection.   PGI 1997

⇨ **Adeno virus:**

► Non enveloped DNA virus.

► Mc manifestation is URTI in children.

► Mc manifestation is RDS in adults.

Causes:

► Diarrhoea   DNB 2011

► <u>Haemorragic</u> cystitis   JIPMER 1993

► <u>Epidemic</u> keratoconjuctivitis   KERALA 1994

⇨ **Picarnovirus:**

- ► Polio virus
- ► Cox sackie A
- ► Cox sackie B
- ► Echo virus
- ► Enterovirus   KERALA 2004
- ► Hepatitis A virus
- ► Rhino virus   PGI 1998

- ► Enterovirus 70 causes: Acute haemorrhagic conjunctivitis   AI 1997
- ► Enterovirus 70 causes: Acute epidemic kerato conjunctivitis   AI 1997
- ► Adeno virus causes: Epidemic keratoconjuctivitis
- ► Heres virus causes: Acute kerato conjuctivitis

⇨ **Commonest cause of meningitis:**

- ➡ Enteroviruses
- ➡ Arboviruses
- ➡ HIV
- ➡ HSV 2
- ➡ Acute encephalitis
- ➡ Arboviruses
- ➡ Enteroviruses
- ➡ HSV 1

⇨ **Coxsackie virus**

↻ **Herpangina** ↞↠
- It is most commonly seen in **infants and children**, though can occur in adults.
- The incubation period lies between 3 and 5 days and fecal infectivity may last for several weeks.
- Local examination of the mouth will usually reveal **hyperemia of the pharynx, and characteristic papulovesicular lesions**, approximately 1-2 mm in diameter and surrounded by an erythematous ring.
- Most commonly the lesions are present over the **tonsillar pillars, soft palate and uvula** though on occasion the tongue may be involved.

↻ **Aseptic meningitis** ↞↠
- is the **most common clinical manifestation** and may result from infection by several different Coxsackie A virus strains
- **Coxsackie virus A7** is the most frequently implicated but other strains such as A9 have also been involved.
- **Severe and fatal encephalitis** has been described in only a small number of cases of Coxsackie A virus infection.

↻ **Hand, foot and mouth disease (HFM)**

5

- Examination of the mouth often shows some **mild ulceration over the tongue and further examination indicates the pearly white vesicles**, sometimes surrounded by a red halo, on the extremities. ☛
- The lesions are mainly found over the ventral surface of the fingers and toes and have a characteristic distribution along the sides of the feet. Some cases also show a **maculopapular rash over the buttocks**.

Polio virus✹✹✹

- Polio virus belongs to **picarnoviradiae family** and has **icosahedral symmetry**.
- Polio virus is **ether "resistant"**.
- Polio virus is a **single stranded, positive sense, RNA Virus**.
- Most common type is **Type 1** Polio virus.
- Mc cause of epidemics: **type 1**
- Most difficult to eradicate: **type 1**
- Mc associated with paralysis: **type 1**
- Mc cause of **vaccine induced paralysis: type III**
- Most **antigenic strain is type 2**.
- Most common manifestation is **subclinical infection.**(90%)   PGI 1980

  Descending assymetrical paralysis is the predominant sign.

  Proximal muscles are more involved than distal

  No sensory loss

  No autonomic disturbance
- Inapparent infections mc feature.transmitted by feco oral route.   PGI 2001
- Spreads by **both haematogeneous and neural route**.   KERALA 2004
- Death in polio is mostly due to **respiratory paralysis**   ORISSA 2005

⇨ **Influenza virus**

Belongs to <u>orthomyxovirus</u> group.

<u>Enveloped</u> RNA virus.

Type A: Causes all pandemics and most <u>epidemics</u>

Type C: Causes <u>endemics</u>

Type B: Causes Reyes syndrome.(mc)   AIIMS 1993

Haemaglutinin and Neuraminidase is strain specific.   AI 1999

Antigenic variation seen as :   PGI 2004

Antigenic drift (minor change) seen. Small mutations in H and N.   MAHE 2007

Antigenic shift (major change) seen.

⊃ The Bird Flu Virus

▶ H5 N1 IS THE "AVIAN FLUE INFLUENZA VIRUS" ALSO CALLED AS "THE BIRD FLU VIRUS." ☞☞   AI 2008

▶ H5N1 **was** previously believed to cause outbreak in birds only. **(enzootic)** ☞

▶ H5N1 is a **highly pathogenic** virus. ☞☞

▶ Risk factor is handling of infected **poultry.** ☞☞

▶ **H** stands for **Haemaglutinin** and **N** in H5N1 Stands for **Neuraminidase.** ☞☞

▶ Virus can pass **vertically** from mother to fetus. ☞☞

⇨ "Swine flu"✳✳✳✳

Occurred in Mexico in may 2009 with threat of a pandemic spreading as far as Newzeland,Australia, Asia, UK etc

Caused by swine influenza virus **(SIV)** ☞☞

SIV **usually infects pigs.** ☞☞

Undercooked pork is a **common cause.** ☞

When infection spreads to humans, it is called **zoonotic flu.** ☞☞☞

Clinical features: chills, fever, sore throat, headache, coughing weakness. ☞☞

SIV subtype: **H1N1 CAUSED 2009 OUTBREAK.** ☞☞

This strain has **human to human transmission.** ☞☞☞

The U.S. Centers for Disease Control and Prevention recommends the use of **"Tamiflu"** (oseltamivir) or **(zanamivir)** for the treatment and/or prevention of infection with swine influenza viruses. ☞☞☞

However, the majority of people infected with the virus make a full recovery without requiring antiviral drugs. ☞☞☞

The virus isolates in the 2009 outbreak have been found **resistant to amantadine and rimantadine.** ☞☞

⇨ Measles:

Paramyxovirus.   PGI 1997

Causes rubeola (measles)

Infective period 4 days before and 5 days after appearance of rash

Kopiloks spots+maculopapular rash a feature

<u>Otitis media</u> is the mc complication.

Hechts pneumonia/ primary giant cell pneumonia is seen in measles.   PGI 1998

SSPE is a late complication.(RARE)   AI 1998

5

⇨ **Mumps:**

Paramyxovirus

Bilateral parotid enlargement seen.

<u>Orchitis</u> is the mc complication in post pubertal males.   AI 2000

Meningoencephalitis can precede parotitis.   AI 2006

One attack gives life long immunity.

Incubation period varies from 2-3 weeks.

Pain and swelling of parotids (ear ache) is a feature.

Orchitis, ovaritis, pancreatitis, meningoencephalitis, throditis, neuritis, hepatitis, myocarditis are a feature.

Mumps is leading cause of parotitis in children

Control of mumps is difficult because disease is infectious before a diagnosis is made.

⇨ **Rubella:**

Toga virus

No carrier state.

Cervical lymphadenopathy + Forschemeirs spots seen.

Congenital rubella causes: cataract+deafness+heart diseases.   TN 1990

⇨ **Arboviruses:**

Chikungunya:	• alpha virus	
Japenese encephalitis	• flavi virus	
West nile	• flavi virus	
Yellow fever	• flavi virus	
Dengue	• flavi virus	PGI 2006
Kyanasaur forest disease	• flavi virus	
Sandfly fever	• bunya virus	
Rift valley fever	• bunya virus	
Hanta virus	• bunyaviridae	

⇨ **Hanta virus:**

Is a RNA virus

Belongs to arbovirus

causes haemorragic fever with nephritis

Causes hanta virus pulmonary syndrome   PGI 2002

⇨ **Rabies Virus:**

Rabies virus has Negative polarity☞
Rhabdoviridae
Bullet shaped, Neurotropic,
Enveloped virus with ss RNA. ☞☞   AI 2003
It is Lyssavirus serotype 1☞
Inactivated by Phenol, UV radiation, Beta propiono lactone ☞☞   PGI 1997

- **Negri bodies***** are present inside **nerve cells**. Most characteristic finding in CNS is the formation of **cytoplasmic inclusionbodies** called Negri Bodies (composed of **fibrillary matrix and rabies virus particles**) within neurons of Ammons horn, Cerebral cortex, Brain stem, Hypothalamus, Cerebellum and Dorsal spinal ganglia.   AI 2007
- Since first described by Negri in 1903, the Negri body has been regarded as a **pathognomonic**
- **Finding signifying the presence of rabies encephalitis.** Negri bodies (light microscope) were found in the brain of a patient with conclusive evidence in favour of the presence of rabies encephalitis.

Brain stem encephalitis is a feature.   AI 1997

Flourscent stains are used for ante mortem diagnosis.   KAR 1995

⇨ **Hepatitis A virus**

- ▶ is a **nonenveloped** 27-nm, heat-, acid-, and
- ▶ ether-resistant RNA virus
- ▶ in the hepatovirus genus of the **picornavirus** family,
- ▶ Previously called **enterovirus 72**   DNB 1989
- ▶ No chronic course.   KERALA 1999
- ▶ Inactivated by boiling, formalin, uv radiation.   AIIMS 1991

⇨ **Hepatitis B virus**

- ▶ is a <u>DNA</u> virus,
- ▶ Hepadenavirus Contains DNA dependent DNA polymerase and RNA dependent reverse transcriptase.
- ▶ Reverse transcriptase is coded by <u>P gene</u>.   AI 2000
- ▶ <u>Dane particle</u> is HBV.   PGI 1987
- ▶ HBV strain in india is <u>Ayw, Adr</u>   Manipal 2006
- ▶ HBV has <u>maximum perinatal transmission risk</u>.   AI 2003
- ▶ **Oncogenicity present** in Hepatitis B especially after neonatal infection.
- ▶ **Carrier state** present in Hepatitis B
- ▶ Hepatitis B virus may present in blood and other body fluids and excretions such as saliva, breast milk, semen, vaginal secretions, urine, bile etc.
- ▶ Feces not known to be infectious

▶ **HBs Ag** is the **first viral marker to appear in blood** after infection; it remains in circulation throughout icteric course of disease. In a typical case it disappear within roughly 2 months but may last for 6 months.

▶ HBcAg is not demonstrable in circulation but antibody, antiHBe appear in serum a week or two after appearance of HbSAg. **JK BOPEE 2011**

▶ **Anti-HbeAg** is the **antibody marker** to be seen in blood.

▶ Serological marker of acute hep B is: HBsAg + core antibody. **AI 1993**

▶ Epidemological marker of Hep B is: core antibody **AI 1997**

▶ HBeAg (HB envelop antigen) appears in blood concurrently with HBsAg.

▶ **HbeAg** is an indicator of intrahepatic viral replication and its presence in blood Indicates
high infectivity. **UPSC 2007**

▶ For diagnosis of HBV infection, simultaneous presence of IgM, HBC indicates **recent infection**

▶ Presence of **IgG; anti H-Be** indicates **remote** infection.

▶ Hep B vaccine is **cell fraction derived.** **AP 1997**

▶ **Hepatitis C virus,**

which, before its identification was labeled "**non-A, non-B hepatitis,**"

is a linear, single-stranded, **positive-sense, RNA virus**; (Enveloped) **PGI 2005**

HCV belongs to family **Flaviviridae.** **AIIMS 2004**

Mc cause of <u>post transfusion hepatitis</u> **AIIMS 1998**

Causes chronic hepatitis. **JIPMER 1999**

▶ **Hepatitis D**

The **delta hepatitis** agent, or HDV, is a **defective RNA virus**

Coinfects with and requires the helper function of HBV (or other hepadnaviruses) for its replication and expression.

Resembles plant viruses

▶ **Hepatitis E**

Previously labeled "**epidemic or enterically transmitted non-A, non-B hepatitis**",

HEV is an enterically transmitted virus. **AI 1993**

Is a **Calci virus.**

— **Mortality in pregnancy is a feature of Hep E virus.** **AIIMS 1998**

— **Hepatic encephalopathy in pregnancy is seen.** **AI 2001**

— **Fulminant hepatic failure can occur with Hep C in pregnancy.** **AI 2004**

► **Hepatitis G**

  Also called GB virus

  R NA virus.

  Blood borne virus

  Resembles Hep C virus.

  Lamuvudine responsive

Spreads by <u>faeco oral</u> route - **hepatitis A and E**   AIIMS 2003

Spreads by <u>percutaneous</u> route - **Hepatitis B,C and D**

► ☞HTLV I cause adult T cell Leukemia/ Lymphoma and Tropical spastic paraplegia. *Other putative HTLV-I-related diseases In areas where <u>HTLV</u>-I is endemic, diverse inflammatory and autoimmune diseases have been attributed to the virus, including uveitis, dermatitis, pneumonitis, rheumatoid arthritis, and polymyositis*

► ☞HTLV II causes **Hairy cell leukemia**

► ☞HTLV III causes **AIDS**

HIV virus ✳✳✳

Important points in <u>HIV Pathology</u>

Never forget the below mentioned paragraph:

  ➡ AIDS is caused by **HIV,**

  ➡ **A human retrovirus belonging to the lentivirus family**

  ➡ **HIV-1 is the more common type** associated with AIDS in the United States, Europe, and Central Africa, whereas HIV-2 causes a similar disease principally in West Africa.

  ➡ The viral particle is covered by a lipid bilayer derived from the host cell and studded with **viral glycoproteins gp41 and gp120.**

  ➡ Like most retroviruses, **the HIV-1 virion is spherical** and contains an electron-dense, cone-shaped core surrounded by a lipid envelope derived from the host cell membrane

  ➡ The virus core contains:

  ❑ <u>major capsid protein p24,</u>

  ❑ <u>nucleocapsid protein p7/p9,</u>

  ❑ <u>two copies of genomic RNA, and</u>

  ❑ <u>three viral enzymes (protease, reverse transcriptase, and integrase).</u>

5

MICROBIOLOGY

➧ *p24 is the most readily detected viral antigen and is therefore the target for the antibodies used to diagnose HIV infection in blood screening.*

➧ *The viral core is surrounded by a **matrix protein called p17**, lying beneath the virion envelope.*

➧ *The viral envelope itself is studded by two **viral glycoproteins (gp120 and gp41)**, critical for HIV infection of cells.*

➧ *The HIV-1 proviral genome contains the **gag, pol, and env genes**, which code for various viral proteins.*

➧ *In addition to these three standard retroviral genes, HIV contains several other genes (given three-letter names such as **tat, rev, vif, nef, vpr, and vpu**) that regulate the synthesis and assembly of infectious viral particles.*

➧ **The product of the tat (transactivator) gene**, for example, is critical for virus replication.

➧ **The nef protein** activates intracellular kinase activity (affecting T-cell activation, viral replication, and viral infectivity) and reduces surface expression of CD4 and MHC molecules on infected cells.

➧ **The two major targets of HIV infection** are the **immune system and the CNS**. The life cycle of the virus is best understood in terms of its interactions with the immune system.

➧ The entry of HIV into cells **requires the CD4 molecule**, which acts as a high-affinity receptor for the virus This explains the tropism of the virus for CD4+ T cells and its ability to infect other CD4+ cells, particularly macrophages and DCs.

➧ However, binding to CD4 is not sufficient for infection; the HIV envelope gp120 must also bind to **other cell surface molecules (coreceptors) to facilitate cell entry. Two cell surface chemokine receptors, CCR5 and CXCR4, serve this role.**

MAH 2012, AIIMS 2011 & AIP 2011

▶ **Positive sense, single stranded , RNA virus**   AI 02

▶ <u>Retro</u>virus.

▶ Diploid

▶ Attacks **T helper cells and macrophages.**

▶ **Non segmented**

▶ Found in semen , saliva and blood   (AMU 1999)

▶ Contains **two copies of ss (+) RNA, RNA dependent DNA Polymerase (Reverse Transcriptase), integrase and protease**
                      AI 2002

▶ **Subtype A** is most prevalent world wide.

▶ **Subtype C** is most prevalent in india.

▶ Seroconversion takes 4 weeks   JIPMER 1993

▶ <u>Heterosexual mode</u> is the mc mode of transmission of HIV.   SGPGI 2004

▶ <u>Male -female</u> transmission>female-male.   PGI 2000

▶ Accidental needle prick for health worker is 1%.   PGI 1999

▶ <u>RNA-DNA-RNA</u> is the retroviral sequence in host cell.   AI 2002

▶ p 24 is used for early diagnosis.

▶ p 24 antigen disappears 6-8 weeks after HIV infection.   AMU 2005

▶ CD 4 cells are attacked.

▶ CD4: CD 8 ratio is reversed.   AI 2002

▶ Macrophages serve as <u>reservoir</u> of infection.   AI 2002

▶ Window period of AIDS: infection to appearance of antibodies in serum.   JIPMER 2004

▶ Both ELISA and western blot are <u>negative</u> in window period.   NIMHANS 1996

✓ **Cryptosporiodosis** is the mc cause of Diarrhoea in AIDS.   UP 2007

✓ Oral ulcer in AIDS is commonly due to **candida.**   ORISSA 2005

✓ MC cause of acute meningitis in AIDS: **Cryptococcus.**   AI 2005

✓ MC cause of tuberculosis in AIDS in tropical countries: **Myc. Tuberculosis**   PGI 2000

✓ Mc Cause of seizures in AIDS: **Toxoplasmosis.**

✓ Multi focal tumor of vascular origin in AIDS is: **Kaposis sarcoma.**

✓ MC opportunistic infection in AIDS in india is: **Tuberculosis**   ORISSA 2004

⇨ **Structural genes of HIV Virus❋❋**.

Gag	(DELHI 96)	▪ Antigens	▶ Proteins
		▪ p 24	▶ Capsid protein
		▪ p 7p9	▶ Core nucleocapsid protein
		▪ p17	▶ Matrix protein
Pol		▪ Reverse transcriptase	▶ Produces ds DNA pro virus
		▪ Integrase	▶ Produces ds DNA integration into host DNA
		▪ Protease	▶ cleaves poly protein
Envelop		▪ gp 120	▶ <u>Surface protein</u> that binds to CD4 on host cell
		▪ gp 41	▶ Transmembrane protein for cell fusion

⇨ **Regulatory genes of HIV virus:**

Tat:	Transactivator protein : activator of transcription
Rev:	Regulator Protein: regulator of transport of RNA to cytoplasm.
Nef:	Negative factor: Decrease MHC on infected T cells.

5

MICROBIOLOGY

⇨ **Negative sense RNA Viruses:**

Para influenza virus	*Croup, common cold, bronchitis*	
Mumps	*Parotitis, pancreatitis, orchitis, memingoencephalitis*	
Measles	*Rubeola*	
	Cough, coryza, conjunctivitis, <u>kopliks spots</u>	
	<u>*Warthin Finkdley cells*</u>	
	SSPE	
RSV	*Bronchiolitis and pneumonia in infants*	PGI 2000
Rabies virus	*Bites of rabid dogs*	
	Negri Bodies	
	Bullet shaped from Rhabdo viridae	
Marburg virus	*Acute Haemmorrhagic fever*	
Ebola Virus	*Acute Haemorrhagic fever*	
Influenza virus	*Segmented*	
	Enveloped nucleocapsid	
	Shows minor variation: antigenic drift	
	Major variation: antigenic shift	
	Shows Von Magnus phenomenon (on serial passing progeny with high haemagluttination titre but low infectivity.	
	Gullian barre and Ryes Syndrome associations	
Lassa Fever virus	▶ Haemorrhagic fever in Africa	

⇨ **Double stranded RNA viruses** ✳

Reo virus	URTI	
Rota virus	Mc cause of infantile Diarrhoea	
	Non cultiviable virus	KERALA 2004
	Detected by antigen in stools	KERALA 2004

⇨ **Rota virus:**

<u>Reoviridae</u> family	
<u>Double stranded RNA</u> virus.	
<u>Group A</u> mc causative agent.	
Does not grow in cell cultures (non cultiviable)	KERALA 2004
Mc cause of Diarrhoea in infants.	AIIMS 1997
Causes <u>destruction of mature enterocyte</u>s.	
Detected by <u>antigen in stools</u>.	KERALA 2004

⇨ **Extra points: Rotavirus**

- Nonenveloped double stranded RNAsegmented
- Double walled, wheel like appearance in electron microscope
- MC cause of diarrheal disease in infants and children <5 yrs
- By Major destruction of mature enterocytes in villous epithelium of Small intestine
- Enterotoxin has Action on enteric nervous system
- Rotavirus undergoes extensive reassortment, both in vivo and in vitro.
- Diagnosis is by Electron microscope, ELISA of faecal sample—Ag detection
- Human rotavirus does not grow readily in cell culture (Only some strains of group A grow)
- Vaccine – Best is genetic reassortment due to segmented genome

⇨ **Diarrhoeas are a feature of:**

Rota virus
Adenovirus
Calcivirus
Entero virus

⇨ **Haemorrhagic fever:**

• African haemorrhagic fever:	▶ Marburg/ ebola virus
• Haemorrhagic fever with renal syndrome:	▶ Hanta virus
• Dengue haemorrhagic fever:	▶ Flavi virus.

⇨ **Oncogenic Viruses**

Virus	Disease
Pox disease	Molluscum contagiosum
Hepatitis B and C	Liver Cancer
EBV COMED 2006	Burkitt's lymphoma (in malaria infested parts of Africa), and other lymphomas in immunosuppression; nasopharangeal carcinomas
Human papilloma virus MP1998	Warts, genital warts, cervical, vulval, penile, anal and perianal carcinoma
HTLV-1	Adult T-cell Leukemia (RNA virus) COMED 2006
HHV 8	Kaposi's sarcoma
Adenovirus, SV40	Malignant neoplasms in mice
Polyomavirus hominis 1 and 2	Are found in the urine of some transplant recipients. COMED 2008

⇨ **Human Pappiloma Virus:**

Deep plantar/palmar warts : ☞ HPV 1

Common warts/Verruca Vulgaris: ☞ HPV 2

Plane warts: ☞ HPV 3

Laryngeal Papillomas: ☞ HPV 6,11,30

Anogenital warts (Condyloma accuminata): ☞ HPV 6,11

Butchers warts: ☞ HPV 7

"Koilocytes" are a feature of HPV infections. ☞

"High oncogenic potential" is with: HPV 16, 18,31,33☞   JIPMER 1998

"Low oncogenic potential" is with: HPV 6,11,42,43☞

⇨ **Viruses and CNS ✳✳**

Acute viral meningitis is most commonly due to enterovirus. ☞☞☞

Fungal meningitis is mostly due to Candida, Aspergillus, Mucor and Cryptococcus. ☞☞

Viral Encephalitis shows:

Perivascular cuffs☞

Microglial nodules☞

Neuronophagia☞

HSV1 particularly effects Temporal lobes, causes haemorrhagic necrosis of temporal lobes) ☞☞

Aspergillus and Mucor causes vasculitis with haemorrhage. ☞

Cryptococcus invades brain via Virchow Robins spaces with soap bubble lesions. ☞☞

Toxoplasmosis presents with ring enhancing lesions. ☞

Kaposi's sarcoma

- Kaposi's sarcoma is common in **homosexuals.**
- KS arises from **cells linning lymph vessels or blood vessels.**
- KS is associated with **HIV, immunosuppression, organ transplants.**
- On skin Kaposis lesions are red/purple blotches which are asymptomatic or tender.
- GIT, liver, lung lesions can prove dangerous.
- Treatment of HIV with HAART reduces KS as well.
- Associated with **HHV 8 virus.**
- Common sites: Skin, GIT, Lymph nodes, Lungs.
- **Classic KS** as originally described was a relatively indolent disease affecting elderly men from the Mediterranean region, or of Eastern European descent.
- **Endemic KS** was described later in young African people, mainly from sub-Saharan Africa, as a more aggressive disease which infiltrated the skin extensively, especially on the lower limbs. This, it should be noted, is unrelated to HIV infection.
- **Transplant Related KS** had been described, but only rarely until the advent of calcineurin inhibitors (such as ciclosporin, which are inhibitors of T-cell function) for transplant patients.

⇨ **Erythema infectiosum (fifth disease, slapped cheek disease)**

Erythema infectiosum is caused by <u>parvovirus B19 (human parvovirus),</u> a small, **single-stranded DNA virus.**

In children the first sign of infection is usually **marked erythema of the cheeks or slapped cheek appearance often with relative circumoral pallor.**

Then 1-4 days after the slapped cheeks an itchy, erythematous, maculopapular rash develops on the trunk and limbs.

As the rash on the limbs clears it leaves a **lacy, reticular pattern.** The rash may fluctuate over the next 1-3 weeks and a hot bath, for example, may lead to recrudescence of an evanescent rash.

Complications

Arthritis or arthralgia is more common in adults, but certainly can occur in children. It usually appears 1-6 days after the rash but there may be no history of rash at all.

Arthritis is characteristically transient and asymmetrical, affecting wrists, knees, ankles, elbows and fingers, though it may persist for weeks or even months.

Children with sickle cell anemia, thalassemia major, hereditary spherocytosis or other hemolytic anemias, may have **severe aplastic crises** with hemoglobin levels falling as low as 1-2 g/dl and no reticulocytes.

Infection during pregnancy can result in hydrops fetalis due to fetal anemia, which may be fatal, but no congenital syndrome has been described in babies of infected mothers who delivered at term.

The diagnosis can be made serologically by **demonstrating parvovirus B19-specific IgM** on an acute serum sampleTreatment

5

Arthritis may require salicylates or non-steroidal anti-inflammatory agents.

Children with aplastic crises may require **blood transfusion** until the red cell aplasia resolves spontaneously after 1-2 weeks.

Herpesvirus 6 (HHV-6) is the main causative agent for Roseola infantum a common disease of infancy, characterized by fever and the appearance of an **erythematous maculopapular rash** as the fever defervesces. It is generally benign. ☞☞

⇨ **Viral hemorrhagic fever:**

Lassa fever

Rift valley fever

Hf with renal syndrome

Hantavirus pulmonary syndrome

Yellow fever

Dengue hemorrhagic fever/dengue shock syndrome

⇨ **Slow viruses diseases:**

► Group A	
Maedi,	
Visna	

► **Group B**

Prion diseases

- Caused By prion Protein ☞☞
- Prions are proteins. — AIIMS 2007
- They are infectious. — AI 2008
- Most common infectious prion disease in humans: CJD. — MAH 2002
- Kuru
- Gerstmann Straussler disease — MAH 2002
- Fatal familial insomnia — UPSC 2001

► **Group C**
- SSPE
- PML

SSPE

*Subacute sclerosing panencephalitis (SSPE), a rare degenerative central nervous system (CNS) disease characterized by behavioral and intellectual deterioration and convulsions, is a result of a persistent **measles** **virus** infection that develops years after the original infection*

PML

*JC virus, a human papilloma virus the etiologic agent of **progressive multifocal leukoencephalopathy (PML)**, is an important opportunistic pathogen in patients with AIDS*

⇨ **Remember**

Nagleria	Primary ameobic meningoencephalitis
Acanthameoba	Keratitis
	Granulomatous amebic encephalitis JK BOPEE 2012
Entameoba histolytica	Ameobiasis with flask shaped ulcers
Giardia lamblia	Giardiasis (malabsorption)
	Habitat: duodenum, jejunem
	Falling leaf motility,
	Tennis racket shape
	Trophozites and cysts seen in man.
	Associated with Common variable immunodeficiency
	May cause travelers Diarrhoea.
Cryptosporidium	Diarrhoea in immunocompromised
Trichomonas vaginalis	Trichomoniasis (frothy vaginal discharge)
Balantidium coli	Dysentery

⇨ **Malaria:**

Plasmodium vivax	Benign tertain malariae
Plasmodium ovale	Benign tertain malariae
Plasmodium malarie	Quartan malaria
Plasmodium falciparum	Malignant malaria

⇨ **Malarial Parasites:**

Species Identification
Mauriers clefts: P. falciparium
Schuffners dots: P. vivax
Zeimmans dots: P. malariae
James dots: P. ovale

Urban Malaria is caused by Anopholes Culcifacies	
Type of malaria **not** seen in India is ovale.	
Size of RBC is increased in vivax malaria	AI 1996
The infective agent of malaria is **sporozite**.	PGI 1990
Gametocytes are seen in PBFof falciparum malaria.	PGI 2005
Shizont is not seen in PBF.	PGI 1999

Relapse of malaria is seen in P. ovale and P. malariae

⇨ **Important features of P. falciparum**

Spleenic rupture is commonest with P. falciparum	AIIMS 1978
Parasitemia is highest with P. falciparum	JIPMER 1981
Most virulent form. P.falciparum.	JK 2005
Exoerythrocytic stage is absent in P. falciparum	PGI 1996
Multiple infection of RBC'S is seen in P. falciparum	KAR 2005
Most Virulent plasmodium species is P. falciparum	AI 1997

⇨ **KALA-AZAR:**

▪ L.donovani	▶ Visceral Lieshmaniasis
▪ L.tropica	▶ Cutaneous Lieshmaniasis
▪ L.major	▶ Cutaneous Lieshmaniasis
▪ L.braziliens	▶ Mucocutaneous Lieshmaniasis

▶ Spleenomegaly is a feature.	
▶ NNN (Novy, mc Neal, Nicolle) medium used.	PGI 2002
▶ Aldehyde test + in 12 weeks	DNB 1991

KALA-AZAR

(Visceral Leishmaniasis; Dumdum Fever)☛☛

Kala-azar occurs in **India, China, southern USSR, Africa, the Mediterranean basin**, and several South and Central American countries.

Children and young adults are particularly susceptible.

The protozoa (L. donovani) invade the bloodstream and localize in the **reticuloendothelial system**, causing fever, pronounced **hepatosplenomegaly, emaciation, and pancytopenia.**

The fever is seldom sustained and recurs irregularly.

Hypergammaglobulinemia is present. ☛☛ TN 1990

The parasite may be found in needle biopsy of the liver, spleen, bone marrow, skin lesions, or lymph nodes or in cultures from these tissues or from blood.

Pentavalent antimony compounds and pentamidine are the drugs of choice. ☞☞

Sodium stibogluconate (sodium antimony gluconate) is given once daily, slowly IV or IM in distilled water. ☞☞

Trypanosoma cruzi	✓ Chagas disease (American Trypanosomiasis,)
	✓ Vector: reduvid bug
	✓ Romana sign +(Swelling around eyelids)
	✓ Megacolon, Megaesophagus, Cardiomyopathy are complications
	✓ Nifurtimox used in treatment
Trypanosoma brucei	✓ Sleeping sickness (African Trypanosomiasis)
	✓ Tse tse fly transmits it.
	✓ Posterior cervical lymphadenopathy (Winter Bottom sign seen) ,
	✓ Suramin and Melarsoprol used in treatment
Babesia microti	✓ Babeiosis
	✓ Seen in immunocompromised/ splenectomized patients.
	✓ Resides in RBC
Toxoplasma gondii	✓ Toxoplasmosis
	✓ Cat: definitive host JK BOPEE 2012
	✓ Oocyst found in cat
	✓ Intracerebral calcifications, chorioretinitis, microcephaly.
	✓ Sabin Feld man test +
	✓ Pyremethamine + sulfadiazine used in treatment
	✓ Frenkels test+

▪ Onchocerca volvolus	River blindness MAH 2012
	▶ Onchocerciasis, most commonly causing skin and eye disease, results from infection with the filarial parasite Onchocerca volvulus.
	▶ Transmission is via the bites of black files (Simulium species) that ingest microfilariae from the skin of an infected person while taking a blood meal. AIMS 2010
	▶ Endemicity of O. volvulus in human populations is dependent upon habitation of fly-infested areas by sufficient numbers of people who are exposed to human-biting flies during daily activities such as farming, fishing, bathing, washing and water collection. Because the flies depend on waterways for egg-laying and reproduction, they concentrate around streams and rivers. hence the term river blindness.
	▶ The disease affects primarily the skin, lymph nodes, and ocular tissues. In the eye, neovascularization and scarring of the cornea lead to loss of transparency and blindness.
	▶ The diagnosis can be made clinically by the presence of onchocercomata,

▪	▶ typical skin changes, or eye findings of onchocerciasis, especially microfilariae visualized by slit-lamp examination of the cornea or anterior chamber in otherwise normal-appearing eyes. Diagnosis is most frequently made by finding microfilariae of O. volvulus in the patient's skin. "Skin snips" are taken ▶ Ivermectin is the drug of choice to treat onchocerciasis. DNB 2011
▪ Wucheria bancrofti	Lymphadenitis Elephantiasis

Genus	Disease produced	
● Taenia solium	▶ Cysticercosis and enteritis	JK BOPEE 2012
● Taenia saginata	▶ Enteritis	
● Entrobius Vermicularis	▶ Pruritis ani	
● Ascaris lumbricoides	▶ Enteritis, cholangitis	

Ent.histolytica	▶ Amoebiasis
Nagleria and Acanthameoba	▶ Meningitis
Cryptosporidium Parvum	▶ Cryptosporidiosis
Giardia lamblia	▶ Giardiasis
Toxoplasma gondi	▶ Intrauterine infection

⇨ **Common Names:**

Fish Tapeworm: Diphyllobotherium latum
Beef Tapeworm: Taenia saginata
PorkTapeworm: Taenia solium
Dwarf Tapeworm: H. nana
Rat Tapeworm: H. diminuta
Dog Tapeworm: Echinococcus granulosus

⇨ **Diphylobothrium latum: Fish tapeworm**

- Lives in small intestine
- Longest intestinal parasite of man
- **Bile stained operrculated eggs (not infective to man)**   KCET 2012
- Humans are **definitive hosts**
- Infective stage for man is pleurocercoid larva from fish
- Inhibits dietary absorption of **Vitamin B12, so can cause megaloblastic anemia.**

Clonorchis sinesis	Chinese liver fluke
Fasciola hepatica	Sheep liver fluke
Fasciola buski	Giant intestinal fluke
Paragonimus westermanii	Lung fluke
Echinococcus granulosus	Hydatid cyst disease
Echinococchus multilocularis	Alveolar hydatid

Parasites causing Autoinfection:
(AIIMS 2009)

- ✓ Taenia solium
- ✓ Strongyloides stercolis
- ✓ Hymenolepsis nana
- ✓ Enterobius vermicularis
- ✓ Cryptosporidium parvum
- ✓ Capillaria philippinesis

Parasites causing malabsorption in adults:

- ➟ Giardia lamblia
- ➟ E.histolytica
- ➟ H. Nana
- ➟ Strongyloides
- ➟ Cycospora

Parasites associated with malabsorption in children:

- ➟ Giardia lamblia
- ➟ Isospora belli
- ➟ Cryptosporidium
- ➟ Ancyclostoma duodenale
- ➟ H. Nana
- ➟ Entamoeba histolytica

Nematode infections:

of medical importance may be broadly classified into those in which the route of infection, larval migration, and disease manifestations are primarily gastrointestinal and those that affect other tissues. Nematode infections include hookworm disease, ascariasis, enterobiasis, and trichuriasis. They are prevalent in temperate and tropical areas of the world, especially those with **overcrowding and poor sanitation.** DNB 2011

The former group includes hookworm

- ▪ (Ancylostoma duodenale, Necator americanus), (small intestine) PGI 2011
- ▪ The roundworm Ascaris lumbricoides, (small intestine) PGI 2011, JK BOPEE 2012
- ▪ The pinworm Enterobius vermicularis, and
- ▪ The whipworm Trichuris trichiuria.

Trichinella spiralis, Strongyloides stercoralis, and Angiostrongylus cantonensis infect humans by the oral route, but disease manifestations are due primarily to migration in other tissues.

Tissue-invasive nematodes include

- Lymphatic filariae (Wuchereria bancrofti, Brugia malayi, and B. timori),

- Skin-dwelling Onchocerca volvulus and Loa loa, and

- The guinea worm, Dracunculus medinensis.

▶ Loa Loa causes **Calabar swellings**	UP 2007
▶ Wucheria bancrofti causes **Lymphatic Filariasis.**	
▶ Strongyloides stercolis **Larva currens**	TN 1998
▶ Toxo caria canis causes **Visceral Larva migrans**	AI 1988
▶ Strongyloides stercolis causes **Cutaneous larva migrans.**	TN 1987

⇨ **Filariasis:**

• **Wucheria bancrofti** causes Filariasis.	AIIMS 1997
• Habitat is **lymph vessels and lymph nodes.**	AIIMS 1997
• **Man** is the definitive host.	
• Innoculation is through **bite of mosquito.**	
• Infective form is **third stage larvae.**	
• Notice the difference in classic Filariasis and occult Filariasis	

Classic Filariasis	Occult Filariasis (Meyer Kouwenaar syndrome)
▪ Caused by **adult worms**	▪ Caused by **microfilariae**
▪ **Epitheloid** granuloma is basic lesion	▪ **Eosinophilic** granuloma is basic lesion
▪ Lymphatic system involved	▪ Lymphatic system ▪ Liver ▪ Lungs involved
▪ Microfilaria present in **blood**	▪ Microfilaria in **tissues**
▪ Complement Fixation test **insensitive**	▪ CFT **Sensitive**

⇨ **TINEA SOLIUM:**

Cysticercosis in muscles➴➴

JK BOPEE 2012

Cysticerci can develop in any voluntary muscle in humans. Invasion of muscle by cysticerci can cause <u>myositis</u>, with **fever**, <u>eosinophilia</u>, and **muscular pseudohypertrophy**, which initiate with muscle swelling and later progress to **atrophy and fibrosis**. In most cases, it is asymptomatic since the cysticerci die and become calcified.

Neurocysticercosis➴➴

Neurocysticercosis presents in many forms, depending on the localization of the cysts and disease activity. 60% of the patients with cysticerci are found to have them in the brain. These cysts increase and slowly leak their antigen into the subarachnoid CSF producing meningitis and can further develop into **arachnoiditis,** which may lead to **obstructive hydrocephalus, cranial nerve involvement, intracranial hypertension, arterial thrombosis and stroke**. In intraventricular cysticercosis, the cysts occur in the lateral, third or fourth ventricles which may be asymptomatic or if they block the flow of CSF, they may cause increased intracranial pressure.

Ophthalmic Cysticercosis➴➴

In some cases, cysticerci may be found in the **globe, subconjunctiva, and extraocular muscles**. Depending on the location, they may cause visual difficulties that fluctuate with eye position, retinal edema, hemorrhage, a decreased vision or even a visual loss.

Subcutaneous Cysticercosis➴➴

Subcutaneous cysts are in the form of firm, mobile nodules, occurring mainly on the trunk and extremities. Subcutaneous nodules are sometimes painful.

⇨ **Echinococciosis:**

Is also known as **hydatid disease. (Echinococcus granulosus)**　　PGI 2001
Hydatid cyst is a **parasitic infection** of humans by the tapeworm of genus echinococcus.
It is a **zoonosis.**

1. **Echinococcus <u>granulosus</u>** causes **Cystic Echinococcuosis**
2. **Echinococcus <u>multilocularis</u>** causing **Alveolar Echinococcuosis**
3. **Echinococcus <u>vogeli</u>** causes **Polycystic disease**

Echinococcus granulosus:

The **liver is the most common organ effected** followed by lungs, muscles, bones and kidneys.

Passage of hydatid membrane in emesis is called **hydatid emesia.**

Passage of hydatid membrane in stools is called **hydatid enterica.**

▶ Echinococciosis is caused by **larval stages of parasite.**
▶ Man is an **accidential intermediate host**. Other intermediate hosts are sheep and cattle.

5

▶ The **dog** is the **definitive host.** (D-D)   **KAR 1994**

▶ **Serological assay** (<u>Weinberg reaction</u>) is specific example of Complement fixation test used in detection.

▶ ELISA is also sensitive.

▶ **ARA C 5** is used in diagnosis.   **JIPMER 1993**

⇨ **Entamoeba Histolytica:**

Amebiasis is an infection with the intestinal protozoan Entamoeba histolytica.

About 90% of infections are asymptomatic, and the remaining 10% produce a spectrum of clinical syndromes ranging from dysentery to abscesses of the liver or other organs.

E. histolytica is **acquired by ingestion of viable cysts** from fecally contaminated water, food, or hands.

Both trophozoites and cysts are found in the intestinal lumen, but only trophozoites of E. histolytica invade tissue.

Cyst has glycogen mass, chromidial bars, eccentric nucleus   **KERALA 1994**

Liver abscesses are always preceded by intestinal colonization, which may be asymptomatic.

The most common type of amebic infection is **asymptomatic cyst passage.**

Amebic Liver Abscess Extraintestinal infection by E. histolytica **most often involves the liver.**   **DELHI 1993**

Pleuropulmonary involvement, which is reported in 20 to 30% of patients, is the **most frequent complication of amebic liver abscess.**

<u>Primary amebic encephalitis</u>: Nagleria fowleria   **SGPGI 2005**

<u>Fulminant</u> amebic meningoencephalitis: Nagleria fowleria   **AP 1996**

<u>Granulomatous</u> amebic encephalitis: Balmuthia mandrallis   **JK 2009**

⊃ **Paracapillaria Philippinensis** 🠔🠔

• It has long been known that the nematode Capillaria hepatica can cause a "visceral larva migrans-like syndrome" in people who have eaten meat (e.g. infected liver) or sand containing the eggs of the worm.

• These children exhibit such symptoms as **fever, eosinophilia, abdominal pain and hepatomegaly**, with large numbers of typical eggs being found in the liver on histological examination. 🠔🠔

• P. philippinensis is **a parasite of the small intestine** and it is believed to be a zoonotic infection involving birds and freshwater fish. Humans become infected by ingestion of eggs or infected raw fish, the usual intermediate host, and loads within the host may increase as a result of autoinfection.

• Diagnosis of capillariasis is based upon **histology or finding eggs and larvae in feces.** 🠔

• These eggs are like those of Trichuris, but the polar plugs are inset and the shells are striated or pitted.

• Treatment for capillariasis is **tiabendazole** 25 mg/kg per day for 30 days or longer. Side-effects and relapses are, however, common. Mebendazole and albendazole are also reported to be effective for the treatment of capillariasis. 🠔

⇨ **Note:**

DISEASES	PARASITE	HOST	
		Primary	Secondary
Malaria	Plasmodium	Anopheles	Man
Tapeworm	Taenia solium	Man	Pigs
Tapeworm	Taenia saginata	Man	Cattle
Guinea worm	Darcunculus medinensis	Man	Cyclops
Filariasis	Wuchereria bancrofti	Man	Culex
Hydatid disease	Echinococcus	Dog	Sheep, cattle, man
Sleeping sickness	Trypanosomes	Man	Tse tse fly

⇨ **Gems never to be forgotten**

Pneumoniae after exposure to **parrots**:	✓ Chlamydiae Psittaci
Pregnant women with **cats**:	✓ Toxoplasmosis gondii JK BOPEE 2012
Muscle pain and **eosinophilia**:	✓ Trichinosis (Trichinella spiralis)
Slaughter house worker with fever:	✓ Brucellosis
Gardener stuck with a **thorn**:	✓ Sporothrix schenckii
Aplastic anemia in Sickle cell Disease:	✓ Parvo virus B 19
Fungus Ball:	✓ Aspergillus

Swollen **jaw** with **sulfur granules**:	Actinomyces israelii
Necrotizing fasciitis:	Sterptococcus pyogenes
Diaper rash with **hyphae** and yeast on **microscopy**:	Candida
Burnt tissue with **blue green pus**, grape like odour:	Pseudomonas aeruginosa
Denuded superficial area of large skin area: SSS.	Staph aureus
Pink umblicate warts with central debris:	Molluscum contagiosum

Virus latent in **sensory ganglia with unilateral reactivation**: ✱	Varicella zoster virus
Virus latent in **trigeminal** ganglia: ✱	Herpes simplex virus **1**, VZV
Virus latent in S2, S3: ✱	Herpes simplex virus **2**

5

MICROBIOLOGY

Conjuctivitis on **first day of life**: ✳	✓ Chemical conjunctivitis
Purulent Conjuctivitis on **day 1-4**: ✳	✓ Gonococcal conjunctivitis
Conjuctivitis on **3-10 days** with inclusion bodies: ✳	✓ Chlamydiae trachomatis
Follicular conjucivitis wit inturned eye lashes, Corneal scarring:	✓ Chlamydiae trachomatis
Chorioretinitis in immunocompromised: ✳	✓ Toxoplasma gondii

Gram positive cocci in clusters: ✳	✓ Staph aureus
Pear shaped trophozites: ✳	✓ Giardia lamblia
Budding yeasts forming germ tubes:	✓ Candida albicans
Yeast within macrophages: ✳	✓ Histoplasma capsulatum
BLOODY E. coli: ✳	✓ E. coli 0157: H7
Scotch tape test positive organism: ✳	✓ Entrobius vermicularis

Cholera toxin : stimulates Gs✳

Ecoli heat labile toxin: Stimulates Gs✳

Pertussis toxin: inhibits Gi✳

Diptheria Toxin: acts on EF: shuts down protein synthesis✳   JK BOPEE 2012

Pseudomonas aeruginosa: acts on EF: shuts down protein synthesis

Man is the definitive host in most of the parasitic infection except the following parasites where it is an intermediate host.

- ✳ Echinococcus granulosus (Hydatid worm)
- ✳ Plasmodium (Malaria)
- ✳ Taenia solium (Man is both definitive an intermediate host)
- ✳ Toxoplasma gondii
- ✳ Sarocysts lindemanii

⇨ **Causative organisms of commonly asked diseases:**

▶ **Progressive post operative Bacterial synergistic gangrene**☞☞	Microaerophillic, non hemolytic Streptococci plus staphylococci
▶ **Malignant Otitis externa**☞	Pseudomonas
▶ **Scleroma** ☞	Klebsiella. rhinoscleromatosis
▶ **Soduku**☞☞	Spirillum minus
▶ **Botryomycosis**☞☞☞	Staph aureus
▶ **Chicleros ulcer**☞☞	Leishmania Mexicana
▶ **Espundia**☞	L.Braziliensis
▶ **Favus**☞☞	Tricophyton Schonleneii
▶ **Erysipeloid**☞	Erysipelothrix rhusiopathia

⇨ **Not so common disease with causative agents**

■ Necrotizing fasciitis:	Group A streptococci
■ Purpureal sepsis:	Group B streptococci
■ Sweaty tennis shoe syndrome:	Pseudomonas
■ Fish handlers disease:	Erysipelothrix rhusiopathiae
■ Granuloma infantisepticum:	Listeria
■ Gay bowel syndrome:	Shigella flexiniri
■ Human monocytic ehrilichiosis:	E. chaffeneensis
■ Human granulocytic ehrilichiosis:	E. equi
■ Rat bite fever:	Spirillum minus DNB 2011
■ Medittarenean spotted fever:	Ricketssia conorii
■ Cat scratch disease:	Bartonella hensla PGI 1988
■ Typhilitis:	Pseudomonas aeruginosa
■ Red leg disease:	Aeromonas PGI 2001

► First disease:	Rubeola, (measles, kopliks spots)
► Second disease:	Scarlet fever, (circumoral pallor, pastias lines, straw berry tongue)
► Third disease:	Rubella, (Forschmiers spots, posterior cervical lymphadenopathy)
► Fourth disease:	SSSS, (Nikolskys sign)
► Fifth disease:	Erythema infectiosum (parvovirus b 19, slapped cheek appearance)
► Sixth disease:	Exanthem subitum, Roseola infantum

⇨ **Chlamydiae**

Species	Serotype	Disease
Chlamydia trachomatis	A, B, Ba, C	➡ Endemic trachoma
Chlamydia trachomatis	D- K	➡ Inclusion conjunctivitis
		➡ Genital chlamydia
		➡ Infant pneumonia
Chlamydia trachomatis	L1, L2, L3	➡ LGV
Chlamydia psittaci	Many serotypes	➡ Psittacosis
Chlamydia pneumoniae	Only 1 serotype	➡ Pneumonia

Ankylostoma duodenale:	Iron deficiency anemia
Babesia:	Hemolytic anemia
Diphyllobithirum latum :	Megaloblastic anemia

MICROBIOLOGY

5

⇨ **Microbiology of sexually transmitted /genital diseases:**

Syphilis: <u>painless ulcer</u> with <u>painless lymphadenopathy</u>
Chancroid: (soft chancre) <u>painful ulcer</u> with <u>painful</u> lymphadenopathy.
LGV: <u>un noticed painless</u> papule with **suppurative lymphadenopathy.**, <u>Groove sign</u>
Donovaniosis (Granuloma inguinale): <u>painless</u> subcutaneous nodules <u>without lymphadenopathy</u> with <u>pseudobuboes.</u>
Herpes genitalis: <u>painful papule</u>, with <u>inguinal lymphadenopathy</u>

The chance of CHANCROID IS **"PAINFUL"** IN CONTRAST TO SYPHILIS WHICH IS **"PAINLESS".** <u>Ducreyi makes you cry</u>. Never forget the lines about Features of Chancroid: <u>Lesions are **multiple** in number in the form of ulcers which are **painful** with **undermined and ragged edges** accompanied **by Tender and suppurative lymphadenopathy** in the form **of inguinal buboes.**</u>

⇨ **Important Microbiological Tests:**

▶ Dick Test: ✳	Scarlet Fever
▶ Freis Test: ✳	Lymphogranuloma venerum
▶ Kahns Test: ✳	Syphilis
▶ Kveims Test: ✳	Sarcoidosis
▶ Mono spot/ Paul Bunnel Test: ✳	Infectious Mononucleosis
▶ Rose waaler Test: ✳	Rheumatoid Arthritis
▶ Sweat Test: ✳	Cystic Fibrosis
▶ Weil Felix Test: ✳	Rickettsial infection
▶. Rumpel leed test (Capillary Fragility Test): ✳	Scurvy

⇨ **Clinical scenarios**

▪ Vomiting 1-6 hours after eating **fried rice:** ☞☞	Bacillus Cereus
▪ Vomiting and Diarrhoea 1-6 hours after eating **contaminated food (Creams)**☞:	Staph aureus
▪ Diarrhoea after ingestion of **raw shell fish:** ☞☞	Vibrio parahaemolyticus
▪ Watery Diarrhoea with or without vomiting **after travel** in developing countries☞☞:	ETEC JK BOPEE 2012
▪ Diarrhoea with **rapid Fluid loss and Dehydration:**☞☞	V. cholera
▪ **Acute** endocarditis: ☞☞	Staph aureus
▪ Endocarditis in **IV Drug abusers:** ☞	Staph aureus
Megaloblastic Anemia with history of **fish ingestion:** ☞☞	Diphyllobothrium latum

⇨ **Bacillus cereus:**

- Gram-positive bacilli
- Motile
- Spore forming
- Noncapsulated
- Not susceptible to gamma phage.
- MYPA (mannitol-egg yolk-phenol red polymyxin agar) is used for cultivation.

⇨ **Tests**

Tube agglutination tests:

- ✓ Widal test for Typhoid
- ✓ Paul Bunnel test for Infectious Mononucleosis

Precipitation tests:

- ✓ Kahns test **(tube precipitation)** for syphilis
- ✓ VDRL **(slide precipitation)** for syphilis
- ✓ Ascolis test **(ring precipitation)** for anthrax
- ✓ Lancefield test **(ring precipitation)** for streptococci.
- ✓ Wasserman reaction **(complement fixation test)** for Syphilis

"Sporothrix schenckii." This organism is responsible for **"Rose Gardener's disease,"** known technically as **sporotrichosis.** The organism enters **through skin breaks in the fingers or hands,** causing a chancre, papule, or subcutaneous nodule with erythema and fluctuance. Ulcerating lesions appear along <u>lymphatic channels, but the lymph nodes are not commonly infected</u>. **Potassium iodide** is the treatment for the subcutaneous manifestations✳

Stressed and asked

A woman who pricked her finger while pruning some rose bushes develops a local pustule that progressed to an ulcer. Several nodules then developed along the local lymphatic drainage. Disease is sporotrichosis.

KCET 2012

Tularemia, which may be spread by handling **rabbits or rabbit skins,** or by bites from ticks that feed on the blood of wild rabbits. The causative organism is **Francisella tularensis, a gram-negative coccobacillus.** The disease begins as a rupturing pustule followed by an ulcer, with involvement of regional lymph nodes. More serious cases can be complicated by bacteremia, splenomegaly, rash, pneumonia, or endotoxemic shock.✳

Borrelia spp. Cause **relapsing fever** (transmitted by ticks and lice) and **Lyme disease** (transmitted by ticks).✳

Brucella causes **brucellosis** after ingestion of **contaminated milk or contact with Infected livestock.**✳

Leptospira causes **leptospirosis and Weil's disease**; the organism is acquired by **ingestion of water** contaminated with animal urine.✱

Listeria causes **listeriosis** after contact with contaminated milk, vegetables, or with transplacental transmission.✱

⇨ **Fungi:**

Characteristics	Fungi
▶ Nucleic Acid ⬅⬅	▶ Both
▶ Nucleus ⬅	▶ Eukaryotic
▶ Ribosomes ⬅	▶ 80S
▶ Mitochondria ⬅	▶ Present
▶ Motility	▶ Nil
▶ Reproduction	▶ Budding✱

- **Dimorphic** ("having two forms") because they are spherical in tissue but grow like molds when cultured at room temperature.　　　　　　　　　　　　　　　　　　　　　　　　　**AIIMS 2009**

  Histoplasmosis,

  Blastomycosis,　　　　　　　　　　　　　　　　　　　　　　　　　　　　　**PGI 2002**

  Sporotrichosis,　　　　　　　　　　　　　　　　　　　　　　　　　　　　**MAHE 2007**

  Coccidioidomycosis,　　　　　　　　　　　　　　　　　　　　　　　　　**AIIMS 2002**

  Paracoccidioidomycosis

  Pencillin marfenii

- Fungi are **Eukaryotic** organisms.⬅⬅
- **Fungal cell wall** contains **Chitin**. (Chitin is a polysaccharide of long chains of N acetyl glucosamine.)⬅
- **Fungal Cell membrane** contains **Ergosterol** in contrast to human cell membrane which contains cholesterol.⬅⬅
- STAINED by PAS　　　　　　　　　　　　　　　　　　　　　　　　　　　　**AI 2010**
- **Most** fungi reproduce **asexually** by forming asexual spore's **conidia.** ⬅
- Fungi without sexual stage: fungi imperfectii　　　　　　　　　　　　　　　**MAHE 2005**
- Fungi are culture in Saboubards medium.　　　　　　　　　　　　　　　　　**PGI 1999**
- NON Culturable fungus: Rhinosporodium　　　　　　　　　　　　　　　　**PGI 2007**
- Candida species other than Candida glabrata appear in tissue as both budding yeasts and tubular elements called **pseudohyphae.**　　　　　　　　　　　　　　　　　　　　　**DELHI 1987**
- Pneumocystis carinii is closer to fungi than to parasites by ribosomal sequences

▶ **Monomorphic** , Hyphal fungi with **dichotomus branching** hyphae at **acute angles**: Aspergillus fumigates➛

▶ Yeasts with **pseudohyphae** and true hyphae : **Candida albicans** ➛

▶ **Monomorphic yeast** with polysaccharide capsule: **Cryptococcus**➛

▶ **Non septate** filamentous fungi: **Mucor, Rhizopus, Absidia**➛

▶ Yeast with **broad based bud** and **double retractile cell wall:** ✳ Blastomyces Dermatitidis

▶ Fungus with **Endospores and spherules :** ✳ Coccidomyces immitis

▶ Filamentous fungi with **Tuberculate Macronidia:** ✳ Histoplasma capsulatum

---

▶ **Mycotoxicosis:** ingestion of fungal toxins produced in food most notably aflatoxin in pea nuts

▶ **Mycetismus:** Illness from toxic ingestion of toxic mushrooms. JK BOPEE 2012

▶ **Fungemia:** Sever disseminated fungal infections in immunocompromised patients

▶ **Sick building syndrome:** Inhalation of volatile fungal toxins which aggreviates allergies

⟳ Candidia

Candidiasis, commonly called yeast infection or thrush, also known as "**Candidosis,**" "**Moniliasis,**" and "**Oidiomycosisis** a fungal infection (mycosis) of any of the Candida species, of which Candida albicans is the most common

Is an endogeneous infection. PGI 1980

In **immunocompetent** persons, candidiasis is usually a very localized infection of the skin or mucosal membranes, including the oral cavity (thrush), the pharynx or esophagus, the gastrointestinal tract, the urinary bladder, or the genitalia (vagina, penis).

Hyphal elements can be observed by direct microscopic examination. Dermatophyte hyphae appear as long, branching, refractile, walled structures;

■ Candida appears as shorter, linear hyphae in association with budding yeast forms. AIPGME 2012

 Differentiate from:

■ *Tinea versicolor is seen as round yeast forms with short, club-shaped hyphae (so-called spaghetti and meatballs pattern).*

 MC fungal infection in neutropenic patients. AIIMS 1999

 Candidiasis is a very common cause of vaginal irritation, or vaginitis, and can also occur on the male genitals.

 In **immunocompromised** patients, Candida infections can affect the esophagus with the potential of becoming systemic, causing a much more serious condition, a fungemia called candidemia.

 Shows **Reynolds Braude phenomenon**- ability to form germ tubes within 2 hours of incubation. COMED 2006

5

⇨ **Candidiasis may be divided into the following types**

▪ Oral candidiasis (THRUSH)	AI 1995
▪ Perlèche (around mouth) ↞↞	
▪ Candidal vulvovaginitis	
▪ Candidal intertrigo	
▪ Diaper candidiasis	
▪ Perianal candidiasis	
▪ Candidal paronychia	
▪ Erosio interdigitalis blastomycetica	
▪ Chronic mucocuntaneous candidiasis	
▪ Systemic candidiasis (Meningitis, endocarditis)	AI 1995

- ■ Candida shows **Reynolds Braude Phenomenon** (ability to form germ tubes within two hours when incubated in human serum at 37 °C.

- ■ Hepatospleenic candidiasis manifests as **Bulls Eye Lesion.**

Types of Dermatophyte Infections

- Dermatophytes infect: skin, nails, hair.   DELHI 1993
- Athlete's foot or tinea pedis ↞↞ T. rubrum, T.mentagrophytes, E. floculossum
- Jock itch or tinea cruris ↞ T. rubrum, T.mentagrophytes, E. floculossum
- Ringworm of the body or tinea corpora ↞
- Facial ringworm or tinea faciei ↞
- Blackdot ringworm or tinea capitis ↞
- ✓ MC agent: T. tonsurans   PGI 2000
- ✓ Favus is other manifestation. Caused by T. schoneilenni   COMED 2008
- ✓ Kerion is caused by T.mentagrophytes and T.verrucosum
- Ringworm of the hands or tinea manuum ↞
- In most cases of tinea manuum, only one hand is involved. Frequently both feet are involved concurrently,

Thus the saying "one hand, two feet".

Ringworm of the nail, **Onychomycosis,** or tinea unguum

⇨ **MYCETOMA:**

> Chronic granulomatous involvement of **subcutaneous and deep tissues.**
>
> Commonly effecting **foot.**
>
> Usually presents with ulcer on leg, indurated margins and discharging sinuses. | AIIMS 1994
>
> Destruction of bone occurs.
>
> **Actinomycetoma** is caused by bacteria: nocardia, actinomadura, streptomyces, actinomyces | AI 1996
>
> **Eumycetoma** is caused by fungus: madurella, pseudoallescheria boydii, philphora

➲ Cryptococcus

- Cryptococcus is **Monomorphic Yeast.** ✒✒
- Has a **Polysacchride** capsule. | PGI 1999
- The environmental source is soil enriched with **pigeon droppings.** ✒
- **Prediliction for brain.** | PGI 1998
- Acute pulmonary infections are common in pigeon breeders. ✒
- **Cryptococcal meningitis** is dominant in AIDS patients and patients with cancers. ✒
- **Latex particle agglutination** test for capsular polysaccharide in CSF is rapid and sensitive | AI 2000
- It is urease **positive** yeast. ✒✒
- **Microscopy on India ink** wet mount is also used for diagnosis. ✒ | PGI 2002

After aerosolized spores are inhaled, <u>most infections begin with an asymptomatic pulmonary focus</u>. In individuals with normal host defense, cryptococci remain localized in the lungs and are eventually eliminated. By contrast, in immunocompromised individuals, there is hematogenous spread to extrapulmonary organs. Neutrophils and later monocytes clear cryptococci from inflammatory sites. Phagocytosis by neutrophils and macrophages appears to be mediated in part by complement and several cytokines including interferon-g, tissue necrosis factor, and GM-CSF. Cryptococcal polysaccharide is a major virulence factor and may be immunosuppressive, inhibit phagocytosis, and impair migration of leukocytes.

KCET 2012

"Late infections" (>6 months after kidney transplantation) include CMV retinitis and a variety of CNS complications. Patients (particularly those whose immunosuppression has been increased) are at risk for "**subacute meningitis due to Cryptococcus neoformans.**" Cryptococcal disease may present in an insidious manner (sometimes as a skin infection before the development of clear CNS findings).

Cryptococcal Meningitis is the mc cause of acute meningitis in AIDS. | AI 2005

Cryptococcal infections of the lung can be seen in patients with AIDS. Patients with pulmonary cryptococcal disease present with "**fever, cough, dyspnea, and in some cases, hemoptysis**". A focal or diffuse interstitial infiltrate is seen on chest x-ray in >90% of patients. In addition, one may see lobar disease, cavitary disease, pleural effusions, and hilar or mediastinal adenopathy.

"**Indium In 111-labeled leukocyte scans**" have become useful as an adjunct to other diagnostic procedures in the detection of gastrointestinal and central nervous system (CNS) infections, such as focal encephalitis, **cryptococcal meningitis,** and cytomegalovirus encephalitis, in acquired immunodeficiency syndrome (AIDS) patients

⇨ **Coccidioides immitis:**

- Grows as a white fluffy mold on most culture media and as a **nonbudding spherical form (a spherule)** in host tissue or under special conditions. ☜   **AIIMS 1984**
- The organism reproduces in host tissue by forming **small endospores** within mature spherules.   **AIIMS 1984**
- After rupture of the spherule, the released endospores enlarge, become spherules, and repeat the cycle. The fungus is identified by its appearance and by the **formation of thick-walled, barrel-shaped spores, called** *arthrospores*, in the hyphae of the mold form.☜
- Causes: **Valley fever / Desert Rheumatism**☜   **AIIMS 1986**

⇨ **Histoplasma capsulatum:**

- It is a **dimorphic fungus**   **PGI 1997**
- Hyphae bear **both large and small spores**, which are used for identification.
- H. capsulatum grows as **a small budding yeast** in host tissue and on enriched agar, such as blood cysteine glucose, at 37°C☜.
- The fungus is **unencapsulated.**☜
- Grows in bird/ bat enriched soil
- Coculture of isolates with opposite mating types can produce different sporulating structures in which genetic recombination occurs.
- When these structures, referred to as a teleomorph or the perfect state, are seen in culture, the name **Ajellomyces capsulatus** is used
- Causes: **Histoplasmosis** ☜☜

⇨ **Blastomyces dermatitidis**

It is a **dimorphic fungus** ☜   **JK BOPEE 2012**

Seen as **broad, based, and budding, round yeast like cells with thick wall.**☜   **JIPMER 1981**

Causes:

Blastomycosis

✓ Has an <u>indolent onset</u> and a chronically progressive course. Fever, cough, weight loss, lassitude, skin lesions, and chest ache are common.

✓ Skin lesions favor exposed areas and enlarge over many weeks from pimples to well-circumscribed, verrucous, crusted, or ulcerated lesions

✓ Pain and regional lymphadenopathy are minimal. Large chronic lesions may undergo central healing with scarring and contracture. Mucous membrane lesions resemble squamous cell carcinoma.

✓ Chest x-ray findings are abnormal in two-thirds of patients, with one or more pneumonic or nodular infiltrate

✓ Remember: Blasts skin, lungs

⇨ **Aspergillus fumigates**

It is the **most common cause of aspergillosis**, but A. flavus, A. niger, and several other species can also cause disease.
One of the Most common opportunistic fungal sinusitls in immunocompromised. **AIPGME 2012**
Has <u>branching hyphae. (septate)</u> **AI 2010**
Mc disease caused: **otomycosis.**
Aspergillus is a mold with **septate hyphae.**
Portal of entry is <u>lungs</u> **DNB 1991**
Aspergillus can colonize the damaged bronchial tree, pulmonary cysts, or cavities of patients with underlying lung disease. **AMU 1985**
CAUSES:
Aspergillomas: Balls of hyphae within cysts or cavities usually in the upper lobe, may reach several centimeters in diameter and may be visible on chest x-ray. Tissue invasion does not occur.
Allergic bronchopulmonary aspergillosis denotes the condition of patients with preexisting asthma who have eosinophilia, IgE antibody to Aspergillus, and fleeting pulmonary infiltrates from bronchial plugging.

⊃ **Phycomycosis/Mucormycosis**

- The Mucorales are morphologically distinct. Their **hyphae are nonseptated, broad, and variable in size and shape. Furthermore, the branching of the hyphae is usually irregular and at right angles.** MAH 2012

- **Species of the genera Rhizopus and Mucor are the common** pathogens of this group.

- Other genera, including <u>**Absidia, Cunninghamella, Rhizomucor, Mortierella, Saksenaea, Syncephalastrum, and Apophysomyces,**</u> have also been reported to cause disease.

- The Mucorales are **ubiquitous saprophytic fungi and are abundant in nature.**

- They have been **recovered from bread, fruits, vegetables, soil, and manure.** These fungi have been isolated from the nose, stool, and sputum of healthy individuals. Despite their widespread distribution, they cause disease infrequently. Fortunately, even in the severely immunocompromised hosts, mucormycosis remains a rare opportunistic infection. The disease is not contagious.

- **Diabetic patients appear to be more frequently colonized.** **AIPGME 2012**

- Whereas normal human serum can inhibit their growth, serum obtained from patients with diabetic ketoacidosis is not inhibitory and may even promote fungal growth. Undefined defects of macrophages and neutrophils contribute to the loss of immunity against this infection in the susceptible host. Corticosteroids weaken normal inhibitors of spore germination in tissue. Unlike most pathogenic fungi, these can grow in theabsence of oxygen.

- **Invasion, thrombosis, and necrosis** are the characteristic findings in this disease. Once the fungal spores havegerminated at the site of infection, **the hyphal elements are very aggressive and tend to invade blood vessels, nerves, lymphatics, and tissues.** The infarction leads to further tissue hypoxia and acidosis, resulting in a vicious circle enhancing rapid growth and infection.

MICROBIOLOGY

5

⇨ **Mucormycosis:**

- Species of *Rhizopus, Rhizomucor,* are the most common causes of **mucormycosis,** ☞

- Is **angio invasive.**   PGI 2002

- *Zygomycosis* is a term that includes **mucormycosis and entomophthoramycosis.**

- *Rhizopus* and *Rhizomucor* species are ubiquitous, appearing on decaying vegetation, dung, and foods of high sugar content.

- **Mucormycosis** is uncommon and is largely confined to patients with serious preexisting diseases. **(Diabetic ketoacidosis)**   JIPMER 1987

- **Mucormycosis** originating in the **paranasal sinuses and nose** predominantly affects patients with poorly controlled diabetes mellitus. ☞

- Patients who have undergone organ transplantation, who have a **hematologic malignancy, or who are receiving long-term deferoxamine therapy**☞☞ are predisposed to **mucormycosis** of either sinus or lung.

- Gastrointestinal **mucormycosis** occurs in a variety of conditions, including uremia, severe malnutrition, and diarrheal diseases. ☞☞

- Pulmonary **mucormycosis** manifests as progressive severe pneumonia accompanied by high fever and toxicity. The necrotic center of large infiltrates may cavitate.

⇨ **Chromoblastomycosis**

Chronic subcutaneous mycosis, presents as a **verrucoid, ulcerated, or crusted skin lesion.**

<u>Cladosporium </u>is causative organism.   AIIMS 1993

The disease follows the introduction of any of several fungi into subcutaneous tissue by thorns or bits of vegetation.

The appearance of thick-walled, dark-colored, rounded forms **("copper pennies")** in histopathologic section is diagnostic./**Sclerotic bodies**   AP 1997

Surgical excision is the treatment of choice

⇨ **Pneumocystis carnii:**

- Obligate <u>extracellular</u> fungus.☞   PGI 2007

- Present in patients with **defects in cell-mediated immunity as with hematologic malignancies, lymphoproliferative diseases, cancer chemotherapy, and AIDS**

- Causes <u>interstitial</u> pneumonia☞

- Traditional stains have included reagents such as **methenamine silver, toluidine blue, and cresyl violet**☞☞, which selectively stain the wall of *P. carinii* cysts, and reagents such as **Wright-Giemsa,** which stain the nuclei of all developmental stages. Other reagents include **nonspecific fluorochrome stains (calcofluor white) and Papanicolaou's stain**☞

⟳ Remember the Associations

☐ **Bartonella henselae is the infective agent of cat scratch disease** which generally presents as regional lymphadenopathy with or without low fevers and headaches. Bartonella is a gram-variable pleomorphic rickettsial organism that is introduced to the skin in a cat bite or scratch. It produces a self-limited granulomatous response in the draining lymph nodes.

☐ **Borrelia burgdorferi** is a spirochetal organism that is transmitted by a tick bite (Ixodes spp.), **producing Lyme disease**. Lyme disease progresses from a skin rash to fevers, headache and pain over about one month. It may produce lymphadenopathy, but is not associated with granuloma formation.

☐ **Chlamydia psittaci** infection occurs after contact with infected bird droppings and produces an **atypical pneumonia**. The central nervous system may also be involved, but lymph nodes are spared. Chlamydia trachomatis is the chlamydial species that typically produces suppurative nodal granulomas (lymphogranuloma venereum).

☐ **Coxiella burnetii infection** is transmitted by inhaling dusts or drinking milk from infected mammals, especially sheep and cows. The disease in humans, **Q fever**, is marked by mild nonspecific symptoms or pneumonia, and may progress to myocarditis or hepatitis.

☐ **Rickettsia prowazekii** produces **epidemic (louse-borne) typhus,** which is transmitted by body lice and produces a rash akin to Rocky Mountain spotted fever. Although the organism may reside in the lymph nodes in dormancy, it does not elicit granuloma formation.

☐ **Parvovirus B19 causes erythema infectiosum, or Fifth disease** has the classic "slapped cheek" appearance. Adults typically do not get the facial rash, but have arthralgias and arthritis. The symmetrical distribution of involved joints is similar to that in rheumatoid arthritis. The onset in adults is typically 3 to 4 weeks after exposure. Parvovirus infections may persist in immunosuppressed patients, resulting in red blood cell aplasia.

⇨ Diarrhoeal Associations

▶ *Campylobacter jejuni* **is a pathogen causing an invasive enteric infection associated with ingestion of raw or undercooked food products,** or through direct contact with infected animals. Unsufficiently cooked food is the most common means of acquiring the infection. The patients typically have bloody diarrhea, abdominal pain, and fever. The presence of fecal leukocytes indicates an invasive infection. The organism is a gram negative rod with a "comma-shape."

▶ *Enterotoxigenic E. coli* **causes the classic traveler's diarrhea.** The infection is non-invasive and is acquired via the fecal-oral route through consumption of unbottled water or uncooked vegetables. The major manifestation is a copious outpouring of fluid from the GI tract presenting as explosive diarrhea. This is due to the action of one of two types of enterotoxins on the GI tract mucosa.

▶ *Shigella sonnei* **produces a syndrome very similar to C. jejuni.** However, the organism appears as a gram-negative rod on Gram's stain. It does not have a comma shape. Transmission is from person to person via the fecal-oral route. Infection requires a low infective dose since the organism is fairly resistant to gastric acidity.

5

MICROBIOLOGY

► _Staphylococcus aureus_ produces food poisoning due to the ingestion of a pre-formed enterotoxin. The organism is present in food that is high in salt content such as potato salad, custard, milk shakes, and mayonnaise. The patient presents with nausea, vomiting, and abdominal pain, followed by diarrhea beginning 1-6 hours after ingestion of the enterotoxin.

► _Vibrio cholerae_ produces a secretory diarrhea due to increases in cAMP in the intestinal cells. The organism is not invasive. The patient presents with the sudden onset of painless, watery diarrhea that becomes voluminous, followed by vomiting. The stool appears nonbilious, gray, and slightly cloudy with flecks of mucus, no blood, and a sweet odor.

☐ **Chickens can harbor Salmonella spp.** producing a gastroenteritis or enterocolitis. Chicken guano is also a favorable environment for the fungus Histoplasma capsulatum. The mycelial phase thrives in the rich soil. The human disease is a granulomatous infection involving the lungs and mimicking tuberculosis.

☐ **Dogs or puppies carry Capnocytophaga canimorsus** as part of the normal flora of the oral cavity. Infections from licking or biting range from a self-limited cellulitis to fatal septicemia. Patients at risk for more severe infections are those with asplenia, alcoholism, or hematologic malignancies. This organism is also associated with cat bites, but the patient develops cellulitis and fulminant septicemia, especially in asplenic patients.

☐ **Pasteurella multocida** is another pathogen that colonizes the nasopharynx and gastrointestinal tract of cats and dogs, and rats. P. multocida most commonly causes a localized soft tissue infection or cellulitis after an animal bite, but systemic symptoms may be present in about 40% of the cases. These symptoms include osteomyelitis, septic arthritis, or tenosynovitis.

☐ **Horses and horse manure** have been associated with a pulmonary opportunistic infection with cavitation caused by Rhodococcus equi that resembles tuberculosis in immunocompromised patients. **Burkholderia mallei (the cause of glanders)** is characterized by non-caseating granulomatous abscesses of skin, lymphadenopathy, and pronounced involvement of the lungs.

☐ **Parrots are associated with psittacosis caused by Chlamydia psittaci.** Psittacosis is associated with a dry, hacking cough productive of scant sputum, an interstitial infiltrate in the lungs, severe headache, and myalgias. A pale macular rash is also seen.

⇨ **Methods of identifying organisms:**

☐ Gram stain: Most bacteria

☐ Acid-fast stain : Mycobacteria, nocardiae (modified)

☐ Silver stains : Fungi, legionellae, pneumocystis

☐ Periodic acid-Schiff : Fungi, amebae

☐ Mucicarmine : Cryptococci

☐ Giemsa: Campylobacteria, leishmaniae, malaria parasites

☐ Antibody probes : Viruses, rickettsiae

☐ DNA probes: Viruses, bacteria, protozoa

⇨ **Occular Microbiology:**

♯ A young man aged 30 years, presents with difficulty in vision in the left eye for the last 10 days.

➡ He is immunocompetent, a farmer by occupation, comes from a rural community and gives history of trauma to his left eye with <u>vegetative matter</u> 10-15 days back.

➡ On examination, there is an ulcerative lesion in the cornea, whose base has raised soft creamy infiltrate.

➡ Ulcer margin is feathery and hyphate. There are a few satellite lesions also.

The most probable etiological agent is: Fusarium   <u>"Question asked in AIIMS 2011"</u>

♯ A 35 year. old male presented with a
➡ 15 day history of proptosis in his right eye and pain on eye movement.
➡ There is difficulty in upwards and down wards gaze movements.
➡ CT scan showed a cystic lesion with a hyperdense opacity within it, located in the superior oblique muscle.

Most probable diagnosis is : Cysticercosis cellulosae

♯ A 25 yr male pt. presented with a
➡ Red eye and complains of pain, photophobia, watering and blurred vision.
➡ He gives a history of trauma to his eye with a vegetable matter.
➡ Corneal examination shows a dendritic ulcer.
➡ A corneal scraping was taken and examined. Microscopy showed macrophages like cells on culturing the corneal scrapings over a non-nutrient agar enriched with E.coli, there were plaque formations.

Organism most likely is : Acanthameoba

♯ A 30 year old male presents with a history of injury to the eye with a leaf 5 days ago and pain, photophobia and redness of the eye for 2 days.

The most likely pathology is: Fungal corneal ulcer.

♯ A 56 year old man has painful weeping Rashes over the upper eyelid and forehead for the last 2 days along with ipsilateral acute punctate keratopathy. About a year back, he had chemotherapy for Non-Hodgkin's lymphoma. There is no other abnormality. Which of the following is.

The most likely diagnosis: Herpes Zoster

⊃ **Bioterrorism (High yield for 2011-2012)**

> The ability of infectious agents to inflict widespread illness and thus to cause societal disruption and panic, together with the relatively low cost of these agents, has led to their being called a "poor man's nuclear arsenal."
>
> Several pathogens have been considered likely candidates for biological warfare.
>
> ✓ **Bacillus anthracis**, which causes the zoonosis anthrax, is widely viewed as the leading contender.
>
> ✓ **Smallpox**, an ancient scourge caused by variola virus, has also been considered as a bioweapon owing to its contagiousness and high mortality rate and to the declining population of immunized persons.
>
> ✓ **Yersinia pestis**, the agent of plague, and
>
> ✓ **Francisella tularensis**, the agent of tularemia.
>
> ✓ **Viral hemorrhagic fever agents** such as the Ebola and Marburg viruses
>
> ✓ **Clostridium botulinum toxin**

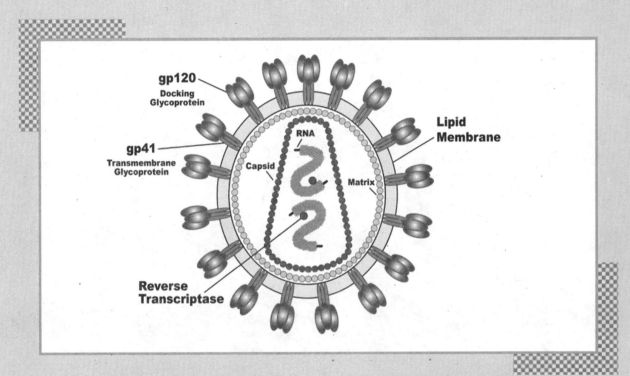

PATHOLOGY

➲ "Different Cell Types (Commonly asked)

☐ Labile cells	✓ Regenerate **throughout life.** (Surface Epithelial Cells, Stem cells, Blood Cells)	
☐ Stable cells	✓ Replicate **at low levels.** (Hepatocytes, Proximal tubule Cells)	
☐ Permanent cells	✓ **Don't Replicate** (Neurons)	KCET 2012
☐ Totipotent cells:	✓ **They can develop into any cell type.** E g: Germ cells	
☐ Pleuropotent cells:	✓ **They are primitive cells and can develop into multiple cell types**	

➲ Growth factors and their Importance (High Yield for AIIMS/AIPGME/DNB 2012-2013)

Epidermal growth factor EGF source is Activated macrophages, salivary glands, keratinocytes, and many other cells

☐ Mitogenic for keratinocytes and fibroblasts; stimulates keratinocyte migration and granulation tissue formation

Transforming growth factor α TGF-α source is Activated macrophages, T lymphocytes, keratinocytes, and many other cells Similar to EGF;

☐ Stimulates replication of hepatocytes and many epithelial cells

Hepatocyte growth factor (scatter factor) HGF source is Mesenchymal cells

☐ Enhances proliferation of epithelial and endothelial cells, and of hepatocytes; increases cell motility

Vascular endothelial cell growth factor (isoforms A, B, C, D) VEGF source is Mesenchymal cells

☐ Increases vascular permeability; mitogenic for endothelial cells

Platelet-derived growth factor (isoforms A, B, C, D) PDGF source is Platelets, macrophages, endothelial cells, keratinocytes, smooth muscle cells

☐ Chemotactic for PMNs, macrophages, fibroblasts, and smooth muscle cells; activates PMNs, macrophages, and fibroblasts; mitogenic for fibroblasts, endothelial cells, and smooth muscles cells; stimulates production of MMPs, fibronectin, and HA; stimulates angiogenesis and wound remodeling; regulates integrin expression.

Fibroblast growth factor source is Macrophages, mast cells, T lymphocytes, endothelial cells, fibroblasts, and many tissues.

☐ Chemotactic for fibroblasts; mitogenic for fibroblasts and keratinocytes; stimulates keratinocyte migration, angiogenesis, wound contraction, and matrix deposition

Keratinocyte growth factor KGF source is Fibroblasts

☐ Stimulates keratinocyte migration, proliferation

➲ Difference in Calcifications (High Yield Topic)

Dystrophic Calcification		Metastatic Calcification
☐ Occurs in "Dying" tissues	JKHND 2006	☐ Occurs in "Normal" tissues
☐ Serum calcium levels are usually Normal	PGI 97	☐ Serum calcium levels are usually elevated

Seen in	Seen in
☐ Atherosclerosis,	☐ Kidneys,
☐ Damaged heart valves,	☐ lungs,
☐ Psammoma bodies☞☞	☐ gastric mucosa☞

An elevated calcium phosphate product, as in secondary hyperparathyroidism, can lead to nodules of **metastatic calcinosis cutis**, which tend to be subcutaneous and periarticular. This form is often accompanied by **calcification** of muscular arteries and subsequent ischemic necrosis (**calciphylaxis**).✱✱

➲ Types of Infarcts✱✱✱

Red Infarct		Pale Infarct	
☐ **Haemorrhagic** infarct☞☞		☐ White Infarct	
☐ Seen in **venous** occlusion☞☞		☐ Occurs in arterial occlusion	
☐ Area of infarct usually has **double blood supply**☞☞		☐ Area of infarct usually has single blood supply	
☐ Seen in		☐ Seen in	
✓ Brain,	KERALA 1994	✓ Kidney,	AI 1995
✓ Gut,	COMED 2005	✓ Myocardium,	AI 1995
✓ Liver☞		✓ spleen	

Inflammation   JK BOPEE 2009

➲ Key Events in Acute Inflammation (High Yield for AIIMS/AIPGME/DNB 2012-2013)

⇨ Vascular Events

☐ Increased Blood Flow
☐ From relaxation of terminal arterioles in the inflammatory lesion
☐ Produces local erythema (**rubor**) and heat (**calor**)
☐ Increased Vascular Permeability
☐ From contraction of capillary endothelial cells
☐ Extravasation of water, low and high molecular weight solutes and blood cells
☐ Leads to local swelling (**tumor**)

➲ Leukocyte Events (Cellular Events)

- **Margination:** neutrophils pass through inflamed vascular beds, attach to vessel wall Mediated by expression of binding sites on activated endothelial cells for neutrophil surface glycoproteins.

- **Diapedesis:** after rolling along endothelial surface, the neutrophil attaches to insinuate itself between 2 endothelial cells and pass through the basement membrane into the extravascular tissues.

- ➡ **Chemotaxis:** once free in the extravascular space, the neutrophil senses minute concentration gradients of chemoattractants, and orients its migration to approach the source of the gradient. Margination, diapedesis, chemotaxis deliver leukocytes to an inflammatory focus within hours.

- ➡ **Phagocytosis:** upon encountering a foreign particle, a neutrophil engulfs the particle and attempts to digest it by releasing enzymes into the phagolysosome.

- ➡ **Degranulation:** even in absence of particles for phagocytosis, an overstimulated neutrophil will release enzymes and other toxic intermediates into the extracellular space (can cause severe tissue damage with temporary or permanent loss of function double edged sword).

➲ Physiological Significance

Mechanisms for the "Cardinal signs" of inflammation

↑ blood flow redness → (rubor) and heat (calor)
↑vascular permeability→ swelling (tumor)
↑nerve stimulation → pain (dolor)
↑tissue destruction → loss of function (functio laesa)

⇨ Leukocyte Defects

☐ Leukocyte adhesion deficiency : defect in 1 β chain of CD11/CD18 integrins
☐ Leukocyte adhesion deficiency: defect in 2 Fucosyl transferase required for synthesis of sialylated oligosaccharide (receptor for selectins)
☐ Chronic granulomatous disease : defect in Decreased oxidative burst
• X-linked NADPH oxidase (membrane component)
• Autosomal recessive NADPH oxidase (cytoplasmic components)
☐ Myeloperoxidase (MPO) deficiency: Absent MPO-H2O2 system
☐ Chédiak-Higashi syndrome : defect in Protein involved in organelle membrane docking and fusion

➲ Acute Phase Reactants

- ➡ The systemic response to tissue injury, regardless of cause, is characterized by a **cytokine-mediated alteration in the hepatic synthesis** of a number of different plasma proteins, known collectively as "acute phase reactants."

- ➡ These proteins, which include **fibrinogen, haptoglobin, ceruloplasmin, a1-antitrypsin, complement components C3 and C4, serum amyloid a protein, and C-reactive protein (CRP)**, rise in proportion to the severity of tissue injury, although the magnitude of rise in each component varies. Fibrinogen and the von Willebrand factor antigen are other acute-phase reactants whose plasma levels frequently are increased in reactive thrombocytosis.

⊃ Positive" Acute Phase Reactants✳✳

✓ CRP	
✓ Mannose binding protein	MAH 2012
✓ Complement factors	
✓ Ferritin	
✓ Cerruloplasmin	
✓ Serum amyloid A	
✓ Haptoglobin	MAH 2012
✓ Alpha 1 antitrypsin	
✓ Alpha2 macroglobulin	

⊃ "Negative" Acute Phase Reactants✳✳

✓ Albumin
✓ Transferrin
✓ Transthyretin
✓ Transcortin
✓ Retinol Binding Protein

⊃ Types of Necrosis (Very Important Topic)

Coagulation Necrosis☞☞	Liquefaction Necrosis☞	Fat Necrosis☞	Caseous Necrosis☞	Gangrenous Necrosis☞
Most Common Type (Kerala 96)	Seen in Brain	Seen in adipose Tissues	Combination of Coagulation and Liquefaction	Due to Ischemia esp to Lower Limb.
Severe ischemia Predisposes	Due to Hydrolytic enzymes	Due to Lipases	"Cottage cheese" appearance	
Examples: ☐ Thermal injury ☐ Myocardial infarction ☐ Tuberculosis (AI 97)	Bacterial infections	Acute Pancreatic Necrosis Trauma to Breast Retroperitoneal fat	Seen in centre of Tuberculous Lesions	More of coagulation leads to Dry gangrene.☞ More of Liquefaction leads to Wet Gangrene☞ (AIIMS 97)

⋑ Reversible Cell Injury

✓	Cellular swelling
✓	Loss of microvilli
✓	Formation of cytoplasmic blebs
✓	ER swelling
✓	Ribosomal detachment
✓	Myelin figures
✓	Clumping of nuclear chromatin.

⋑ Irreversible Cell Injury

✓	Flocculent , amorphous densities in mitochondria	AI 2005
✓	Swelling and disruption of lysosomes	AI 2005
✓	Plasma membrane damage	
✓	Nuclear changes :	
✓	Pyknosis (nuclear condensation)	
✓	Karryorexhis(nuclear fragmentation)	
✓	Karyolysis (nuclear dissolution)	

⋑ Apoptosis (High Yield for AIIMS/AIPGME/DNB 2012-2013)

(Programmed cell death). Features are (Try To remember all Latest Concepts about this topic)

✓ Regulated mechanism of cell death that serves to eliminate unwanted and irreparably damaged cells, with the least possible host reaction.

✓ Characterized by: enzymatic degradation of proteins and DNA, initiated by caspases; and recognition and removal of dead cells by phagocytes

✓ Initiated by two major pathways:

✓ Mitochondrial (intrinsic) pathway is triggered by loss of survival signals, DNA damage and accumulation of misfolded proteins (ER stress); associated with leakage of pro-apoptotic proteins from mitochondrial membrane into the cytoplasm, where they trigger caspase activation; inhibited by anti-apoptotic members of the Bcl family, which are induced by survival signals including growth factors.

✓ Death receptor (extrinsic) pathway is responsible for elimination of self-reactive lymphocytes and damage by cytotoxic T lymphocytes; is initiated by engagement of death receptors (members of the TNF receptor family) by ligands on adjacent cells.

- ☐ Lack of Inflammation.🔶🔶
- ☐ Cell shrinkage.🔶🔶
- ☐ "Condensation of nuclear chromatin" followed by fragmentation. 🔶   (PGI 2007)
- ☐ "Intranucleosomal cleavage" of DNA is characteristic.✱
- ☐ Formation of cytoplasmic /Membrane blebs 🔶   (PGI 2007)
- ☐ Cytoplasmic chromophilia is a feature   AI 2010
- ☐ "Apoptotic" bodies.🔶
- ☐ "bcl$_2$ " <u>inhibits</u> Phagocytosis 🔶   MAH 2012 (SGPGI 04)
- ☐ "p53" <u>stimulates</u> phagocytosis🔶

➲ Proapoptotic Factors

- ▶ Apaf 1
- ▶ Cytochrome C
- ▶ AIF
- ▶ p53
- ▶ Caspaces <u>(INITIATORS/EXECUTIONERS)</u>   JK BOPEE 2012, AI 2010, AIIMS 2007
- ▶ TNFRI
- ▶ FAS (CD 95)

- ▶ Apoptosis inhibiting gene is: bcl2   MAH 2012
- ▶ Detection of Apoptosis:
- ▶ DNA fragmentation analysis🔶
- ▶ Capsase activity assays🔶
- ▶ Annexin V Assay🔶   DNB 2011
- ▶ Propium Iodide assay🔶🔶

⇨ Autoimmune Diseases are:

- ➥ SLE   AIPGMEE 2011
- ➥ Grave's disease   AIPGMEE 2011
- ➥ Myasthenia gravis   AIPGMEE 2011
- ➥ Rheumatoid arthritis
- ➥ Sjogrens syndrome

Diseases with ↑ apoptosis:	autoimmune diseases✱✱	cancers
Diseases with ↓ apoptosis:	ischemic injury	AIDS✱✱
	neurodegenerative diseases	

⇨ Sepsis, Severe sepsis, Septic shock, Systemic Inflammatory Response Syndrome (SIRS)

The **host's reaction to invading microbes** involves a rapidly amplifying polyphony of signals and responses that may spread beyond the invaded tissue. Fever or hypothermia, tachypnea, and tachycardia often herald the onset of **sepsis,**

The systemic response to microbial invasion. When counter regulatory control mechanisms are overwhelmed, homeostasis may fail, and dysfunction of major organs may supervene **(severe sepsis).**

Further regulatory imbalance leads to **septic shock**, which is characterized by **hypotension as well as organ dysfunction.** As sepsis progresses to septic shock, the risk of dying increases substantially. Sepsis is usually reversible, whereas patients with septic shock often succumb despite aggressive therapy.

Systemic Inflammatory Response Syndrome (SIRS):✳✳✳
- ✓ **Temp >38^{0}C or <36^{0}C**
- ✓ **HR>90 bpm**
- ✓ **RR>20 breaths/min**
- ✓ **WBC >12000cells/mm^3 or <4000 cells/mm^3**

- ► Monocytes arise from precursor cells within bone marrow and circulate with a half-life ranging from 1 to 3 days.
- ► Common locations where tissue macrophages (and certain of their specialized forms) are found are lymph node, spleen, bone marrow, perivascular connective tissue, serous cavities such as the peritoneum, pleura, skin connective tissue, lung (alveolar macrophage),
- ✓ **liver (Kupffer cell),**
- ✓ **bone (osteoclast),**
- ✓ **central nervous system (microglia),**
- ✓ **and synovium (type A lining cell).**

⊃ **(High Yield for AIIMS/AIPGME/DNB 2012-2013)**

- ❑ **Lymphocytes:** are the mediators of adaptive immunity and the only cells that produce specific and diverse receptors for antigens.
- ❑ **T (Thymus-derived) lymphocytes:** Express antigen receptors called T cell receptors (TCRs) that recognize peptide fragments of protein antigens that are displayed by MHC molecules on the surface of antigen-presenting cells.
- ❑ **B (Bone marrow-derived) lymphocytes:** Express membrane-bound antibodies that recognize a wide variety of antigens. B cells are activated to become plasma cells, which secrete antibodies.

□ **Natural Killer (NK) Cells:** Kill cells that are infected by some microbes, or are stressed and damaged beyond repair. NK cells express inhibitory receptors that recognize MHC molecules that are normally expressed on healthy cells, and are thus prevented from killing normal cells.

□ <u>**Antigen-presenting Cells (APCs):**</u> Capture microbes and other antigens, transport them to lymphoid organs, and display them for recognition by lymphocytes. The most efficient APCs are dendritic cells, which live in epithelia and most tissues.The cells of the immune system are organized in tissues, some of which are the sites of production of mature lymphocytes (the generative lymphoid organs, the bone marrow and thymus), and others are the sites of immune responses (the peripheral lymphoid organs, including lymph nodes, spleen, and mucosal lymphoid tissues).

⊃ Dendritic/Langerhans Cells (High Yield for 2011/2012)

▶ Dendritic/Langerhans cells are **bone marrow-derived**

▶ They generally lack the standard T, B, NK, and monocyte cell markers but do **express CD83**

▶ **CD 1 is the marker**   AI 2011, AI 2010

▶ Dendritic cells are **referred to as Langerhans cells** when they are present in the skin and beneath the mucosal surface.

⊃ Mediators of Shock: (High Yield for AIIMS/AIPGME/DNB 2012-2013)

Clinical finding	Mediator	
□ Fever	▶ Interleukin 1	MAH 2012
□ Hypotension	▶ Bradykinin, Nitric Oxide	
□ Inflammation	▶ C3a, C5a	
□ DIC	▶ Hageman Factor	AIIMS 1999
REMEMBER Bradykinin also causes pain, vasodilation and cough		AI 2010

➡ CVC Lungs: Brown induration of lungs	
➡ CVC Liver: "Nut meg" liver	JK 2011
➡ CVC Spleen: "Gamma Gandy" bodies	JK BOPEE 2008

⊃ Cytokines (High Yield for 2011/2012)

Cytokines are **soluble proteins** produced by a wide variety of hematopoietic and non hematopoietic cell types Cytokines are involved in the regulation of the growth, development, and activation of immune system cells and in the mediation of the inflammatory response.

1. **Immunoregulatory cytokines** involved in the activation, growth, and differentiation of lymphocytes and monocytes, **e.g., IL-2, IL-4, IL-10, , and transforming growth factor (TGF)**

2. **Proinflammatory cytokines** produced predominantly by mononuclear phagocytes in response to infectious agents **(e.g., IL-1, TNF- and IL-6)** and the chemokine family of inflammatory cytokines, within which are included IL-8, monocyte chemotactic protein (MCP)-1, MCP-2, MCP-3, macrophage inflammatory protein and regulation-upon-activation, normal T expressed and secreted (RANTES)

3. Cytokines that regulate **immature leukocyte growth and differentiation**, e.g., IL-3, IL-7, and GM-CSF.

⊃ Prostaglandins

LTA_4:

✓ Produced in leucocytes, platelets, mast cells, vascular tissue.

LTC_4, LTD_4, LTE_4:

✓ contraction of smooth muscle

✓ Bronchoconstriction

✓ Vasoconstriction   PGI 1995

✓ ↑vascular permeability

✓ Components of SRSA.

LTB_4:

✓ ↑Chemotaxis

✓ Adhesion of WBC   COMED 2006

✓ Release of lysosomal enzymes

Thromboxanes:

✓ Produced mainly in **platelets**

✓ **Promotes** platelet aggregation

✓ Vasoconstriction

✓ Smooth muscle contraction.

Prostacyclins:

✓ Produced by **endothelium of vessels**

✓ Vasodilation

✓ **Inhibits** platelet aggregation   PGI 1992

▶ Cortisol inhibits	**Phospholipase** A_2
▶ Aspirin, Indomethacin, Phenylbutazone inhibit Both	**COX 1 and COX 2.**
▶ Coxibs are selective	**COX 2** inhibitors (Celecoxib)

✓ Cells involved first in tissue injury are **neutrophils.**   AI 2007

✓ **Heart failure cells** are seen in: lung.   JK BOPEE 2012

✓ **Lines of Zahn** are found in **thrombus.**   JKHD 2005

✓	Chicken fat clot is post mortem thrombus.	JKHD 2006
✓	Shock lung is other name for ARDS.(Diffuse alveolar damage)	AIIMS 2008
✓	Macrophages are derived from monocytes.	JKHD 2003
✓	Epitheliod and multi nucleated giant cells are derived from monocyte -macrophages.	AI 2002
✓	Wound contraction is mediated by myofibroblasts.	JKHD 2005
✓	C5a is the most important mediator of chemotaxis.	Delhi 2005

◯ Procoagulant States:

▶	Factor V (Leidein mutation)	AIIMS 2003
▶	Protein C deficiency	PGI 2003
▶	Protein S deficiency	PGI 2003
▶	Homocystenemia	
▶	Antiphospholipid antibody	

◯ Anti coagulant factors

▶	Antithrombin III
▶	Protein C
▶	Protein S
▶	Prostacyclin
▶	Nitric oxide

⇨ Hyperviscosity

▶	Multiple myeloma	PGI 2004
▶	Cryoglobinemia	PGI 2003
▶	Myeloproliferative disorders	

Remember: Virchow's triad:

▶	Endothelial injury
▶	Alteration in blood flow
▶	Hypercoagulability

⇨ Virchow's triad describes three factors that lead to thrombosis

Endothelial injury

▶ Endothelial cell injury exposes highly **thrombogenic subendothelial extracellular matrix** which allows platelet to adhere to the collagen of ECM.

▶ This effect is due to increased production of Von willebrand factor by endothelium, an essential cofactor for of platelet binding to collagen.

Disturbance in blood flow

▶ Normal blood flow is laminar such that the platlets flow centrally in the vessels lumen, separated from the endothelium by a slower moving clear zone of plasma.

Stasis and turbulence leads to thrombosis because:-

▶ Disruption of laminar flow brings platelet into contact with endothelium

▶ Prevent dilution of activated clotting factors by fresh flowing blood

▶ Retard the inflow of clotting factor inhibitors

▶ Turbulence can cause endothelial injury or dysfunction.

⟳ Stains:

▶ Von kossa: calcium

▶ Toluidine blue: mast cells

▶ Alician blue: mucins

▶ Congo red: amyloid

▶ Masons trichome: collagen, connective tissue

▶ Orcein: elastic fibres

Major Histocompatibilty complex

⟳ (High Yield for 2011/2012)

The human major histocompatibility complex (MHC), commonly called the human leukocyte antigen (HLA) complex, is a 4-megabase (Mb) region on **chromosome 6✱✱**   JK BOPEE 2011

Class I MHC✱✱

➡ They are glycoproteins

➡ present on surface of all <u>nucleated</u> cells↼↼

➡ Presents antigen to **CD 8 positive cells**↼

➡ Have <u>only one chain</u> encoded by MHC locus.

➡ Antigen binding site on MHC I is proximal end of alpha subunit of 1 and 2   AI 2010

Class II MHC✱✱

➡ They are glycoproteins present on the surface of **Macrophages, B cells, Dendritic cells of spleen and Langerhans cells.**↼

➡ Presents antigen to **CD 4 positive cells**↼

➡ Not Present on surface of nucleated cells

➡ **Have both chains encoded by MHC** locus. ↼

6

PATHOLOGY

⊃ Important HLA Associations (Frequently asked) (High Yield for 2011/2012)

- ❏ A3 HAEMACHROMATOSIS✳
- ❏ B5 BEHCETS DISEASE✳
- ❏ B 27 ANKYLOSING SPONDYLITIS, RIETERS SYNDROME, PSORIATIC ARTHRITIS✳
- ❏ DR2 MULTIPLE SCLEROSIS, NARCOLEPSY✳
- ❏ DR3 DERMATITIS HERPETIFORMIS, SJOGRENS SYNDROME, MYASTHENIA GRAVIS, IDDM✳
- ❏ DR4 IDDM,RHEUMATOID ARTHRITIS✳
- ❏ DR5 PERNICIOUS ANEMIA✳
- ❏ DR7 COELIAC DISEASE✳

⊃ Natural Killer Cells: (High Yield for AIIMS/AIPGME/DNB 2012-2013)

- ▶ Are part of "innate" immunity✳✳ — AI 2007
- ▶ Are "large granular lymphocytes"✳
- ▶ Lack T cell receptor, surface IgM and IgD.✳
- ▶ Express CD 16 and CD 56.✳ — DELHI 2009
- ▶ The classic NK cells are CD2+, CD3+, CD4+, CD56+, and CD16+.
- ▶ Thymus is not required for their development
- ▶ Activity not enhanced by prior sensitization. NK cells do not require sensitization to express the killer function. ✳
- ▶ NK cells constitute 2 to 10% of normal peripheral blood lymphocytes.✳
- ▶ Contain Azurophilic granules.
- ▶ Kill virus infected cells and cancer cells — JIPMER 1993
- ▶ Kill by producing perforins, granzymes.

- ➡ Killing is non specific.
- ➡ NK cells are not MHC-restricted--they will kill certain autologous, allogeneic, and even xenogeneic tumor cells whether or not these targets express MHC.
- ➡ NK cells do not use the TCR, CD3 complex to recognize target cells.
- ➡ Killing is not dependent on foreign antigen presentation.(MHC Independent) — DNB 1991

⊃ Important Translocations: ✳✳✳(High Yield for 2011/2012)

- ➡ t(8;14) Burkitts Lymphoma — JK BOPEE
- ➡ t(9;22) CML — DNB 2001
- ➡ t(15;17) AML
- ➡ t(11;22) Ewings sarcoma — UPSC 01
- ➡ t(X;18) Synovial cell Ca

➲ Basic terminology (High Yield for AIIMS/AIPGME/DNB 2012-2013)

> ► Atrophy: decreae in cell size/ function.
>
> ► Hypertrophy: increase in cell size/ function.
>
> ► Hyperplasia: increase in number of cells in tissues/organs
>
> ► Metaplasia: reversible change of epithelial transformation.
>
> ► Anaplasia: hallmark of malignant transformation
>
> ► Dysplasia: reversible abnormal proliferation of cells. Intact basement membrane

⇨ Molecular Basis of Carcinogenesis:

> 1. Self-sufficiency in growth signals
>
> 2. Insensitivity to growth-inhibitory signals
>
> 3. Evasion of apoptosis
>
> 4. Limitless replicative potential (i.e., overcoming cellular senescence and avoiding mitotic catastrophe)
>
> 5. Development of sustained angiogenesis
>
> 6. Ability to invade and metastasize
>
> 7. Genomic instability resulting from defects in DNA repair

> ❏ Oncogenes that Promote Unregulated Proliferation (Self-sufficiency in Growth Signals)
>
> ❏ Proto-oncogenes: normal cellular genes whose products promote cell proliferation
>
> ❏ Oncogenes: mutant versions of proto-oncogenes that function autonomously without a requirement for normal growth-promoting signals

➲ Insensitivity to Growth-Inhibitory Signals

> Tumor suppressor genes encode proteins that inhibit cellular proliferation by regulating the cell cycle. Unlike oncogenes, both copies of the gene must be lost for tumor development, leading to loss of heterozygosity at the gene locus.In cases with familial predisposition to develop tumors, the affected individuals inherit one defective (nonfunctional) copy of a tumor suppressor gene and lose the second one through somatic mutation. In sporadic cases both copies are lost through somatic mutations

➲ Oncogenic Viruses: (USMLE Favourite)

> ➥ HPV has been associated with benign warts, as well as cervical cancer.The oncogenic ability of HPV is related to the expression of two viral oncoproteins, E6 and E7; they bind to RB and p53, respectively, neutralizing their function; they also activate cyclins.
>
> ➥ E6 and E7 from high-risk HPV (that give rise to cancers) have higher affinity for their targets than E6 and E7 from low-risk HPV (that give rise to low-grade tumors).

- EBV has been implicated in the pathogenesis of **Burkitt lymphomas, lymphomas in immunosuppressed individuals with HIV infection or organ transplantation**, some forms of Hodgkin lymphoma, and nasopharyngeal carcinoma. All except the nasopharyngeal cancers are B-cell tumors.

- **The oncogenic effects of HBV and HCV are multifactorial**, but the dominant effect seems to be immunologically mediated chronic inflammation, hepatocellular injury, stimulation of hepatocyte proliferation, and production of reactive oxygen species that can damage DNA. **The HBx protein of HBV and the HCV core protein** can activate a variety of signal transduction pathways that may also contribute to carcinogenesis.

H. pylori infection has been implicated in both **gastric adenocarcinoma and MALT lymphoma.** The mechanism of H. pylori-induced gastric cancers is multifactorial, including immunologically mediated chronic inflammation, stimulation of gastric cell proliferation, and production of reactive oxygen species that damage DNA. H. pylori pathogenicity genes, such as CagA, may also contribute by stimulating growth factor pathways. It is thought that H. pylori infection leads to polyclonal B-cell proliferations and that eventually a monoclonal B-cell tumor (MALT lymphoma) emerges as a result of accumulation of mutations.

⇨ **Viruses Causing Lymphoma:**

✓ EBV	JK BOPEE 2012
✓ HTLV1	
✓ HHV8 (Kaposi Sarcoma)	

⇨ **Chemical Carcinogens:**

- ❏ Chemical carcinogens have highly reactive eletrophile groups that directly damage DNA, leading to mutations and eventually cancer.

- ❏ Direct-acting agents do not require metabolic conversion to become carcinogenic, while indirect-acting agents are not active until converted to an ultimate carcinogen by endogenous metabolic pathways.

- ❏ Hence polymorphisms of endogenous enzymes like cytochrome P-450 may influence carcinogenesis. Following exposure of a cell to a mutagen or an initiator, tumorigenesis can be enhanced by exposure to promoters, which stimulate proliferation of the mutated cells.

- ❏ Examples of human carcinogens include direct-acting (e.g., alkylating agents used for chemotherapy), indirect-acting (e.g., benzopyrene, azo dyes, and aflatoxin), and promoters/agents that cause pathologic hyperplasias of liver, endometrium

⇨ **Immune Surveillance:**

- ❏ Tumor cells can be recognized by the immune system as non-self and destroyed. Antitumor activity is mediated by predominantly cell-mediated mechanisms. Tumor antigens are presented on the cell surface by MHC class I molecules and are recognized by CD8+ CTLs.

☐ The different classes of tumor antigens include products of mutated proto-oncogenes, tumor suppressor genes, overexpressed or aberrantly expressed proteins, tumor antigens produced by oncogenic viruses, oncofetal antigens, altered glycolipids and glycoproteins, and cell type-specific differentiation antigens.Immunosuppressed patients have an increased risk of cancer. In immunocompetent patients, tumors may avoid the immune system by several mechanisms, including selective outgrowth of antigen-negative variants, loss or reduced expression of histocompatibility antigens, and immunosuppression mediated by secretion of factors (e.g., TGF-β) from the tumor.

➲ Premalignant Forms of SCC: (High Yield for AIIMS/AIPGME/DNB 2012-2013)

- ✓ Actinic keratosis, or solar keratoses ☛☛
- ✓ Actinic cheilitis☛
- ✓ Bowen's disease☛
- ✓ Erythroplasia of Queyrat☛
- ✓ DLE ☛
- ✓ Xeroderma Pigmentosa☛
- ✓ UV Radiation -UV B ☛
- ✓ Hypertrophic lichen planus ☛

▶ **Actinic keratoses and cheilitis** are hyperkeratotic papules and plaques that occur on sun-exposed areas. While the potential for malignant degeneration is low in any individual lesion, the risk of SCC increases with larger numbers of lesions. ✱✱

▶ **Bowen's disease** presents as a scaling, erythematous plaque, which may develop into invasive SCC in up to 20% of cases. Treatment of premalignant and in situ lesions reduces the subsequent risk of invasive disease ✱✱

➲ The following oral lesions are Premalignant Lesions: ✱✱✱

☐ Leucoplakia	
☐ Erythroplakia	JKBOPEE 2012
☐ Chronic hyperplastic candidiasis.	
☐ Oral submucous fibrosis	
☐ Syphilitic glossitis;	
☐ Sideropenic dysphagia.	

➲ Environmental Risk Factors and Cancers (High Yield for AIIMS/AIPGME/DNB 2012-2013)

Cancer Type	Environmental Risk Factor	
▶ Lung:☛☛	Smoking, Asbestos, Nickel, Radon, Coal, Arsenic , Chromium , Uranium✱✱✱	
▶ Mesothilioma:☛	Asbestos(Crocodilite fibres) ✱✱	MAH 2012
▶ Bladder Ca☛	Smoking, Aniline dyes, Schistomiasis✱	

6

► Skin Ca: ☞	UV light exposure, coal , Tar, Arsenic✳	
► Liver: ☞	**Alcohol, Vinyl chloride, Aflatoxins✳✳**	
► Pancreas: ☞☞	Smoking✳	
► Renal Cell Carcinoma: ☞	Smoking✳	
► Stomach: ☞	Alcohol, Nitrosamines	

➲ Hereditary DNA Repair Disorders (High Yield for AIIMS/AIPGME/DNB 2012-2013)

☐ **Xeroderma pigmentosum:**   **AIIMS 2005**

Hypersensitivity to sunlight/UV, resulting in increased skin cancer incidence and premature aging ✳✳

☐ **Cockayne syndrome:**

hypersensitivity to UV and chemical agents ✳

☐ **Trichothiodystrophy:**

sensitive skin, brittle hair and nails ✳

☐ **Werner's syndrome:**

Defect in DNA helicase   **JK BOPEE 2012**

premature aging and retarded growth ✳✳

☐ **Bloom's syndrome:**   **COMED 2004**

Sunlight hypersensitivity, high incidence of malignancies (especially leukemias). ✳

☐ **Ataxia telangiectasia:** ·

Sensitivity to ionizing radiation and some chemical agents ✳

All of the above diseases are often called **"segmental progerias" ("accelerated aging diseases")** because their victims appear elderly and suffer from aging-related diseases at an abnormally young age.

Other diseases associated with **reduced DNA repair function** include

► **Fanconi's anemia,**		**AIIMS 2005**
► **Hereditary breast cancer and**		
► **Hereditary colon cancer.**		**AIIMS 2005**

➲ Important Tumor Markers: (High Yield for AIIMS/AIPGME/DNB 2012-2013)

Marker	Cell Type/Tumor
✓ **Mucin**	**Adeno carcinoma**
✓ **Keratin**	**Epithelium**
✓ **Gremilius**	**Neuroendocrine**
✓ **Lymphocyte**	**Common Antigen Lymphoma**
✓ **S-100**	**Melanoma**

✓ Vimentin	Sarcoma
✓ Desmin	Sarcoma

Alpha feto protein	➥ Hepato cellular carcinoma	PGI 2011
	➥ Endodermal sinus tumor.	COMED 2008
	➥ Yolk Sac tumors	JK BOPEE 2011
	➥ Hepatoblastoma	
	➥ Cirrhosis of liver	
	➥ Hepatitis	PG1 2011
PSA	➥ Prostate cancer	
Neuron Specific enolase	➥ Small cell lung cancer, Neuroblastoma	
LDH	➥ Lymphoma	
Cathecolamines	➥ Phaeochromocytoma	
Beta 2 microglobulin	➥ Multiple Myeloma	
	➥ Lymphoma	
Gastrin	➥ Pancreatic neuroendocrine tumors	AIIMS 2005
Bladder Tumor Antigen	▶ Bladder Tumor, UTI, Renal Calculi	
CA27.29	▶ Breast Cancer	
CA 72.4	▶ Ovarian and Pancreatic Cancer	
LASA -P (Lipid Associated Sialic Acid)	▶ Ovarian Cancer	
Keratin	▶ Cacervix	AI 1992
NMP 22	▶ Bladder Cancer	
HCG	➥ Gestational Trophoblastic Disorders	
CA 125	➥ Ovarian Cancer	
Placental Alkaline Phosphatase	➥ Seminoma	
S100	➥ Melanoma, Neural Tumors	

➔ Mesenchymal Tumors: (High Yield for 2011/2012)

▶ Endothelial tumors: FACTOR VIII, CD 34
▶ Melanoma: HMB 45, S 100
▶ Fibrohistiocytic tumors: Lysosyme, HAM 56
▶ Muscle tumors: Desmin, Myoglobin

6

⇨ **Prognostic Variables in Breast Cancer used in Pathology✱✱✱**

- The most important prognostic variables are provided by **Tumor staging.**

- The **size of the tumor and the status of the axillary lymph nodes** provide reasonably accurate information on the likelihood of tumor relapse

- **Estrogen and progesterone receptor status** are of prognostic significance. Tumors that lack either or both of these receptors are more likely to recur than tumors that have them.

- **S-phase analysis using flow cytometry** is the most accurate measure, and the **indirect S-phase assessments** using antigens associated with the cell cycle, such as **PCNA (Ki67)**

- Several studies suggest that tumors with a high **proportion (more than the median) of cells in the S phase** pose a greater risk of relapse and that chemotherapy offers the greatest survival benefit for these tumors.

- Assessment of **DNA content in the form of ploidy** is of modest value, with non diploid tumors having a somewhat worse prognosis.

➲ **Hypersensitivity Reactions (High Yield for AIIMS/AIPGME/DNB 2012-2013)**

⇨ **Type I Hypersensitivity reactions: IgE Mediated✱**   AI 2007

❏ Theobald phenomenon	
❏ Prusnitz reaction (PK)	**AIIMS 1984**
❏ **Casonis Test (hydatid cyst)**	**AIPGME 2012**
❏ Anaphylaxis	
❏ Local: Asthma, Hay fever, Angioedema, Eczema, Urticaria, Atopy	**JK BOPEE 2011**

⇨ **Type II Hypersensitivity Reactions: IgG or IgM Mediated✱**

❏ Graves disease (ALSO TYPE V)	**AP 1985**
❏ Good Pausters Syndrome	**UP 2001**
❏ Myasthenia Gravis	**AIPGME 2012**
❏ Blood transfusion reactions.	**PGI 2006**
❏ Immune hemolytic anemia	**JK BOPEE 2011**
❏ Immune Thrombocytopenic purpura	**DNB 2001**

⇨ **Type III Hypersensitivity reactions: Immune complex Mediated✱**

❏ Arthus reaction	**AI 2007**
❏ Serum Sickness	**AP 1998**
❏ SLE	
❏ Schiks test	**COMED 2003**
❏ Post Streptococcal Glomerulonephritis	

⇨ **Type IV Hypersensitivity Reactions: Delayed Hypersensitivity✱**

☐	Tuberculin test	
☐	Lepromin Test	
☐	Contact dermatitis	PGI 2006
☐	Pernicious anemia	

⇨ **Immune-Complex-Dependent Reactions /Serum sickness**   AIIMS 2009

Serum sickness is produced by **circulating immune complexes** and is characterized by

✓ Fever,

✓ Arthritis,

✓ Nephritis,

✓ Neuritis,

✓ Edema, and anurticarial, papular, or purpuric rash.

► Serum sickness was first described following administration of foreign sera, but drugs are now the usual cause.

► **TYPE III hypersensitivity reaction**.

► Drugs that produce serum sickness include the

✓ **Penicillins,**

✓ **Sulfonamides,**

✓ **Thiouracils,**

✓ **Cholecystographic dyes,**

✓ **Phenytoin, aminosalicylic acid,**

✓ **Heparin, and antilymphocyte globulin.**

► In classic serum sickness, symptoms develop 6 days or more after exposure to a drug, the latent period representing the time needed to synthesize antibody. The antibodies responsible for immune-complex-dependent drug reactions are largely of the IgG or IgM class.

► Vasculitis, may also be a result of immune complex deposition.

Collagen

☐	Collagen is the **main protein of connective tissue** in animals and
☐	The **most abundant protein in mammals**, making up about 25% to 35% of the whole-body protein content.
☐	In muscle tissue it serves as a major component of Endomysiun.

Type I

This is the **most abundant collagen** of the human body.   MAH 2002

It is present in **scar tissue**, the end product when tissue heals by repair. It is found in

- ✓ Tendons,
- ✓ Skin,
- ✓ Artery walls,
- ✓ The endomysium of myofibrils,
- ✓ Fibrocartilage and the organic part of bones and teeth. ☞ ☞

Type II

- ✓ **Hyaline cartilage** makes up 50% of all cartilage protein.
- ✓ **Vitreous humour** of the eye. ☞

Type III

This is the collagen of granulation tissue, and is produced quickly by young fibroblasts before the tougher type I collagen is synthesized. Also found in

- ✓ Artery walls,
- ✓ Skin,
- ✓ Intestines and the
- ✓ Uterus,
- ✓ Reticular fiber. ☞

Type IV

Present in

- ✓ Basal lamina;   COMED 2005
- ✓ Eye lens.
- ✓ Filtration system in capillaries and the
- ✓ Glomeruli of nephron in the kidney. ☞

Remember:

- ❑ **Their disruption results in characteristic disturbances**
- ❑ Osteogenesis imperfecta [type I collagen],
- ❑ Chondrodysplasia [type II collagen],
- ❑ Ehlers-Danlos syndrome or arterial aneurysms [type III collagen]

Amyloidosis

⊃ **(High Yield for 2011/2012) Remember the Type of Amyloidosis and the Protein Type Associated✳✳✳**

Type of Amyloidosis	Amyloid protein	
❏ **Primary** Amyloidosis, Myeloma	AL☞☞	AI07, PGI 1989
❏ **Secondary** Amyloidosis	AA☞☞	UP 2007, TN 1990
✓ Tuberculosis		
✓ Rheumatoid arthritis		
✓ Hodgkins ltymphoma		
❏ **Familial** Medittarean Fever	AA☞	
❏ **Hemodialysis** associated Amyloidosis	Aβ2M☞	
❏ **Cerebral** (Alzhiemers) Amyloidosis	Aβ☞	
❏ **Cardiac** Amyloidosis	ATTR☞	AIIMS 2007

▶	Amyloidosis is deposition of an **"extracellular protein"**.✳	
▶	Individual subunits form **"β pleated sheets."**✳	
▶	**Kidney** followed by liver is the commonest sites involved.	PGI 1988
▶	Deposits stain **"red"** with Congo red.✳	
▶	**"Apple green birefrigerence"** is seen on Congo red stain under <u>polarized light.</u>✳	
▶	Amyloid is composed of **"<u>fibrillary protein</u>**, amyloid P Component and Glycosaminoglycans".✳	
▶	Thyroid cancer with amyloid stroma. : MTC(Medullary ca thyroid)	PGI 1988
▶	**Rectal biopsy is the best diagnostic method.**	AI 2007

❏	On **light microscopy**: Eosinophilic amorphous substance✳	
❏	Congo red in **ordinary light**: Pink color✳	AIIMS 1983
❏	Congo red on **polarizing microscope**: Yellow green birefringence✳	
❏	**Electron microscopy**: Non branching fibrils✳	
❏	**X ray crystallography**: Crossed β pleated configuration✳	

Pathology and Genetics: Autosomal Dominant Traits: (High Yield for AIIMS/ AIPGME/ DNB 2012-2013)

Are fully manifest in the presence of a gene in the heterozygous state, i.e., when only one abnormal gene (mutant allele) is present and the corresponding partner allele on the homologous chromosome is normal. The following features are characteristic:

- ☐ Each affected individual has an affected parent (unless the condition arose by a new mutation in a germ cell that formed the individual);
- ☐ An affected individual usually bears an equal number of affected and unaffected offspring;
- ☐ Males and females are affected in equal numbers;
- ☐ Each gender can transmit the trait to male and female;
- ☐ Normal children of an affected individual have only normal offspring;
- ☐ When the trait does not impair viability or reproductive capacity, vertical transmission of the trait occurs through successive generations. Three or more generations of male-to-male transmission argues against X-linkage of a rare gene.

⇨ Autosomal Recessive Triats: (High Yield for AIIMS/AIPGME/DNB 2012-2013)

Autosomal recessive conditions are clinically apparent only in the homozygous state, i.e., when both alleles at a particular genetic locus are mutant alleles. The following features are characteristic:

- ☐ The parents are clinically normal;
- ☐ Only siblings are affected;
- ☐ Males and females are affected in equal proportions;
- ☐ If an affected individual marries a homozygous normal person, none of the children is affected but all are heterozygous carriers;
- ☐ If an affected individual marries a heterozygous carrier, one half of the children are affected, and the pedigree pattern superficially suggests a dominant trait;
- ☐ If two individuals who are homozygous for the same mutant gene marry, all of their children are affected;
- ☐ If both parents are heterozygous at the same genetic locus, one fourth of their children are homozygous affected, on average one fourth are homozygous normal, and one half are heterozygous carriers of the same mutant gene; and
- ☐ The less frequent the mutant gene is in the population, the greater the likelihood that the affected individual is the product of consanguineous parents.

⇨ X-Linked Recessive Triats:

- ☐ Diseases or traits that result from genes located on the X chromosome are termed X-linked. Because the female has two X chromosomes, she may be either heterozygous or homozygous for the mutant gene, and the trait may exhibit recessive or dominant expression. The terms X-linked dominant and X-linked recessive refer only to expression of the trait in females. The male has only one X chromosome and therefore is hemizygous for X-linked traits. Males can be expected to express X-linked traits regardless of their recessive or dominant behavior in the female. This accounts for the large numbers of X-linked diseases.
- ☐ Males transmit their X chromosome to all of their daughters, making them all obligate carriers of an X-linked disease trait.
- ☐ Affected males do not transmit an X chromosome to their sons; thus, an important feature of X-linked inheritance is the absence of male-to-male transmission.

⊃ **X-Linked Dominant Traits:**

This mode of inheritance is uncommon. Its characteristic features are as follows:
❏ Females are affected about twice as often as males;
❏ Heterozygous females transmit the trait to both genders with a frequency of 50%;
❏ Hemizygous affected males transmit the trait to all of their daughters and none of their sons; and
❏ The expression is more variable and generally less severe in heterozygous females than in hemizygous affected males. Examples of X-linked dominant inheritance include the vitamin D-resistant (hypophosphatemic) rickets and pseudohypoparathyroidism.

The following conditions are inherited as:

⇨ **Asked innumerable times in AIIMS, PGI, NIMHANS, AP, COMED.**

Autosomal Dominant	Autosomal Recessive	X linked recessive
Huntington's disease✱✱	Cystic fibrosis✱	Becker
Marfans syndrome✱	Ataxia telengectasia DNB 2011	Colour blindness✱✱
Adult polycystic kidney disease✱	Freidrechs ataxia	Duchenne muscular dystrophy✱ KCET 2012
Familial hypercholestremia✱✱	Infantile polycystic kidney disease✱✱	Fabry's disease✱
AIIMS 2011	Wilsons disease✱	G6PD deficiency✱
Osteogenesis imperfecta✱	Alkaptonuria✱✱	Haemophilia A,B✱
Neurofibromatosis✱	Haemochromatosis AIPGE 2011	Hunter's disease✱✱
Achondroplasia✱	Sickle cell anemia	Lesch-Nyhan syndrome✱
Myotonic dystrophy	phenyl ketonuria	Nephrogenic diabetes insipidus✱
Von Willebrands disease✱	beta thalessemia	Ocular albinism✱
HNPCC	alpha 1 antitrypsin deficency	Retinitis pigmentosa✱
BRCA1, BRCA2 Breast cancer		Testicular feminization syndrome
Otosclerosis		Wiskott-Aldrich syndrome
Tuberous sclerosis		Color blindness
MC group of mendelian disorders		Affects males more. AI 2010

⇨ **X linked dominant:**

▶ Hypophosphatemic type of vitamin D resistant rickets.
▶ Incontenentia pigmentii
▶ Orofaciodigital syndrome

▶ Hereditary spherocytosis is AD.	AI 2002
▶ Achondroplasia is AD.	AI 1996
▶ Familial hypercholestrelemia is AD.	AI 2004
▶ Retinoblastoma is AD.	AI 2000
▶ Von willebrands disease is AD.	AI 1998
▶ Homocystinuria is AR.	AI 1998

⇨ **Y-Linked Disorders**

> ▶ Only a few genes are known on the Y chromosome.
>
> ▶ One such gene, the sex-region determining Y factor (SRY), or testis-determining factor (TDF), is crucial for normal male development. ✴✴
>
> ▶ Men with **oligospermia/azoospermia** frequently have microdeletions on the long arm of the Y chromosome that involve one or more of the azoospermia factor (AZF) genes.

⮣ **Genetic Imprinting (High Yield for AIIMS/AIPGME/DNB 2012-2013)**

> **Imprinting disorders result from an imbalance of active copies of a given gene, which can occur for several reasons**
>
> ✴ Prader-Willi syndrome and Angelman's syndrome are classical, e.g. diseases of genomic imprinting.
>
> ✴ Involves different mechanism:
>
> ✴ Microdeletions of chromosome 15q11-12:
>
> ✴ The microdeletion in **Prader-Willi syndrome** is always on the <u>paternally</u> derived chromosome 15.

> **The Prader-Willi syndrome** is a congenital disorder due to a **deletion in chromosome 15,** which includes **mental retardation, hypogonadism, and hyperphagia, (With raised Gherlin levels) often with massive obesity.** It is characterized by **hypotonia, obesity, short stature, mental deficiency, hypogonadism, and small hands and feet.** About half have a chromosome 15 deletion.   **AIIMS 2011**
>
> ✴ **Whereas in Angelman syndrome it is on the <u>maternal</u> copy.**

> **Increasing maternal age leads** to an increased risk of chromosomal anomalies in the fetus.
> These anomalies include
>
> ⇀ Trisomy 13,
> ⇀ Trisomy 18, and
> ⇀ Trisomy 21
> ⇀ Increased rates of the sex chromosome aneuploidies 47 XXY and 47 XXX
>
> Paternal age has not been shown to be related to chromosomal anomalies. There is evidence that **advanced paternal age is linked to an increased risk** of autosomal dominant mutations, which lead to diseases such as
>
> ⇀ Neurofibromatosis,
> ⇀ Achondroplasia,
> ⇀ Apert syndrome, and
> ⇀ Marfan syndrome.
> ⇀ X chromosome mutations that are transmitted through carrier daughters to affected grandsons.

| Trinucleotide repeat disorders: |

⊃ (High Yield for 2011/2012)

✓ A number of diseases are caused by a mutation that is an expansion of a repetitive sequence of three nucleotides which is genetically unstable.

✓ When repeat length increases from one generation to the next, disease manifestations may worsen or be observed at an earlier age; this phenomenon is referred to as **anticipation.**✱✱

Conditions include:

☐ Huntington's disease   PSC 2002

☐ Myotonic dystrophy

☐ Fragile X Syndrome   UP 01

☐ Kennedys Syndrome

☐ Some forms of Spino cerebellar Ataxia

⊃ Mitochondrial DNA: (High Yield for 2011/2012)

▶ **Mutation rate about ten times greater** than nuclear DNA."

▶ This is because there are no introns and a mutation invariably strikes a coding sequence (axon)."

▶ Tissues with **greatest ATP requirement** (CNS, Skeletal muscle, Heart muscle, Kidney, Liver) are most affected.

▶ Mitochondrial DNA is **maternally inherited** because mitochondria from sperms do not enter the fertilized egg.

▶ Mitochondrial DNA is Closed and **circular** and 16.5 kb in length.   AI 2006

▶ **MELAS** (Mitochondrial Encephalopathy, Lactic Acidosis and Stroke like episodes) are attributed to

Mitochondrial mutations. Other diseases associated with mt DNA are:

➥ Lebers Hereditary Optic Neuropathy.

➥ MELAS (mitochondrial encephalopathy with lactic acidosis and stroke like episodes)

➥ Myopathy✱

➥ MERRF Syndrome :(myoclonic epilepsy and ragged red fibres.)

➥ Cardiomyopathy

➥ Strokes

➥ Lactic acidosis

➥ External Ophthalmoplegia

➥ Optic atrophy

➥ NARP (Neuropathy, ataxia and retinitis pigmentosa)   AIPGMEE 2011

➥ Pearsons syndrome.

➥ Sensorineural deafness

➥ Diabetes mellitus

⊃ **"Commonly" asked Terminology (High Yield for 2011/2012)**

☐ **"Allelic Heterogeneity"** refers to the fact that <u>different mutations in the same genetic locus</u> can cause an <u>identical or similar phenotype</u>. For example, many different mutations of the b-globin locus can cause b-thalassemia ✶✶   **COMED 2003**

☐ **"Phenotypic Heterogeneity"** occurs when **more <u>than one phenotype is caused by allelic mutations (e.g., different mutations in the same gene).</u>** Eg: Similarly, identical mutations in the FGFR2 gene can result in very distinct phenotypes: Crouzon syndrome (craniofacial synostosis), or Pfeiffer syndrome (acrocephalo polysyndactyly).✶✶   **KAR 01**

☐ **"Locus or Nonallelic Heterogeneity"** and Phenocopies: refers to the situation in which a <u>similar disease phenotype results from mutations at different genetic loci.</u> For example, osteogenesis imperfecta can arise from mutations in two different procollagen genes (COL1A1 or COL1A2) that are located on different chromosomes ✶

☐ **"Variable Expressivity"** and Incomplete Penetrance: The <u>same genetic mutation causes a phenotypic spectrum illustrating the phenomenon of variable expressivity</u>.eg:. MEN-1 illustrates several of these features. Families with this autosomal dominant disorder develop tumors of the parathyroid gland, endocrine pancreas, and the pituitary gland. However, the pattern of tumors in the different glands, the age at which tumors develop, and the types of hormones produced vary among affected individuals, even within a given family✶✶

☐ **Penetrance:** is the **probability of expressing the phenotype given a defined genotype**; it can be complete or incomplete. For example, hypertrophic obstructive cardiomyopathy (HOCM) caused by mutations in the myosin heavy chain b gene is a dominant disorder with clinical features in only a subset of patients who carry the **mutation. Patients who have the mutation but no evidence of the disease** can still transmit the disorder to subsequent generations. In this situation, the disorder is said to be nonpenetrant or incompletely penetrant.✶✶

⊃ **Isotype Sswitching High Yield for 2011/2012**

➡ Isotype switching is a **biological mechanism that changes a B cell's production of antibody from one class to another, for example IgM in primary response to IgG in secondary response.**

➡ During this process the **constant region portion of the antibody heavy chain is changed,** but the variable region of the heavy chain stays the same.

➡ **Complement binding site on heavy chain of IgG IS CH2**   **JK BOPEE 2012**

➡ Since the variable region does not change, **class switching does not effect antigen specificity.**

➡ Instead, the antibody retains affinity for the same antigen, but can interact with different effector molecules.

⇨ **Sequence of events in activation of B and T cells respectively**

- Immature dendritic cells in the epidermis are called <u>langerhan cells.</u>
- These **immature dendritic** cells capture the antigen in the epidermis.
- After capturing the antigen these cells secrete cytokines.
- These cytokines cause loss of adhesiveness of dendritic cells.
- Dendritic cells separate from each other and **migrate into lymphatic vessels.**
- In lymphatic vessels **maturation of dendritic cells** take place.
- These mature dendritic cells reach naive T cells in the lymph nodes and present antigen to these cells and activate them.

Superantigen mediated Diseases

✓ Staphylococcal toxic shock syndrome
✓ Streptococcal toxic shock syndrome
✓ Scarlet fever
✓ Atopic Dermatitis
✓ Kawasaki Disease
✓ SIDS (Sudden Infant Death Syndrome)
✓ Crohns Disease

<u>Autoimmune Disorders</u>

- Rheumatoid Arthritis
- -Rheumatic fever
- -Multiple Sclerosis
- -SLE
- -Sjogrens Syndrome
- -Myasthenia Gravis

⇨ **Cluster Designation (CD) Markers:**

CD 3	Pan T cell marker
CD 10	Immature B cell marker
CD 19	Pan B Cell marker — AIIMS 2000
CD 20, 21, 22	B cell markers — AIIMS 2007
CD 16 and CD 56	NK Cells

6

PATHOLOGY

Chromosomal Involvements (High Yield for 2011/2012)		
☐ Chromosome 1	Neuroblastoma✱✱	
☐ Chromosome 2	Cystinuria ✱	
☐ Chromosome 3	RCC	
☐ Chromosome 4	Huntingtons Chorea✱✱	UPSC 2001
☐ Chromosome 5	FAP, Cri Du Chat✱	KCET 2012
☐ Chromosome 6	HLA/MHC Antigens✱	
☐ Chromosome 7	Cystic Fibrosis✱	AIIMS 1996
☐ Chromosome 8	Osteopetrosis✱	
☐ Chromosome 9	Freidreichs Ataxia✱	
☐ Chromosome 11	Wilms Tumor✱	UP 2005
☐ Chromosome 13	Retinoblastoma✱	

➲ **Chromosomal Disorders: (Higher Magnification for Extra Edge)**

Chromosome 14:

- Krabbes disease
- Niemann pick disease
- Multiple myeloma
- Alpha 1 antitrypsin deficiency
- Familial HOCM
- Congenital hypothyroidism

Chromosome 15:

- Albinism
- Angelman syndrome
- Prader willi syndrome
- Tay Sachs disease.
- Xeroderma pigmentosum
- Marfans syndrome
- Bloom syndrome

Chromosome 16:

- ADPKD
- Alpha thalesemia
- Pseudoxanthoma elasticum

Chromosome 17:

- p53 gene
- Neurofibromatosis 1
- BRCA 1gene
- Medulloblastoma
- Ovarian tumour

6

Chromosome 18:

- De Gruchy syndrome
- Bipolar disorder

Chromosome 19:

- Myotonia dystrophica
- Malignant hyperthermia
- Familial hypercholesterolemia
- Peutz jeghers syndrome

Chromosome 20:

- Severe Combined immunodeficiencydisease (SCID)

Chromosome 21:

- Amyloidosis
- Homocystinuria
- Down syndrome

Chromosome 22:

- Meningioma
- Acoustic neuroma
- Neurofibromatosis 2
- Di George syndrome
- Velocardiofacial syndrome

▶ Gene for **Major Histocompatibility** is carried on chromosome 6.	AIIMS 2008
▶ Gene for **Folate carrier protein** is carried on chromosome 21.	AIIMS 2008
▶ **Cystic fibrosis transmembrane conductance regulator gene** is carried on chromosome 7	UP 2005
▶ **Short arm** of chromosome is p arm	DELHI 2008
▶ **Long arm** of chromosome is q arm.	DELHI 2008
▶ Genes regulating morphogenesis: homeobox genes(HOX)	AIIMS 2002
▶ APC gene is located on chromosome 5	AIIMS 2008
▶ BRCA 1 gene is located on **chromosome 17**	AIIMS 2008

➲ **"Important Points" about Antibodies High yield for AIPGME/AIIMS/PGI 2012- 2013**

IgM,	
➥ **The first Ab formed after primary immunization** (exposure to new Ag), ✳✳	COMED 2008
➥ <u>First antibody</u> to be synthesized by fetus.	JK BOPEE 2011
➥ Exists in a **monomeric or pentameric form** ✳✳and protects the intravascular space from disease.	
➥ The large IgM molecules readily activate complement and serve as opsonizers and agglutinators to assist the phagocytic system to eliminate many kinds of microorganisms.	

6

- Fixes **complement**

- Isohemagglutinins and many Abs to gram-negative organisms are IgM.

- **IgG,**

- **The most prevalent type of Ab**, is found in plasma and extravascular spaces; it is produced when IgM titers begin to decrease after primary immunization. ✳

- IgG is the **major Ig produced after <u>re immunization</u>** (the memory immune response or secondary immune response). ✳

- IgG is the **prime mediator of the memory response** and protects the tissues from bacteria, viruses, and toxins. ✳

- It is the **only Ig that crosses the placenta.** ✳

- IgG subclasses neutralize bacterial toxins, activate complement, and enhance phagocytosis by opsonization.

- **Commercial gamma globulin is almost entirely IgG**, with small amounts of other Igs.✳

- **IgA (secretory Ab)**

- Is found in **mucous secretions (saliva, tears, respiratory, GU and GI tracts, and colostrum)**, where it provides an early antibacterial and antiviral defense. ✳✳

- Secretory IgA is synthesized in the subepithelial regions of the **GI and respiratory tracts** and is present in combination with locally produced secretory component (SC). ✳

- **IgD**

- Is not known to have much biologic activity. Present in serum in extremely low concentrations, it appears on the surface of developing B cells and may be important in their growth and development.

- **IgE**

- **(reaginic, skin-sensitizing, or anaphylactic Ab)**, like IgA, is found primarily in respiratory and GI mucous secretions.✳

- In serum, IgE is present in very low concentrations.

- IgE is elevated in atopic **diseases (eg, allergic asthma, hay fever, and atopic dermatitis)**, parasitic diseases, far-advanced Hodgkin's disease, and IgE-monoclonal myeloma. ✳

- IgE may also have a beneficial role in the **defense against parasites.**

- ☐ IgE - Mediates **reagenic hypersensitivity**☞

- ▶ IgG: This is **major** serum immunoglobulin. ☞☞

- ▶ IgG: is only maternal immunoglobulin that is normally transported **across the placenta** and provides natural passive immunity in newborn. ☞☞

- ▶ IgA: It is the **second most abundant** class of immunoglobulin seen in body fluids such as colostrums, saliva and tears.☞

- ▶ IgM: Is called **'millionaire" molecule**. It is not transported across the placenta hence presence of IgM in the foetus or newborn indicates diagnosis of congenital infection such as syphilis, rubella, HIV and toxoplasmosis.☞

▶ IgM antibodies are short lived, hence their presence in serum indicates **recent infection.**☞

▶ IgE:- greatly elevated in **atopic (Type I allergy) conditions** such as asthma, hay fever, eczema, and also in children having high load of intestinal parasites. ☞

Interferons

⇨ **IFN-Alpha**

❑ Produced by **leucocytes**☞☞	AP 2006
❑ Antiviral action	
❑ Useful in **hepatitis B & C, Kaposi's sarcoma, metastatic renal cell cancer, hairy cell leukaemia**✱✱✱	

⇨ **IFN-beta**

❑ Produced by **fibroblasts**☞☞	AI PGEE 2001
❑ Antiviral action	
❑ Reduces the frequency of exacerbations in patients with **relapsing-remitting MS**	

⇨ **IFN-gamma**

❑ Produced by **T lymphocytes & NK cells**☞☞	AI 2005
❑ Weaker antiviral action, more of a role in immunomodulation particularly macrophage activation	
❑ May be useful in **Chronic granulomatous disease**	

➲ **Interleukins**

▶ **IL1 causes fever**☞☞	MAH 2012
▶ **IL2 T cell stimulation**☞☞	
▶ **IL3 Bone Marrow stimulation**☞☞	
▶ **IL4 IgE Stimulation**☞	
▶ **IL5 IgA Stimulation**☞	

⇨ **Functions of Different Complement Components:**

❑ Opsonization (C3 b)☞☞	JK BOPEE 2011
❑ Chemotaxis (C5a)☞	JK BOPEE2007
❑ Anaphylotoxin (C3a,C4a,C5a)☞	
❑ Cytolysis (insertion of C5b, 6,7,8,9 into the cell membrane)☞	
❑ enhancement of antibody production (C3b)☞	

⇨ **Complement System:**

Functions of Complement
➡ Lysis of cells, bacteria, and viruses
➡ Opsonization
➡ Binding to specific complement receptors on cells of the immune system,
➡ Triggering specific cell functions, inflammation, and secretion of immunoregulatory molecules.
➡ Immune clearance, which removes immune complexes from the circulation and deposits them in the spleen and liver.

Oncogenes
➡ Oncogenes are regulatory genes
➡ Activity is abnormally increased after a genetic alteration
➡ Oncogene activation may occur after
• Chromosomal translocation
• Gene amplification
• Mutation within coding sequence of oncogene
➡ Oncogenes act in a dominant fashion
➡ Examples of oncogenes include:
➡ ras on chromosome 11 - mediates signal transduction
➡ erbB2 on chromosome 7 - growth factor receptor
➡ src on chromosome 20 - tyrosine kinase
▶ myc on chromosome 8 - transcription factor

Tumour suppressor genes
➡ Code for inhibitory proteins
➡ Normal function is to prevent cell growth
➡ In cancer, suppressor function is lost
➡ Most tumour suppressor genes are recessive
➡ Inactivation of tumour suppressor genes can occur by
• Gene mutation causing loss of gene product
• Prevention of binding of a gene product to its target site
• Inactivation by other proteins
➡ Examples of tumour suppressor genes include
▶ Rb on chromosome 13 - control of cell cycle
▶ p53 on chromosome 17 - DNA repair and apoptosis
▶ Bcl2 on chromosome 18 - apoptosis

- ▶ APC on chromosome 5 - regulation of co-transcriptional activators
- ➡ Mutation of tumour suppressor genes is seen in many familial cancers
- ▶ Rb - childhood retinoblastoma
- ▶ p53 - Li-Fraumeni syndrome
- ▶ APC - familial colon cancer
- ▶ BRCA1/2 - familial breast cancer

➲ Tumor Suppressor Genes: (High Yield for 2011/2012)

Tumor suppressor gene	Tumors	
▶ VHL ☞	☐ Von hippel landau disease	COMED 03
▶ WT 1 and 2 ☞	☐ Wilms tumor	
▶ Rb ☞	☐ Retinoblastoma, Osteosarcoma	AI 2005
▶ P53 (Guardian of genome) ✴	☐ Lung, colon, breat Ca ...	
▶ BRCA1 ✴	☐ **Hereditary breast and ovarian ca**	
▶ BRCA2 ✴	☐ **Hereditary breast ca**	MAH 2012
▶ APC ✴	☐ Adenomatous polyps and colon ca	
▶ DCC ✴	☐ Colon ca	
▶ NF1 and NF2 ✴	☐ Neurofibromas	

➲ Protein 53 High Yield for AIPGME/AIIMS/PGI 2012- 2013

- ☐ p53 also known as **protein 53** or **tumor protein 53** is a **transcription factor which in humans is encoded by the TP53 gene.** ☞   AIIMS 2005

- ☐ p53 is important in multicellular organisms, where it **regulates the cell cycle** and thus functions as a **tumor suppressor** that is involved in preventing cancer. ☞☞

- ☐ Acts at G1 S Phase.   AIIMS 2005

- ☐ As such, p53 has been described as
  - ➡ "the guardian of the genome,"
  - ➡ "the guardian angel gene," and the   JIPMER 2003
  - ➡ "master watchman," referring to its role in conserving stability by preventing genome mutation. ☞☞

- ☐ The name p53 is in reference to its **apparent molecular mass**: it runs as a **53 kilodalton (kDa) protein** on SDS-PAGE. ☞

- ☐ In humans, p53 is encoded by the **TP53 gene** (guardian of the cell) located on the short arm of **chromosome 17 (17p13.1).** ☞

- ☐ p53 has many anti-cancer mechanisms:

- ▶ It can activate DNA repair proteins when DNA has sustained damage. ☞

> ► It can induce growth arrest by **holding the cell cycle at the G1/S regulation point** on DNA damage recognition (if it holds the cell here for long enough, the DNA repair proteins will have time to fix the damage and the cell will be allowed to continue the cell cycle.) ☞

> ► It can initiate apoptosis, the programmed cell death, if the DNA damage proves to be irreparable. ☞

⊃ Oncogenes: (High yield for 2011/2012)

✓ RAS: (Signal Transducing Proteins)	AIIMS 2008/ JK BOPEE 2011

- ► K RAS: colon , lung, pancreatic tumors
- ► N RAS: melanoma, AML
- ► H RAS: Bladder, kidney tumors
- ✓ ABL
- ✓ MYC

► C – MYC: Burkitts lymphoma	KCET 2012

- ► N-MYC: Neuroblastoma
- ► L-MYC: Small cell lung cancer
- ► WNT 1
- ► ERB -B2
- ► FOS
- ► JUN
- ► AKTI, AKT2
- ► BRAF

⇨ Immunology

Most potent activator of T cells: Mature dendritic cells AIPGEE 2011 (From Platinum 2010)

- ➥ Dendritic cells: myeloid and/or lymphoid lineage antigen-presenting cells of the adaptive immune system. Immature dendritic cells, or dendritic cell precursors, are key components of the innate immune system by responding to infections with production of high levels of cytokines. Mature Dendritic cells are key initiators both of innate immune responses via cytokine production and of adaptive immune responses via presentation of antigen to T lymphocytes.

- ➥ Large granular lymphocytes: lymphocytes of the innate immune system with azurophilic cytotoxic granules that have NK cell activity capable of killing foreign and host cells with little or no self major histocompatibility complex (MHC) class I molecules.

- ➥ Natural killer cells: large granular lymphocytes that kill target cells that express little or no HLA class I molecules, such as malignantly transformed cells and virally infected cells. NK cells express receptors that inhibit killer cell function when self MHC class is present.

Primary immunodeficiency disorders may be classified according to which component of the immune system they affect

Neutrophil disorders

☐ Chronic granulomatous disease☞☞

☐ Chediak-Higashi syndrome☞

☐ Leukocyte adhesion deficiency☞

B cell disorders

High yield for AIPGME/AIIMS/PGI 2012- 2013

☐ Common variable immunodeficiency☞

☐ Bruton's congenital agammaglobulinaemia☞

☐ IgA deficiency☞

T cell disorders

☐ Di George syndrome☞(Thymic and Parathroid aplasia)   JK BOPEE 2011, 2012

☐ Paracortical hyperplasia of lymph nodes.   JK BOPEE 2012

Combined B and T cell disorders

☐ Severe combined immunodeficiency☞

☐ Ataxic telangiectasia☞

☐ Wiskott-Aldrich syndrome

⇨ **Job's syndrome /Hyperimmunoglobulin E-recurrent infection syndrome**

▶ The hyperimmunoglobulin E-recurrent infection (HIE) syndrome or **Job's syndrome** ☞

▶ Is a rare multisystem disease in which the immune system, bone, teeth, lung and skin are affected. **"Abnormal chemotaxis"** is a variable feature. ☞

▶ The **"cold abscesses"** have been considered a reflection of impaired chemotaxis with too few phagocytes arriving too late, perhaps due to a lymphocyte factor inhibiting chemotaxis. ☞

▶ Serum **IgE elevated**. Other immunoglobulins normal.   **DELHI 2009**

➲ **Abnormal Neutrophil Function (High Yield for 2011/2012)**

⇨ **Disorders of Adhesion**

▶ Two types of **leukocyte adhesion deficiency (LAD)** have been described.☞

▶ **Both are autosomal recessive traits** and result in the inability of neutrophils to exit the circulation to sites of infection, leading to leukocytosis and increased susceptibility to infection Neutrophils (and monocytes) from patients with LAD 1 adhere poorly to endothelial cells and protein-coated surfaces and exhibit **defective spreading, aggregation, and chemotaxis**.

▶ **LAD 1** Patients **have** recurrent bacterial and fungal infections involving skin, oral and genital mucosa, and respiratory and intestinal tracts; persistent leukocytosis (neutrophil counts of 15,000 to 20,000/uL) because **cells do not marginate; and, in severe cases.**

6

▶ A history of delayed separation of the umbilical stump. UPSC 2002

▶ Infections, especially of the skin, may become necrotic with progressively enlarging borders,

▶ Slow healing, and development of dysplastic scars.

▶ The most common bacteria are Staphylococcus aureus and enteric gram-negative bacteria.

▶ LAD 2 is caused by an **abnormality of** <u>CD15,</u> the ligand on neutrophils that interacts with selectins on endothelial cells.☞

⇨ **Disorders of Neutrophil Granules**

▶ The **most common neutrophil** defect is **Myeloperoxidase deficiency**, a primary granule defect inherited as an autosomal recessive trait☞

▶ **Microbicidal activity of neutrophils is delayed** but not absent.

▶ Myeloperoxidase deficiency may make other acquired host defense defects more serious.

▶ An acquired form of myeloperoxidase deficiency occurs in **myelomonocytic leukemia and acute myeloid leukemia.**

⊃ **Chediak-Higashi Syndrome (CHS) (High Yield for 2011/2012)**

▶ **Autosomal recessive inheritance** due to defects in the **lysosomal transport protein LYST, encoded by the gene CHS1 at 1q42.** This protein is required for normal packaging and disbursement of granules☞.

▶ Neutrophils (and all cells containing lysosomes) from patients with CHS characteristically have **large granules.** Patients with CHS have an increased number of infections resulting from many agents.

▶ **CHS neutrophils and monocytes have impaired chemotaxis** and **abnormal rates of microbial killing due to slow rates of fusion of the lysosomal granules with phagosomes.** ☞

▶ <u>NK</u> cell function is also impaired.

▶ Specific granule deficiency is a rare autosomal recessive disease in which the production of secondary granules and their contents, as well as primary granule component defensins, is defective.

▶ The defect in bacterial killing leads to **severe bacterial infections.** ☞

⊃ **Chronic Granulomatous Disease (High Yield for 2011/2012)**

▶ Disorders of **granulocyte and monocyte oxidative metabolism**☞☞

▶ There is **defective neutrophil oxidative metabolism.** ☞

▶ MOST Effective bactericidal system in neutrophils is H_2O_2 MPO HALIDE system. JK BOPEE 2012

▶ Most often CGD is inherited as an **X-linked recessive trait**; 30% of patients inherit the disease in an **autosomal recessive pattern.**

▶ Leukocytes from patients with CGD have **severely diminished hydrogen peroxide production.** AIIMS 1998

▶ Patients with CGD characteristically have increased **numbers of infections due to catalase-positive microorganisms** (organisms that destroy their own hydrogen peroxide). ☞

▶ When patients with CGD become infected, they often have extensive **inflammatory reactions, and lymph node suppuration is common despite the administration of appropriate antibiotics.** ☞☞

- Persistent Neutrophilia with cell counts of 30,000 to 50,000 /microlitreor higher is called "Leukemoid reaction".
- In leukemoid reaction the circulating neutrophils are mature and not clonally derived.

Cyclic Neutropenia: ✳✳

- Is decrease in neutrophils counts at **intervals of 3 weeks** (13-45) days with normal periods in between.➟➟
- Patients develop **overwhelming infections**.
- It is inherited as **Autosomal Dominant trait.**➟
- It is due to **Neutrophil elastase** gene defect.➟➟

"Hereditary neutropenias" are rare and may manifest in early childhood as a profound constant neutropenia or agranulocytosis.✳✳

Congenital forms of neutropenia include :

- **Kostmann's syndrome** (neutrophil count <100/uL), which is often fatal; more benign chronic idiopathic neutropenia (neutrophil count of 300 to 1500/uL); ✳

Cartilage-hair hypoplasia syndrome; Shwachman's syndrome✳:

- associated with pancreatic insufficiency; myelokathexis, a congenital disorder characterized by neutrophil degeneration, hypersegmentation, and myeloid hyperplasia in the marrow associated with decreased expression of bcl-XL in myeloid precursors and accelerated apoptosis;
- **Neutropenias associated with other immune defects** (X-linked agammaglobulinemia, ataxia telangiectasia, IgA deficiency). ✳
- The presence of immunoglobulin directed toward neutrophils is seen in **Felty's syndrome: a triad of rheumatoid arthritis, splenomegaly, and Neutropenia**✳

➲ Wiskott - Aldrich Syndrome

- Is an **X-linked recessive syndrome.**
- Is characterized clinically by the **triad of eczema, thrombocytopenic purpura, and undue susceptibility to infection.** **DNB 2011**
- Infections are caused by pneumococci and other bacteria with **polysaccharide capsules**, resulting in episodes of otitis media, pneumonia, meningitis, and sepsis.
- The earliest evidence of immunodeficiency is an **impaired humoral immune response to polysaccharide antigens.**
- The predominant dysgammaglobulinemias are a **low IgM, elevated IgA and IgE, and a normal or slightly low IgG concentration.** The molecular basis of this defect, which had been mapped to a gene encoding a proline-rich protein restricted to cells of lymphocytic megakaryocyte lineages. This protein, named **WASP**, is likely to be a key regulator of lymphocyte and platelet.
- The thrombocytopenia is due to an intrinsic platelet abnormality. **Megakaryocytes are present in normal number in the bone marrow, but platelet size is small.**

Feulgen reaction detects DNA	AIIMS 1984
Downs syndrome: Trisomy 21	NIMHANS 1987
Edwards syndrome: Trisomy 18	AIIMS 1985
Pataus syndrome: Trisomy 13	AIIMS 1986

⇨ **Vessel Disorders**

Large vessel arteritis✱✱
- Giant cell arteritis,
- Takayasus arteritis☛☛

Medium sized vessel arteritis✱✱ COMED 2004
- Poly arteritis nodosa,
- Kawasaki disease☛☛

Small sized vessel arteritis✱✱
- Essential cryoglobinemia,
- Churg strauss syndrome☛
- HSP,
- Microscopic poly angitis,
- Wegners Granulomatosis☛

⇨ **Takayasus Arteritis**

- Also called as "Pulseless Disease" or "Aortic Arch Syndrome"☛☛
- Is a **vasculitis** common in **Asia** especially in **young and middle aged females**, affecting medium to large size arteries including Aorta And its branches.☛
- Characterised by **granulomatous Inflammation leading to arterial thrombosis, stenosis or aneurysm.**☛
- Clinical features are:
- Loss of pulse in upper extremities. (Radial Pulse not felt)☛
- Systemic features: fever, weight loss, arthalgias, fatigue☛
- Anemia and increased ESR.☛
- Visual loss or field defects, retinal heamorrhages☛
- Neurological abnormalities like Headache, plus Chest Pain, Hypertension.☛

⊃ **Polymyositis/Dermatomyositis**

A systemic connective tissue disease characterized by inflammatory and degenerative changes in the **muscles (polymyositis)** and frequently also in **the skin (dermatomyositis),** leading to **symmetric weakness and some degree of muscle atrophy, principally of the limb girdles.**✱✱

⊃ Reiter's Syndrome (RS): High Yield for AIPGME/AIIMS/PGI /KCET 2012-2013

REITER'S SYNDROME (RS)
➥ Arthritis associated with nonbacterial **urethritis or cervicitis, conjunctivitis, and mucocutaneous lesions.**
➥ RS is classified with the **seronegative** spondyloarthropathies
▶ Joint involvement generally is **asymmetric and polyarticular,** occurring in the large joints of the lower extremities as well as the toes. Back pain may occur, usually with more severe disease.
▶ **Enthesopathy** (inflammation at tendinous insertion into bone) is common in RS and other seronegative arthritides; eg., **plantar fasciitis, digital periostitis, Achilles tendinitis.**☞☞
▶ Mucocutaneous lesions--small, painless superficial ulcers--are commonly seen on the oral mucosa, tongue, and glans penis **(balanitis circinata).**☞
▶ Patients may also develop hyperkeratotic skin lesions of the palms and soles and around the nails **(keratoderma blennorrhagica).** ☞
▶ Cardiovascular involvement with **aortitis, aortic insufficiency, and conduction defects** occurs rarely.☞☞

⊃ Temporal Arteritis: (High Yield for AIPGME/AIIMS/PGI/JKBOPEE 2012-2013)

TEMPORAL ARTERITIS (Giant Cell Arteritis; Cranial Arteritis) JK BOPEE 2012
A **chronic inflammatory** disease of large blood vessels, particularly those with a **prominent elastica**, occurring primarily in the elderly.
▶ Giant cell arteritis most often involves **arteries of the carotid system**, particularly the cranial arteries.
▶ Segments of the aorta, its branches, the coronary arteries, and the peripheral arteries may also be affected.
▶ The disease has a predilection for arteries containing elastic tissue; it is rarely seen in veins.
▶ The histologic reaction is a **granulomatous inflammation** of the intima and inner part of the media;
Presentations are diverse, depending on the distribution of the arteritis, but typically include
✓ **severe headache (especially temporal and occipital),** ☞
✓ **scalp tenderness,** ☞
✓ **visual disturbances (amaurosis fugax, diplopia, scotomata, ptosis, and vision blurring).** ☞
✓ **Claudication of the masseter, temporalis, and tongue muscles** are characteristic. ☞
➥ **Blindness due to ischemic optic neuropathy** probably occurs in <= 20% of patients but is infrequent after high dose corticosteroid treatment. On physical examination, there may be **swelling and tenderness** with nodularity over the temporal arteries **and bruits over the large vessels.**✻✻
➥ **ESR is usually markedly elevated** (often >100 mm/h, Westergren) during the active phase, but is normal in about 1% of patients. ✻ UPSC 2001
➥ **Normochromic and normocytic anemia** is often present and, at times, profound. Alkaline phosphatase may be elevated. Other nonspecific findings include "**polyclonal hyperglobulinemia and leukocytosis.**"✻

PATHOLOGY

6

- ▶ Wegners granulomatosis: necrotizing lesions in upper respiratory tract and kidney.
- ▶ Henon scholein purpura: IgA deposits with vasculitis
- ▶ Churg strauss syndrome: asthma plus blood eosinophilia
- ▶ Kawasakis disease: in children
- ▶ Takayasus arteritis: in young patients
- ▶ Giant cell arteritis: in older patients

Pathological feature of malignant hypertension: fibrinoid necrosis.	APGI 1986

⊃ Aneurysms

Pseudo aneurysm also known as **false aneurysm** is usually as a result of trauma to all the three layers of the artery resulting in hametaoma. ✱✱ **JK BOPEE 2009**

- ➥ This haematoma **must communicate** with artery to be considered as a pseudoaneurysm.
- ➥ Pseudoaneurysm differs from true aneurysm in that it **does not contain** any vessel wall.
- ➥ **Penetrating trauma** is the most common cause of pseudoaneurysm.

⇨ Other Causes are:

- ➥ Marfans syndrome
- ➥ Fibromuscular Dysplasia
- ➥ Vasculitis

⇨ Pulsatile mass is the most common manifestation. Locations of Pseudoaneurysms:

- ➥ Femoral artery
- ➥ Left Ventricular Pseudoaneurysm
- ➥ Abdomonal Aorta Pseudoaneurysm
- ➥ Carotid Pseudoaneurysm

- ▶ The most common type of "**true aneurysm**" is fusiform type. ➹➹
- ▶ The most common site of **arterial aneurysm** is <u>Infra renal</u> part of Abdominal Aorta. ➹➹
- ▶ Popliteal Aneurysms are the **most common Peripheral** aneurysms. ➹
- ▶ The most common site for **dissecting aneurysms** is Ascending Aorta. ➹
- ▶ "Cirsoid aneurysms" are common in superficial temporal artery. ➹
- ▶ Atherosclerosis is the mc cause of Abdominal aneurysms   **AIIMS 1991**
- ▶ Atherosclerosis is the mc cause of any aneurysm   **AI 1998**

Types of aneurysms:

- ☐ **Berry aneurysm**: occurs in circle of willis➹➹
- ☐ **Micro aneurysms**: seen in Diabetes and Hypertension➹
- ☐ **Mycotic aneurysms**: are seen in <u>bacterial</u> infections.➹➹➹

6

☐ Aortic dissecting Aneurysms: Due to degeneration of tunica media	
Occur in Marfans Syndrome and Hypertension.	
☐ Syphilitic aneurysms or Luetic aneurysms: involve **ascending Aorta**	AI 1988
☐ **Tree bark** calcification is seen in syphilis	JIPMER 1993

⇨ **Pericarditis:**

— **Fibrinous and serofibrinous pericarditis** may follow acute myocardial infarction (Dressler's syndrome) and can be seen in uremia, chest radiation, rheumatic fever, systemic lupus erythematosus, and following chest trauma (including chest surgery) or chest radiation.

— **Caseous pericarditis** is generally due to tuberculosis.

— **Hemorrhagic pericarditis** can be seen with tuberculosis, malignant tumors, patients with bleeding diatheses, and following chest surgery.

— **Purulent pericarditis** is seen when pyogenic infections involve the pericardium, e.g., after cardiothoracic surgery.

— **Serous pericarditis** is seen in non-infectious inflammations (rheumatic fever, lupus, scleroderma, tumors, and uremia).

⇨ **Rheumatic Heart Disease:**

▶ Preceded by **streptococcal pharyngitis.**	
▶ **Aschoff bodies** are a feature.	PGI 2007
▶ **Anitschowk cells/ caterpillar cells** are seen.	DELHI 2006
▶ Pancarditis	
▶ **Bread and butter** pericarditis.	
▶ Vegetation along **line of closure of valves.**	
▶ Sub endocardial **Mc Callums** patches present.	
▶ Mc cause of mitral stenosis.	
▶ ASLO titers used in diagnosis.	DNB 2004
▶ Tricuspid valve is least commonly involved.	DNB 2008
▶ MC cause of MS is rheumatic fever.	UP 2002

☐ Mc Callums Patch	▶ Lesions of Mural endocardium ▶ Deposition of Aschoff Bodiies occurs here ▶ Site of Thrombus formation
☐ Aschoff Bodies JKHND 2003	▶ Present in Perivascular connective tissue ▶ Feature of Rheumatic heart disease
☐ Anitschow myocytes	▶ Modified cardiac mesenchymal cells with caterpillar nuclei, ↑cytoplasm.
☐ Aschoff cells	▶ Multinucleated giant cells

⊃ Feature of Rheumatization: High Yield for AIPGME/AIIMS/PGI/DNB 2012-2013

➡ Fusion and shortening of chordae tendinae	PGI 2011
➡ Calcification of valve	
➡ Annular involvement	AIIMS 2011

▶ **Chronic RHD** is characterized by organization of the acute inflammation and subsequent scarring.

▶ The cardinal anatomic changes of the mitral (or tricuspid) valve include **leaflet thickening, commissural fusion and shortening, and thickening and fusion of the chordae tendineae.**

▶ Fibrous bridging across the valvular commissures and calcification create "fish mouth" or "buttonhole" stenoses.

▶ Microscopically there is neovascularization with diffuse fibrosis that obliterates the normal leaflet architecture. Aschoff bodies are replaced by fibrous scar, so diagnostic forms of these lesions are rarely seen in chronic RHD.

⇨ Myocarditis

Can be caused by a variety of conditions such as a virus, sarcoidosis, and immune diseases (such as systemic lupus, etc.), pregnancy, and others. The most common cause of myocarditis is infection of the heart muscle by a virus. **Coxsackievirus B is the most common** culprit in the United States. Viruses capable of causing myocarditis include.

JK 2009

▶ **Coxsackievirus types A and B (especially type B)**
▶ Adenovirus (most commonly types 2 and 5)
▶ Cytomegalovirus
▶ Echovirus
▶ Epstein-Barr virus
▶ Hepatitis C virus
▶ Herpes virus
▶ Human immunodeficiency virus
▶ Influenza and parainfluenza
▶ Measles
▶ Mumps, associated with endocardial fibroelastosis (EFE)
▶ Parvovirus B19
▶ Poliomyelitis virus
▶ Rubella
▶ Varicella

HIV infection - About 10 percent of people with HIV develop myocarditis,

➡ **Bacterial infection** - Rarely, myocarditis occurs as a complication of endocarditis, an infection of the heart valves and the lining inside the heart's chambers caused by bacteria. Some common bacteria responsible for myocarditis include Staphylococcus aureus, enterococci and **Corynebacterium diphtheriae**   **KAR 2005**

➡ **Chagas' disease** - This infection, caused by the protozoan Trypanosoma cruzi, is transmitted by an insect bite. In the United States, myocarditis caused by Chagas' disease is most common among travelers or immigrants from Central and South America. In up to one-third of people with Chagas' disease, a form of chronic myocarditis develops many years after the initial infection. This chronic myocarditis leads to significant destruction of heart muscle with progressive heart failure.

➡ **Lyme myocarditis** - Lyme disease, an infection caused by the tick-borne bacterium Borrelia burgdorferi, causes myocarditis or other heart problems in about 10 percent of patients.

➡ **Giant cell myocarditis** - This rare form of myocarditis takes its name from large, abnormal giant cells that are found when a piece of the affected heart muscle is examined under a microscope. Giant-cell myocarditis is most common among patients suffering from thymoma, **systemic lupus erythematosus** (SLE or lupus), or thyrotoxicosis   **KAR 2005**

Other agents - Myocarditis also can be caused by :

Alcohol, radiation, chemicals (hydrocarbons and arsenic), and drugs, including doxorubicin Adriamycin, cyclophosphamide emetine, chloroquine and sulfonamides

"Diphtheria causes myocarditis by virtue of it **exotoxin**. The **flabby, stretched out heart muscle is characteristic of diphtheria** .Because of flabby nature of heart muscle, the myocardial pumping activity is significantly reduced as a result if which **congestive heart failure** occurs within **three weeks** of illness."

➲ Myxoma: High Yield for AIPGME/AIIMS/PGI/KCET/DNB 2012-2013

➡ Myxomas are the **most common type of primary cardiac tumor** in all age groups   **DNB 2004**

➡ **Female** predilection.

➡ Most myxomas are sporadic

➡ <u>NAME syndrome</u> (nevi, atrial **myxoma**, myxoid neurofibroma, and ephelides) or the

➡ <u>LAMB syndrome</u> (lentigines, atrial **myxoma**, and blue nevi).

➡ <u>Carney complex</u>

➡ Pathologically, myxomas are gelatinous structures consisting of **myxoma** cells imbedded in a stroma rich in glycosaminoglycans.

➡ The majority are solitary and located in the atria.

➡ Myxomas commonly present with obstructive, embolic, or constitutional signs and symptoms.

⇨ **Remember the Rare Cardiac Tumors:**

Papillary fibroelastoma: This lesion is not neoplastic, despite the sound of the name.

* It probably results from organized thrombi forming on the endocardial surfaces of the mitral valve or left ventricular cavity.
* Papillary fibroelastomas are usually clinically silent and are discovered at autopsy as an incidental finding.
* The growth consists of a small mass of finger-like projections attached to the mitral valve, without associated valvular or other cardiac abnormalities.
* Histologically, each papillary structure is composed of a core of fibrous tissue lined by thickened endothelium.

Rhabdomyoma is a benign tumor of muscle origin. It can occur as a primary cardiac tumor, typically in infants and children, in whom it may be associated with tuberous sclerosis. It usually occurs in the ventricles.

Rhabdomyosarcoma is a malignant neoplasm that can also occur as a rare primary cardiac tumor. It is of muscle origin and usually affects the right heart.

⇨ **Myocardial Infarction:**

▶ LAD is the mc artery involved.	UP 2006
▶ Enzyme elevated in first two hours is: CPK MB	
▶ Waviness of fibres is the earliest change.	BHR 2003
▶ Coagulation necrosis and neutrophilic infiltration is seen within 1-3 days	DNB 2008
▶ Granulation tissue is seen within 1 week.	AI 2002
▶ Scarring in MI is completed by 3 months.	RJ 2000
▶ Troponin T is a marker of MI	AIIMS 2004/ JK BOPEE 2011

▶ Hyaline arteriosclerosis: benign hypertension	JK BOPEE 2011
▶ Hyperplastic arteriosclerosis: malignant hypertension.	
▶ MC Primary tumor of heart myxoma.	DNB 2004
▶ Libman sacks endocarditis is found in SLE.	UP 2001
▶ Dresselers syndrome is autoimmune.	RJ 2000

⇨ **Respiratory Pathology:**

▶ Pores of Kohn are present in Alveoli.		
▶ Charcoat layden crystals:	Feature of asthma	AIIMS 1985
▶ Curschmanns spirals:	Feature of asthma	AIIMS 1985
▶ Creola bodies:	Feature of asthma	
▶ Reid index is used for	Chronic bronchitis	JIPMER 2001
▶ Blue bloaters:	Chronic bronchitis	
▶ Pink puffers:	Emphysema	

▶ **Emphysema** is defined anatomically as a permanent and destructive enlargement of airspaces distal to the terminal bronchioles without obvious fibrosis and with loss of normal architecture.

▶ α_1 antitrypsin (α_1AT) deficency is associated with **panacinar** emphysema.   AIIMS 1999

▶ Smoking is a cause of emphysema.   TN 2002

⇨ **Sarcoidosis:**

➡ Non caseating granulomas with bilateral hilar lymphadenopathy   AI 1997

➡ Berrylium inhalation mimicks sarcoidosis.   COMED 2005

➡ Is an end stage lung disease.   PGI 2004

➡ Epitheloid cells with no caseation Seen   JIPMER 1998

➡ Sarcoidosis does not involves brain   RJ 2004

➡ Kveim test is used for sarccoidosis   KAR 2006

➤ **Schaumann bodies** (conchlike structures),

➤ **Asteroid bodies** (stellate-like structures), and   DNB 2011

➤ **Residual bodies** (refractile calcium-containing inclusions).

➡ Two syndromes have been identified in the acute group.

➤ **Lofgren's syndrome** includes the complex of **Erythema nodosum** and x-ray findings of **bilateral hilar adenopathy,** often accompanied by joint symptoms, including arthritis at the ankles, knees, wrists, or elbows.

➤ **The Heerfordt-Waldenstrom syndrome** describes individuals with **fever, parotid enlargement, anterior uveitis, and facial nerve palsy**

⊃ **Silicosis: High Yield for AIPGME/AIIMS/PGI/KCET 2012-2013**

✓ Mc occupational disorder.

✓ Crystalline form mc cause.

✓ Upper lobes involved.

✓ **"Eggshell"** pattern.   COMED 2004

✓ Patients with silicosis are at greater risk of acquiring Mycobacterium tuberculosis infections (silicotuberculosis) and atypical mycobacterial infections.   KCET 2012

⊃ **Asbestosis: High Yield for AIPGME/AIIMS/PGI/DNB 2012-2013**

▶ **Asbestos** is a generic term for several different mineral silicates, including chrysolite, amosite, anthophyllite, and crocidolite

▶ **Asbestosis** is a diffuse interstitial fibrosing disease of the lung

▶ Physiologic studies reveal a restrictive pattern with a decrease in lung volumes.

▶ Lower lobes affected commonly.

▶ Asbestos bodies

6

▶ Ferruginous bodies

▶ Laryngeal and colonic cancers associated

▶ **Mesotheliomas,** both pleural and peritoneal, are also associated with asbestos exposure.

Remember:

Asbestos is a generic term that refers to six minerals divided into two groups. Chrysotile belongs to the **serpentine group,** while crocidolite, amosite, anthophyllite, tremolite, and actinolite compose the **amphibole group.** Studies demonstrate that carcinoma of the lung and severity of asbestosis also correlate with lung burden of crocidolite and amosite fibers, supporting the amphibole hypothesis, namely, **that amphibole fibers (crocodilite) are significantly more pathogenic than chrysotile fibers especially for mesotheliomas.** Whereas cigarette smoking and asbestos act synergistically in causing carcinoma of the lung, cigarette smoking does not increase the risk of mesothelioma.   MAH 2012

▶ Intense fibrosis is a pathological feature of mesotheliomas.   PGI 2001

⊃ Coal Worker's Pneumoconiosis (CWP): High Yield for AIPGME/AIIMS/PGI 2012-2013

▶ Coal dust is associated with CWP,

▶ Much of the symptomatology associated with simple <u>CWP</u> appears to be similar and additive to the effects of cigarette smoking on the development of chronic bronchitis and obstructive lung disease

▶ With prolonged exposure, small, rounded, regular opacities, 1 to 5 mm in diameter (nodular pattern). Calcification is generally not seen,

▶ Complicated <u>CWP</u> is manifested by the appearance on the chest radiograph of nodules ranging from 1 cm in diameter to the size of an entire lobe, generally confined to the upper half of the lungs.

▶ Particle size of **1-5 micrometer** is dangerous for pneumoconiosis.   COMED 2008

⊃ Caplan's Syndrome High Yield for AIPGME/AIIMS/PGI 2012-2013

First described in coal miners but subsequently found in patients with a variety of

▶ **Pneumoconioses,**

▶ **Seropositive Rheumatoid arthritis with**

▶ **Characteristic progressive massive fibrosis**

▶ **Beryllium** may produce an acute pneumonitis or, far more commonly, a chronic interstitial pneumonitis. **(BERYLLIOSIS)** Radiodense dusts include iron and iron oxides from welding or silver finishing **(Siderosis)** tin oxide used in metallurgy, color stabilization, printing, and the manufacture of porcelain, glass, and fabric **(Stannosis)** and barium sulfate used as a catalyst for organic reactions, drilling mud components, and electroplating **(Baritosis)**

○ GIT Pathology

Esophageus: High Yield for AIPGME/AIIMS/PGI 2012-2013

► The metaplasia of esophageal squamous epithelium to columnar epithelium (**Barrett's esophagus**) is a complication of severe reflux esophagitis, and it is a risk factor for esophageal adenocarcinoma.   **MAH 2012**

► Barrett's epithelium progresses through a dysplastic stage before developing into adenocarcinoma.

► The etiology of **squamous cell esophageal cancer** is related to   **PGI 05**

► **Excess alcohol consumption and/or cigarette smoking.** ☞

► Ingestion of **nitrites, smoked opiates, and fungal toxins** in pickled vegetables, as well as mucosal damage caused by such physical insults as long-term exposure to **extremely hot tea, the ingestion of lye, radiation-induced strictures, and chronic achalasia.** ☞☞

► The presence of an esophageal web in association with glossitis and iron deficiency(i.e., **Plummer-Vinson or Paterson-Kelly syndrome**) and congenital hyperkeratosis and pitting of the palms and soles (**i.e., tylosis palmaris et plantaris**) have each been linked with squamous cell **esophageal cancer,** ☞☞

► Dietary deficiencies of **molybdenum, zinc, and vitamin A.**

► **Viral Esophagitis Herpes simplex virus (HSV) type 1** occasionally causes esophagitis in immunocompetent individuals, but either **HSV type 1 or HSV type 2** may afflict patients who are immunosuppressed.

► Herpetic vesicles on the nose and lips may provide a clue to the diagnosis. Barium swallow is inadequate to detect early lesions and cannot reliably distinguish HSV infection from other types of infections. Endoscopy shows vesicles and small, discrete, **punched-out superficial ulcerations** ✳✳with or without a fibrinous exudate. In later stages, a diffuse erosive esophagitis develops from enlargement and coalescence of the ulcers. Mucosal cells from a biopsy sample taken at the edge of an ulcer or from a cytologic smear show ballooning degeneration, **ground-glass changes** ✳in the nuclei with eosinophilic intranuclear inclusions (Cowdry type A)✳, and giant cell formation on routine stains.

Viruses causing esophagitis:

► HSV1   **DELHI 2009**

► HSV2

► Varicella zoster   **DELHI 2009**

► CMV   **DELHI 2009**

► HIV

Varicella-zoster virus (VZV) sometimes produces **esophagitis in children with chickenpox** and **adults with herpes zoster.** ✳Esophageal VZV also can be the source of disseminated VZV infection without skin involvement. In an immunocompromised host, VZV esophagitis causes vesicles and confluent ulcers and usually resolves spontaneously, but it may cause necrotizing esophagitis in a severely compromised host.

Cytomegalovirus (CMV) infections occur only in immunocompromised patients. CMV is usually activated from a latent stage or may be acquired from blood product transfusions.

CMV lesions initially appear as <u>serpiginous ulcers</u> in an otherwise normal mucosa. ✳

These may coalesce to form giant ulcers, particularly in the distal esophagus.

► H. **pylori** colonization induces chronic superficial gastritis, which includes both mononuclear and polymorphonuclear cell infiltration of the mucosa.

► Progression to atrophy when H. **pylori** is present. ☞

► Most H. **pylori**-colonized persons do not develop clinical sequelae. ☞

► The two major disease-associated H. **pylori** virulence factors are a <u>vacuolating cytotoxin, VacA</u>, and a group of genes termed the **cag pathogenicity island (cag PaI).** ☞

► H. **pylori** colonization diminishes the number of somatostatin-producing cells; somatostatin-mediated inhibition of gastrin release leads to hypergastrinemia. ☞

► H .pylori is tested by **urease test, culture and biopsy. KCET 2012**

➲ Gastrointestinal Stromal Tumor (GIST)

GIST Tumors: (High Yield for 2011/2012)

- ➼ Originate from the **interstitial cell of cajal (intestinal pacemaker cells)**
- ➼ 70% spindle cells and 30% epithelial cells.
- ➼ **Benign are more frequent** than malignant.
- ➼ Lymph node metastasis is rare.
- ➼ Liver is involved in metastasis.
- ➼ Manifest in fourth decade.
- ➼ Bleeding is the main presentation in gastric GIST, bleeding and obstruction in small intestinal.
- ➼ Expresses **CD117 and CD34.**   JK 2010
- ➼ Treatment margin negative resection and adjuvant therapy with **Imatinib Mesylate.**

Carneys triad:

Gastric GIST+Para ganglioma+pulmonary chondroma.

➲ Intestinal Polyposis and Associations

(This table has been repeated in surgery for revision) V. imp✳: High Yield for AIPGME/AIIMS/PGI 2012-2013

- ☐ **Bessauds-Hillmand-Augier Syndrome.** Sexual infantilism associated with intestinal polyposis.
- ☐ **Carter-Horsley-Hughes Syndrome.** Diffuse polyposis of the small and large intestine.
- ☐ **Cowden's Disease or** <u>Multiple Hamartoma Syndrome</u>.   COMED 2003
- ✓ **Hamartomatous, juvenile, lipomatous, or inflammatory polyps are present mainly in the stomach and colon but are also present in the small intestine.** Benign and malignant breast and thyroid disease are also found in these patients, as well as mucocutaneous lesions, tricholemomas, acral keratoses, and oral papillomas.

❑ **Cronkhite-Canada Syndrome.** This syndrome is characterized by

✓ Generalized gastrointestinal polyposis and

✓ <u>"Ectodermal defects," such as alopecia, excessive skin pigmentations, and nail atrophy.</u> DNB 2001

✓ In the intestinal polyps, dilated cystic glands are found in an edematous lamina propria. Loss of protein from the gut, along with calcium, magnesium, and potassium deficiencies, may occur.

❑ **Familial Polyposis of the Colon.** This syndrome is customarily associated with polyps of the colon, but cases of generalized polyposis have been recorded, with associated malignancy.

❑ **Gardner's Syndrome.** This syndrome is generally characterized by **rectal and colonic polyposis,** but generalized Polyposishas been recorded. These polyps are involved in the development of adenocarcinoma. The syndrome also includes JK BOPEE

✓ **cysts of the skin, ✱✱**

✓ **osteomas, ✱**

✓ **fibrous and fatty tumors of the skin and mesentery,✱**

✓ **follicular odontomas, ✱**

✓ **dentigerous cysts and**

✓ **Changes in the bony structures of the jaws. ✱**

✓ This syndrome is familial and is transmitted as an **autosomal dominant trait. ✱**

❑ **Gordon's Disease.** This is a **protein-losing gastroenteropathy,** usually manifested as Ménétrier's disease, which involves ✱✱✱

✓ **mucosal hypertrophy,**

✓ **hyperplasia of the superficial epithelium,**

✓ **degeneration in the glandular layer, and**

✓ **Hypoproteinemia** due to leakage of proteins through the mucous membranes. A diffuse gastrointestinal polyposis associated with protein loss has also been reported.

❑ **Juvenile Polyposis.** Juvenile polyposis is most commonly found in the colon and rectum, but isolated examples of generalized gastrointestinal polyposis have been reported with and without family history or other congenital abnormalities.

❑ **Muir-Torre Syndrome.** This syndrome was described to include

✓ **sebaceous adenomas,**

✓ **epidermoid cysts, fibromas, desmoids, lipomas, fibrosarcomas, and**

✓ **Leiomyomas with visceral cancers.**

❑ **Peutz-Jeghers Syndrome.** This syndrome is characterized by <u>hamartomatous polyps</u> KAR 2008

❑ Of the gastrointestinal tract (stomach, small bowel, colon) that are associated with **mucocutaneous pigmentation (lips, oral mucosa, fingers, forearm, toes, umbilical area).** The skin pigmentation may fade after puberty, but that of the mucous membrane is retained. UPSC 2003

- ❑ **Rendu-Osler-Weber Disease.** This disease is described as <u>telangiectasia</u> of the nasopharynx or gastrointestinal tract.

- ❑ **Turcot's Syndrome.** Malignant <u>brain tumors</u> are associated with inherited intestinal adenomatous polyposis.

- ❑ **Von Recklinghausen's Disease.** Generalized **neurofibromatosis** with café au lait skin pigmentation may also include **neurofibromas of the gastrointestinal tract.**   PGI 2001

➲ Pathology of Intestinal Diseases: High Yield for AIPGME/AIIMS/PGI 2012-2013

- ❑ **Celiac sprue** is gluten sensitive enteropathy or **non tropical** sprue.✳✳

- ▶ Hypersensitivity to **gluten/gliadin** occurs with **loss of villi and Malabsorption.**✳

- ▶ Genetic predisposition:

- ▶ HLA B8 ,

- ▶ DR 3 and

- ▶ DQ2   AI 2003

- ▶ Pathology: **Loss of villi, increased intraepithelial lymphocytes**

- ▶ **Increased plasma cells in lamina propria**

- ▶ Presentation: Malabsorption, abdominal distension, bloating, diaorrhea, steatorrhea, weight loss.

- ▶ Association with **"dermatitis herpetiformis"**

- ❑ **Tropical sprue:**

- ❑ Malabsorptive disease in tropical regions with unknown etiology.✳✳

Similar features to celiac sprue and **responds to antibiotics, Vitamin B$_{12}$, Folate.**✳

- ❑ **Whipple disease:** Malabsorptive disease caused by **Trophermyma whippeli**✳

- ▶ **PAS positive** ,rod shaped bacilli fill lamina propria ✳

- ▶ Treatment is with **antibiotics**

➲ Inflammatory Bowel Diseases: High Yield for AIPGME/AIIMS/PGI 2012-2013

Ulcerative Colitis	Crohns Disease
❑ Involves rectum always	❑ Involves ileum mostly (JIMPER 91)
❑ **Pipe stem colon** (AI 89)	❑
❑ May cause **"pancolitis"**	❑ Non diffuse involvement
❑ **diffuse involvement**	❑ Called **"regional enteritis"**
❑ Retrograde spread to ileum is **backwash ileitis**	
❑ Disease of continuity	❑ Skip lesions (JIMPER 91)
❑ **Pseudopolyps present** (PGI 88)	❑ Pseudopolyps absent
❑ Limited to mucosa and submucosa	❑ **Transmural inflammation** (JIMPER 98)

☐ Non caseasting granulomas not seen	☐ Non caseasting granulomas seen **JK BOPEE 2012**
☐ Creeping fat not seen	☐ Creeping fat seen **(JK BOPEE)**
☐ Strictures, ulcerations , fistula less frequent	☐ Strictures, ulcerations , fistula frequent
☐ Toxic megacolon occurs	☐ Rare
☐ Malignant transformation +++	☐ Malignant transformation +

➲ **Typhoid Ulcer (AIIMS 87, AI 09)**

▶ Ulceration of **peyers patches**

▶ It is a **longitudinal** ulcer.

▶ Perforates

▶ Stricture formation is **rare**

▶ Mallory bodies are composed of <u>eosinophilic intracytoplasmic inclusions</u>   **UP 2007**

▶ are seen in :

✓ Alcholism,

✓ **Primary** Biliary Cirrhosis,

✓ Wilsons Disease.✱✱

▶ **Mallory Hyaline is absent in:**   **SGPGI 2005**

✓ Hepatitis,

✓ **Secondary** Biliary Cirrhosis,

✓ Fibrosis✱✱✱

▶ **Ito cells** are a source of collagen in Cirrhosis of liver.✱✱

▶ **Nut meg Liver** is due to Chronic passive congestion✱

⇨ **Hepatitis**

☐ **Acute infection:**	HBsAg+, IgM antiHBc+ ☛☛☛
☐ **Resolved infection:**	HBsAg-, IgG antiHBc+ ☛☛
☐ **Vaccination:**	HBsAg-, anti HBs+ ☛☛☛
☐ **Inactive carrier:**	

☛ HBsAg+ Greater than 6 months, ✱✱✱☛

☛ HBeAg-, anti HBe+

☛ HBV DNA < 10^5 copies/ml

☛ Normal liver enzymes

☐ **Chronic Hepatitis:**

☛ HBV DNA> 10^5 copies/ml✱✱✱☛

☛ ↑liver enzymes

☛ Necro inflammation on liver biopsy

⇨ **Features of Acute Hepatitis:**   PGI 2002

- ➥ Zonal necrosis↢↢
- ➥ Bridging hepatic necrosis↢↢
- ➥ Hepatic cell necrosis↢
- ➥ ↑liver size
- ➥ ↑liver redness
- ➥ Kuffer cell hypertrophy and hyperplasia↢
- ➥ Lobular disarray↢
- ➥ Focal necrotic spot
- ➥ Councilman / apoptotic bodies are seen in acute hepatitis.↢↢↢

⇨ **Features of Chronic Hepatitis:**

Chronic <u>Active</u> Hepatitis:

- ➥ <u>Piece meal</u> necrosis↢↢↢
- ➥ <u>Bridging</u> necrosis↢↢
- ➥ Rossette and Pseudo lobule formation↢
- ➥ Ground glass appearance of Hepatocytes
- ➥ Concilman Bodies↢
- ➥ Kuffer cell Hyperplasia↢↢

Chronic <u>Persistent</u> Hepatitis:

- ▶ No piece meal necrosis↢
- ▶ Mononuclear infiltrate confined to portal tract.↢
- ▶ Septae into parenchyma↢

Hepatitis C

The Characteristic lesion is:

- ✓ Paucity of inflammation,↢
- ✓ Increase in activation of sinusoidal linning, ↢
- ✓ Lymphoid aggregates ↢
- ✓ Bile duct damage in portal tracts↢↢
- ✓ Mc cause of <u>post transfusion hepatitis</u>   AIIMS 1998
- ✓ Causes chronic hepatitis.   JK BOPEE 2012

Hepatitis D

- ➥ HDV is "Defective" because it does not have genes for its proteins. ↢↢
- ➥ HDV can replicate in cells only infected with HBV.↢
- ➥ HDV uses surface antigen of HBV (HBsAg) as its envelop protein.↢
- ➥ HBV is a helper virus for HDV.↢

✓ HDV is an enveloped virus.✱

✓ HDV is an RNA virus.✱

✓ Genome of HDV is small and encodes only one protein the delta antigen.✱

✓ HDV genome is a Ribozyme ie has ability to self cleave and self ligate.✱

✓ Infection with hepatitis D can be prevented by vaccinating susceptible persons with hepatitis B vaccine.✱

✓ MC cause of sporadiac cases of hepatitis in adults: hep E	AI 97
✓ Worst prognosis in pregnancy: hep E.	AIIMS 97, AIIMS 95, AI 2000
✓ Most common route of spread of hep E is feco oral.	AI 95

⊃ Alcoholic Hepatitis:

Features of alcoholic hepatitis:

☐ Liver cell necrosis,

☐ Perivenular distribution,

☐ Pericellular fibrosis, infiltration by neutrophils, and Mallory's hyaline.

➡ Neutrophil accumulation is relatively unique to alcoholic injury (most forms of hepatitis display mononuclear cells predominantly) and may contribute to hepatocellular injury. Mallory's hyaline is an eosinophilic intracellular inclusion composed of condensed cytoskeletal filaments.　　MAH 2012

➡ While most typically associated with alcoholic hepatitis, Mallory's hyaline may occasionally be seen in other forms of liver injury, including Indian childhood cirrhosis, morbid obesity, primary biliary cirrhosis, Wilson's disease, and following jejunoileal bypass.

➡ Other common pathologic findings of alcoholic hepatitis include steatosis, bridging necrosis, bile duct proliferation, cholestasis, and mitochondrial enlargement within hepatocytes.

☐ Angiosarcoma liver: ☛☛	Vinyl chloride, Aflatoxin, Thorotrast	JIPMER 1988
☐ Peliosis hepatitis: ☛☛	Steroids, Danazol	
☐ Hepatic vein thrombosis: ☛	OCP, cytotoxic drugs	
☐ Veno occlusive disease: ☛	Pyrozziline alkaloids, cytotoxic drugs	

⇨ Renal System

Renomegaly:✱✱✱　　PGI 2002

► Diabetic nephropathy

► Amyloidosis

► Scleroderma

► Polycystic kidney

► Acute Glomerulonephritis

Contracted Kidney:✳✳✳	
▶ **Chronic** Glomerulonephritis	
▶ Chronic Pyelonephritis	
▶ Benign Nephrosclerosis(B/L)	AI 2005

Flea Bitten Kidney:✳✳✳	AI 1996
▶ Acute Post Streptococcal Glomerulonephritis	
▶ RPGN	
▶ HUS	
▶ TTP	
▶ HSP	
▶ SABE	
▶ Malignant Hypertension	AI 1996

⊃ Differentiate

Nephritic syndrome	Nephritic syndrome
▶ Haematuria	▶ Severe proteinuria
▶ Hypertension	▶ hypoalbumenemia
▶ oliguria	▶ hyperlipidemia
▶ proteinuria	

⊃ Glomerulopathies (High Yield for 2011/2012)

☐ The most frequent cause of nephrotic syndrome in children is **minimal change disease (lipoid nephrosis)**,	
☐ Is characterized by an absence of findings by light microscopy, and	AIIMS 2001
☐ Fusion of epithelial foot processes by electron microscopy. ☛	
☐ **Dense deposits** are seen in type II membranoproliferative glomerulonephritis.☛	
☐ **Mesangial deposits** are a prominent feature of IgA nephropathy and are seen to a lesser degree inseveral other glomerulonephritides.☛	
☐ **Subendothelial** deposits are seen in type I membranoproliferative glomerulonephritis. ☛☛	
☐ **Diffuse involvement is seen in PSGN.**	UP 2001
☐ **Anti GBM antibodies are seen in Good pasteurs syndrome.**	Kol 2005
➡ **Focal segmental glomerulosclerosis is a feature of HIV associated nephropathy.**	
➡ **Collapsing variety of FSGS has worst prognosis.**	AIIMS 2008
➡ **Hypertrophy and necrosis of epithelium are a feature.**	AIIMS 2007

☐ **Sub epithelial humps: PSGN**	JK 2001
☐ **Sub epithelial spikes with M spike: Membranous GN.**	AP 2001

- □ Sub endothelial deposits: lupus nephritis
- □ Spike and dome pattern: Membranous glomeruolonephritis
- □ Lumpy bumpy deposits: RPGN
- □ Tram track appearance: Membranoproliferative GN. ⟶ AP 2005
- □ Crescents: epithelial cells+fibrin+macrophage. SEEN in RPGN ⟶ JK BOPEE 2011 JK BOPEE 2012

⮂ Causes of Low Complement: (High Yield for 2011/2012)

- ▶ Post streptococcal GN. (NON PERSISTENT) — AIIMS 2006
- ▶ Lupus nephritis
- ▶ Cryoglobinemia — AI 2004
- ▶ Bacterial endocarditis — AI 2004
- ▶ Shunt nephritis — AI 2003
- ▶ MP GN
- ▶ Cresentric GN
- ▶ Idiopathic Proliferative GN.
- ▶ Lupus nephritis
- ▶ Shunt nephritis
- ▶ Endocarditis(bacterial) — PGI 2006
- ▶ Sepsis
- ▶ Cryoglbenemia.

⮂ Alports Syndrome (High Yield for 2011/2012)

- ▶ Hereditary Nephritis — PGI 2003
- ▶ Nerve Deafness
- ▶ Eye disorders(Lens Dislocation, Corneal Dystrophy, Posterior cataracts)
- ▶ Foamy cells in interstitium. — PGI 2005
- ▶ Thining of Base ment membrane<100 nm.
- ▶ Mutation in alpha 5 chain of collagen type IV. — AIIMS 2006

⇨ Xanthogranulomatous Pyelonephritis✳

- ▶ Rare type of chronic pyelonephritis
- ▶ Accumulation of **foamy macrophages, plasma cells,lymphocytes**

⇨ Analgesic Nephropathy✳✳

- ▶ Chronic disease due to excessive use of analgesics.
- ▶ Pathological ;lesions: Papillary Necrosis with Chronic Tubulointerstitial nephritis

►	But mc cause of renal pappilary necrosis is **Diabetes mellitus.**	UP 2000
►	**Diabetes mellitus, Analgesics, sickle cell disease** cause necrotizing pappilitis.	AI 2002

6

PATHOLOGY

⊃ **Fibronectin Nephropathy: High Yield for 2011/2012**

- ➥ **Autosomal dominant** mode of inheritance.
- ➥ Presents with **proteinuria and slowly progressive loss of renal function.**
- ➥ The principal light microscopic change is **glomerular enlargement and lobulation resulting from PAS and trichrome-positive mesangial deposits and mild mesangial proliferation.**
- ➥ No specific changes in the **renal tubules, interstitium, and blood vessels.**
- ➥ Special stains for amyloid are negative.
- ➥ By immunofluorescence microscopy, the glomeruli <u>do not stain</u> for immunoglobulin or complement components.
- ➥ The most consistent ultrastructural finding is **large (giant), mesangial and subendothelial electron-dense deposits that mirror the location of the PAS-positive, fibronectin deposits.**
- ➥ Plasma levels of <u>fibronectin are not elevated.</u>

⊃ **Polycystic Kidneys:**

Autosomal Dominant Polycystic Kidney Disease (High Yield for 2011/2012)

❑	**ADPKD-1** accounts for 90% of cases, and the gene has been localized to the <u>short arm</u> of **chromosome 16.** ☞☞	
❑	**ADPKD-2** has been mapped to the <u>long arm</u> of **chromosome 4.** ☞☞	PGI 2001

The protein products of the two genes form the **"Polycystin complex"**, which may regulate cell-cell or cell-matrix interactions. ✻

Pathology :

- ❑ The kidneys are **grossly enlarged**, with multiple cysts studding the surface of the kidney. ✻
- ❑ The cysts contain **straw-colored fluid** that may become hemorrhagic. ✻
- ❑ The cysts are spherical, vary in size from a few millimeters to centimeters, and are distributed evenly throughout the cortex and medulla
- ❑ The remaining renal parenchyma reveals **varying degrees of tubular atrophy, interstitial fibrosis, and nephrosclerosis.**
- ❑ **Colonic diverticulae**
- ❑ **Cysts in other organs**
- ❑ **Berry aneurysm**
- ❑ **Mitral valve prolapsed+Aortic Regurgitation.**

AUTOSOMAL RECESSIVE POLYCYSTIC KIDNEY DISEASE

- ➥ The gene for ARPKD has been localized to **chromosome 6.** ☞☞
- ➥ Hepatic cysts with hepatic fibrosis

➲ Tuberous Sclerosis (High Yield for 2011/2012)

Patients with this multisystem disease most commonly present with skin lesions and benign tumors of the central nervous system).

► **Renal involvement is common;**

► **Angiomyolipomas**✱ are the most frequent abnormality and are usually bilateral.

► **Renal cysts** ✱may be present as well and can give an appearance similar to that of <u>ADPKD</u>.

Histologically, the cysts are unique.

The cyst lining cells are large with an eosinophilic staining cytoplasm and may form hyperplastic nodules that can fill the cyst space.

⇨ Von Hippel-Lindau Disease

This autosomal dominant disease is characterized by

✓ **Hemangioblastomas of the retina and the central nervous system.**

✓ **Renal cysts** ✱occur in the majority of cases and are usually bilateral.

✓ The VHL gene is a tumor-suppressor gene and has been localized to chromosome 3. It is the same gene that is mutated in **sporadic renal cell carcinoma**✱, which may be found in up to 25% of patients with von Hippel-Lindau disease and is frequently multifocal. **COMED 2008**

➲ Medullary Sponge Kidney

❑ Medullary sponge kidney (MSK) is a **congenital disorder.** ☛☛

❑ Although some cases have apparent autosomal dominant inheritance, **most are sporadic.**

❑ **Males and females are affected equally.** ☛

❑ The pathologic lesion is **cystic dilation of the inner medullary and papillary collecting ducts, with collecting diameters ranging from 1 to 5 mm.** ☛

❑ **Bilateral renal involvement is present in 70% of cases**, but not all papillae are equally affected.

❑ **The dilated ducts are lined by cuboidal epithelium** with areas of pseudostratified and stratified squamous epithelium. ☛

❑ **Calculi are frequently found** in the dilated collecting ducts.

➲ Juvenile Nephronophthisis/Medullary Cystic Disease✱✱✱

High Yield for AIPGME/AIIMS/PGI 2012-2013

❑ Juvenile nephronophthisis (JN) and medullary cystic disease (MCD) have similar pathologic findings but differ in inheritance pattern and age of onset.

❑ <u>JN</u> is inherited as an **autosomal <u>recessive</u> disease;**

❑ <u>MCD</u> is an **autosomal <u>dominant</u> disease.**

☐ In both conditions,

▶ The kidneys tend to be <u>small, with cysts throughout the medulla</u>;

▶ The <u>cortex and papilla rarely have cysts</u>.

▶ The cysts originate in the collecting ducts, distal convoluted tubules, and loops of Henle and range in size from 1 to 10 mm.

▶ Sclerotic glomeruli, tubule atrophy, and interstitial fibrosis are frequent findings on biopsy.

JUVENILE NEPHRONOPHTHISIS

☐ Patients with <u>JN</u> present during **childhood** with symptoms of **polyuria, growth retardation, anemia, and progressive renal insufficiency**

☐ Most patients develop <u>ESRD</u> prior to the age of 20;

☐ JN accounts for 2 to 10% of renal failure in children.

☐ **Hepatic fibrosis and cerebellar ataxia** has been reported in association with JN.

☐ JN with **retinal degeneration** is termed the **Senior-Loken syndrome**

MEDULLARY CYSTIC DISEASE

☐ <u>MCD</u> presents in the **third or fourth decade**, though some cases may be diagnosed in the elderly population. Presenting symptoms in MCD are the same as in JN **except for growth retardation**. In addition,

☐ MCD **does not have extrarenal abnormalities.** Severe salt wasting can be seen

☐ Other features of tubule damage are often found, including hyperkalemia and hyperchloremic metabolic acidosis. Proteinuria is mild, and hematuria is rare.

☐ **Renal cell neoplasia** represents a heterogeneous group of tumors with distinct histopathologic, genetic, and clinical features ranging from benign to high-grade malignant.

Categories Include

✓ **Clear cell carcinoma** (MC)   AP 2003
✓ **Papillary**
✓ **Chromophobic tumors**
✓ **Oncocytomas**
✓ **Collecting or Bellini duct tumors**

☐ Clear cell tumors are characterized by tumor cells with clear cytoplasm and consistently show **a deletion of 3p.** ✱

☐ Papillary tumors tend to be **bilateral and multifocal.** Trisomy 7 and/or 17 is most frequent genetic markers. ✱

☐ Chromophobic tumors are characterized by multiple chromosomal losses but **do not exhibit 3p deletions**

☐ **Oncocytomas** have a characteristic morphology including a deeply **eosinophilic cytoplasm, do not exhibit 3p deletions or trisomy 7 or 17, and are considered benign neoplasms.** ✱

☐ **Bellini duct carcinomas are very rare** and are thought to arise from the collecting ducts within the renal medulla. They tend to afflict **younger patients** and are very aggressive tumors. ✱

⊃ **Wegners Granulomatosis**

High Yield for AIPGME/AIIMS/PGI 2012-2013

Wegners Granulomatosis

❑ **Necrotizing vasculitis of <u>small</u> arteries and veins** together with **granuloma formation** that can be either intravascular or extravascular.✹✹

❑ **Lung** involvement: bilateral **nodular cavitary infiltrates**, demonstrate **necrotizing granulomatous vasculitis.**   **PGI 2003**

❑ **The renal biopsy** lesion is that of a <u>pauci-immune necrotizing</u> and crescentic GN.✹   **PGI 2003**

❑ **Lung, nose, kidneys involved.**   **PGI 2006**

❑ **Anti-GBM disease** commonly presents with **hematuria, nephritic urinary sediment, subnephrotic proteinuria,**

❑ **Rapidly progressive renal failure over weeks, with or without pulmonary hemorrhage.**✹

When pulmonary hemorrhage occurs, it usually predates nephritis by weeks or months.

Hemoptysis can vary from fluffy pulmonary infiltrates on Chest x-ray and mild dyspnea on exertion to Life-threatening pulmonary hemorrhage.

❑ **Renal biopsy** is the **gold standard** ✹ for diagnosis of anti-GBM nephritis.

❑ The typical morphologic pattern on light. Microscopy is diffuse proliferative glomerulonephritis, with focal necrotizing lesions and crescents in >50% of glomeruli (**crescentic glomerulonephritis**).

❑ **Immunofluorescence microscopy** reveals **linear ribbon-like deposition of IgG along the GBM** ✹✹

⇨ **Catheter-Associated UTIs**

❑ Bacteriuria develops in at least **10 to 15% of hospitalized patients** with indwelling urethral catheters.✹

❑ **E. coli, Proteus, Pseudomonas, Klebsiella, Serratia, staphylococci, enterococci, and Candida** usually **cause these infections**✹

❑ Infection occurs when bacteria reach the bladder by one of two routes: by migrating through the column of urine in the catheter lumen (**intraluminal route**) or by moving up the mucous sheath outside the catheter (**periurethral route**).

❑ Clinically, most catheter-associated infections cause minimal symptoms and no fever and often resolve after withdrawal of the catheter.

❑ Catheter-associated <u>UTIs</u> can sometimes be prevented in patients catheterized for 2 weeks by use of a **sterile closed collecting system**, by attention to **aseptic technique during insertion** and **care of the catheter**, and by measures to minimize cross-infection. Other preventive approaches, including ✐✐

✓ **short courses of systemic antimicrobial therapy,**

✓   topical **application of periurethral antimicrobial ointments,**

✓ **use of preconnected catheter-drainage tube units,**

✓   **use of catheters impregnated with antimicrobial agents,** and

✓ addition **of antimicrobial drugs to the drainage bag,**

6

PATHOLOGY

▶ Bilateral renal cell carcinomas can be a feature of Von Hippel Lindau disease.   **COMED 2008**

▶ Kimlstein wilson lesions: feature of diabetic nephropathy.   **AI 1988**

Finnish type of nephritic syndrome is due to mutation of nephrin.   **AI 2006**

MC gene defect in steroid resistant nephritic syndrome is: NPHS 2.   **AIIMS 2007**

Michaels Guttaman bodies are seen in: Malakoplakia.   **AIIMS 2007**

Salt losing nephritis is interstitial nephritis.   **UP 2000**

Thin membrane disease is benign familial haematuria.

⇨ **Thyroid pathology**

Primary hyperthyroidism: TSH ↓, T4↑

Secondary hyperthyroidism: TSH ↑

Hypothyroidism: TSH ↑

⇨ **Hashimotos Thyroiditis:**

Mc type

Mc cause of hypothyroidism

Mc in females

▶ Anti TSH receptor antibodies

▶ Anti thyroglobulin antibodies

▶ Anti thyroid peroxidase antibodies

Hurthle cells seen.

⇨ **Malignant Solitary Thyroid Nodule:**

▶ Male

▶ Young

▶ Solitary nodule

▶ Cold on radioactive scan

▶ Radiation exposure to head and neck.

⇨ **Pappilary ca Thyroid:**

▶ Mc type

▶ Spread by lymphatics   **KOLK 2005**

▶ Psammoma bodies seen   **AP 2002**

▶ Orphan annie eyed nuclei seen

▶ Develops in thyroglossal tract

▶ Associated with dystrophic calcification

▶ Least malignant

⇨ **Follicularhca Thyroid:**

▶ Second mc tumor of thyroid

▶ Haematogeneous spread

▶ Diagnosis by biopsy not FNAC

▶ Hurthle cell ca is a variant.   KOL 2005

⇨ **Medullary ca thyroid:**

▶ Arises from <u>parafollicular cells C cells</u>   Kolk 2005

▶ Secrete <u>calcitonin</u>

▶ Associated with <u>MEN II</u>   AI 2003

▶ Amyloid stroma   JK BOPEE 2012

▶ RET protooncogene involved   AI 2004, AIIMS 2005

⊃ **Anaplastic Ca:**

Worst Prognosis

⇨ **Struma Ovary:**

▶ Is composed of mature thyroid tissue,   KAR 2006

▶ Usually a teratoma

▶ May present with hyperthyroidism

⇨ **Phaeochromocytoma:**

Sweating, tachycardia, palpitations, hypertension are features.

MC site: adrenal glands

<u>Zellaballen</u>(Cluster of Cell nests is a feature)   MAH 2012

▶ Bilaterality: 10%   AP 2006

▶ Extraadrenal: 10%

▶ Malignant: 10%

▶ Children : 10%

▶ Familial: 10%

Immunomarkers:

✓ Chromogranin

✓ Synaptophysin

✓ S 100

Associations:

- ✓ MEN I
- ✓ MEN II
- ✓ MEN III
- ✓ Sturge weber syndrome
- ✓ Von Hippel Landau syndrome
- ✓ Neuro fibromatosis

Diagnosis:

► Tumor location must be known in order to plan the proper surgical route.

► Ninety-five per cent of pheochromocytomas are in the abdomen, and the great majority of these can be visualized by one of three modalities: computed tomographic (CT) scan, magnetic resonance imaging (MRI), or metaiodobenzylguanidine (MIBG) scintigraphy.

► CT and MRI are highly sensitive, although nonspecific, because they visualize any mass lesion, not just pheochromocytomas.

► MIBG scanning is highly specific for chromaffin tissue, although somewhat less sensitive than CT or MRI.

► MIBG, a radiolabeled analogue of guanethidine, is transported into chromaffin cells by the reuptake cell membrane catecholamine carrier. Because it accumulates in chromaffin cells, an MIBG abnormality is extraordinarily specific (about 98%) for pheochromocytoma, although somewhat less sensitive (85 to 90%).
PGI 2011

► MIBG imaging is especially useful for metastatic, recurrent, or extra-adrenal tumors. Indeed, arteriography or venography of the tumor may trigger hypertensive crises.
PGI 2011

➲ Haematology: High Yield for AIPGME/AIIMS/PGI 2012-2013

❏ Uraemia	➥ Burr cells are seen
❏ G6PD deficiency	➥ Bite cells (JIPMER 05)
❏ Hemet cells	➥ Hemolytic Uremic Syndrome (AIIMS 80)
❏ Cirrhosis	➥ Spur cells are seen
❏ Iron depletion	➥ Seen in Iron deficiency anaemia, polycythemia vera
❏ Thalassemia minor	➥ Decreased osmolysis, microcytic hypochromic anaemia, increased HbA2.
❏ Sickle cell anaemia	➥ Tactoids and sickling seen.
❏ Acquired spherocytosis	➥ Schistocytes present, Coombs positive (Orrisa 05)
❏ Hereditary spherocytosis	➥ Coombs negative
❏ Aplastic anaemia	➥ Platelets maximum affected and last to recover, Pancytopenia present

☐ Pernicious anaemia and Folate deficiency anaemia	➡ Anisocytosis, poikilocytosis, fragmented RBC, neutrophil lobes increased, platelets normal. Absolute reticulocyte count low.
☐ Sideroblastic Anaemia	▶ **Ring Sideroblasts** present (These are Iron granules in mitochondria around the nucleus)　　**COMED 2005** Microcytic, hypochromis RBC Macrocytic hypo or normochromic RBC
☐ Polycythemia vera	➡ Increased RBCs, platelets and Leukocytes Splenomegaly Present
☐ Myeloid metaplastia and Myelofibrosis	➡ Giant Platelets Macrocytic Anaemia **'Tear Drop' poikilocytes**　　**DNB 2001** Leukoerythroblastic picture
☐ Megakaryocytosis marrow seen in	➡ Idiopathic Thrombocytopenic purpura Myeloid Metaplasia Polycythemia vera

Remember:

➲ High Yield for AIPGME/AIIMS/PGI 2012-2013

☐ **Faggot Cell:** Is a term used for cells normally found in the hypergranular form of acute promyelocytic leukemia. This term is applied to these blast cells because of the presence of numerous Auer rods in the cytoplasm. The accumulation of these Auer rods gives the appearance of a bundle of sticks, from which the cells are given their name. They are also seen in AML type M3.

☐ **Dohle Bodies:** Irregular grayish or greenish inclusions in the peripheral cytoplasm of neutrophils. They are nuclear remnants that are often seen in association with toxic granules and vacuoles. They may be present in association with burns, trauma, acute or systemic infections, and may be present with exposure to cytotoxic agents (i.e., chemotherapy). They may also be seen during a normal pregnancy.

☐ **Toxic Granulation:** Large dark blue granules in the cytoplasm, associated with severe infection, chemical poisoning, and other toxic states.

☐ **Auer Bodies (Auer Rods):** Unique, pink or red rod-shaped inclusions that are seen in very immature granulocytes ("blasts") in patients with acute non-lymphocytic leukemias (i.e., Acute Myeloid leukemia; AML).

☐ **Pelger-Huet Anamoly:** Hereditary anomaly where neutrophils appear with fewer than two lobes. The nucleus is often in the shape of a peanut or dumbbell, or may consist of two lobes connected with an obvious filament.

☐ **Pseudo-Pelger-Huet anomaly:** An acquired or pseudo-Pelger-Huet anomaly is seen in myelodysplastic disorders and following drug therapy, and may accompany leukemia and certain infections

☐ **Alder-Reilly Granules:** Large, dark leukocyte granules that stain purple. They are indicative of mucopolysaccharidosis (an inherited enzyme deficiency disorder, Hurler's and Hunter's syndromes).

⇨ **Post Spleenectomy Changes:**

▶ Anisocytosis, poikilocytosis	
▶ Macrocytosis	
▶ Howell jolly bodies	RJ 2002
▶ Heinz bodies	UPSC 2001
▶ Target cells	
▶ Pappanhemeir bodies	

▶ Burr cell is seen in uremia	JKHND 2003
▶ Acanthocytes are seen in abetalipoproteinemia.	JKHND 2003
▶ Macroploycytes are seen in megaloblastic anemia	KAR 2004
▶ Hypersegmented neutrophils are seen in megaloblastic anemia.	RJ 2000
▶ Spurr cells are seen in chronic liver disease.	UP 2003

▶ Sickle cell anemia is due to structurally abnormal Hb.	UP 2001
▶ Sickle cell anemia is due to replacement of glutamate by valine.	AI 2003
▶ Hereditary spherocytosis is due to spectrin deficiency.	UP 2001
▶ Basically a CELL MEMBRANE DEFECT.	JK BOPEE 2011
▶ Proteins defective in hereditary spherocytosis are ankyrin, paladin, anion transport protein.	AI 2007
▶ Hereditary spherocytosis is Autosomal dominant.	

❑ Subleukaemic Leukaemia	➡ Abnormal cells present White cell count normal or decreased
❑ Aleukaemic leukaemia	➡ No abnormal cells WBC Count usually decreased below normal Diagnosis from marrow aspiration
❑ Hairy cell leukaemia (B CELL)	➡ **Neutropenia, Splenomegaly, hairy cells seen.** (AI 99)
❑ Acute non- lymphocytic Leukaemia Lymphoblasts Myeloblasts	▶ Total count usually more than 1, 00, 000 Macrocytic Normochromic Anaemia Severe Thrombocytopenia PAS Positive, Sudan black positive, stains with Romanowski stain.
❑ CML	➡ All series of cells seen Myeloblasts greater than 10, ➡ Increased Basophils, eosonophils, thrombocytes
❑ C.L.L (B Cell disease)	➡ Small lymphocytes increased. Blasts are rare. Auto immune hemolytic anaemia present.
❑ Pro- lymphocytic Leukaemia	➡ Large lymphocytes with prominent nucleolus
❑ Eosinophillic Leukaemia	➡ Eosnophils increased
❑ Burkit's lymphoma	➡ "Starry sky" appearance in Lymphnode biopsy

⇨ Causes of Aplastic Anemia:

✓	Drugs(chloramphenicol)	PGI 2003
✓	Viruses	AI 1995
✓	PNH	
✓	Pregnancy	AI 1995
✓	Idiopathic	
✓	Fanconis anemia	
✓	Schwaman Diamond syndrome	
✓	PNH	PGI 2003

⇨ Hemolytic Anemias are Classified As:

— **Intrinsic (intracorpuscular) abnormalities of red cells**

Hereditary

1. **Disorders of red cell membrane cytoskeleton** e.g. spherocytosis
2. **Red cell enzyme deficiencies**
a) Glycolytic enzymes: Pyruvate kinase, hexokinase
b) Enzymes of HMP shunt: G6PD, glutathione synthetase
3. **Disorders of hemoglobin synthesis**
a) Deficient globin synthesis: thalassemia syndrome
b) Haemoglobinopathies: sickle cell, unstable hemoglobin

Acquired

1. Membrane defect: Paroxysmal nocturnal hemoglobinuria

— **Extrinsic (extracorpuscular) abnormalities**

1. **Antibody mediated**
a) Isohemagglutinins: transfusion reaction, erythroblastosis foetalis
b) Autoantibodies: idiopathic(primary), drug associated, SLE
2. **Mechanical trauma to red cells**
a) Microangiopathic hemolytic anemias: TTP, DIC
b) Cardiac traumatic hemolytic anemia
3. **Infections: malaria**

◑ Autoimmune Acquired Hemolytic Anemia

High Yield for AIPGME/AIIMS/PGI 2012-2013

Idiopathic 50%

Secondary 50% They include

— Drugs
— Infections-M Pneumonia, inf. Mononucleosis, CMV
— Chronic lymphocytic leukemia
— Malignant lymphoma
— SLE
— Other autoimmune diseases like RA, chr. Active hepatitis, UC, Ankylosing, Spondylitis
— Miscellaneous- Carcinoma, sarcoidosis

6

⇨ Pan Cytopenia with Hypocellular Marrow:

▶ Acquired aplastic anemia
▶ Fanconis anemia
▶ Aleukemic leukemia

⇨ Pan Cytopenia with Hypercellular Marrow:

▶ Myelodysplastic syndrome	AI 2008
▶ PNH	AII 2007
▶ Megaloblastic anemia.	AIIMS 2007
▶ Myelofibrosis	
▶ Hairy cell leukemia	
▶ Myelopthisis.	

Spleenomegaly is absent in aplastic anemia.	PGI 2005
BMT (bone marrow transplant) is the most effective treatment.	AI 2002

⊃ **Leukemia: High Yield for AIPGME/AIIMS/PGI 2012-2013**

⇨ **Acute Myeloid Leukemia**

☐ **Heredity:** Certain syndromes with somatic cell chromosome aneuploidy, e.g., **Down** (chromosome 21 trisomy), **Klinefelter** (XXY and variants), and **Patau** (chromosome 13 trisomy), are associated with an increased incidence of AML. Inherited diseases with excessive chromatin fragility, e.g.,

▶ Fanconi anemia,	
▶ Bloom syndrome,	JIPMER 1988
▶ Ataxia telangiectasia, and	
▶ Kostmann syndrome, are also associated with AML	

☐ **Radiation Survivors of the atomic bomb explosions** in Japan had an increased incidence of myeloid leukemias that peaked 5 to 7 years after exposure. Therapeutic radiation alone seems to add little risk of AML but can increase the risk in people exposed to alkylating agents

☐ **Chemical and Other Exposures** Exposure to **benzene**, which is used as a solvent in the chemical, plastic, rubber, and pharmaceutical industries, is associated with an increased incidence of AML. **Smoking and exposure to petroleum products, paint, embalming fluids, ethylene oxide, herbicides, and pesticides,** have also been associated with an increased risk of AML.

☐ **Drugs** Anticancer drugs are the leading cause of treatment-associated AML. **Alkylating agents, Topoisomerase II inhibitors, Chloramphenicol, phenylbutazone,** and, less commonly, **chloroquine and methoxypsoralen** can result in bone marrow failure that may evolve into AML.

☐ Chloroma occurs in AML.	PGI 1999
☐ Auer rods seen	PGI 1989

►	Non specific esterase is positive.	PGI 1997
☐	Non specific esterase is NOT positive IN M 6 Type only.	AI 2007
☐	AML with gum infiltration is M4	AIIMS 2008
☐	DIC is seen in APML.	AIIMS 2007
☐	t (15: 17) is seen in APML.	UP 2003
☐	MC type is pre B cell ALL.	

6

PATHOLOGY

➲ CML

- ☐ The diagnosis of CML is established by identifying a clonal expansion of a hematopoietic stem cell possessing a reciprocal translocation between **chromosomes 9 and 22.**
- ☐ This translocation results in the head-to-tail fusion of the breakpoint cluster region (BCR) gene on chromosome 22q11 with the ABL (named after the abelson murine **leukemia** virus) gene located on chromosome 9q34.
- ☐ Basophilic leukocytosis occurs. \hfill UP 2007
- ☐ Untreated, the disease is characterized by the inevitable transition from a chronic phase to an accelerated phase and on to blast crisis.

➲ Chronic Lymphoid Leukemia (CLL)

- ☐ Is the **most prevalent form** of leukemia in western countries.
- It occurs most frequently in **older adults** and is exceedingly rare in children.
- **CLL** is more common in men than in women and more common in whites than in blacks.

➲ Acute Lymphoid Leukemias (ALLs)

- ☐ Acute lymphoid leukemias (ALLs) are **predominantly cancers of children and young adults.**
- ☐ The L3 or Burkitt's leukemia occurring in children in developing countries seems to be associated with infection by the **Epstein-Barr virus (EBV)** in infancy.
- ☐ Childhood ALL occurs more often in **higher socioeconomic** subgroups.
- ☐ Children with **trisomy 21 (Down's syndrome)** have an increased risk for childhood acute lymphoblastic leukemia as well as acute myeloid leukemia.
- ☐ Exposure to **high-energy radiation** in early childhood increases the risk of developing T cell acute lymphoblastic leukemia.

➲ FAB Classification of All:

- ► **L 1** Lymphoblasts with uniform, round nuclei and scant cytoplasm
- ► **L 2** More variability of lymphoblasts; nuclei may be irregular with more cytoplasm than L 1
- ► **L 3** Lymphoblasts have finer nuclear chromatin and blue-to-deep-blue cytoplasm with cytoplasmic vacuolization

➲ FAB Classification of AML:

▶ **M 1** **Undifferentiated myeloblastic**; no cytoplasmic granulation

▶ **M 2** **Differentiated myeloblastic**; a few to many cells may have sparse granulation

▶ **M 3** **Promyelocytic**; granulation typical of promyelocytic morphology

▶ **M 4** **Myelomonoblastic**; mixed myeloblastic and monocytoid morphology

▶ **M 5** **Monoblastic**; pure monoblastic morphology

▶ **M 6** **"Erythroleukemic;"** predominantly immature erythroblastic morphology, sometimes megaloblastic appearance

▶ **M 7** **Megakaryoblastic**; cells have shaggy borders that may show some budding

➲ B Cell Neoplasms:

▶ **CLL**

▶ **Hairy cell leukemia**   **AIIMS 2006**

▶ **Promyelocytic leukemia**

▶ **NHL**

▶ **Mantle cell lymphomas**   **AIIMS 2006**

▶ **Burkitts lymphoma**

➲ T Cell Neoplasms:

▶ **Mediastinal lymphatic leukemia**

▶ **Adult T cell leukemia**

➲ Infectious Mononucleosis: High Yield for AIPGME/AIIMS/PGI 2012-2013

➡ Is the cause of **"heterophile-positive"** infectious mononucleosis (IM), which is

➡ characterized by

✓ fever,

✓ sore throat,

✓ lymphadenopathy, and

✓ **Atypical lymphocytosis.**

➡ The **EBV receptor (CD21)**, present on the surface of B cells and epithelial cells, is also the receptor for the C3d component of complement.

➡ Lymphadenopathy most often affects the posterior cervical nodes but may be generalized. Enlarged lymph nodes are frequently tender and symmetric but are not fixed in place. Pharyngitis, often the most prominent sign, can be accompanied by enlargement of the tonsils with an exudate resembling that of streptococcal pharyngitis.

▶ **A morbilliform or papular rash**, usually on the arms or trunk, develops in about 5% of cases. Most patients treated with **ampicillin** develop a macular rash.

▶ **Erythema nodosum and erythema multiforme** ✱

▶ **Downey cell**✱

▶ **Atypical lymphocytes**✱

▶ **Paul Bunnel test+** ✱   PGI 1986

▶ **Monospot Test +**✱

▶ **Called Kissing Disease**✱

⮑ Other Diseases Associated With EBV Infection

The **X-linked lymphoproliferative syndrome (Duncan's disease)** is a recessive disorder of young boys who have a normal response to childhood infections but develop fatal lymphoproliferative disorders after infection with EBV. ✱✱✱✱

✓ Oral hairy leukoplakia.   AI 2006

✓ Chronic fatigue syndrome

✓ Burkitt's lymphoma   MAHE 2007, KERALA 1997

✓ Anaplastic nasopharyngeal carcinoma EBV has been associated with Hodgkin's disease, especially the mixed-cellularity type   KERALA 1997

✓ Tonsillar carcinoma,

✓ Angioimmunoblastic lymphadenopathy,

✓ Angiocentric nasal NK/T cell immunoproliferative lesions,

✓ T cell lymphoma,

✓ Thymoma,

✓ Gastric carcinoma, and

✓ CNS lymphoma from patients with no underlying immunodeficiency.

⮑ Plasma Cell Dyscrasiasis: KAR 2005

<u>Multiple myeloma:</u>

✓ Mc symptomatic monoclonal gammopathy

▶ <u>Russel bodies</u>   JK BOPEE 2012

▶ <u>Flame cells</u>   JIPMER 1995

▶ <u>Mott cells</u>

▶ <u>Dutcher bodies(Globular inclusions in cytoplasm)</u>   JK BOPEE 2012

✓ Pathological fractures with hyercalcemia with M spike with Bence jones proteins

✓ IL 6 associated with poor prognosis.

✓ Bence Jones proteins are light chains.   AIIMS 1991

- ✓ ↑ Ca
- ✓ ↑ uric acid
- ✓ urea↑   **PGI 1998**
- ► Waldenstroms macroglobunemia: hyperviscocity with ↑IgM
- ► Heavy chain disease
- ► Immune associated amyloidosis
- ► Monoclonal gamma pathy of undetermined significance(MGUS) is the common plasma cell dyscrasia

  JK BOPEE 2012

➲ Recent Hot Topics: High Yield for AIPGME/AIIMS/PGI 2012-2013

Mantle cell lymphoma

- ❏ Makes up ~6% of all **non-Hodgkin's lymphomas.**☞
- ❏ These lymphomas have a characteristic chromosomal translocation, **t(11;14)** ☞
- ❏ The tumor is **a B cell lymphoma**.
- ❏ Mantle cell lymphoma and small lymphocytic lymphoma share a **characteristic expression of CD5. AIIMS 2001**

Present CD 20, CD 43 also.   **AI 2006**

- ❏ Mantle cell lymphoma usually has a **slightly indented nucleus.**☞
- ❏ Express bcl 1 protein called **cyclin D**
- ❏ The most common presentation of mantle cell lymphoma is with **palpable lymphadenopathy, frequently accompanied by systemic symptoms.** ☞☞

Hairy cell leukemia

- ✓ Is a rare disease that presents **predominantly in older males.**☞
- ✓ **B cell neoplasm**   **AI 1999**
- ✓ Typical presentation **involves pancytopenia,** although occasional patients will have a leukemic presentation.
- ✓ **Splenomegaly is usual.** ☞   **AI 2004**
- ✓ The malignant cells appear to have "**hairy**" projections on light and electron microscopy ☞
- ✓ The cells are **tartrate-resistant acid phosphatase positive (TRAP)+.** ☞   **AI 2004**
- ✓ Bone marrow is typically not able to be aspirated, and biopsy shows a pattern of fibrosis with diffuse infiltration by the malignant cells.
- ✓ Patients with this disorder are prone to unusual infections including infection by Mycobacterium avium intracellulare, and vasculitic syndromes have been described.
- ✓ Hairy cell leukemia is responsive to chemotherapy with **interferon, pentostatin, or**
- ✓ **Cladribine** being the usually preferred treatment. (DOC)☞   **AI 1995**

- ❐ **Castleman's disease**, which can present with **localized or disseminated lymphadenopathy**; some patients have systemic symptoms. ✳✳
- ▶ The **disseminated form** is often accompanied by **anemia and polyclonal hypergammaglobulinemia**, and the condition seems to be related to an **overproduction of interleukin 6**, possibly produced by human **herpesvirus 8.**

- ❐ **Rosai-Dorfman's disease** ✳✳
- ▶ **Sinus histiocytosis with massive lymphadenopathy** (usually presents with bulky lymphadenopathy in children or young adults. The disease is usually nonprogressive and self-limited, but patients can manifest autoimmune hemolytic anemia

- ❐ **Mycosis fungoides** is also known as **cutaneous T cell lymphoma.**➤➤
- ▶ Mycosis fungoides is an indolent lymphoma with patients often having **several years of eczematous or dermatitic skin** lesions. The skin lesions progress from **patch stage to plaque stage to cutaneous tumors.** ➤➤➤

- ❐ A particular **syndrome** in patients with this lymphoma involves erythroderma and circulating tumor cells. This is known as **Sezary**'s syndrome.

➲ Hodgkin's Disease:

- ▶ **Bi modal** age distribution. (late 20 and after 50 years)
- ▶ The commonest presentation of Hodgkins Lymphoma is **painless** enlargement of Lymph nodes.
- ▶ Prognosis is **directly proportional** to number of RS cells and **inversely proportional** to number of lymphocytes.
- ▶ Spread is to contigious to **adjacent lymph nodes.**
- ▶ Extranodal spread **is uncommon.**
- ▶ Malignant cell is **Reed Stenberg Cell.** (Owl eyed, bilobed nucleus with prominent nucleoli)
- ▶ RS cells are positive for **CD 15 and CD 30.** (except Lymphocyte Predominant)   **AIPGMEE 2008**
- ▶ CNS involvement is uncommon.   **AI 2000**

- ▶ **Starry sky appearance:** Burkitts Lymphoma   **UP 2007**
- ▶ **Lacunar cells** are seen in nodular sclerosis type of lymphoma.   **MAHE 2007**
- ▶ **Stomach** is the mc site for extranodal NHL.   **TN 2003**
- ▶ **Hilar lymphadenopathy** is a feature of nodular sclerosis type.   **PGI 1981**

➲ Nodular Sclerosing HL

- ✓ **Most common** type   **AI 96**
- ✓ **Most common type** in females

6

PATHOLOGY

✓ <u>Mediastinal involvement</u> common.

✓ <u>Lacunar</u> cell present

➲ Antiphospholipid Antibody Syndrome: High yield for AIPGME/AIIMS/PGI 2012-2013

Antiphospholipid syndrome	**AIIMS 2009**

Arterial thromboses, recurrent fetal loss and thrombocytopenia.

It may occur as primary disorder or secondary to other conditions, **most commonly systemic lupus erythematous(SLE)**

A key point for the exam is to appreciate that antiphospholipid syndrome causes a **paradoxical rise in the APTT.** This is due to an ex-vivo reaction of the lupus anticoagulant autoantibodies with phospholipids involved in the coagulation cascade

Features: can be assymptomatic

➥ Venous/arterial thrombosis NOT BLEEDING	**AIIMS 2009**
➥ Recurrent fetal loss (2nd trimester abortions)	**AIIMS 2009**
➥ Livedo reticularis	
➥ Thrombocytopenia	
➥ Prolonged APTT , Normal PT	**AIIMS 2009**
➥ Other features: pre-eclampsia,	
➥ Pulmonary hypertension	

CNS Pathology:

✓ Macrophage of Brain is	Microglia	**JIPMER 1990**
✓ Complex granular corpuscles are produced by	Microglia	**AI 1991**
✓ Cell not participating in repair after brain infarction is	Fibroblast	

➲ Bacterial Meningitis is Due to:

✓ **In Neonates:** Group B streptococci, E. Coli ☛

✓ **Infants:** H. Influenza ☛☛

✓ **Youg Adults :** Nisseria meningitides ☛

✓ **Elderly:** Strep. pneumoniae ☛☛☛

"Bacterial Meningitis Score" = determined that patients had a very low risk for bacterial meningitis if all of the following were absent: ✳✳✳

▶ Positive CSF gram stain,

▶ CSF absolute neutrophil count (ANC) of ≥ 1000,

▶ CSF protein of ≥ 80 mg/dL, a circulating ANC of ≥ 10,000 cells/microliter (mcL), or a seizure as part of the presentation.

▶ CSF findingsin Tubercular meningitis: increased protein decreased sugar, increased lymphocytes.

AI 2007

▶ CSF findings in pyogenic meningitis: increased protein, decreased sugar.

AI 1998

✓ Features of viral encephalitis:

▶ Perivascular cuffing,

▶ microglial nodules,

▶ neuron loss,

▶ neuronophagia✳

✓ **Viral Meningitis** (Aseptic) is most commonly due to **Enteroviruses.**✳

✓ HSV Virus usually affects **Temporal Lobes.**✳

✓ Negri bodies in **Hippocampus** in Rabies✳

PGI 1991

➲ HIV

☐ Cerebral involvement: AIDS dementia complex☛

☐ Multinucleate giant cells☛

☐ Vacuolar myelopathy☛

⇨ Progressive Multi Focal Leukoencephalopathy

☐ Is due to **Polyoma JC Virus**☛

☐ Is mostly due to immunocompromised states.

☐ **Demyelination and Astrogliosis** are a feature☛

➲ Creutz Feldt Jackobson Disease

☐ **Caused By prion Protein** ☛☛

☐ **Prions are** proteins.

AIIMS 2007

☐ **They are** infectious.

AI 2008

☐ **Most common infectious prion disease in humans**

☐ On light microscopy, the pathologic hallmarks of **CJD** are **spongiform degeneration and astrogliosis.**☛

☐ The lack of an inflammatory response in **CJD** and other prion diseases is an important pathologic feature of these degenerative disorders. ☛☛

☐ Spongiform degeneration is characterized by many 1- to 5-um **vacuoles in the neuropil between nerve cell bodies**☛

☐ **In (New variant) nvCJD,** a characteristic feature is the presence of "**florid plaques.**" These are composed of a central core of PrP amyloid surrounded by vacuoles in a pattern suggesting petals on a flower.☛

⇨ **CJD can Occur Following these Procedures:**

- Corneal transplants
- EEG electrodes
- Dura mater grafts
- Human growth hormones from human pituitaries

⇨ **Diffuse Axonal Injury,**

- Deep white matter lesion consists of widespread **acute disruption, or "shearing,"** of axons at the time of impact.
- Pathologically there are **small areas of tissue disruption in the corpus callosum** and dorsolateral pons.
- The presence of widespread **axonal** damage of both hemispheres, a state called **Diffuse axonal injury**, has been proposed as the explanation of persistent coma or vegetative state, but **small ischemic-hemorrhagic lesions in the midbrain and low diencephalon are as often the cause.**
- Only severe shearing lesions that contain blood are visualized by CT, usually in the corpus callosum and centrum semiovale however, within days of the injury,
- MRI scan demonstrates such lesions throughout the white matter, especially with the use of **gradient echo MRI sequences.**

⇨ **CNS Tumors (Gems about Tumors) (Never Forget)**

Astrocytoma	Oligodendroglioma	Ependymoma
- Origin From astrocytes - **Most common primary brain tumor in adults.** - **GFAP Positive** - **Glioblatoma multi forme** is **grade IV** astrocytoma - **Crosses midline** - **(Butterfly Glioma)** - **Pseudopallisading Necrosis** - Common in white matter	- Origin From oligodendrocytes - **Fried Egg Appearance** - **Chicken wire pattern of capillaries** - Slow growing	- Usually in ventricular system - **Ependymal rosettes** - **Perivascular pseudorossettes** - Often causes hydrocephalus

⇨ **Pathologically Important about Brain Tumors**

- **Oligodendroglioma:** features are: **"fried egg" cells**, which are tumor cells with round nuclei (the "yolk") and cleared cytoplasm (the "white"). These tumors may contain areas of calcification, hemorrhage, or cysts. They tend to occur in the cerebral hemispheres of middle-aged patients of both sexes, and have a better prognosisthan astrocytomas.
- **Choroid plexus papilloma:** features are a **papillary growth in a ventricle.**
- **Ependymoma :** features are **pseudorosettes** and structures resembling ependymal canals.(blephroplasts-remanants of basal body of cilia)

* Glioblastoma multiforme: features are extreme **butterfly** shape, pleomorphism, necrosis, and hemorrhage.

* Pilocytic astrocytoma: features are **bipolar cells**, and location in the cerebellum of young children.

Meningioma	Schwanomma	Craniopharyngioma
➡ Most common **benign brain** tumor	➡ From schwann cells	➡ From **Odontogenic epithelium**
➡ Origin from arachnoid cells	➡ Eighth cranial nerve	➡ Affects young/children
➡ **Whorled pattern**	➡ At **CP angle**	➡ **Calcium deposits** seen
➡ **Psommoma bodies**	➡ **Antoni A and Antoni B areas**	
➡ Good prognosis	➡ **Verocay Bodies**	
	➡ **S 100 positivity**	
	➡ Bilateral →NF 2	

➲ Medulloblastomas High Yield for AIPGME/AIIMS/PGI 2012-2013

➡ Are primitive neuro ectodermal tumors **(PNET)**✸

➡ Arise in cerebellar vermis**(midline)**✸

➡ Responsive to **radiotherapy**✸

➡ These highly cellular malignant tumors are thought to arise from **neural precursor cells.**✸

➡ They are the **most frequent malignant brain tumor of children.**

➡ These tumors frequently disseminate along **CSF pathways.**✸

Remember:

✓ Mc primary brain tumor: glioma.	AIIMS 1994
✓ Mc brain tumor in adults: astrocytoma	AIIMS 1993
✓ Mc type of glial tumor: astrocytoma.	AI 2006
✓ Mc site of brain tumors in children: infratentorial(cerebellar)	
✓ Mc site of brain tumor in neonates: supratentorial.	
✓ Mc posterior fossa tumor in children: cerebellar astrocytoma.	AIIMS 1995
✓ Second mc posterior fossa tumor in children. Medulloblastoma.	

▶ Pseudo rosettes: Neuroblastoma	AP 2002
▶ Enamel like structures: Craniopharyngioma	AP 2001
▶ Glial fibrillary proteins: Astrocytoma	RJ 2006
▶ Verocay bodies: Schwannoma	
▶ Butterfly tumor: Glioblastoma multi forme	
▶ Fried egg appearance: Oligiodendroglioma	

6

➲ High Yield for AIPGME/AIIMS/PGI 2012-2013

Alzhiemers disease	Picks Disease	Lewy Body Disease	Parkinsonism
❑ **Neurofibrillary tangles** are intracytoplasmic filamentous inclusions found in Alzheimer disease and, to a lesser extent, in normal aging brains✳ ❑ **Granulovacuolar degeneration** ✳ ❑ **Hirano Bodies:** They are Specific protein deposits associated with **AGE**(Advance Glycosylation End products) localised within soma of neurons✳ ❑ **Amyloid Plaques:** They represent fragmented accumulations of proteins which are normally broken down but accumulate in Alzheimer's disease.✳ ❑ **Alzhiemers Cells(Special cells)**✳ ❑ **Neurofibrillary tangles:** are insoluble twisted fibrils composed of **Tau proteins** ✳ UP 2007 COMED 2006 PGI 2005 DELHI 1998 JK BOPEE 2006 UPSC 2005	**Swollen or ballooned neurons** contain silver-staining cytoplasmic inclusions referred to as **Pick bodies**✳✳ ▶ walnut brain ▶ knife blade atrophy ▶ balloning degeneration. AI 2004	Lewy bodies are **intraneuronal cytoplasmic inclusions** that stain with **periodic acid-Schiff and ubiquitin.** They contain epitopes recognized by antibodies against phosphorylated and nonphosphorylated neurofilament proteins, ✳**ubiquitin**, and a ✳presynaptic protein called α synuclein AIIMS 2003 SGPGI 03 COMED 2004	**Lewy bodies** ✳are **filamentous inclusions** that appear **brightly eosinophilic** on hematoxylin and eosin stain and accumulate in the cytoplasm of dopaminergic neurons in the **substantia nigra** in Parkinson disease.

Marinesco bodies are also present in the dopaminergic neurons of substantia nigra. They are intranuclear. These inclusions are found occasionally in normal brains, and their significance is unknown.

⇨ Abnormal Protein Aggregates:

▶ Alzhiemers disease:	A beta , tau
▶ Picks disease:	tau
▶ Parkinsons disease, multiple systems atrophy:	alpha synuclein

6

▶	Huntigtons disease:	huntingtin
▶	Spinocerebellar ataxia:	ataxin
▶	Prion disease:	prion protein

⇨ **Berry Aneurysm✱**

☐	Thin walled Saccular out pouching of Tunica intima and adventitia.	
☐	**Most frequent cause of SAH.✱**	
☐	Most frequent site: **Anterior circle of willis✱**	
☐	Least frequent site: posterior circulation.	MAHE 2005
☐	Association with:	
▶	Marfans syndrome,	
▶	Ehler danhlos Syndrome,	
▶	**Adult Polycystic Kidney Disease✱✱**	

⇨ **Multiple Sclerosis**

Multiple sclerosis (MS) is characterized by

(1) A relapsing-remitting or progressive course and

(2) A pathologic triad of <u>CNS</u> **inflammation, demyelination, and gliosis (scarring). ✱**

MS derives its name from the **multiple scarred areas visible on macroscopic examination of the brain.** These lesions, termed **plaques,** are sharply demarcated gray or pink areas easily distinguished from surrounding white matter.☛☛

☐	The acute MS lesion, rarely found at autopsy, consists of **perivenular cuffing** by inflammatory mononuclear cells, predominantly T lymphocytes and macrophages, which also infiltrate white matter tissue and appear to orchestrate demyelination. At sites of inflammation, the blood-brain barrier is disrupted but the vessel wall itself is preserved, distinguishing the MS lesion from vasculitis☛☛
☐	**The correspondence between number and size of plaques ("Plaque burden")** and the severity of clinical symptoms is imprecise. ☛
☐	Axonal loss and cavitation are particularly prominent in the subtype of MS known as **"Neuromyelitis Optica"** or **"Devic's syndrome "**☛☛

⇨ **Clinical Scenarios**

☐	A doctor is concerned about a disease in a child from india affecting **alpha motor neurons** in ventral horn of spinal cord	**Poliomyelitis**
☐	A pathologist is concerned **about an acute , inflammatory disease** causing **demyelination** of peripheral nerves after an infection	**Gullian Barre Syndrome**
☐	A patient is concerned about a disease which causes demyelination of upper motor neurons with a pathologic triad of <u>CNS</u> inflammation, demyelination, and gliosis (scarring) who presented with weakness of muscles and optic neuritis .	**Multiple Sclerosis**

➲ Breast Pathology: High Yield for AIPGME/AIIMS/PGI 2012-2013

▶ MC disorder of breast:	✓ Fibroadenosis ☞☞
▶ MC tumor of breast:	✓ Fibroadenoma ☞
▶ MC carcinoma of breast:	✓ Ductal/ Schirrous carcinoma ☞
▶ Mc bilateral tumor	✓ Lobular carcinoma of breast ☞☞ PGI 2002
▶ Mc inviolved Lymph nodes are	✓ Axillary group.
▶ MC cause of breast discharge:	✓ Duct ectasia ☞
▶ Mc cause of bloody discharge:	✓ Duct pappiloma
▶ Mc site of metastasis of breast ca:	✓ Bone ☞
▶ Mc site of breast ca:	✓ Upper outer quadrant
▶ FIRST INVESTIGATION FOR BREAST LUMP:	✓ FNAC ☞
▶ BEST INVESTIGATION FOR BREAST LUMP:	✓ BIOPSY ☞
▶ BRCA 1 gene is located on chromosome	✓ 17 AIIMS 2008
▶ BRCA 2 gene is located on chromosome	✓ 13
▶ Marker for breast cancer	✓ CA 15-3

➲ Ovarian Tumors

PRIMARY EPITHELIAL TUMOURS 80% MAHE 2007, UPSC 2007	NON-EPITHELIAL TUMORS	HORMONE-PRODUCING TUMOURS
❑ Mucinous Cystadenoma or Cystadenocarcinoma ☞☞	❑ Fibroma	❑ Estrogen- producing ☞☞
❑ Serous Cystadenoma or Cystadenocarcinoma ☞☞	❑ Dysgerminoma	✓ Granulosa cell tumour
❑ Endometrioma or Endometriod Carcinoma ☞☞	❑ Teratoma	✓ Thecoma
	❑ Gonadoblastoma	❑ Androgen -producing ☞☞
❑ Clear cell carcinoma ☞☞	❑ Yolk-sac tumour	✓ Sertoli-Leydig cell tumour
❑ Brenner Tumour ☞☞		✓ (Arrhenoblastoma)
		✓ Hilar cell tumour
		✓ Lipoid cell tumour
		(Ovoblastoma,Musculinovoblastoma,
		✓ Adrenal-like tumour)
		❑ OTHERS
		✓ Carcinoid(Seratonin- producing)
		✓ Thyroid tumour(Struma Ovarii)
		✓ Choriocarcinoma of the ovary

Granulosa cell tumor is a non germ cell tumor. It is a sex cord tumor.

Other sex cord tumors are:

Thecoma and Sertoli Leyding cell tumor.

Tumors may arise from any of the major components of the ovary:

- Surface epithelium, ovarian stromal and follicle lining granulosa cells, or germ cells.
- Epithelial tumors are the most common malignant ovarian tumors and are more common in women older than 40 years of age.
- The major types of epithelial tumors are serous, endometrioid, and mucinous.
- Germ-cell tumors (dysgerminoma), (embryonal), (endodermal sinus tumor), (choriocarcinoma), (teratoma).
- Sex cord stromal tumors may display differentiation toward granulosa, Sertoli, Leydig.

Call Exner Bodies:	PGI 2003	
Renkies Crystals: ☞☞		
Signet ring cells: ☞☞		
Schiller Duval bodies:	UP 2007	
Psommoma bodies: ☞☞		
Meigs syndrome: ☞☞		
Pseudomeigs syndrome: ☞☞		
Walthard cell nest: ☞☞		
Rokintansky bodies: ☞☞		

- Granulosa cell tumor — AIIMS 2001
- Hilus cell tumor — AIIMS 1995
- Krukenbergs tumor
- Endodermal sinus tumor — AMU 2005
- Pappillary Serous tumors
- Fibroma ovary
- Brenner cell tumor
- Brenner tumor
- Teratoma — AMU 2005

➲ Testicular Cancer: High Yield for AIPGME/AIIMS/PGI 2012-2013

- Primary germ cell tumors (GCTs) of the testis constitute 95 percent of all testicular neoplasms. ☞Infrequently, GCTs arise from an extragonadal site, including the
- Mediastinum,
- Retroperitoneum and, very rarely,
- Pineal gland. (Remember the sites).
- Cryptorchidism is associated with a several fold higher risk of GCT. ☞ PGI 2002
- Abdominal cryptorchid testes are at a higher risk than inguinal cryptorchid testes. ☞
- Orchiopexy should be performed before puberty, if possible. ☞
- Testicular feminization syndromes increase the risk of testicular GCT, and ☞ PGI 2002
- Klinefelter's syndrome is associated with mediastinal GCT. PGI 2002
- An isochromosome of the short arm of chromosome 12 is pathognomonic for GCT ☞
- A painless testicular mass is pathognomonic for a testicular malignancy.
- Commonest testicular malignancy is : seminoma
- Most malignant testicular cancer is: Choriocarcinoma
- MC in infants however is yolk sac tumor. JK BOPEE 2012

⊃ Seminoma

- ☐ Has a median age in the **fourth decade,**☞
- ☐ Generally follows a more **indolent clinical course.**
- ☐ Seminomas are **radiosensitive.**☞
- ☐ Seminomas metastasize by **lymphatics.**☞
- ☐ Seminomas correspond to **dysgerminomas of ovary.**   (PGI 99)

⊃ Miscellaneous Hot Topics asked In Previous Examinations

NEUROFIBROMATOSIS TYPE 1 (VON RECKLINGHAUSEN'S DISEASE)

⇨ NF1

- ☐ **Cutaneous neurofibromas,** pigmented lesions of the skin called **cafe au lait spots,** freckling in non-sun exposed areas such as the axilla, **hamartomas** of the iris termed **Lisch nodules,** and **pseudoarthrosis of the tibia.** ☞☞

                                                                      JK BOPEE 2012
- ☐ Neurofibromas are **benign peripheral nerve tumors** composed of **proliferating Schwann cells and fibroblasts.** They present as **multiple, palpable, rubbery, cutaneous tumors.** ☞☞
- ☐ Mutation of the NF1 gene on **chromosome 17** causes von Recklinghausen's disease. ☞
- ☐ **The NF1 gene is a tumor suppressor gene**; it encodes a protein, neurofibromin, which modulates signal transduction through the ras GTPase pathway.
- ☐ Patients with NF1 are at **increased risk of developing nervous system neoplasms,** including plexiform **neurofibromas, optic gliomas, ependymomas, meningiomas, astrocytomas, and pheochromocytomas.** ☞☞
- ☐ Neurofibromas may undergo **secondary malignant degeneration** and become sarcomas.☞☞
- ☐ **Optic nerve glioma** is the one of the mc tumor associated with NF 1.   **AIIMS 2003**

NEUROFIBROMATOSIS TYPE 2

⊃ NF2

- ☐ Is characterized by the development of **bilateral vestibular schwannomas** in 90% of individuals who inherit the gene☞☞.
- ☐ Patients with NF2 also have a predisposition for the development of **meningiomas, gliomas, and schwannomas of cranial and spinal nerves.** ☞
- ☐ In addition, a characteristic type of cataract, **juvenile posterior subcapsular lenticular opacity,** occurs in NF2. Multiple cafe au lait spots and peripheral neurofibromas occur rarely.
- ☐ In patients with NF2, vestibular schwannomas usually present with progressive unilateral deafness early in the third decade of life.
- ☐ Bilateral vestibular schwannomas are generally detectable by MRI.☞
- ☐ The NF2 gene on chromosome 22q codes for a protein called neurofibromin 2, schwannomin, or merlin.☞☞

TUBEROUS SCLEROSIS (BOURNEVILLE'S DISEASE)

- ❑ Is characterized by **cutaneous lesions, seizures, and mental retardation.** ☞☞
- ❑ The cutaneous lesions include
- ✓ **Adenoma sebaceum** (facial angiofibromas, ☞
- ✓ **Ash leaf-shaped hypopigmented macules** (best seen under ultraviolet illumination with a Wood's lamp),
- ✓ **Shagreen patches** (yellowish thickenings of the skin over the lumbosacral region of the back), and
- ✓ **Depigmented nevi.** ☞☞
- ❑ On neuroimaging studies, the presence of subependymal nodules, which may be calcified, is characteristic.
- ❑ Patients inheriting the tuberous sclerosis gene are at increased risk of developing **ependymomas and childhood astrocytomas**, of which 90% are subependymal giant cell astrocytomas. ☞
- ❑ **Rhabdomyomas** of the myocardium and angiomyomas of the kidney, liver, adrenals, and pancreas may also occur. ☞

VON HIPPEL-LINDAU SYNDROME

- ◼ This syndrome consists of **retinal, cerebellar, and spinal hemangioblastomas**, which are slowly growing cystic tumors. ☞
- ✓ **Hypernephroma,**
- ✓ **renal cell carcinoma,**
- ✓ **Pheochromocytoma, and**
- ✓ **Cysts of the kidneys, pancreas, epididymis, or liver may also occur.** ☞
- ◼ Erythropoietin production by hemangioblastomas may result in polycythemia.
- ◼ The von Hippel-Lindau (VHL) is a tumor suppressor gene on chromosome 3p. ☞

⮂ Sturge Weber Syndrome

✓ Port wine stain	DELHI 1996
✓ Cavernous hemangioma	
✓ Seizures	AIIMS 1994
✓ Hemiatrophy of cerebral cortex	AIIMS 1994
✓ Rail road calcifications of cerebral cortex	

Appendegeal tumors

- ❑ Adenexal or Appendegeal tumors arise from **cutaneous appendages.** ☞
- ❑ They may serve as **markers for internal malignancies.**
- ❑ They are mostly in the form of solitary or multiple nodules/papules.
- ❑ <u>**Eccrine porcoma**</u> is seen on palms and soles. ☞☞

- ❏ <u>Cylindroma or turban tumor</u> is seen on forehead and scalp.☞

- ❏ <u>Syringomas</u> are seen in vicinity of lower eyelids☞

- ❏ <u>Trichoepitheliomas and Tricolemmoma</u> arise from hair follicles and are seen on face, scalp, neck and upper trunk.☞

- ❏ <u>Sebaceous adenoma</u> arises from sebaceous glands.☞

- ❏ <u>Brookes tumor</u> from hair follicles   AIIMS 1981

- ▶ Benign fibrous histiocytoma on the other hand is a benign dermal neoplasm.

- ▶ Most common presentation is a dermatofibroma.

- ▶ They are most common in adults with indolent behaviour and appear as tan to brown firm papules

⇨ **Important Pathological Eponyms related to Fruits/ Vegetables**

- ▶ **Potato Nodes:** Sarcoidosis☞ ☞

- ▶ **Potato Tumor:** Chemodectoma☞

- ▶ **Potato / oyster ovary:** PCOD☞

- ▶ **Strawberry Cervix:** Trichomonas Vaginalis☞

- ▶ **Straw berry tongue:** Scarlet fever☞

- ▶ **Strawberry hemangioma:** Nevus vasculosus

- ▶ **Barley coloured fluid cyst:** Spermatocele☞

- ▶ **Apple jelly nodules:** Lupus Vulgaris☞

- ▶ **Apple core lesion:** Ca Colon☞

- ▶ **Raspberry tumor:** Umbilical adenoma☞

- ▶ **Raspberry thorn sign:** Crohns disease☞

- ▶ **Peau de Orange appearance of breast:** Breast Cancer

- ▶ **Orange Tonsils :** Tangiers disease☞

⊃ **Kindly Memorize**

Antibody Target	Disease
❏ Nicotinic acetyl choline receptor	❏ Myasthenia Gravis☞☞
❏ Intrinsic factor	❏ Pernicious Anemia☞
❏ Proiteinase 3 (ANCA)	❏ Wegners Granulomatosis☞
❏ Alpha 3 chain of Collagen Type IV	❏ Good Pasteurs Syndrome☞
❏ Thyroid Peroxidase	❏ Hashimotos Thyroiiditis☞

➲ High Yield for AIPGME/AIIMS/PGI 2012-2013

❏ ANA: SLE✳✳
❏ Anti Smith, anti ds DNA: specific for SLE✳
❏ Anti Histone: Drug induced SLE✳
❏ Anti centromere: CREST Syndrome✳
❏ Anti Scl 70: Scleroderma✳
❏ Anti SSA, Anti SSB: Sjogrens syndrome✳
❏ Anti Jo 1: Polymyositis✳   **AIIMS 2008**
❏ Anti mitochondrial: Primary Biliary Cirrhosis✳
❏ Anti glidian, Anti transglutaminase: Celiac disease✳
❏ Anti GIL: Hemolytic transfusion reactions✳
❏ Anti sacchromyces cervessiae: Crohns disease✳
❏ Anti epithelial cell: Pemphigus vulgaris✳✳
❏ Anti IgG: Rheumatoid Arthritis✳✳

Anti-Ri is the least common of the paraneoplastic autoantibodies. Detection of Anti-Ri antibody in serum or spinal fluid identifies an otherwise unexplained neurological disorder as autoimmune and paraneoplastic. A positive result prompts a search for an underlying occult malignancy. Anti-Ri antibodies are detected most commonly in postmenopausal women who usually present with signs of midbrain, brain stem, cerebellar and/or spinal cord dysfunction. Ocular opsoclonus-myoclonus may be a prominent symptom. Most patients have a primary carcinoma of the breast. Lung and gynecological cancer are less frequently associated with this syndrome. Treatment of the cancer can lead to decreased antibody titer and improvement of the neurological disorder. A negative result does not rule out cancer.

Anti-Hu is one of several antibodies detected in the serum of patients with neurologic paraneoplastic syndromes. Anti-Hu antibody causes either a syndrome of encephalomyelitis or sensory neuropathy. The underlying cancer is usually small cell cancer of the lung.

Anti-Yo polyclonal IgG autoantibody directed against Purkinje's cells and associated with paraneoplastic cerebellar degeneration in oat cell carcinoma of the lung and cancer of the breast or ovary. Also called anti-Purkinje cell antibody.

➲ HIV

▶ **HIV** is an RNA virus whose hallmark is the reverse transcription of its genomic RNA to DNA by the enzyme reverse transcriptase
▶ **Window period is time between infection and detection of antibodies against HIV.**   **AIIMS 2007**
▶ HIV is transmitted by
▶ Homosexual
▶ Heterosexual contact;

▶ By blood and blood products;

▶ By infected mothers to infants either intrapartum, perinatally, or via breast milk.

▶ HIV can be transmitted to individuals who receive HIV-tainted blood transfusions, blood products, or transplanted tissue.

▶ The hallmark of HIV disease is a profound immunodeficiency progressive quantitative and qualitative deficiency of the subset of T lymphocytes referred to as helper T cells, or inducer T cells.   AIIMS 1998

AIDS related neoplasms are: JK BOPEE 2009

▶ Kaposis sarcoma

▶ B cell non Hodgkins lymphoma

▶ Primary lymphoma of brain.

Kaposis Sarcoma

⮑ High Yield for AIPGME/AIIMS/PGI 2012-2013

❑ Kaposis sarcoma is common in homosexuals. ✳

❑ Kaposis sarcoma (KS) is asociated with HHV 8 virus.🠖🠖

🠖 KS arises from cells linning lymph vessels or blood vessels. KS actually arises as a cancer of lymphatic endothelium ✳   AIIMS 2005

❑ KS is associated with HIV, immunosuppression, organ transplants.✳   JK BOPEE 2011

❑ On skin Kaposis lesions are red/purple blotches which are asymptomatic or tender.✳

❑ GIT, liver, lung lesions are dangerous.✳

❑ Treatment of HIV with HAART reduces KS as well.

❑ **Common sites:** Skin, GIT, Lymph nodes, Lungs.

Pathologically KS lesions contain tumor cells with a characteristic abnormal elongated shape, called "spindle cells". ✳

The tumor is highly vascular, containing abnormally dense and irregular blood vessels, which leak red blood cells into the surrounding tissue and give the tumor its dark color. Inflammation around the tumor may produce swelling and pain.

🠖 Although KS may be suspected from the appearance of lesions and the patient's risk factors, a definite diagnosis can only be made by biopsy and microscopic examination, which will show the presence of spindle cells.

🠖 Detection of the "KSHV protein LANA"✳ in tumor cells confirms the diagnosis.

➲ Histiocytosis X: (Important Features) High Yield for AIPGME/AIIMS/PGI 2012-2013

☐ Birbeck granules with tennis racket appearance✱✱	UP 2006
☐ Immunostaining for S 100 protein✱	
☐ CD 1 a positivity✱	
☐ Express HLA DR✱	

➲ Histiocytosis X

► This condition is rare

► Cells involved are Langerhans' cells ✱

► Cells contain Birbeck granules ✱

► Cells express CDI markers. ✱✱

Letterer-Siwe disease

☐ Discrete yellow-brown papules develop on the scalp, face, upper trunk and flexures, with a distribution mimicking seborrheic eczema. Purpura and crusting of the lesion may become evident. In some children mucous membranes are also involved, with gingivitis and oral and genital ulceration.

☐ <u>Floating teeth sign</u> are a feature of Histiocytosis.   MAH 2012

☐ Signs of systemic involvement become manifest, with **hepatosplenomegaly, lymphadenopathy and anemia.** Chest X-ray shows miliary shadowing and bone scans may show osteolytic areas.

Hand-Schüller-Christian disease

☐ This is a more benign form of histiocytosis X, which usually presents within the first 5 years of life and follows a chronic non-fatal course. The usual manifestations are **radiological bone defects, exophthalmos and diabetes insipidus.**

Eosinophilic granuloma

☐ This is the **most benign form of histiocytosis** X. It commonly presents within the first 5 years of life, and skin involvement is rare. When it does occur, **yellowish or brownish papules are found on the scalp and trunk** in a distribution similar to the other forms of histiocytosis X.

☐ Solitary lesion is commonest in skull.   AIIMS 1986

☐ **Spontaneous resolution** usually occurs.

➲ Pathological Condirions Related to Term "X"

<u>Cardiac syndrome X:</u> occurs when a patient has all of the symptoms of angina pectoris without coronary artery disease or spasm. These spasms can occur either at rest or with exertion. Cardiac syndrome X, the triad of

✓ angina pectoris,

✓ a positive exercise electrocardiogram for myocardial ischaemia and

✓ angiographically smooth coronary arteries

The main cause of this syndrome is coronary microvascular dysfunction, as indicated by an abnormal response of coronary microcirculation to both vasoconstrictor and vasodilatory stimuli (microvascular angina)

Syndrome X :

Is a term used to describe a constellation of metabolic derangements that **includes**

✓   insulin resistance,

✓   hypertension,

✓   dyslipidemia,

✓   **central or visceral obesity,**

✓   **endothelial dysfunction, and**

✓   **Accelerated cardiovascular disease.**

X-Linked agammaglobulinemia

✓   Males with this **syndrome** often begin to have **recurrent bacterial infections** late in the first year of life, when maternally derived immunoglobulins have disappeared.

✓   Affected individuals have very few immunoglobulin-bearing B lymphocytes in their circulation and lack primary and secondary lymphoid follicles.

✓   Mutations of **Bruton's tyrosine kinase (Btk) gene** are responsible for X-linked agammaglobulinemia.

✓   **Sinopulmonary bacterial infections** constitute the most frequent clinical problem.

✓   Treatment with **intravenous immunoglobulin.**

Fragile X syndrome:

✓   It is now recognized as the **second commonest cause** of mental handicap in males after Downs syndrome

✓   Fragile X males have

▶   a **large forehead,**

▶   **large head,**

▶   **long nose,**

▶   **prominent chin and**

▶   **Long ears.**

✓   Fragile X males tend to be **larger at birth.**

✓   **Macro-orchidism is present.** The size of the **testes may be considerably enlarged.**

✓   There is a slight increase in the frequency of mitral valve prolapse, aortic root dilatation and hernias. More striking clinically is the soft skin and joint hypermobility, which may be helpful diagnostically. The range of intellectual handicap in fragile X males varies but most are moderately to severely retarded.

The X-linked lymphoproliferative syndrome (Duncan's disease)

✓   Is a X LINKED recessive disorder of young boys who have a normal response to childhood infections but develop fatal lympho proliferative disorders after infection with EBV.

⇨ **Enzyme Markers used in Pathology:**

Serum Enzyme	Diagnostic Use	
❏ Aminotransferases	❏ Viral Hepatitis(AST>ALT)	
	❏ Alcoholic Hepatitis(ALT>AST)	
❏ Amylase	❏ Acute Pancreatitis	
❏ Cerulloplasmin	❏ Wilsons DiseaseAutosomal recessive)	JK 2011
❏ CPK	❏ Muscular Dystrophies, MI	
❏ LDH	❏ MI(LDH 1>LDH2)	
❏ Lipase	❏ Acute Pancreatitis	
❏ Alkaline Phosphatase	❏ Pagets disease(of bone)	
	❏ Obstructive Liver Disease	

⇨ **Remember (How to Identify Tricky Questions)**

❏ Burkitts lymphoma:	**Starry skin pattern**
❏ Mycosis fungoides:	**Pautriers abscess**
❏ Hairy cell leukemia:	**TRAP Positive**
❏ Histiocytosis X :	**Birbeck granules**
❏ Multiple Myeloma:	**Lytic bony lesions**
❏ Waldenstroms Macroglobunemia:	**Non -lytic lesions**

⊃ **Pathologically Important Bodies: (Viral)**

High Yield for AIPGME/AIIMS/PGI 2012-2013

▶ Guarneri bodies :	❏ Vaccinia
▶ Bollinger bodies:	❏ Fowl pox
▶ Paschen bodies:	❏ Small pox
▶ Torres Bodies:	❏ Yellow fever
▶ Cowdry Type A:	❏ Herpes Virus
▶ Cowdry Type B:	❏ Adeno virus, Polio virus

⊃ **Some other Important Bodies are:**

High Yield for AIPGME/AIIMS/PGI 2012-2013

▶ HP (Halber staedtler) bodies:	❏ Trachoma
▶ Levinthal Colle Bodies:	❏ Psittacosis
▶ Moosers bodies:	❏ Endemic Typhus
▶ Miyagawa bodies:	❏ Chlamydia Trachomatis

▶ Asteroid Bodies:	☐ Sarcoidosis	DNB 2011
▶ Babes Ernest Bodies:	☐ Diptheria	
▶ Verocay Bodies:	☐ Neurilemmoma	
▶ Civatte Bodies:	☐ Lichen Planus	KERALA 1998
▶ Donavan Bodies:	☐ Kala Azar	
▶ Hassal bodies:	☐ Thymus	

▶ Zebra bodies:	☐ metachromatic leukodystrophy
▶ Winkler bodies:	☐ syphilis
▶ Ross bodies:	☐ Syphilis
▶ Moot bodies:	☐ multiple myeloma
▶ Creola bodies:	☐ asthma
▶ Citron bodies:	☐ Clostridium septicum

➲ **Psamomma Bodies are seen in: High Yield for 2011/2012**

- ➡ Papillary thyroid carcinoma
- ➡ Papillary renal cell carcinoma
- ➡ Papillary serous cystadenocarcinoma of ovary
- ➡ Papillary serous carcinoma of endometrium
- ➡ Papillary adenocarcinoma of lung
- ➡ Meningioma
- ➡ Mesothelioma
- ➡ Somatostatinoma
- ➡ Endosalpingosis
- ➡ Melanotic variants of schwannoma

➲ **SRBCTS (Small Round Blue Cell Tumors)**

High Yield for AIPGME/AIIMS/PGI 2012-2013

Are characterised by sheets of cells with rounded, small nuclei. They include

▶ Neuroblastoma	JK BOPEE 2009
▶ Ewings sarcoma	AIIMS 2005
▶ Rhabdomyosarcoma	
▶ Burkitts lymphoma	
▶ Lymphobalstic lymphoma	

► Wilms tumor

► Retinoblatoma

► Medulloblastoma

⊃ Types of Erythema: High Yield for AIPGME/AIIMS/PGI 2012-2013

- ❏ ☞**Erythema chronicum migrans: Lymes Disease**
- ❏ ☞**Erythema Ab Agne**: reticulate pigmentation due to long term heat exposure.
- ❏ ☞**Erythema Gyratum Repens**: Internal malignancies
- ❏ ☞**Erythema Nodosum**: multisystemic disorders eg sarcoidosis
- ❏ ☞**Erythema multiforme**: mucosal involvement with viral, bacterial, rickettsial diseases with target lesions
- ❏ ☞**Erythema toxicum neonatorum** This is a transient condition of unknown etiology occurring in up to **70% of neonates**. The onset is from birth to 14 days but most cases start between day 1 and day 4. The commonest lesions are **erythematous macules and papules** but in some cases pustules appear.
- ❏ ☞**Erythema marginatum**: present in acute rheumatic fever, pink/red non prurtitic rash on trunk and upper limbs in associasion with carditis
- ❏ ☞**Erythema necrolyticum migrans: Glucagonoma**
- ❏ ☞**Erythema infectiosum: Parvo virus**
- ❏ ☞**Erythema arthriticum epidemicum Haver hill fever, sterptobacillus monoliformis**

⊃ More Associations with Fruits, Vegetables etc: High Yield for AIPGME/AIIMS/PGI

"Pear" shaped bladder:	❏ Pelvic lipomatosis
"Doughnut"sign:	❏ Circumferential thickening of bowel wall in carcinoma of colon
"Coffee bean" sign:	❏ Dilated air filled sigmoid colon in sigmoid volvolus.
"Rice grain" calcification:	❏ Calcified cystercii in muscles.
"Onion"skin periostealreaction:	❏ Ewings sarcoma JK BOPEE 2012
"Salt and pepper" skull:	❏ Hyperparathyroidism
"Pop corn" calcification:	❏ Pulmonary Hamartoma
"Miliary" shadowing:	❏ Miliary tuberculosis
"Grape" like vesicles	❏ Hydatid mole

⇨ Pathologically Types of Common Cancers:

► Mc type of Stomach Ca:	**Adeno carcinoma**
► Mc type of Lung Ca:	**Adeno Carcinoma**
► Mc type of Pancreatic Ca:	**Ductal cell Adeno carcinoma**
► Mc type of Breast Ca:	**Intra ductal Adeno carcinoma**

☐ **Pelger Huet anamoly**: A benign inherited condition in which <u>neutrophils fail to segment properly</u>. Majority of circulating neutrophils have only two discrete equal sized lobes connected by thin chromatin bridge.

☐ **Pseudo pelger cells** have hypogranular, often irregular nuclear pattern.

⇨ <u>"Smudge cells"</u> seen in CLL	KAR 2009
⇨ Mallory bodies are composed of "<u>intermediate filaments</u>."	KAR 2009
⇨ "<u>Infantile</u> "polyarteritis nodosa: Kawasaki disease	KAR 2009
⇨ "Commonest" endocrine tumor of pancreas: <u>insulinoma(beta cell tumor)</u>	KAR 2009
⇨ Classic karyotype of Kleinfielters syndrome: <u>"47 XXY"</u>.	KAR 2009
⇨ Leprosy has "<u>non necrotizing</u>" epitheliod cell granulomas.	DELHI 2009
⇨ In Myeloperoxidase deficiency (MPO) infection is inability to produce "<u>hydroxyl-halide radicles</u>".	DELHI 2009
⇨ "<u>Aschoff nodules</u>" are pathogonomic of acute rheumatic fever.	DELHI 2009
⇨ "<u>Lacunar type</u>" Reed Sternberg cell is seen in Nodular sclerosis lymphoma.	DELHI 2009
⇨ "<u>Extensive nodular</u>" pulmonary fibrosis is seen in silicosis.	DELHI 2009
⇨ Distended macrophages with "<u>PAS positive</u>" granules in lamina propria are seen in Celiac disease.	DELHI 2009

⮂ Important Clinical Scenarios: High Yield for 2012/2013

⇨ **New Topics Incorporated**

☐ Liver biopsy in an adolescent with cirrhosis revealed hepatocytes containing round to oval 'PAS distase resistant' globular inclusions. The most likely cause of cirrhosis in this patient is: **(MH 07)**
Alpha-1 antitrypsin deficiency

☐ In a case of diarrhea with histopathological feature of intestinal mucosal clefts studded with copious thick secretions and inflammatory cells, characteristic of pseudomembranous colitis, the likely cause is:
(MH 05)

Clostridium Deficile

☐ A 34 years old person has rapidly developing cough, dyspnoea, expectoration and blood tinged sputum. He is febrile, cyanosed, and toxic. Chest examination reveals crepitations and ronchi. The most likely diagnosis is:
Pneumonic plague   **(Delhi 2005)**

☐ In a 40 year old man following tooth extraction developed oral local infection with draining discharge, which on examination showed gram positive branching roads and leucocytes. Anaerobic growth was absent. The most likely organism responsible for this is: **(MH 06)**
Actinomyces

- ❏ In a poultry farm, many chickens developed diarrhea, emaciation and mucopurulent discharge. After about 2 hours the farmer developed fever, chills, headache, and Breathlessness. The most likely diagnosis is: (MH 06)
  Ornithosis

- ❏ A gardener receives a thorn bite. KoH culture mount shows fine branching hyphae & pear shaped conidia borne in rosette like clusters typically. The features are suggestive of: Sporotrichosis
  (Nimhans 1994, TN 1990) (AP 2002)

- ❏ A person presents with hemoptysis and hematuria with anti basement membrane antibodies Diagnosis is:
  Good Pasteur's Syndrome (Delhi 2005)

- ❏ Males who are
- ➡ sexually under developed with rudimentary testes and prostate glands,
- ➡ sparse pubic and facial hair, long arms and legs and large hands & feet are likely to have the chromosome complement of: Klienfilters disease

- ❏ A 70 year old male who has been
- ➡ Chewing tobacco for the past 50 years presents with a six months history of a large, fungating, soft papillary lesions in the oral cavity.
- ➡ The lesion has penetrated into the mandible. Lymph nodes are not palpable.
- ➡ Two biopsies taken from the lesion proper show benign appearing papillomatosis with hyperkeratosis and acanthosis infiltrating the subjacent tissues.
The most likely diagnosis is : Verrucous carcinoma

- ❏ A sarcoma appears
- ➡ Like a malignant melanoma, which arises in the sof tissue.
- ➡ It usually is found on the tendons of extremities of young patients.
- ➡ Histologically, the cells can have pigment or clear cytoplasm. It is associated with t(12,22)
The sarcoma is: Clear Cell sarcoma

- ❏ A disease is characterized by osteolysis, producing patchwork areas of
- ➡ Bone resorption with bizarre, large osteoclasts.
- ➡ In the middle stage of the disease, secondary osteoblastic activity compensates with new bone formation, producing the mosaic pattern.
- ➡ In late Paget's, the bones are dense and osteosclerotic. A mosaic pattern is a feature.
The Pathology represents:Pagets Disease

- ❏ Intracytoplasmic spherules composed of
- ➡ Paired helical filaments stained with silver stains are seen in frontal lobe with
- ➡ Severe neuronal loss and astrocytosis.
The condition most likely is: Picks Disease (Pick's bodies)

❑ **Testicular tumours** having an increased elevation of **placental alkaline phosphatase in the serum** as well as a positive immunohistochemical staining for **placental alkaline phosphatase: Seminoma**

❑ **A 60 year old man** presented with **fatigue, weight loss and heaviness in left hypochondrium for 6 months.**

The hemogram showed

- Hb. 10gm/dL,
- TLC 5 lakhs/mm^3,
- platelet count 4 lakhs/mm^3,
- DLC; neutrophil 55%, lymphocutes 4%, monocytes 2%, basophils 6%,
- Metamyelocytes 10%, myelocytes 18%, promyelocytes 2% and blasta 3%.

The most likely diagnosis is :**CML**

❑ A **renal biopsy from a 56 year** old woman with

- **Progressive renal failure** for the past 3 years shows **glomerular and vascular deposition of pink amorphous material.**
- It **shows apple-green birefringence under polarized light after Congo red staining.**
- These deposits are positive for lambda light chains.

Likely diagnosis is: **Multiple myeloma**

❑ On sectioning of an organ at the time of autopsy,

- A **focal, wedge-shaped firm area is seen accompanied by extensive hemorrhage, with a red appearance.**
- The lesion has a base on the surface of the organ.

This findings is typically of **Lung with pulmonary thromboembolism**

❑ A **young lady presented with**

- **Bilateral nodular lesions** on shins.
- She was also **found to have bilateral hilar lymphadenopathy** on chest X-ray.
- Mantoux test reveals indurations of **5 mms.**
- Skin biopsy would reveals **Non caeseating Granuloma.**

Likely diagnosis is: **Sarcoidosis.**

❑ An elderly 77 year old man comes to oncology clinic with

- **Anemia** and **multiple infections.**
- **Physical examination is remarkable for** marked hepatosplenomegaly.
- Blood counts demonstrates **pancytopenia.**
- Peripheral smear by a hematologist demonstrates rare, distinctive,
- **Neoplastic white cells covered by fine,** hairlike **projections.**

Most likely disease is: **Hairy cell leukemia**

❑ A 52-year-old man presents to Gastro clinic with a complaint of

➥ **Nonbloody diarrhea** and right **lower quadrant pain with a palpable mass and tenderness.**

➥ He states that this "**flare-up**" is one of the worst he has ever experienced.

➥ Radiographic examination reveals **evidence of ulceration, stricturing, and fistula development of the colon and small bowel.**

The most likely diagnosis is: **Crohn's disease**

❑ A disease occurs with

➥ Prolonged **exposure to dust** during glass production which can progress to respiratory failure and death, and is associated with **increased risk for tuberculosis.**

➥ Classic x-ray findings include calcified **lymph nodes that produce an "eggshell" pattern.** Pleural involvement creates **dense fibrous plaques and adhesions** that may obliterate the pleural cavities.

Most likely disease is: **Silicosis**

❑ It is seen that **vasa vasorum of the aorta undergoes obliterative endarteritis,**

➥ Leading to atrophy of the muscularis and elastic tissues of the aorta and dilatation.

➥ **Linear calcifications are often seen in the ascending aorta by X ray.**

➥ The intimal wrinkling is seen.

The disease most likely represents: **Syphilis infection (The intimal wrinkling or "tree barking" is also a common feature.)**

❑ A boy presents with a

➥ **purple, flat vascular ectasia** on the **head and along distribution of the trigeminal nerve, mental retardation,**

➥ **seizures,** and

➥ **hemiplegia**

The most likely disease is: **Sturge-Weber syndrome**

❑ A patient presents with

➥ **Respiratory symptoms i.e. cough, hemoptysis and glomerulonephritis.**

➥ **His C-ANCA levles in serum were found to be raised.**

The most lkely diagnosis is **Wegener's granulomatosis.**

❑ A 35 year old female presented

➥ With one **year history of menstrual irregularity and galactorrhea.**

➥ She also had off-and-on headache.

➥ Her examination revealed bitemporal superior quadrantopia.

➥ Her fundus examination showed primary optic atropy.

The most likely diagnosis in this case: **Pituitary macroadenoma**

PATHOLOGY

❑ A four year old boy was admitted with a history of **abdominal pain and fever** for two months, **maculopapular rash for ten days, and dry cough, dyspnea and wheezing for three days**. On examination, **liver and spleen were enlarged** 4 cm and 3 cm respectively below the costal margins. His **hemoglobin was** 10.0 g/dl, platelet count 37x 10^9/L and total leukocyte count 70 x 10^9/L, which included 80% **eosinophils**. Bone marrow examination revealed a cellular marrow comprising 45% blasts and 34% Eosinophils and eosinophilic precursors. The **blasts stained negative for myeloperoxidase and non -specific esterase** and were **positive for CD19, CD10, CD22 and CD20.**

The most likely diagnosis **Acute lymphoblastic leukemia with hypereosinophilic syndrome**

❑ **CD 19 positive, CD22 positive, CD103 positive** monoclonal B-cells with bright **kappa positivity** were found to comprise 60% of the **peripheral blood lymphoid cells** on flow cytometric analysis in a 55 year old man with massive splenomegaly and a total leucocyte count of 3.3 x 10^9/L.

The most likely diagnosis**Hairy cell leukemia.**

❑ A 30 year old male, Kallu, with a history of sexual exposure comes with a **painless indurated ulcer over the penis with everted margins.**

The diagnosis is : **Syphilis**

❑ **A HIV** positive female
- Presents with an **indurated ulcer over the tongue.**
- Laboratory findings show **growth in corneal agar at 20 degree celcius, microscopy showing hyphae** and growth in human serum at 37 degree celcius show **budding yeasts.**

The probable cause is : **Candida albicans**

❑ A 6 year old boy has been complaining of
- Headache, ignoring to see the objects on the sides for four months. On examination, he is not mentally retarded, his grades at school are good, and visual acuity is diminished in both the eyes. Visual charting showed significant field defect.
- CT scan of the head showed **suprasellar mass with calcification.**

The most probable diagnosis: **Craniopharyngioma**

❑ A 25-year-old man presented with fever and cough for two months.
- CT chest showed bilateral upper lobe fibrosis and mediastinal enlarged necrotic nodes with peripheral rim enhancement.

The most likely diagnosis: **Tuberculosis**

☐ A 30-year-old male patient presents with complaints of

➡ **Weakness in right upper and both lower limbs** for last 4 months.

➡ He developed **digital infarcts** involving 2nd and 3rd fingers on right side and 5th finger on left side. On examination, **BP was 160/140 mm Hg**, all **peripheral pulses were palpable** and there was asymmetrical neuropathy.

➡ Investigations showed Hb **12 gm%**, TLC **12,000 per cu. mm**, Platelets **4,30,000** and ESR **49 mm**. Urine examination showed Proteinuria and RBC-10-15/hpf with no casts.

The most likely diagnosis : **Polyarteritis nodosa**

☐ A 45 year old coal mine worker presents with

➡ **Cutaneous nodules, joint pain** and occasional **cough with dyspnoea.**

➡ His chest radiograph shows **multiple small (1-4 cm) nodules** in bilateral lung fields.

➡ Some of the nodules show **cavitation and specks of calcification.**

Most likely these features are diagnostic of : **Caplan's syndrome**

☐ Two identical specimen of the intestine obtained following colectomy shows on examination **hemorrhagic cobblestone appearance**, One of them however, shows **longitudinal grooving**. it is likely to be a specimen of: **(Kolkata 2002)**

Crohn's disease

☐ Salivary gland tumors having propensity for perineural spread and tendency for recurence along the nerve is most likely : **(MH 08)**

Adenoid cystic carcinoma

☐ The antigen/organism responsible in a farmer for fever, chills, malaise, cough, and dyspnoea, but without wheezing with likely exposure to "mouldy hay" and grains is most likely :

Thermophilic actinomycetes

☐ Megalolastic anemia resistant to treatment is seen with **Hepatic cirrhosis:** (MHPGMCET 2007) (MH 2010)

☐ Ganglion of tendons is an example of: **Myxomatous degeneration** (MHPGMCET 2006) (MH 2010)

☐ **Chromosome 13** is involved in Patau syndrome (MH 2010)

☐ Myocarditis can be caused by: **Trichinella spiralis** (MHPGMCET 2008) (MH 2010)

☐ **"Groundglass hepatocytes"** are seen in **Hepatitis B**

☐ **"Acrodermatitis enteropathica"** is seen in deficiency of: **Zinc** (MHPGMCET 2006)(MH 2010)

☐ Compared to the other leukemias, Hairy cell leukemia is associated with infections of **Mycobacterium kansasi** (MH 2010)

6

- Arthropods are vectors for following ricketsial infections except **Q-fever**   (MHPGMCET 07)(MH 2010)

- Spontaneous regressison can occur with: **Strawberry angioma**   (MHPGMCET 2007) (MH 2010)

- Patients with Hashimoto's thyroiditis are at increased risk of developing **B-cell lymphoma:**   (MH 2010)

- Ovarian counterpart of testicular seminoma **Dysgerminoma**

- Munro Microabscesses are seen in: **Psoriasis**   (MH 2010)

- High mitotic activity with rapid cellular turnover and characteristic "Starry sky" appearance is seen in: **Burkitt's lymphoma**   (MH 2010)

- **CLUE Cells:** bacterial vaginosis   (AIIMS 2010)

- Wegners granulomatosis on renal biopsy shows: **focal necrotizing glomerulonephritis.**   AIIMS 2010

- INCLUSION BODIES in oligodendroglia are seen in **PML.**   AIIMS 2010

- **Pale Infarcts** are seen in: Spleen, kidney, heart.   AIIMS 2010

- **OSTEOID mineralization:** Is detected by: tetracycline labelling.   AIIMS 2010

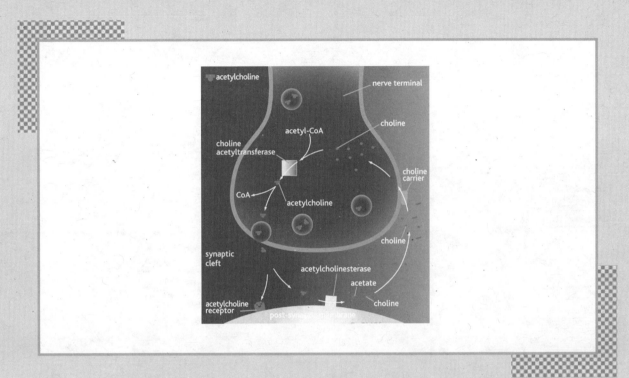

PHARMACOLOGY

- Pharmaco<u>kinetics</u>: is quantitative **study of drug movement in through and out of the body.** PGI 1995
- What the <u>body does to a drug</u>.
- Pharmaco<u>dynamics</u>: is what the <u>drug does to a body</u>.
- Pharmac<u>ogenetics</u>: study of <u>genetic basis for variability in drug response.</u>
- Pharmaco<u>genomics: use of genetic information to guide choice of drug and dose on individual basis.</u>
- Pharmaco<u>vigilance: science and activities related to detection, assessment, understanding and prevention of adverse effects of drug or other drug related problems.</u>

⊃ Clinical Trials: (High Yield for AIIMS/AIPGME/DNB 2012-2013)

Clinical trials:✱ Determine:

- ▶ Phase I: Human pharmacology and safety
- ▶ PhaseII: Theraupatic exploration and dose ranging, Determines efficacy   AI 2008
- ▶ PhaseIII: Theraupatic confirming
- ▶ Phase IV: Post marketing surveillance. No ethical clearance required.   AI 2004
- ▶ Good clinical practice is not needed for <u>pre clinical tials</u> but is needed for phase I – IV   AIIMS 2007
- ▶ Preclinical study is done in <u>animals</u>
- ▶ Clinical trial is done in <u>humans</u>
- ▶ Unwanted effect at <u>theraupatic doses</u>: <u>Side effect</u>   PGI 1999
- ▶ Unwanted effect <u>due to overdose</u> <u>Toxic dose</u>

⊃ Terms Frequently Asked in Examinations

- ▶ Affinity: ability of a drug to <u>combine</u> with receptor
- ▶ Intrinsic activity (efficacy):   ability of drug to <u>activate</u> receptor
- ▶ Agonist: have affinity and <u>maximal</u> efficacy   Delhi 1987
- ▶ Antagonist: have affinity and no maximal efficacy   Delhi 1990
- ▶ Partial agonist: have affinity and <u>sub maximal</u> efficacy
- ▶ Inverse agonist: have affinity and <u>opposite</u> efficacy

7

⊃ Important Terminology ✳ (High Yield for 2011-2012)

▶ <u>Clearance</u>, a measure of the **body's ability to eliminate drug**; Clearance is a measure of the rate at which the organs that eliminate drug from the body remove drug from the blood. ☞   **KAR 2006**

▶ <u>Volume of distribution,</u> an indication of the **extent to which the drug is distributed outside of the blood compartment;** ☞☞

▶ <u>Bioavailability</u>, the **fraction of the administered dose that reaches the systemic circulation.** ☞

▶ **Steady state** is achieved when the **rate of drug elimination equals the rate of drug delivery into the systemic circulation,** which, if bioavailability is complete, corresponds to the rate at which the drug dose is administered:☞

▶ <u>Therapeutic index</u>: the ratio of the toxic dose to the therapeutic dose. LD_{50}/ED_{50} **AI 2008, UP 2007**

  If absorption is too rapid, then the resulting high concentration may cause adverse effects not observed with a more slowly available formulation. At the other extreme, slow absorption is deliberately designed into "slow-release" or "sustained-release" drug formulations in order to maintain plasma concentrations essentially constant during the dosage interval, because the drug's rate of elimination is offset by an equivalent rate of absorption controlled by formulation factors. ☞☞   **JK 2005**

▶ <u>Half-Life</u>: Half-life ($t_{1/2}$) is the time that it takes for the plasma concentration or amount of drug in the body to decline by 50%. ☞☞. **Time taken for a drug to reach plateau level in plasma after repeated doses also depends on its plasma half life.**   **JK BOPEE 2012**

▶ **Drug Potency**: Relative concentrations of two or more drugs that elicit same effect. **Refers to amount of drug needed to produce a certain response.** ☞☞

▶ <u>Drug Efficacy</u>: **Maximal effect** that a particular drug may elicit. ☞☞   **PGI 1998**

▶ **More important than potency in determining choice of drug.** ☞

▶ <u>Theraupatic window phenomenon</u>: Optimal theraupatic response of drug is exerted only over a narrow range of plasma drug concentration. e.g.: TCA, clonidine, glipize   **PGI 1995**

⇨ $t_{1/2}$ can determine: ☞☞   **AIIMS 1992**

- ✓ Elimination time☞
- ✓ Steady state plasma concentration☞
- ✓ Dosing rate☞
- ✓ Maintainance dose☞

▶ First pass metabolism is seen with oral route and rectal route. ☞   **AI 1994**

▶ <u>More</u> first pass metabolism is seen with oral route. ☞

▶ Bioavailability by <u>IV route</u> is 100%.☞

▶ **Sublingual route bypasses** first pass metabolism.☞

⊃ **Drug Metabolism Occurs in Two Phases: ✶✶ (High yield for 2011-2012)**

■ **Phase I:** ☞☞
✓ Oxidation☞
✓ Reduction☞
✓ Hydrolysis☞
✓ Cyclization, Decyclization ☞

MFO (Mixed Function Oxidases) in Liver participate.☞

■ **Phase II:** ☞☞Conjugation with
✓ Glucronide, ☞
✓ Sulfate☞
✓ Glutathione, Acetylation, Methylation☞   PGI 2002
✓ Conjugation **does not** occur in metabolism of xenobiotics. ☞   AIIMS 2008

⇨ **Drugs with high first pass metabolism: ✶**

✓ Beta blockers (propranolol), ☞   PGI 2003
✓ Lignocaine, ☞   PGI 2003
✓ Salbutamol, ☞   PGI 2003
✓ Verapamil,☞
✓ Nitroglycerine, ☞
✓ Testosterone, ☞
✓ Morphine, ☞
✓ Hydrocortisone☞

⇨ **Drug Montoring is useful in drugs with low safety margin:**

1. Lithium
2. Diagoxin
3. Antiepileptics
4. Antiarrhythmics
5. Theophylline
6. Aminoglycosides.

Drug deposited in retina: chloroquine	UP 2007
Drug deposited in muscle: digoxin.	UP 2007

⇨ **Factors governing volume of distribution of a drug are: ✳✳**

▶ Lipid: water coefficient of drug. ☜	UP 2007
▶ pKa: value of a drug. ☜	
▶ Degree of Plasma protein binding☜	UP 2007
▶ Degree of blood flow. ☜	
▶ Affinity for different tissues. ☜	UP 2007
▶ Fat: Lean body mass ratio☜	
▶ Diseases like CHF, Uremia,Cirrhisis☜	
▶ Pregnancy☜	

⊃ **The cytochrome P450 superfamily (CYP): (High yield for 2011-2012)**

- Is a **large and diverse group of enzymes**.
- The function of most CYP enzymes is to **catalyze the oxidation of organic substances.**
- The substrates of CYP enzymes include metabolic intermediates such as **lipids and steroidal hormones, as well as xenobiotic substances such as drugs and other toxic chemicals.**
- CYPs are the major enzymes involved in drug metabolism and bioactivation, accounting for ~75% of the total metabolism.
- The most common reaction catalyzed by cytochromes P450 is a monooxygenase reaction.
- Cytochromes P450 (CYPs) belong to the superfamily of proteins containing a heme cofactor and, therefore, are hemoproteins.
- CYPs use a variety of small and large molecules as substrates in enzymatic reactions.
- Often, they form part of multi-component electron transfer chains, called P450-containing systems.
- Cytochromes P450 have been named on the basis of their cellular location and spectrophotometric characteristics (chrome): when the reduced heme iron forms an adduct with CO, **P450 enzymes absorb light at wavelengths near 450 nm, identifiable as a characteristic Soret peak.**
- CYP enzymes have been identified **in all kingdoms of life**, i.e. in animals, plants, fungi, protists, bacteria, archaea, and viruses.

⊃ **Never Forget: (High Yield for AIIMS/AIPGME/DNB 2012-2013)**

☐ Plasma protein binding occurs with many drugs. ☜	
☐ Highly plasma protein bound drugs are <u>restricted mainly to vascular compartment</u>. ☜	
☐ Displacement of protein bound drug↑ plasma levels of drug.	PGI 2000
☐ Have <u>lower volumes of distribution</u>. ☜	

- ❑ <u>Bound fraction</u> is not available for action.
- ❑ In hypoalbumenemia binding may be reduced and high concentration of free drug may be available☞
- ❑ Binding sites are <u>non specific</u> and one drug can displace other. AI 2000

⇨ **Drugs bound to albumin are:** ☞☞

✓ barbiturates☞	
✓ benzodiazepenes☞	
✓ phenytoin☞	PGI 1986
✓ pencillins☞	
✓ sulfonamides☞	
✓ tetracycline☞	
✓ tolbutamide☞	
✓ warfarin ☞	PGI 1986

⇨ **Drugs bound to α acid glycoprotein are:** ☞☞ JK BOPEE

→ Prazosin☞	→ Methadone☞
→ Lidocaine☞	→ Imipramine☞
→ Verapamil☞	→ Bupivicaine☞
→ Diisopyramide☞	→ Quinidine☞

⇨ **List of "Pro drugs":** ☞(High Yield for AIIMS/AIPGME/DNB 2012-2013)

■ Enalapril: Enalaprilate☞☞	AIIMS 2006 NIMHANS 2001
■ Sulfasalazine:5 Aminosalisylic acid☞☞	
■ Flourouracil:Flourouracil monophosphate☞☞	
■ Dipivefrine: Epinephrine☞☞	
■ Predsnisone: Prednisolone☞☞	
■ Levodopa: Dopamine☞☞	

⇨ **Other pro drugs**☞☞(High Yield for AIIMS/AIPGME/DNB 2012-2013)

❑ Methyl dopa☞	
❑ Terfenadine☞	
❑ Zidovudine☞	
❑ Bitolterol	PGI 2011

PHARMACOLOGY

7

☐ Sulindac☛	**PGI 2011**
☐ Cyclophosphamide☛	
☐ Bacampacillin☛	
☐ Fluorouracil, mercaptopurine☛	
☐ Ticlopidine, Clopidregel	**AIIMS 2007**

➲ Orphan Drugs✳

When a drug is not developed into a usable medicine because the costs will not be recovered by the developer then it is called an **orphan drug** and the disease as **orphan disease** and sufferer as **health orphan**☛☛

(High yield for 2011-2012)

Remember the terms:

- ▪ <u>Theraupatic window phenomenon</u>: best possible theraupatic effect is exerted by a drug only in narrow range of drug concentrations. Exhibited by: <u>**tricyclic antidepressants, clonidine, and glipizide.**</u> ☛

- ▪ <u>Hit and run drugs</u>: drugs **whose effects last much longer** than the drug itself.**reserpine, guanethidine, MAO Inhibitors, omperazole.** ☛

- ▪ <u>Drugs with zero order kinetics</u>: **phenytoin, aspirin, ethanol, Theophylline, propafenone, warfarin, tolbutamide**☛

- ▪ <u>Drugs with First-order kinetics</u>, the time required to achieve steady-state levels can be predicted from the half-life, because accumulation is a first-order process with a half-life identical to that for elimination. Thus, accumulation reaches 90% of steady-state levels at the end of three to four half-lives☛

➲ Drugs Undergoing Enterohepatic Circulation:

- — Erythromycin,
- — Ampicillin,
- — Rifampicin,
- — Tetracycline,
- — OCPS,
- — Phenopthalein.☛

- ▶ Placebo: inert substance given in the form of medicine with no pharmacological effect but pshycological Effect. ☛

- ▶ Nacebo: is <u>reverse of placebo</u>: refers to <u>negative pshycodynamic</u> effect evoked by loss of faith in Medication or physician prescribing medication. ☛

➲ In Zero Order Reaction: ☛☛ (High Yield for AIIMS/AIPGME/DNB 2012-2013)

- A "constant <u>amount</u> "of drug is eliminated per unit time. ☛

- Rate of elimination is <u>independent</u> of plasma concentration. ☛

- Drugs with zero order elimination have no fixed half life. (t $_{1/2}$ is variable) ☛

- **Phenytoin, Ethanol and Salicylates** show zero order kinetics. ☛   AI 1996

➲ In First Order Reaction: ☛☛ (High Yield for AIIMS/AIPGME/DNB 2012-2013)

- A "Constant <u>fraction</u> "of drug is eliminated per unit time. ☛

- Rate of elimination is <u>directly dependent</u> on plasma concentration. ☛   COMED 2008

- Drugs with first order elimination have fixed half life. (t $_{1/2 \text{ is constant}}$) ☛

- <u>Most drugs</u> show first order kinetics. ☛

Zero order: Elimination rate constant ☛

    t $_{1/2}$ variable ☛

First order: Elimination rate variable ☛

    t $_{1/2}$ Constant ☛

"Some drugs follow first order kinetics but at higher doses follow zero order kinetics. This is actually known as "<u>Pseudo zero order</u>". **Phenytoin, Tolbutamide, Warfarin and Theophylline** follows both zero as well as first order kinetics."

➲ Important Points:

▶ In ist t$_{1/2}$ ☛	50% drug eliminated	
▶ In 2 nd t$_{1/2}$ ☛	75% drug eliminated	
▶ In 3 rd t$_{1/2}$ ☛	87.5% drug eliminated	
▶ In 4 th t$_{1/2}$ ☛	93.7% drug eliminated	COMED 2003
▶ In 5 th t$_{1/2}$ ☛	97% drug eliminated	

- ▶ <u>Loading</u> dose is governed by <u>volume of distribution</u>.

- ▶ Maintainance dose is governed by clearance of drug and half life (t ½).

7

- ☐ Acidic drugs ionize more at <u>alkaline pH</u>. ☞
- ☐ Basic drugs ionize more at <u>acidic pH</u>. ☞
- ☐ <u>Unionized drugs</u> are lipid soluble and diffusible. ☞
- ☐ <u>Ionized </u>drugs are lipid insoluble and non diffusible. ☞
- ☐ Ionized drugs are excreted mainly by kidney.   AI 2006
- ☐ <u>Acidic drugs are absorbed in stomach.</u>(are unionized in acidic medium and hence difusable) ☞
- ☐ <u>Basic drugs are absorbed from intestine.</u> ☞(Proximal)   AI 1991

- ▶ Ionized drugs poorly pass across placenta. ☞
- ▶ Ionized drugs poorly pass across blood brain barrier☞
- ▶ Ionized drugs poorly pass across renal tubules (easily excreted) ☞

➲ Microsomal Enzyme Inducers☞☞ (High yield for 2011-2012)

✓ Barbiturates☞
✓ Carbamezapine, clofibrate ☞
✓ DDT☞
✓ Ethanol☞
✓ Griseofulvin☞
✓ Phenytoin, phenobarbitone☞   AIIMS 1991
✓ Primidone, ☞

✓ Rifampicin, ritonavir ☞   AIIMS 1991
✓ Phenobarbitone☞
✓ Smoking, **chronic** alcohol intake☞

➲ Microsomal Enzyme Inhibitors✱

✓ Quinolones☞
✓ Erythromycin☞
✓ Quinidine☞
✓ Grape Fruit juice☞
✓ Cimetidine☞
✓ Allopurinol☞
✓ Ketocanazole☞

✓ Omperazole

✓ Sulfonamides

✓ MAO inhibitors

⊃ Acteylation and why it is an Important Reaction: (High yield for 2011-2012)

❏ **Isoniazid, hydralazine, sulfonamides, procainamide,** and a number of other drugs are metabolized by **acetylation** of a hydrazino or amino group. **AIPGME 2012**

❏ This reaction is catalyzed by **N-acetyl transferase-2 (NAT-2)**, an enzyme in the liver cytosol that transfers an acetyl group from acetyl coenzyme A to the drug.

❏ Individuals differ markedly in the rate at which drugs are acetylated, because of polymorphisms in the NAT-2 gene, resulting in a bimodal distribution of the population into **"rapid acetylators" and "slow acetylators."**

⊃ Features Related to Nephrotoxicity:

▶ **Most** nephrotoxic cephalosporine: **cephaloridine**

▶ **Most** nephrotoxic aminoglycoside: **gentamycin.**

▶ **Least** nephrotoxic antitubercular: rifampicin

▶ **Least** nephrotoxic aminoglycoside: tobramycin.

▶ Tetracycline **safe** in renal failure: doxycycline.

⊃ Drugs affecting liver ✳

(Repeated In 2008, 2009, 2010, 2011)

Causing "Hepatitis"

• Halothane   PGI 2003

• MAO inhibitors

• Anti convulsants

• Methyl dopa

• Rimapicin, Isoniazid, Pyrizanamide

Causing "Intrahepatic Cholestasis"

• Phenothiazines

• TCA

• NSAIDS

• Erythromycin, Carbencillin, Sulfonamides

Hepatotoxins

- Tetracycline☞
- CCL₄☞
- Paracatemol☞
- Methotrexate☞
- Alfatoxin☞

➲ Remember Hepatotoxic Drugs and Type of Hepatotoxicity

Acetaminophen hepatotoxicity (direct toxin)

Halothane hepatotoxicity (idiosyncratic reaction)

Methyldopa hepatotoxicity (toxic and idiosyncratic reaction)

Isoniazid hepatotoxicity (toxic and idiosyncratic reaction)

Sodium valproate hepatotoxicity (toxic and idiosyncratic reaction)

Phenytoin hepatotoxicity (idiosyncratic reaction)

Chlorpromazine hepatotoxicity (cholestatic idiosyncratic reaction)

Amiodarone hepatotoxicity (toxic and idiosyncratic reaction)

Erythromycin hepatotoxicity (cholestatic idiosyncratic reaction)

Oral contraceptive hepatotoxicity (cholestatic reaction)

17, a-alkyl-substituted anabolic steroids (cholestatic reaction)

Trimethoprim-sulfamethoxazole hepatotoxicity (idiosyncratic reaction)

Hydroxymethylglutaryl-coenzyme (HMG-CoA) reductase inhibitors ("statins") (idiosyncratic mixed hepatocellular and cholestatic reaction)

Total parenteral nutrition (steatosis, cholestasis)

➲ Cardiotoxic Drugs: ☞☞(High Yield for AIIMS/AIPGME/DNB 2012-2013)

- ✓ Doxarubicin, ☞
- ✓ Daunorubicin, ☞
- ✓ Vincristine☞
- ✓ Halothane☞
- ✓ Alcohol☞

➲ Drugs Causing Pulmonary Fibrosis: ☞☞(High Yield for AIIMS/AIPGME/DNB 2012-2013)

- ❑ Busulfan☞
- ❑ Bleomycin☞
- ❑ Methotrexate☞
- ❑ Nitrofurantoin☞
- ❑ Sulfasalazine☞
- ❑ Practolol☞
- ❑ Amiadarone☞

7

⊃ **Drugs Causing Osteoporosis: (High Yield for AIIMS/AIPGME/DNB 2012-2013)**

→ Glucocorticoids

→ Anticonvulsants

→ Cytotoxic drugs

→ Cyclosporine

→ Lithium

→ Heparin

→ GnRH analouges

→ Almunium

→ Throxine in increased doses

⊃ **Drugs with Low Safety Margin:** ✳

✓ Digoxin☞

✓ Anticonvulsants☞

✓ Antiarrythhmics☞

✓ TCA (tricyclic antidepressants) ☞

✓ Lithium☞   **AIIMS 1982**

✓ Aminoglycosides☞

⊃ **Teratogens**

(High Yield for AIIMS/AIPGME/DNB 2012-2013)

❑ Carbamezapine:	→	Cleft Lip, cleft palate.✳✳	
❑ Valproic acid:	→	Neural tube defects. ✳	
❑ Warfarin:	→	Chondrodysplasia punctata☞☞☞	
❑ Carbimazole:	→	Fetal cutis Aplasia☞☞☞	
❑ Lithium:	→	Ebsteins Anomaly☞☞	
❑ Thalidomide:	→	Phocomelia✳✳	
❑ Chloramphenicol:	→	Grey baby syndrome	
❑ DES:	→	Clear cell cancer. ✳	

7

PHARMACOLOGY

⊃ ↑Age Related Changes in Body Which Effect Drug Action:✳✳

- Body fat ↑ ☜☜
- Volume of distribution↑☜☜

→ Total body water↓☜
→ Lean body mass↓☜
→ Baroreceptor sensitivity↓☜
→ Renal function↓☜
→ Serum albumin↓☜
→ Hepatic blood flow↓☜

⊃ Drugs Produced by DNA Recombinant Technology:✳

- ► Human insulin☜
- ► Growth hormone☜
- ► Interferons☜
- ► Interleukins☜
- ► Monoclonal antibodies☜
- ► Vaccines ☜

⊃ Pharmacology of Autonomic Nervous System:

- ► Neuro transmitter in all pre ganglionic nerves is acetyl choline.
- ► Neuro transmitter in all ganglia is acetyl choline.
- ► Neuro transmitter in all post ganglionic parasympathetic nerves is acetyl choline.
- ► Neuro transmitter in almost all post ganglionic sympathetic nerves is noradrenaline except renal, Mesenteric beds and sweat glands.

Botulinium inhibits ACH release.	AIIMS 1991
ACH use is not possible because it is rapidly degraded.	JIPMER 1992

⊃ Receptor Agonists: (High Yield for AIIMS/AIPGME/DNB 2012-2013)

→ Contraction of sphincter puppilae:	➡ Miosis
→ Contraction of ciliary muscle:	➡ Accomodation

→ Heart:	➡ ↓ Heart rate↓ conduction velocity
→ Lungs:	➡ Bronchoconstriction
→ GIT:	➡ ↑motility, cramps
→ Urinary bladder:	➡ Contraction
→ Glands:	➡ Secretion
→ Blood vessels:	➡ Dilatation

▶ Ach:	✓ No clinical use
▶ Bethanacol:	✓ Treatment of <u>ileus, urinary retention</u>
▶ Methnachol:	✓ Diagnosis of <u>bronchial hyperreactivity</u>
▶ Pilocarpine:	✓ Treatment of <u>glaucoma, xerostomia</u>

Acetyl cholinesterase inhibitors:

▶ Edrophonium: diagnosis of myasthenia gravis   AI 2001

▶ Physostigmine: tertiary amine antidote in atropine poisoning

▶ Neostigmine/pyridostigimine: treatment of ileus, urinary retention, reversal of NM blockade. AIIMS 1998

▶ Donepezil: treatment of Alzhiemers disease

Organophosphates: used as insecticides

⊃ **OP Poisoning: (DUMB-BELLS) (High Yield for 2011-2012)**

▶ Diarrhoea
▶ Urination
▶ Pin point pupils   TN 1989
▶ Miosis
▶ Bradycardia
▶ Bronchoconstriction
▶ Excitation of muscles and CNS (Nicotinic)
▶ Lacrimation
▶ Salivation
▶ Sweating

Atropine is used in OP Poisoning.(Antidote)	KERALA 1995
Atropine is also used for amantia (mushroom) poisoning.	AI 2007
Pralidoxime is used in conjuction and reactivates cholinesterase.	AI 2008, AI 2007

Pralidoxime:

PAM is <u>an acetylcholinesterase (AChE) reactivating agent</u>. It is only useful for counteracting AChE inhibitors which act by phosphorylating the enzyme (organophosphates). Pralidoxime can remove the phosphate group from AChE, thus regenerating the enzyme. This must be done in a timely fashion because normally after the phosphate group is bound to the enzyme, it undergoes a chemical reaction known as "aging." Once this bond ages, pralidoxime will no longer be effective.

Atropine:

<u>It is a nonselective muscarinic antagonist.</u> Although atropine would be an appropriate agent for this patient, it acts by preventing the excess ACh from stimulating muscarinic receptors rather than altering the activity of AChE.

⊃ Atropine Uses (Asked)

► Atropine is used in OP Poisoning.

► Atropine is used as mydriatic.

► Atropine is used in mushroom poisoning   **JK BOPEE 2012**

► Atropine is used in preanaesthetic medication

► Atropine is used in treating Brady arrhythmias.   **PGI 1998**

⇨ Nicotinic receptor antagonists:

Ganglion blockers:
- ✓ Hexamethonium and Mecamylamine.
- ✓ Reduce autonomic tone.
- ✓ Prevent baroreceptor reflex changes in heart rate

α 1 agonists: uses
- ✓ <u>Phenyl epherine</u>: Nasal decongestant, Mydriatic
- ✓ <u>Methoxamine</u>: Paroxysmal atrial tachycardia

α 2 agonists:
- ✓ <u>Clonidine and methyl dopa</u>: used in hypertension.

⊃ Alpha-Methyldopa is Used Most Commonly in: Pregnancy induce Hypertension

- ➥ Methyldopa is a 'sympatholytic drug'.
- ➥ It is the member of family of alpha-2 agonists that act centrally and reduce sympathetic output.
- ➥ The drug has a good safety record in pregnancy and is used for hypertension in pregnancy
- ➥ Side effects of the drug are sedation and dry mouth.
- ➥ Prolonged use can cause
- ✳ Mental depression
- ✳ Hemolytic anemia (Coombs +ve),
- ✳ Hepatitis

7

➲ β Agonists: (High yield for 2011-2012)

▶ <u>Isoproterenol</u>: β1 =β2, used in bronchospasm, heart block, bradyarrythmias

▶ <u>Dobutamine</u>: β1>β2

Selective β ₂ agonists:

▶ <u>Salmeterol, albuterol, terbutaline</u> : used in asthma   <u>MAH 2012</u>

▶ <u>Ritodrine</u>: used in premature labour

■ Isoprenaline	β 1 ,β2	Diastolic BP↓, HR↑
■ Noradrenaline	α1,α2,β1	Systolic BP↑, Diastolic BP↑, HR↓
■ Adrenaline	α1,α2,β1,β2	Systolic BP↑, Diastolic BP↓, HR↑
■ Dopamine	D1,D2,α1,α2,β1	Improves renal perfusion

➲ Remember Noradrenaline, Adrenaline, Dopamine act Through Seven Pass Receptors. AIIMS 2011

α 1 blockers:
✓ prazosin,
✓ doxazosin,
✓ terazosin,
✓ tamsolusin   ROHTAK 1997
α 2 blockers:
✓ yohimbine,
✓ mirtazapine (antidepressant)   TN 2004

⇨ Beta blockers:

▶ β 1 blockers:
✓ Acebutolol,
✓ Atenolol,
✓ Metoprolol
▶ Combined β1 β2 blockers:
✓ Labetelol,
✓ Cardeivelol,
✓ Dilevelol   PGI 2007, PGI 2005

➲ Timolol:

▶ Used mainly for glaucoma.   ROHTAK 1997

▶ No miosis   AIIMS 1987

- ► No accomdative spasm
- ► Timolol can cause
- ✓ AV Block,
- ✓ Bradycardia,
- ✓ Hypotension,
- ✓ Asthma.   PGI 2001
- ► Contraindicated in asthma, heart block.   PGI 2005

⮞ Esmolol:

- ► Is cardioselective.   PGI 2006
- ► Esmolol is shortest acting beta blocker.
- ► It has no intrinsic activity.   PGI 2003

⮞ Carvedilol:

- ► Combined α1, β1,β2 Blocker   PGI 2003
- ► Antioxidant

⮞ Serotonin: 5HT

5HT Agonists:

- ► $5HT_{1A}$ Agonist: ✳✳ buspirone, ipsapirone, gepirone: antianxiety
- ► $5HT_{1B}$ Agonist: ✳ sumitriptan migrane
- ► $5HT_4$ Agonist: ✳ cisapride ↑gastric motility

5HT Antagonists:

- ► $5HT_{2A}$ Antagonist : ✳ cyproheptadine, ketansarein,   AI 1994
- ► $5HT_{2A/2\,C}$ Antagonist:✳ clozapine   AI 1994
- ► $5HT_3$ Antagonist: ✳ ondansteron, granisteron, tropisteron   JK BOPEE 2012

⮞ Anti Migrane Drugs (High Yield for 2011-2012)

- ► Triptans act on $5HT_{1B}$ receptors. (agonists)   AIIMS 2007
- ► Sumitriptan is <u>shortest</u> acting triptan.
- ► Frovatriptan is <u>longest</u> acting triptan
- ► Rizatriptan is <u>fastest</u> acting triptan

Ergotamine or methysergide toxicity may cause severe vasospasm, which may affect the large arteries and diminish pulses.   AIIMS 2011

✓ DOC for <u>acute</u> migrane: aspirin, paracatemol

✓ DOC for <u>acute severe</u> migrane: sumitriptan.　　PGI 1999

Drugs used in **prophylaxis of migrane:**

— Beta blockers: propranolol　　NIMHANS 2K

— TCA: amytriptiline

— Calcium channel blockers(flunarazine)　　NIMHANS 2K

— Valproic acid,cyproheptadine　　NIMHANS 2K

— Methyl sergide

— Papaverin

⊃ Prostaglandins:

✓ Cytoprotective for stomach.　　PGI 1998

✓ Dilate renal vasculature

✓ Contract uterus　　KERALA 1995

✓ Maintain ductus arteriosus

PGE 1:

▶ Misoprostol: treatment of NSAID induced ulcer. maintains ductus arteriosus　　COMED 2008

▶ Alprostadil: used in male impotence,

PGE 2:

▶ Dinoprostone: used in cervical ripening, abortifacient

PGF 2 α:

▶ Carboprost: abortifacient

▶ Latanoprost: treatment of glaucoma

PGI 2:

▶ Prostacyclin: vasodilator, platelet stabilizer

7

PGE2 and PGF2:

▶ Mediate dysmenorrhea

Thrombaxanes:

Platelet aggregator	JIPMER 2003

➲ Drugs Used for Glaucoma:

Acetazolamide is a **carbonic anhydrase inhibitor** used firstly as **IV** followed by **Oral dose**.

Mannitol is also used as an **IV Solution**

Topical drugs to be used are:

- Topical Pilocarpine 2 %☞☞
- Topical Timolol☞
- Topical Dorzolamide☞
- Topical Brinzolamide☞

Anti glaucoma drugs:

▶ Binatoprost, ☞

▶ Travoprost,☞

▶ Iravoprost

▶ Unoprostone

➲ Aspirin:

▶ Irreversible COX inhibitor: **PGI 2002**

▶ Antiplatelet

▶ Analgesia

▶ Antipyretic

▶ Anti-inflammatory

- Aspirin has an **anti thrombotic effect.**

- It **inhibits** TXA$_2$ synthesis in platelets by irreversible acetylation and inhibition of COX 1.   **JK BOPEE 2008**

- **Platelets are annucleate** and can't overcome this inhibition **but endothelial cells are nucleate** and can overcome this acetylation by regenerating more enzyme.(**these points are gems, so try to remember not just for exams**)

- This is a theraupatic effect finding use of aspirn in prophylaxis for stroke and MI management.

▶ **Causes respiratory alkalosis and metabolic acidosis in high doses.**

▶ GIT ulceration, bleeding, salicylism: tinnitus vertigo

▶ Bronchoconstrction

▶ Reyes syndrome

▶ ↑BT

⊃ Other NSAIDS: (High Yield for 2011-2012)

▶ <u>Non selective COX 2 inhibitors</u>
- — Ibuprofen
- — Naproxen
- — Indomethacin
- — Ketorolac
- — Sulindac

▶ <u>Selective COX 2 inhibitors:</u>
- ✓ Celecoxib,
- ✓ Etorocoxib,
- ✓ Valdecoxib,
- ✓ lumiracoxib,
- ✓ Rofecoxib   PGI 2002

▶ <u>Preferential</u> COX 2 inhibitors:
- ✓ Nimesulide,   JK 2001
- ✓ Meloxicam,
- ✓ Namebutone   AIMS 1998

- — Selective COX 2 inhibitors <u>don't have antiplatelet action</u>.   PGMCET 2007

- — NSAID with good tissue penetration/good concentration in synovial fluid : <u>Ketorolac</u>   UP 2007

- — Ketorolac is <u>non narcotic, non steroidal </u>but acting on opoid receptors.   MP 1998

- — <u>Misoprostol</u> is effective in NSAID induced Gastric ulcer.   AI 2007

- — <u>Nefopam </u>doers not inhibit prostaglandins.   MANIPAL 2006

7

➲ **Acetaminophen: (High yield for 2011-2012)**

> ▶ No antiplatelet action
>
> ▶ No Reyes syndrome
>
> ▶ No bronchospasm
>
> ▶ Lesser GIT effects
>
> ✓ Increased doses cause hepatotoxicity due to depletion of glutathione
>
> ✓ N acetyl cysteine is used in acetaminophen toxicity   AI 1996

➲ **Diuretics✶**

Sites of action of Diuretics: (High yield for 2011-2012)

Thiazides➛➛	
• Chlorthiazide	*Distal tubule*➛
• Hydrochlorthiazide	*Distal tubule*➛
• Chlorthalidone	*Distal tubule*➛
• Indapamide	*Distal tubule*➛
• Metolazone	*Proximal and distal tubules*➛
Loop diuretics➛➛	
• Frusemide	*Loop of Henle*➛
• Bumatenide	*Loop of Henle*➛
• Ethacrynic acid	*Loop of Henle*➛
Carbonic anhydrase inhibitors➛➛	
• Acetazolamide➛	*Proximal tubule*✶
Potassium sparing diuretics➛➛	
• Spironolactone➛	*Distal tubule and collecting duct*
• Triamterene➛	*Distal tubule and collecting duct*
• Amiloride➛	*Distal tubule and collecting duct*

➲ **Thiazides**➥

> ► Chlorthalidone➥
>
> ► Indapamide➥
>
> ► Chlorthaiazide➥
>
> ► Inhibit <u>Na⁺/Cl⁻</u> transporter in DCT. ➥(compare with loop diuretics below)
>
> ► With K+ sparing diuretics are first choice treatment of essential hypertension. ➥
>
> ► "<u>Excretion</u>" of sodium and potassium increases while as that of calcium decreases.　　AIIMS 2011
>
> ► Thiazides are drugs used for" idiopathic Hypercalciuria."(Dents Disease) "But not" Hypercalcemia. ➥
>
> Uses: ➥➥
>
> > — CHF➥
> >
> > — Hypertension➥
> >
> > — Nephrogenic Diabetes Insipidus➥
>
> Side effects/ Cause: ➥➥
>
> ✓ Hyperglycemia➥　　　　　　　　　　　　　　　　　AIIMS 2007
>
> ✓ Hyperurecemia➥
>
> ✓ Hypercalcemia➥　　　　　　　　　　　　　　　　　UP 2007
>
> ✓ Kindly understand the point:
>
> ✓ Thiazides are used in treatment of hypercalciuria but themselves causes hypercalcemia and renal stones.　　　　　　　　　　　　　　　UP 2007

➲ **Loop Diuretics:** ✷✷

> ► **Furesmide** is basically a **diuretic** which acts **rapidly. (high ceiling, loop diuretics)** ➥
>
> ► is a sulphamoyl derivative　　　　　　　　　　　　AP 1986
>
> ► (Furosemide, bumetanide, toresamide, ethacrynic acid.) ➥
>
> ► Furesmide acts on <u>thick ascending limb</u> of loop of Henle. ➥
>
> ► Inhibit Na⁺/K⁺/2Cl⁻ transporter. ➥ (compare with thiazides above)
>
> ► Can be used in renal failure. ➥
>
> ► It is the **drug of choice** for: **Acute Hypercalcemia**➥
>
> ► Second drug of choice after morphine for **Acute Pulmonary edema.** ➥

Uses:

▶ Heart Failure

▶ Pulmonary edema   **AIIMS 2007**

▶ Acute Renal Failure

▶ Hypertension

▶ Anion Overdose

Side effects:

✓ Hyperuricemia   **AI 1994**

✓ Hypocalcemia   **AI 1994**

✓ Hyperlipidemia   **AI 1994**

✓ Hyperglycemia

✓ Acute saline depletion

Ethacrynic acid among the group is more ototoxic.   **AIIMS 1980**

➲ Spironolactone and Eplerenone ✴✴ (High yield for 2011-2012)

Spironolactone **antagonizes the sodium retaining effect of aldosterone**   **TN 2003**

and is used to treat

• **Cirrhotic edema,**

• **Nephrotic syndrome**

• **CHF and**

• **Hyperaldosteronism**

• **Hirusitism**   **DNB 2011**

      JK BOPEE 2012

✓ It also acts as a diuretic. (pottasium sparing)   **AIIMS 1986**

✓ **Caneronone** is its active metabolite.   **APGEE 2004**

✓ Spironolactone reduces potassium loss and in combination with other potassium sparing diuretics, **fatal hyperkalemia** can occur.   **JIPMER 1995**

Side effects are:

▶ Rashes,

▶ Abdominal pain,

▶ Amenorrhea.   **JK BOPEE 2012**

▶ Gynaecomastia   **JK BOPEE 2012**

➲ Triameterene and Amiloride: ➜➜

✓ Pottasium sparing diuretics. ➤	PGI 2001
✓ Saluretic effect is greater than thiazides	PGI 1999
✓ Block Na+ channels in collecting duct. ➤	
✓ Amiloride is more potent. ➤	

➲ Acetazolamide: ✱✱

Carbonic anhydrase inhibitors(CA) ✱✱

♯ Acetazolamide➤

♯ Dorazolamide➤

♯ Brinzolamide ➤

CA is present in renal tubular cells, gastric mucosa, exocrine pancreas, brain, rbc and ciliary body of eye.

Brinzolamide is a highly specific competitive and reversible inhibitor of CA II.   AIIMS 2011

Uses: ➜➜

- ✓ Glaucoma➤
- ✓ Acute mountain sickness➤
- ✓ Epilepsy➤
- ✓ Not given in "sulfonamide sensitivity"

➲ Mannitol✱✱

▶ Primary site of action of Mannitol is **proximal tubule.** ➤

▶ Mannitol Increases **blood viscosity** and increases perfusion. ➤   JK 2009

▶ Mannitol is **not metabolized.** ➤

▶ Mannitol is given **parentally**➤

▶ On **oral administration** mannitol causes **Osmotic diarrhoea.** ➤

Uses: ➜➜

- • Reduce ICT (Intra Cranial Tension) ➤
- • Reduce IOT(Intra Ocular Tension) ➤
- • Increase Urine volume in Renal Compromise. ➤
- • <u>Should not</u> be given in **ATN, anuria, pulmonary edema,**   KERALA 2002

Toxicity: ➜➜

- • Extracellular volume Expansion➤
- • Dehydration and Hyper natremia. ➤

➲ Raised ICT: Treatment

- ✓ IV mannitol
- ✓ Furosemide
- ✓ Hyperventilation
- ✓ Fluid restriction
- ✓ Osmotic agents
- ✓ Corticosteroids (dexamethasone) for vasogenic edema

⊃ <u>Antidiuretics:</u> ✱✱

☐ <u>Vasopressin</u>☛
☐ <u>Lypressin</u>☛
☐ <u>Terlipressin</u>☛
☐ <u>Desmopressin</u>☛
✓ Given intranasally,
✓ "DOC for <u>Diabetes insipidus</u>".   MAHE 2001, AIIMS 1986
✓ Lithium☛
✓ Demeclocycline ☛ "<u>DOC for SIADH</u>"   AIIMS 2005

⊃ **Desmopressin**

▬ Drug of choice for **Central Diabetes Insipidus** is: Desmopressin   AIPGMEE 2011
Desmopressin is a modified form of human hormone <u>arginine vasopressin</u>, a peptide containing nine amino acids.
▬ Desmopressin binds to <u>V2 receptors</u> in <u>renal</u> <u>collecting ducts</u>, increasing water reabsorption.

⊃ **SIADH**

Can be caused by many factors, such as ectopic ADH production and release from neoplastic tissue (small cell carcinoma of lung, pancreatic carcinoma, lymphosarcoma, Hodgkin's disease, reticulum cell sarcoma, thymoma, and carcinoma of duodenum or bladder) or by drugs that release or potentiate the action of ADH, such as

▶ Carbamazepine,   AIIMS
▶ Vincristine,   PGI
▶ Vinblastine,   PGI
▶ Cyclophosphamide,
▶ Chlorpropamide
▶ Tricyclic antidepressants.

⊃ **Antidiabetic Drugs:** ✱

Metformin ☛☛

▶ ↑Glycolysis
▶ ↓Gluconeogenesis   PGI 1997
▶ Diarrhoea and metallic taste in mouth are adverse features. ☛

✓ It is ***particularly used in obese*** patients☛ Obesity <u>is not a</u> contraindication.   JK BOPEE 2011
✓ It does not cause weight gain ☛

✓ **Lactic acidosis** is a feared complication of Metformin use.   AIIMS 1995
✓ Metformin should **not** be used in Renal impairment. ☛   AI 2004
✓ Causes Malabsorption of Vit B 12. ☛
✓ Metformin is a **biguanide**☛

Acarbose and Miglitol

Are **alpha glucosidase inhibitor.**

Decreases progression of impaired glucose tolerance to overt disease. along with (metformin, orlistat)

reduces fibrinogen levels also **AIIMS 2008**

Are euglycemics. Do not cause hypoglycemia. **AI 2004**

✓ Side effects are: GIT Discomfort, Flatulence, Diarrhoea. ☞

✓ Also known as **starch inhibitor.** ☞

✓ Potential Hepatotoxicity has been demonstrated. ☞

➲ Acarbose

✓ Is a **glucosidase inhibitor** and thus it prevents the postprandial digestion and absorption of starch and disaccharides and the postprandial rise in plasma glucose is blunted in both normal and diabetic subjects.

✓ Acarbose reduces postrandial plasma glucose levels in **Type 1 and TypeII** diabetes mellitus patients. (HbAc)

✓ It **significantly improves Hemoglobin Ac** levels in severely hyperglycemic type 2 DM patients.

✓ α Glucosidase inhibitors do not stimulate insulin release and therefore **do not result in hypoglycemia.** These agents may be considered as monotherapy in elderly patients with post prandial hyperglycemia.

✓ α Glucosidase inhibitors **reduce the progression of Type II diabetes** in patients with impaired glucose tolerance. **AIIMS 2009**

Hypoglycemia occurs with sulfonylureas (Tolbutamide) and can be severe, prolonged for days and fatal especially in elderly and in heart failure.

➲ Thiazolidinediones (High Yield for 2011-2012)

Thiazolidinediones or TZDs act by **binding to PPARs (peroxisome proliferator-activated receptors),** a group of receptor molecules inside the cell nucleus, specifically PPARγ (gamma). ☞

The ligands for these receptors are free fatty acids (FFAs) and eicosanoids. When activated, the receptor migrates to the DNA, activating transcription of a number of specific genes. By activating PPARγ: ☞☞

✓ Insulin resistance is decreased ☞

✓ Insulin sensitivity ↑ **PGI 2002**

✓ Adipocyte differentiation is modified ☞

✓ VEGF-induced angiogenesis is inhibited ☞

✓ Leptin levels decrease (leading to an increased appetite) ☞

✓ Levels of certain interleukins (e.g. IL-6) fall ☞

✓ Adiponectin levels rise ☞

Chemically, the members of this class are derivatives of the parent compound thiazolidinedione, and include: ☞☞

☐ Rosiglitazone ☞

☐ **Pioglitazone** ☞   JK 2005 PGI 2002

☐ Troglitazone, which was withdrawn from the market due to an increased incidence of **drug-induced hepatitis.** ☞

☐ Ciglitazone. ☞

Piaglitazone and rosiglitazone are anti hyperglycemics which bind to PPAR (Peroxisome Proliferator Activating Receptors) increase insulin sensitivity, increase insulin receptor numbers and decrease hepatic gluconeogenesis. ☞

Side effects: ☞☞

Hypoglycemia, Weight gain, edema☞

Repaglinide and Nateglinide: ☞☞

✓ Stimulate **insulin release** from Pancreatic Beta cells☞

✓ Used in Type II DM as an adjunct just before meals. ☞

✓ Have rapid onset, short duration. ☞

Glucagon Like Peptide- Exenatide, Liraglutide

✓ It is an **incretin released from small intestine.** ☞

✓ Glucagon like peptide. (GLP 1 analouge) ☞

✓ **Augments insulin secretion**☞

✓ Degraded by enzyme dipeptidyl peptidase **DPP4**☞

✓ **Sitasgliptin** inhibits DPP4 and hence **augments action of exenatide**☞

✓ It is a full agonist and used as a combination☞

➲ **Pramalinitide:** ☞☞**(High Yield for AIIMS/AIPGME/DNB 2012-2013)**

• **Synthetic amylin analogue:** ☞
• <u>Reduces glucagon secretion</u> from alpha cells of pancreas.☞
• **Useful in both type 1 and type 2 DM.** ☞

○ Glucomannan: ☛☛(High Yield for AIIMS/AIPGME/DNB 2012-2013)

✓ Powdered extract from konjar. ☛
✓ Promoted as a dietary fiber for diabetics. ☛
✓ Dietary adjunct for diabetes. ☛
▶ ↓Appetite, ☛
▶ ↓Serum lipids☛
▶ ↓Blood sugar, ☛
▶ ↓Constipation☛

○ Insulin: ☛☛

▶ t ½ of insulin in blood is: 5 minutes.	Orissa 2k
▶ Insulin causes potassium entry into cell.	AIPGMEE 2005
▶ Insulin has 51 amino acids. Human insulin differs from pork insulin by 1 amino acid.	PGI 1987
▶ Humulin is human insulin.	AMU 1987
Insulin R has the same amino acid sequence as endogenous human insulin.	JK BOPEE 2012

▶ Rapid acting: ☛ insulin aspartate, lispro insulin, insulin glusuline	PGI 2004
▶ Short acting : ☛ semilentene, soluble insulin (SSS)	
▶ Intermediate acting: ☛ insulin zinc suspension, isophane insulin	
▶ Long acting: ☛ protamine zinc insulin, insulin glargine	Kar 1990
✓ Shortest acting sulfonyl urea: tolbutamide☛	
✓ Longest acting oral hypoglycemic: chlorpropamide☛	
✓ Shortest acting oral hypoglycemic: nateglinide☛	
✓ Safest in elderly tolbutamide ☛	
✓ Oral hypoglycemic causing cholestatic jaundice: chlorpropamide.	AIIMS 1995

○ Diabetes Insipidus (High Yield for AIIMS/AIPGME/DNB 2012-2013)

Thiazides paradoxically exert an antidiuretic effect in diabetes insipidus.

DRUGS USED IN DI:

❑ Vasopressin (Neurogenic DI)
❑ Amiloride (Lithium induced DI)
❑ Indomethacin
❑ Chlorpropamide
❑ Carbamazepine
❑ Clofibrate

7

PHARMACOLOGY

➲ Corticoids

▶ Maximum mineralocorticoid activity: Aldosterone☞   TN 2001

▶ Maximum glucocorticoid activity: Dexamethasone☞

(Ozurudex is a intravitreal implant containg 0.7% dexamethasone used for treating CRVO, BRVO (Central retinal vein occlusion and branched retinal vein occlusion))   AIIMS 2011

▶ Glucocorticoids with <u>maximum mineralocorticoid</u> activity: Hydrocortisone☞

▶ Glucocorticoids with <u>minimum gluco ocorticoid activity</u>: Hydrocortisone☞

➲ Anti Androgens: ☞☞(High Yield for 2011-2012)

☐ <u>Flutamide</u>☞   AIIMS 2002

☐ <u>Biclutamide</u>☞

☐ <u>Nilutamide</u>

✓ Finasteride☞   AIMS 2002

✓ Dutasteride☞

✓ Danazol☞

✓ Cyproterone☞(Androgen receptor blocker)   NIMHANS 2006

Androgen Receptor Antagonists: Flutamide, Bicalutamide, and Nilutamide

• Used primarily in conjunction with a GnRH analogs in the treatment of metastatic prostate cancer

Spironolactone

• Aldosterone receptor antagonist which also is a weak androgen receptor antagonist/inhibitor of testosterone synthesis (inhibits CYP17)   JK BOPEE 2012

Cyproterone acetate

• Progestin and a weak anti-androgen receptor agent

5 ALPHA Reductase Inhibitors

• Finasteride

• Dutasteride

➲ Important Table: (High Yield for 2011-2012)

▶ **Danazol:** anabolic, progestational anti androgenic with weak androgenic activity☞☞

▶ **USES:** Fibrocystic disease, Endometriosis, menorrhagia, precocious puberty, infertility, gynaecomatia.

▶ **Side effects:** Acne, weight gain, hot flushes occasionally   JK BOPEE 2011

▶ **Flutamide:** used in metastatic prostate cancer. ☞☞

▶ **Has fast action in case of BHP.**   COMED 2008

▶ **Biclutamide:** longer acting and more potent analogue of flutamide☞☞

▶ **Finasteride:** selective 5 α reductase <u>type 1 inhibitor</u>.   MAHE 2007

▶ Uses BHP, hirusitism,   AI 2010

▶ Male pattern baldness.   Manipal 2001

► **Dutasteride:** 5 α reductase <u>type 1 and type 2 inhibitor</u>.longer acting ✍✍

► **Cyproterone:** used in PCOD, Precocious puberty, ✍✍

► **Clompihene** is anti estrogen.   AI 1998

⊃ Tamoxifen

(Repeated In 2008, 2009, 2010, 2011)

► Tamoxifen is an **"oral selective estrogen receptor modulator".**   PGI 2002

► ↓FSH.   PGI 2000

► It is used for the **"treatment of early and advanced breast cancer"** in <u>both pre</u>- and post-menopausal women.

► It is also **"approved by the FDA"** for the **"reduction of the incidence of breast cancer"** in women at high risk of developing the disease. **It has been further approved for the reduction of contralateral (in the opposite breast) breast cancer. "<u>Does not cause</u>"**   AIIMS 2011

► It has **"benefit throughout the whole spectrum of breast cancer":** In the treatment of non-invasive ductal carcinoma in situ (DCIS) it has been shown to be effective as adjuvant to surgery and radiotherapy. In early breast cancer adjuvant treatment with tamoxifen has been shown to significantly reduce the risk of disease recurrence and death, and reduce the risk of new primary tumours developing in the contralateral breast.

► These benefits appear to **"apply to both node-negative and node-positive disease"** and irrespective of the menopausal status of the patient. Five years of treatment with tamoxifen is currently recommended in the adjuvant setting.

► Tamoxifen is a well-established endocrine treatment for advanced breast cancer, providing effective palliative treatment in hormone-responsive breast cancer **"at all stages of the disease and irrespective of the age of the patient".**

► Given orally once daily, it is relatively **well tolerated** , most side effects being of an antioestrogenic nature – hot flushes, tachycardia,

► However, as a **partial agonist the drug also** displays some oestrogenic properties. Whilst these can confer some benefits in postmenopausal women, such as protection against osteoporosis and cardiovascular disease, they can also have detrimental effects in a small number of women, notably an **increase in the risk of** **"endometrial hyperplasia and carcinoma".**

► **Exemastine, latrazole** are other hormonal agents used for breast cancer.   AI 2004

► **Latrazole** is an aromatase inhibitor.   AIIMS 2006

⊃ **Anti Asthmatics:** ✳

Theophylline and Doxophylline ☞☞

Mechanism of Action: ☞

▶	Inhibits phosphodiesterase 4 and increases c AMP concentration. ☞	AI 2006
▶	Blocks **adenosine receptors**☞	AI 2005
▶	**Releases calcium** from Sarcoplasm ☞	
▶	BETA 2 Agonist	AI 2010
▶	Mucociliary movement stimulator	AI 2010

Important points about metabolism: ☞☞

- It has **low therapeutic index**☞
- At high doses **kinetics changes from First order to zero order.** ☞
- Erythromycin **inhibits** metabolism of Theophylline (Increases Theophylline levels) ☞
- Crosses placenta and is sereted in milk. ☞
- **Smoking , phenytoin, rifampicin, phenobarbitone** ↓ **plasma levels of Theophylline**☞   AIIMS 1992
- **Erythromycin, ciprofloxacin, cimetidine, allopurinol** ↑ **plasma levels of theophylline**☞   AI 1997

Theophylline in asthma

- — Simulates mucociliary movements   **AIPGMEE 2010**
- — PDE-4 inhibitor
- — Beta-2 agonist
- ✳ Relaxes bronchial smooth muscles,
- ✳ Increases mucociliary movements that help to clear the respiratory secretions.
- ✳ It also boosts diaphragmatic contractility.

⊃ **Sodium Chromoglycate:** ✳✳

▶	Inhibits mast cell degranulation. ☞	PGI 1997
▶	**Ineffective** in **acute** attack. ☞	
▶	Used for **prophylaxis**☞	
▶	Not absorbed orally, given as aerosol. ☞	

⊃ **Monteleukast**

- Monteleukast is a **LTRA (Leukotriene receptor antagonist)** used in maintainence therapy of asthma and relief of seasonal allergies. ☞   AI 2007
- It is **not useful in acute attacks.** It is usually administered orally. ☞   JK BOPEE 2012
- Montelukast is a **CysLT1 antagonist**; that is it blocks the action of leukotriene D4 on the cysteinyl leukotriene receptor CysLT1 in the lungs and bronchial tubes by binding to it. This reduces the bronchoconstriction otherwise caused by the leukotriene, and results in less inflammation.

Because of its method of operation, it is not useful for the treatment of acute asthma attacks. Again because of its very specific focus of operation, it does not interact with other allergy medications such as theophylline.

Side effects; ☞☞

Side effects include gastrointestinal disturbances, hypersensitivity reactions, sleep disorders and increased bleeding tendency, aside from many other generic adverse reactions. Its use is associated with a higher incidence of **Churg-Strauss syndrome**☞

- Another leukotriene receptor antagonist is **zafirlukast** taken once daily. ☞   **SGPI 2005, JIPMER 2003**

- 5 lipo oxygenase inhibitor is Zileuton   **COMED 2006**

➲ Beta 2 Sympathatomimetic Bronchodilators:

▶ Salbutamol, Terbutaline : short acting: used in acute attacks☞

▶ Salmeterol, Bambuteral, Formoterol: long acting: used for prophylaxis☞

▪ <u>Most effective</u> bronchodilators☞

▪ No anti-inflammatory effects☞

Side effects: ☞☞
- ✓ Hypokalemia☞
- ✓ Hyperglycemia☞
- ✓ Tolerance, tacchyphylaxis☞

➲ Ipratropium and Tiotropium:

— **Anticholinergic** broncho dilators☞   **AI 1993**

— Broncho dilators of choice in COPD/ COAD☞

➲ Steroids: ☞☞(High Yield for AIIMS/AIPGME/DNB 2012-2013)

- ✓ Are **anti-inflammatory**☞.
- ✓ ↑Lipocortin levels.   **PGI 2006**
- ✓ Block phospholipid breakdown.   **JK 2005**
- ✓ Not bronchodilators☞
- ✓ Have **no role in acute attacks or status asthamaticus**☞
- ✓ Reduce airway inflammation.   **PGI 2006**
- ☐ Beclomethasone,
- ☐ Budesonide,   **AI 1995**
- ☐ Fluticasone,   **AI1995**
- ☐ Flunisolide
- ☐ Triamicinolone.   **AI 1995**
- ☐ Ciclesonide are commonly used steroids☞

> ▶ Inhalational steroids cause **oropharyngeal candidiasis**   AP 1996
> ▶ Topical steroids cause: glaucoma   MP 1998
> ▶ Parentral steroids cause cataract.   AIIMS 1986
> ▶ Commonest type of stertoid induced cataract is **posterior subcapsular cataract.**   CUPGEE 1996
> ▶ Steroids are contraindicated in **hepetic corneal ulcer.**

➲ Newer Drugs ☞☞ (High Yield for AIIMS/AIPGME/DNB 2012-2013)

> ▶ Omalizumab. ☞
>
> ▶ Humanized <u>IgE antibody</u>
>
> ▶ Reduces frequency of Asthma exacerbations
>
> ▶ Ciclesonide: ☞
>
> ▶ Inhalational steroid
>
> ▶ Prodrug
>
> ▶ Cilomilast, Roflumilast ☞
>
> ▶ PGE 4 inhibitors

➲ First Generation Antihistaminics: ☞☞

- ✓ Diphenhydramine ☞
- ✓ Dimenhydrinate ☞
- ✓ Promethazine ☞
- ✓ Hydroxyzine ☞
- ✓ Meclizine ☞
- ✓ Pheniramine ☞
- ✓ Chlorphenaramine ☞
- ✓ Cyclazine ☞

➲ Second Generation Antihistaminics: ☞☞

- ✓ Terfenadidine ☞
- ✓ Astemizole ☞
- ✓ loratidine ☞
- ✓ Cetrizine ☞
- ✓ Fexofenadine ☞
- ✓ Rupatidine ☞
- ✓ Azelastine ☞
- ✓ Acrivastin ☞

An antiemetic drug that also decreases acid secretion due to its action on H1 receptors:

Promethazine:

Promethazine is an H1 antihistaminic drug of promethazine class. It has a wide variety of uses :

- o Sedative-Hypnotic
- o Antiemetic
- o Antiallergic
- o Antimotion sickness
- o Morning sickness
- o Antiurticaria
- o As a potentiating agent for meperidine (pethidine)

▶ *Slowest acting:*	✓ Astemizole
▶ *Fastest acting:*	✓ Terfenadine
▶ *Maximum topical activity:*	✓ Azelastine
▶ *Additional PAFantagonistic activity:* ☞	✓ Rupatidine
▶ *Banned drug:*	✓ Astemizole
▶ *Active metabolite of terfenadine:*	✓ Fexofenadine

⊃ Antibiotics

Mechanism of action of Antibiotics: ✱

Inhibition of Cell Wall synthesis: ☞☞   AIIMS 2008, 2006

- ▶ **Inhibition of crosslinking (Transpeptidase): Pencillins**, Cephalosporins, Vancomycin, Imipinem, Aztreonam☞   AIIMS 2008, 2006
- ▶ **Inhibition of Peptidoglycan synthesis: Cycloserine**, Bacitracin☞   DNB 2011 KCET 2012
- ▶ **Inhibition of β glucan synthesis:** Caspofungin☞

⊃ Penicillin-Binding Proteins (PBPs)

- ➡ **Penicillin-binding proteins (PBPs)** are a group of proteins that are characterized by their affinity for and binding of penicillin.
- ➡ All **beta-lactam antibiotics** bind to PBP to have their effect of preventing cell wall construction by the bacterium.
- ➡ PBPs are target site of beta lactam antibiotics.
- ➡ PBPs **mediate the final step in peptidoglycan synthesis** which is a critical step in biosynthesis of cell wall of bacteria.
- ➡ Beta lactam antibiotics kill bacteria by this mechanism.
- ➡ **Mutation** in PBP leads to development of **Resistance.**

Inhibitors of Protein Synthesis:

► Aminoglycosides, Tetracyclines bind to ☞ 30 S Ribosomal subunit.   AIIMS 2005

► Chloramphenicol, erythromycin, clindamycin bind to ☞ 50 S Ribosomal subunit.

Inhibition of Nucleic Acid Synthesis

► Rifampin blocks RNA Synthesis RNA polymerase. ☞

► Quinolones inhibit DNA Synthesis DNA gyrase (topoisomerase) ☞

► Sulfonamides and trimethoprim inhibit Nucleotide synthesis of tetrahydrofolic acid. ☞   KERALA 1884

Alteration of Cell Membrane:

► Anti Bacterial Polymyxin☞

► Anti Fungal Azoles (Ketoconazole,Flucanozole, Itracanazole) inhibit ergostreol synthesis

► Amphoterecin disrupts fungal cell membrane by binding to ergosterol. ☞ AI 2003

Metranadizole acts as an electronic sink taking away electrons that organisms need for survival.

Highly Effective against anaerobes.   JK BOPEE 2012

Drugs Inhibiting Cell Wall Synthesis:

☐ Pencillins☞
☐ Cephalosporins
☐ Cycloserine☞   AIIMS 2009
☐ Vancomycin☞
☐ Bacitracin☞

Drugs Acting on Cell Membrane:

✓ Amphotercin,☞
✓ Nystatin ☞
✓ Polymyxin, ☞
✓ Colistin☞

Drugs Interfering with Metabolism:

✓ Trimethoprim☞
✓ Sulfonamides☞
✓ Ethambutol, Pyrimethamine☞
✓ PAS☞

⊃ Mechanism of Action of Antimicrobials☜☜

▶ **Aminoglycoside, Tetracyclines** Block protein synthesis at the **30S ribosomal Subunit.**☜   PGI 2005

▶ **Chloramphenicol** Blocks protein synthesis at the **50S ribosomal subunit.** ☜

▶ **Clindamycin** Blocks protein synthesis at the **50S ribosomal subunit.** ☜

▶ **Macrolides** Block protein synthesis at the **50S ribosomal subunit.**☜

▶ **Penicillin** along with the cephalosporins, imipenem and actreonam, penicillin inhibits **peptidoglycan cross-linking.** ☜

▶ **Quinolones** Block **DNA topoisomerases.** ☜   AIIMS 1993

▶ **Rifampin** Blocks **mRNA synthesis.** ☜

▶ **Sulfonamides** Block **nucleotide synthesis.**☜

▶ **Vancomycin** Blocks **peptidoglycan synthesis**☜

▶ **Bacteriostatic drugs:**
  → Erythromycin,
  → Clindamycin,
  → Chloramphenicol,
  → Streptomycin,
  → Tetracycline,
  → Trimethoprim
▶ **Bacteriocidal drugs:**
  → Pencillin,
  → Cephalosporin,
  → Aminoglycosides (most),
  → Metronidazole

▶ Aminoglycosides and tetracyclines bind to *30 S Ribosomal subunit.* ☜

▶ Chloramphenicol, erythromycin, clindamycin bind to *50 S Ribosomal subunit.* ☜

▶ Chloramphenicol inhibits bacterial protein synthesis by *blocking peptidyl transferase.* ☜

- ▶ Isoniazid *inhibits synthesis of* **mycolic acid.** ☞
- ▶ Metranadizole acts as an *electronic sink taking away electrons that organisms need for survival.* ☞
- ▶ Rifampin blocks *RNA polymerase.* ☞
- ▶ Quinolones inhibit *DNA gyrase (topoisomerase)* ☞
- ▶ Sulfonamides and trimethoprim *inhibit synthesis of* **tetrahydrofolic acid.** ☞
- ▶ Azoles (Ketoconazole, Flucanozole, Itracanazole) *inhibit* **ergostreol synthesis.** ☞
- ▶ Amphoterecin disrupts fungal cell membrane by **binding to ergosterol.** ☞
- ▶ Vancomycin *inhibits* **transpeptidases.** ☞
- ▶ Capsofungin *blocks synthesis of B glucan.* ☞

⊃ **Penicillinase-Resistant Penicillins are able to Resist Degradation by Staphylococcal Penicillinase**☞☞   **AI 2005**

- ✓ <u>Methicillin,</u> ☞(Acid labile)   **JIPMER 1991**
- ✓ <u>Nafcillin,</u> ☞
- ✓ <u>Oxacillin,</u> ☞
- ✓ <u>Cloxacillin,</u> ☞   **PGI 2004**
- ✓ <u>Dicloxacillin</u> ☞
- ✓ <u>Flucloxacillin</u> ☞

⊃ **Cephalosporins** ☞☞

Ist Gen: effective against gram+organisms☞

Cefazolin	Cephalothin	Cephapirin	Cephalexin	Cefadroxil	Cephradine

2nd Gen: effective against gram- organisms☞

Cefamandole,	Cefuroxime, Cefoxitin, Cefotetan,Cefmetazole, Cefaclor,Cefprozil, Cefpodoxime,
Loracarbef	

3rd Gen: effective against gram- enterobacteriacea☞

Cefotaxime	Ceftriaxone	Ceftizoxime	Ceftazidime	Cefoperazone	Cefixime AIIMS 2009	AIIMS 2004

*The third-generation cephalosporins and the carbapenems are the two classes that include potential candidates for empirical single-agent therapy. Ceftazidime has been the most extensively studied of the third-generation cephalosporins as monotherapy because of its **superior activity against P. aeruginosa**.ceftazidime and cefepime possess **significant antipseudomonal activity**,The third-generation cephalosporin ceftazidime is now likely the drug of choice, with imipenem, piperacillin, or amoxicillin-clavulanic acid as reasonable alternatives.*   **MAH 2012**

4th Gen: ☞

Cefipime	AIIMS 2004
Cefpirome	

⊃ Cefepime

✓ The fourth-generation cephalosporin **cefepime** is **more resistant to hydrolysis by beta-lactamases** than are the third-generation cephalosporins ☞

✓ **It is stable against plasmid-encoded beta-lactamase** and is also relatively resistant to the inducible chromosomally encoded beta-lactamases ☞

✓ **Penetrates rapidly into gram-negative bacteria** ☞

✓ **Targets multiple essential penicillin-binding proteins** ☞

✓ **Cefoxitine is effective against anaerobes. AIIMS 2009**

✓ **Cephaperazone has antipseudonmonal activity. AIIMS 2009**

✓ **Cefepime** is **inactive** against, methicillin-resistant staphylococci, penicillin-resistant pneumococci, most strains of *Clostridium difficile*, and most strains of enterococci such as *Enterococcus faecalis* ☞

Quinupristin and dalfopristin ☞☞

◻ Quinupristin and dalfopristin are used in treatment of <u>vancomycin-resistant Enterococcus faecium (VREF)</u> ☞

◻ **Bind 50 S ribosome. Dalfopristin inhibits the early phase** of protein synthesis in the bacterial ribosome and **quinupristin inhibits the late phase** of protein synthesis ☞

◻ Quinupristin and dalfopristin are **bacteriostatic against Enterococcus faecium** and **bacteriocidal against strains of methicillin-susceptible and methicillin-resistant staphylococci.** ☞   **AI 2006 PGI 2005**

◻ Quinupristin and dalfopristin combination, a **streptogamin** antibacterial agent for intravenous administration, is a sterile lyophilized formulation of two semisynthetic pristinamycin derivatives. ☞

◻ **Quinupristin is derived from pristinamycin I, while**

◻ **Dalfopristin is derived from pristinamycin IIA**

⊃ Carbapenams: ☞☞(High Yield for AIIMS/AIPGME/DNB 2012-2013)

    ◻ <u>Imipenem,</u> ☞

    ◻ <u>Meropenem,</u> ☞

    ◻ <u>Faropenem,</u> ☞

    ◻ <u>Ertapenem</u> ☞

▶ Effective against gram +, gram-, anaerobic pathogenic bacteria. ☞☞

▶ Beta lactamase resistant ☞☞

▶ Imipenem is inhibited by dehydropeptidase and hence given along with cilastatin. ☞☞

                                        COMED 2007/JK BOPEE 2011

7

➲ Aztreonam: ☞

- Is a **monobactam.** ☞
- No activity against gram+ and anaerobes. ☞
- Can be **safely used in patients allergic to pencillin** and related group of drugs because of lack of cross reactivity. ☞

COMED 2008

➲ Linezoild

is a synthetic antibiotic used for the treatment of serious infections caused by multi-resistant Gram-positive bacteria, including ☞☞

- ✓ **Streptococci,** ☞
- ✓ **Vancomycin-resistant enterococci (VRE),** ☞
- ✓ **Methicillin-resistant Staphylococcus aureus (MRSA).** ☞

PGI 2006

- ► **Linezolid is a protein synthesis inhibitor:** ☞
- ► Unlike most other protein synthesis inhibitors, which inhibit elongation, linezolid appears to work on the first step of protein synthesis ie **"initiation"** ☞
- ► Linezolid binds to the **23S portion** of the 50S subunit (the center of peptidyl transferase activity) ☞
- ► Linezolid is effective against all clinically important Gram-positive bacteria, notably Enterococcus faecium and Enterococcus faecalis **(including vancomycin-resistant enterococci)**, Staphylococcus aureus (including methicillin-resistant Staphylococcus aureus, MRSA), Streptococcus agalactiae, Streptococcus pneumoniae, and Streptococcus pyogenes☞
- ► It has **almost no effect on Gram-negative bacteria.** ☞

➲ Macrolides:✸

Three important macrolides are: ☞☞

- ☐ *Erythromycin,* ☞☞
- ☐ *Azithromycin and* ☞☞
- ☐ *Clarithromycin*☞☞
- — Azithromycin is effective against **Chlamydia, Mycoplasma, Ureaplasma. Legionella** ☞   PGI 1997
- — **Mycobacterium avium intercellulare.** ☞
- — Azithromycin is excreted by **kidneys.** ☞
- — Azithromycin does not inhibit cytochrome P450 **(IS NOT AN ENZYME INHIBITOR)** ☞
- — Azithromycin is **safe** in pregnancy. ☞
- ► **Clarithromycin** is most effective against **H.Pylori.** ☞
- ► Macrolides stimulate **motilin recptors** and cause GIT distress. ☞   MP 2000 AI 1999
- ► **Erythromycin estolate** causes **cholestatic** jaundice. ☞
- ► **Erythromycin is used in pencillin allergics.**   AI 2010
- ► **In meningitis and pencillin allergy Chloramphenicol is used**   AI 2010

➲ **Telithromycin**☛☛**(High yield for 2011-2012)**

- ☐ Is the **first ketolide antibiotic** to enter clinical use. ☛
- ☐ It is used to treat **mild to moderate respiratory infections.** ☛
- ☐ Telithromycin is a <u>semi-synthetic erythromycin</u> derivative☛
- ☐ Telithromycin **prevents bacteria from growing**, by interfering with their protein synthesis. ☛
- ☐ Telithromycin binds to the <u>subunit 50S</u> of the bacterial ribosome, and blocks the progression of the growing polypeptide chain. ☛
- ☐ Telithromycin has over **10 times higher affinity** to the subunit 50S than erythromycin☛
- ☐ Telithromycin is metabolized mainly in the **liver**, the main elimination route being the bile, a small portion is also excreted into the urine. ☛

➲ **Glycopeptides Antibiotics: Vancomycin, Teicoplanin: ✳**   **PGI 1998**

⇨ **Vancomycin:** ☛☛

- ✓ Inhibits bacterial cell wall. ☛
- ✓ Ototoxicity, nephrotoxicity, **Red man syndrome**☛   **KAR 2004**
- ✓ It is **DOC for MRSA infection** and used for pseudomembranous colitis☛

➲ **Teicoplanin**☛☛**(High yield for 2011-2012)**

- ✓ **Teicoplanin** is an antibiotic used in the prophylaxis and treatment of serious infections caused by Gram-positive bacteria, including MRSA. **methicillin-resistant Staphylococcus aureus and Enterococcus faecalis.** ☛
- ✓ It is a **glycopeptide antibiotic** extracted from Actinoplanes teichomyceticus, with a similar spectrum of activity to vancomycin. ☛
- ✓ Its mechanism of action is to **inhibit bacterial cell wall synthesis**☛

➲ **Clindamycin:** ☛☛

- ▶ Lincosamide antibiotic. ☛
- ▶ Inhibits protein synthesis. ☛   **AIIMS 1996, 1998**
- ▶ Binds to 50 S ribosomal subunit. ☛
- ▶ Implicated in pseudomembranous colitis. ☛
- ▶ DOC for <u>streptococcal necrotizing fasciitis</u>.

➲ **Tetracyclines:** ☛☛

- ▶ Group I: Tetracycline, oxytetracycline, Chlortetracycline☛
- ▶ Group II : Demeclocycline☛
- ▶ Group III: Minocycline, Doxycycline ☛

- Are bacteriostatic. ☞
- Tetracyclines bind to ☞ 30 S Ribosomal subunit.   **AIIMS 2005**
- All tetracyclines are" **nephrotoxic** "<u>except Doxycycline</u>. ☞
  → Doxycycline is metabolized and excreted via liver in bile. ☞
  → Doxycycline is not excreted via kidneys and hence is not nephrotoxic. ☞
  → All tetracyclines except doxycycline "accumulate" in renal failure. ☞
  → All tetracyclines except doxycycline "enhance "renal failure. ☞
- Contraindicated in pregnancy, lactation. ☞
- Outdated tetracyclines cause <u>Fanconis syndrome</u>. ☞   **JK 2005**
- Doxycycline causes photodermatitis.   **JIPMER 1998**
- Are teratogenic   **AI 2008**
- cause super infections   **AI 2008**
- Cause tooth discoloration   **AI 2008**
- Mibnocycline causes pigmentation   **AI 2010**

Tetracyclines. Tetracyclines have been an important class of antibiotics with significant antianaerobic activity. In addition to activity against anaerobes, tetracyclines possess modest activity against easy gram-negative rods and many gram-positive cocci.

Bind to 30 S ribosomal subunit.	**PGI 2011**
Are hepatotoxic	
Can cause pseudotumor cerebri	**PGI 2011**
Can cause vertigo, dizziness, nausea. (vestibular symptoms)	**PGI 2011**
Are used in malignant pleural effusions.	

Uses: ☞☞

- ▶ Doxycycline is indicated for use in the treatment of **chronic adult periodontitis** in order to increase clinical attachment, reduce probing depth, and reduce bleeding upon probing☞
- ▶ **Endocervical, rectal, or urethral infection**, uncomplicated, caused by Chlamydia trachomatis☞
- ▶ **Epididymo-orchitis** caused by C. trachomatis or Neisseria gonorrhoeae or☞
- ▶ **Nongonococcal urethritis** caused by C. trachomatis or Ureaplasma urealyticum☞
- ▶ **Gonococcal infections**, uncomplicated (except anorectal infections in men) ☞
- ▶ **Lyme disease**☞
- ▶ **Malaria prophylaxis** ☞
- ▶ **Syphilis (early)**, for penicillin-allergic patients☞
- ▶ **Syphilis (of > 1 year's duration)**, for penicillin-allergic patients☞

➲ Chloramphenicol: (Re Emergence) (High yield for 2011-2012)

- ▶ Binds **50 S** subunit. ☛
- ▶ **Bacteriostatic** ☛
- ▶ Blocks elongation of peptide chain. ☛   ICS 1998
- ▶ Undergoes **extensive enterohepatic circulation.** ☛
- ▶ Causes **aplastic anemia** ☛
- ▶ Causes **grey baby syndrome.** ☛

➲ Aminoglycosides: ☛☛

▪ **Bactericidal** ☛	AIIMS 2008
▪ **Inhibit translation.**	AI 1999
▪ Do not show <u>Post antibiotic effects</u>.	PGI 2011
▪ Active against **gram - bacilli.** ☛	
▪ Ineffective against anaerobes ☛	
▪ Used synergestic with pencillins. ☛	
▪ **Distributed only extra cellularly**	AIIMS 2008
▪ Streptomycin was discovered by **Waksman.** ☛	
▪ **Netlimicin is least ototoxic.** ☛	
▪ **Framycetin, sisomycin are aminoglycosides.**	MAHE 2007
▪ Streptomycin is used in treatment of **plague/ tularemia.**	KERALA 1990
▪ **Teratogenic**	AIIMS 2008
▶ **Ototoxic,**	
▶ **Vestibulotoxic (especially) GENTAMYCIN**	PGI 2011
▶ **nephrotoxic**, cause neuromuscular blokade ☛	AIIMS 1985
▶ **Ototoxicity is due to damage to stereocilia.**	
▪ **Should not be used in myasthenia gravis**	PGI 1989
▪ **Resistance is due to enzyme production.**	
▪ **Amakacin is one of the most resistant to bacterial inactivating enzymes.**	KAR 1995

➲ Quinolones: ☛☛

Ist generation:

✓ Norfloxacin, ciprofloxacin, ofloxacin, pefloxacin. ☛

2nd generation:

✓ Lomefloxacin, levofloxacin, sparfloxacin, gatifloxacin, moxifloxacin ☛

7

PHARMACOLOGY

✓ Pefloxacin: attains high CSF concentration☞

✓ Levofloxacin: highest oral bioavalibility☞

✓ Pefloxacin: highest first pass metabolism☞

✓ Sparfloxacin: longest acting, phototoxic   **KERALA 2003**

✓ Moxifloxacin: most potent, active against gram positive organisms☞

▶ Are contraindicated in children   **CUPGEE 1999**

▶ Cause arthopathy in children   **CUPGEE 2001**

▶ Temafloxin: causes immune hemolytic anemia☞☞

▶ Trovafloxacin: hepatotoxic. ☞☞

⇨ **(High yield for 2011-2012)**

■ DOC in brucella: ☞	✓ Doxycycline+rifampicin	
■ DOC in cholera: ☞	✓ Doxycycline	
■ DOC in gonorrhea: ☞	✓ Ceftriaxone	**JIPMER 1992**
■ DOC in MRSA: ☞	✓ Vancomycin	
■ DOC in VRSA: ☞	✓ Linezolid	
■ DOC in toxoplasmosis:	✓ Cotrimoxazole	
■ DOC in Lymes disease: ☞	✓ Doxycycline	
■ DOC in p. carnii: ☞	✓ Cotrimoxazole	**AIIMS 1997**
■ DOC in syphilis: ☞	✓ Pencillin G	
■ DOC in Actinomycosis: ☞	✓ Pencillin G	**AIIMS 2002**
■ DOC in legionella: ☞	✓ Azithromycin/ levofloxacin	
■ DOC in LGV: ☞	✓ Azithromycin	
■ DOC in plague: ☞	✓ Streptomycin	**CUPGEE 1995**
■ DOC in kala azar	✓ Pentamidine	**MP 2000**
■ Oral Drug for Kala Azar	✓ Miltefosine	**JK BOPEE 2011**

➲ **Chemo Prophylactic Agents of Choice:** ☞☞

▶ Cholera:☞	Tetracycline	**KERALA 1996**
▶ Plague:☞	Tetracycline	
▶ P. carnii: ☞	Cotrimoxozole	
▶ Whooping cough: ☞	Erythromycin	
▶ Diphtheria: ☞	Erythromycin	
▶ TB: ☞	INH	
▶ MAC: ☞	clathiromycin, azithromycin	
▶ Leptosporiosis:	Tetracyclines	**AIPGME 2012**
▶ Malaria:☞	Chloroquine	
▶ Rheumatic fever	Benzathine pencillin	**KARNATKA 2005**

⊃ Parasitology

Antimalarials

Treatment of	
Chloroquine sensitive malaria: chloroquine	
Chloroquine resistant malaria: mefloquine	MANIPAL 2006
Mefloquine resistant malaria: sulfadoxine+pyremethamine	
Quinine	
► It is the DOC for cerebral malaria.	PGI 1993
► Causes hypoglycemia	PGI 1999
► Can be given safely in pregnancy along with chloroquine	PGI 2002
Primaquine	
► It is the only anti malarial active in <u>exoerythrocytic stage</u>	
► Primaquine is <u>ineffective</u> against p. falciparum	UPSC 1984
► Primaquine is effective for <u>radical cure of pl. vivax</u>	PGI 1986
► Can cause <u>G6PD deficiency</u>.	AP 1988
Halofantrine	
is effective against Chloroquine resistant p. falciparum and p. vivax.	AIIMS 1997
Causes prolonged QT	
Artemensin derivatives:	
► (Artesunate, artemether, arteheter) are fastest acting erythrocytic schizontocides	
► Lumefantrine is an anti malarial.	AI 2005
► Pyronaridine is an antimalarial.	AIIMS 2003

⊃ Chloroquine:(High yield for 2011-2012)

- ► Chloroquine is an **antimalarial** drug.
- ► Chloroquine is also an **immunosuppressant** drug.
- ► Chloroquine is **lysomotrophic** (accumulates in lysosomes)
- ► It is widely distributed in **adipose tissue.**
- ► It also has
- ► Anti tumor,
- ► Anti viral,
- ► DMARD Properties.
- ► It is used in treatment of SLE, Rheumatoid arthritis

Chloroquine is known to cause lots of side effects.

7

PHARMACOLOGY

Occular manifestations:

▶ Keratopathy,

▶ Retinal toxicity,   APGEE 2004

▶ Blurred vision,   PGI 1989

▶ Corneal deposits,   AP 1997

▶ Central serous retinopathy ,

▶ Pigmentary bulls eye retinopathy,

▶ Optic atrophy

• Myopathy   APGEE 2004

• Retinopathy

⊃ Drugs Acting on GIT:

▶ Prokinetics are- metocloperamide, domeperidone, Plus

    ☐ Cisapride,

    ☐ Mosapride

    ☐ Renzapride

    ☐ Prucalopride

    ☐ Tegaserod

Primary indication is Gastroesphageal Reflux Disease (**GERD**)

▶ Anti ulcer drugs.

▶ Ranitidine, Roxatidine, famotidine, – H_2 antagonist

▶ Omeprazole, esmoperazole, rabeperazole, pentaperazole –**proton pump inhibitor**

▶ Are long acting   AI 2010

▶ Are long lasting   AI 2010

▶ Have high first pass metabolism

▶ Sucralfate – **ulcer protectant.**

▶ H. pylori gastritis responds to: omperazole, clathiromycin,amoxicillin, metronadizole therapies, bismutith

▶ OMPERAZOLE HAS ADDITIONAL ENZYME INHIBITING ACTION   AI 2010

▶ Triple therapy : (lansoprazole, clarithromycin, and amoxicillin)

▶ Triple therapy: (bismuth subsalicylate, tetracycline, and metronidazole).

➲ Drugs Effective in:

- Morning sickness : Promethazine
- Mountain sickness : Acetazolamide
- Motion sickness : Hyoscine
- Sea sickness: Meclizine

⇨ Omeprazole:

Omeprazole is a potent enzyme inhibitor of CYP family. The drug can inhibit metabolism of warfarin and therefore can lead to bleeding.

- Proton pump inhibitors are long acting sulphonamide derivatives.
- These act by blocking the enzyme **Na+K+ ATPase**.
- The drugs are **well absorbed orally**
- The drugs have **high first pass** metabolism.
- These drugs produce **prolonged acid suppression**
- PPI with enzyme inhibiting activity is: Omeprazole   AIPGME 2010

Dexlansoperazole is a Newly developed PPI with novel delivery system for GERD.

➲ Antifungal Drugs:

ANTIFUNGAL	MECHANISM OF ACTION
■ Amphotericin B	Affinity for ergosteol, forms micropores in fungal cell membrane. AI 2003
■ Griseofulvin	Interferes with mitosis, disorients microtubules.
■ Ketoconazole AI 2008	Inhibits fungal lanosterol 14-demethylase, impairing ergosterol synthesis.
■ Flucytosine	KAR 04
	Inhibits thymidilate synthetase (after being converted to active form; 5-fluorouracil)

- **Polyenes**- amphotericin b, nystatin, hamycin, natamycin
- **Heterocyclic benzofuran**- griseofulvin.
- **Azoles:**
  - ☐ **Miconazole,**
  - ☐ **Clotrimazole,**
  - ☐ **Ketoconazole,**
  - ☐ **Fluconazole ,**
  - ☐ **Voricanazole,**
  - ☐ **Itracanazole,**
  - ☐ **Posacanazole,**
  - ☐ **Rabucanazole.**

Echinocandins: (inhibit synthesis of 3 glycan, a component of fungal cell wall)

- ☐ Capsofungin
- ☐ Anidulafungin
- ☐ Micafungin

Newer One:

Terbenafine (FOR ONCHOMYCOSIOS)   MAH 2012, JK BOPEE 2012

Nicomycins:

- ☐ Inhibit chitin synthesis

Aspergillosis (treatment): <u>Itraconazole</u> is indicated in the treatment of aspergillosis caused by *Aspergillus* species in patients who are intolerant of or refractory to amphotericin B therapy.   **PGI 2011**

<u>Voricanazole</u> is also used in treatment of Aspergillosis.   **PGI 2011**

Blastomycosis (treatment) itraconazole is indicated for the treatment of pulmonary and extrapulmonary blastomycosis caused by *Blastomyces dermatiditis* in immunocompromised and nonimmunocompromised patients

Candidiasis (prophylaxis) Fluconazole is indicated for the prophylaxis of candidiasis in patients undergoing bone marrow transplant who receive cytotoxic chemotherapy and/or radiation therapy. ☜

⊃ **Amphoterecin: ✳✳✳(High yield for 2011-2012)**

- ▶ Polyene derivative☜☜
- ▶ Derived from streptomyces nodosus
- ▶ Fungicidal as well as fungistatic.☜
- ▶ High affinity for <u>ergosterol</u>.☜   St. Johns 2002
- ▶ Given IV. With glucose solution☜   COMED 2005
- ▶ Given as lipid bound preprations:
- — Amphotercin B lipid complex
- — Amphotercin B colloid suspension
- — Liposomal Amphotercin Decreases toxicity   AI 2010
- — Is not mixed with saline.   COMED 2007
- ▶ Causes hypokalemia   AIIMS 2004

⇨ **Parenteral amphotericin**

- ▶ **Parenteral amphotericin B is indicated in the treatment of aspergillosis caused byAspergillus fumigates**
                    PGI 2011
- ▶ Parenteral **amphotericin** B is indicated in the treatment of **disseminated candidiasis** caused by *Candida* species C

▶ Parenteral **amphotericin** B is indicated in the treatment of **coccidioidomycosis** caused by *Coccidioides immitis*. C

▶ Parenteral **amphotericin** B is indicated in the treatment of **cryptococcosis** caused by *Cryptococcus neoformans C*   **HP 2006 AIIMS 2002**

▶ Parenteral **amphotericin** B is indicated in the treatment of **fungal endocarditis**

▶ Parenteral and intraocular administration of **amphotericin** B are used in the treatment of candidal endophthalmitis

▶ Parenteral ˙**amphotericin** B is indicated in the treatment of **histoplasmosis** caused by *Histoplasma capsulatum*

▶ Parenteral **amphotericin** B is indicated, with or without concurrent administration of flucytosine, in the treatment and suppression of **cryptococcal meningitis** caused by *Cryptococcus neoformans*   **AIIMS 2002**

▶ Parenteral **amphotericin** B is also indicated in the treatment of fungal meningitis caused by organisms such as *Coccidioides immitis, Candida* species,*Sporothrix schenckii*, and *Aspergillus* species

▶ Parenteral **amphotericin** B is indicated in the treatment of **mucormycosis (phycomycosis)** caused by*Mucor, Rhizopus, Absidia, Entomophthora*, and *Basidiobolus* organisms

▶ Parenteral **amphotericin** B is indicated in the treatment of **fungal septicemia**   **TN PSC 2000**

▶ Parenteral **amphotericin** B is indicated in the treatment of **disseminated sporotrichosis** caused by *Sporothrix schenckii*

Anti virals:

▶ **Acyclovir** is a highly potent and selective inhibitor of the replication of certain herpesviruses, including herpes simplex virus (HSV) types 1 and 2, varicella-zoster virus (VZV), and Epstein-Barr virus (EBV).✱

AI 1995/ JK BOPEE 2011

▶ **Valacyclovir,**

▶ The L-valyl ester of **acyclovir,**

▶ Is converted almost entirely to **acyclovir** after oral administration.

▶ Valacyclovir has pharmacokinetic advantages over orally administered **acyclovir:**

▶ It exhibits **significantly greater oral bioavailability**

▶ **Results in higher blood levels, and**

▶ **Can be given less frequently** than acyclovir.✱

▶ **Cidofovir:** Cidofovir is a phosphonate nucleotide analogue of cytosine.

▶ Its major use is in CMV infections, particularly retinitis, but it is active against a broad range of herpesviruses, including HSV, human herpesvirus (HHV) type 6, HHV-8✱

▶ **FOMIVIRSEN:** Fomivirsen is the first antisense oligonucleotide ✱

▶ Fomivirsen has been approved for intravitreal administration in the treatment of CMV retinitis in AIDS patients who have failed to respond to other treatments or cannot tolerate them

PHARMACOLOGY

7

▶ **Ganciclovir:**

▶ An analogue of **acyclovir**, ganciclovir is active against HSV and VZV and is markedly more active than **acyclovir** against **CMV**. ✲   **AIIMS 1993, AIMS 1987**

▶ **FAMCICLOVIR AND PENCICLOVIR**

▶ **FOSCARNET:** Foscarnet (phosphonoformic acid) is a pyrophosphate-containing compound that potently inhibits herpesviruses, including CMV.

▶ **Idoxuridine:** analogue of thymidine   **KAR 1993**

▶ Idoxuridine inhibits the replication of herpesviruses and poxviruses.

▶ **Cannot be given orally**   **KERALA 2000**

▶ **TRIFLURIDINE:** Trifluridine is a pyrimidine nucleoside active against HSV-1, HSV-2, and CMV.

▶ **VIDARABINE:** Vidarabine is a purine nucleoside analogue with activity against HSV-1, HSV-2, VZV, and EBV.

⊃ **Other Antiviral Drugs (High Yield for 2011-2012)**

▶ <u>Lamivudine</u> is a pyrimidine nucleoside analogue that is used primarily in combination therapy against HIV infection.

It is also active against <u>HBV</u> through inhibition of the viral DNA polymerase and has been approved for the treatment of chronic HBV infection✲

▶ <u>Lobucavir</u> is a synthetic cyclobutane nucleoside analogue with activity against a broad range of herpesviruses, HIV, and <u>HBV</u>. ✲

▶ <u>Pleconaril</u> is an investigational drug active in vitro against picornavirus replication, including over 90% of the most commonly isolated enterovirus types and 80% of rhinovirus serotypes

▶ <u>INTERFERONS</u>

Interferons are cytokines that exhibit a broad spectrum of antiviral activities as well as immunomodulating and antiproliferative properties✲

⊃ **Anti HIV Drugs:**

Nucleoside reverse transcriptase analogues:✲✲

— Zidovudine, ☞
— Didanosine,
— Zalcitabine,
— Stavudine, ☞
— Lamivudine,
— Abacavir   **AI 2006**

Nonnucleoside reverse transcriptase inhibitors ✽

—	Nevirapine, ☞	AI 2007
—	Delavirdine, and	
—	Efavirenz ☞	PGI 2005
		AIIMS 2011

Nucleotide reverse transcriptase inhibitors ✽

—	Tenofovir

Protease inhibitors:

—	Saquinavir ☞	JK BOPEE 2012
—	Nelfanavir	JK BOPEE 2012
—	Indinavir	
—	Atazanavir ☞	
—	Ritonavir ☞	JK BOPEE 2012
—	Tipranavir	

Fusion inhibitor

Enfuvertide ✽

➲ Side Effects Commonly Asked (High yield for 2011-2012)

▪ Stavudine, didanosine, zalcitibine:	✓ *Peripheral neuropathy* ☞☞	AI 2007
▪ Indinavir:	✓ *Nephrolithiasis* ☞	
▪ Efavirenz:	✓ *Rash, liver enzymes ↑, CNS effects*	
▪ Zidovudine :	✓ *Myelosuppression, Megaloblastic anemia*	PGI 2006
▪ Didanosine:	✓ *Pancreatitis* ☞☞	AIIMS 1991
▪ Abacavir:	✓ *Severe hypersensitivity* ☞	
▪ Ritonavir:	✓ *Dyslipidemias*	AIPG 2011

Elvitegravir: ✽

HIV integrase inhibitor

Interferes with HIV replication by blocking activity of virus to integrate into genetic material.

7

Emtricitabine: NRTI ✱

Lobucavir is a synthetic cyclobutane nucleoside analogue with activity against a broad range of **herpesviruses, HIV, and HBV**. It is currently under investigation in clinical trials. Its mechanism of action is through "**inhibition of viral DNA synthesis**". Lobucavir is initially phosphorylated by virus-induced kinases, and lobucavir triphosphate is a potent inhibitor of HSV, CMV, and HBV DNA polymerases.✱

⮕ **Drugs Against HIV (Quick wrap up) (High yield for 2011-2012)**

Attachment inhibitor
- ➡ **Dextrin 2 SO4 (D2S)** Inhibit the binding of HIV-1 gp 120 with CD4 cells.

Co receptor antagonists CCR5 is a co-receptor involved in the entry of the HIV virus into the cell
- ➡ **Maraviroc** Binds to CCR5, preventing HIV from binding to this receptor.
- ➡ **Vicriviroc**
- ➡ **Aplaviroc**

Fusion inhibitors
- ➡ **Enfuvirtide** - targets multiple sites in gp 41 and gp 120.
- ➡ **Tifuvirtide** - 2nd generation HIV fusion inhibitor.

Integrase inhibitors

- ➡ **Raltegravir** first integrase inhibitor (FDA approved)   AIIMS 2011
- ➡ **Elvitegravir**

Maturation inhibitors Inhibits the development of HIV's internal structures in a new virus.
- ➡ **Bevirimat**
- ➡ **Vivecon**

Zinc finger inhibitors
- ➡ **Azodicarbonamide**

Monoclonal antibodies Restrict HIV entry - CD4 blocker:
- ➡ **Ibalizumab**

Pleconaril is an investigational drug active *in vitro* against **picornavirus replication** including over 90% of the most commonly isolated **enterovirus types and 80% of rhinovirus** serotypes.

Neuaminidase Inhibitors :

Neuraminidase inhibitors **zanamivir and oseltamivir** for both **influenza A and influenza B.**

Oseltamivir is indicated for the treatment of uncomplicated acute infection caused by influenza A virus in patients older than 1 year of age

Oseltamivir is indicated for the treatment of uncomplicated acute infection caused by influenza B virus in patients older than 1 year of age

Specific antiviral therapy is available for influenza: **Amantadine and Rimantadine for influenza A**

Antituberculous Drugs:

First-line agents for the treatment of tuberculosis:

- ▶ Isoniazid,
- ▶ Rifampin,
- ▶ Pyrazinamide,
- ▶ Ethambutol, and streptomycin ☞☞

Second-line drugs are used only for the treatment of patients with tuberculosis resistant to first-line drugs. Included in this group are the injectable **drugs**

- ▶ **Kanamycin, amikacin, and capreomycin and the oral agents**
- ▶ **Ethionamide, cycloserine, and PAS, ofloxacin, levofloxacin and sparfloxacin.**
- ▶ **Other second-line drugs include clofazimine, amithiozone (thiacetazone)**☞

The treatment regimen of choice for virtually all forms of tuberculosis in both adults and children consists of a **2-month initial phase of isoniazid, rifampin, and pyrazinamide** followed by a **4-month continuation phase of isoniazid and rifampin**

Except for patients who seem unlikely on epidemiologic grounds to be initially infected with a drug-resistant strain, ethambutol (or streptomycin) should be included in the regimen for the first 2 months or until the results of drug susceptibility testing become available.

Tuberculo*cidal** drugs	Isoniazid, Rifampin, Pyrazinamide, Streptomycin	**UPSC 2004**
Tuberculo*static** drugs	Ethambutol, Thiacetazone, PAS, Ethionamide, Cycloserine.	

➲ Mechanism of Action:

ISONIAZID	▶ *Inhibits mycolic acid synthesis*	**ORISSA 2005**
RIFAMPIN	▶ *Inhibits RNA polymerase*	
ETHAMBUTOL	▶ *Inhibits mycolic acid incorporation into cell wall*	
STREPTOMYCIN	▶ *Inhibits protein synthesis*	

SIDE EFFECTS:

INH - Remember as

- ▶ I - Irritation (epigastric distress)
- ▶ N- Neuritis (peripheral neuritis – common in slow acetylator)
- ▶ H- Hepatotoxicity (Rare in children, common in elderly & alcoholics) **NIMHANS 2006**

Rifampin – Remember as *Syndromes*

► Respiratory syndrome

► Cutaneous syndrome

► Flu like syndrome   CUPGEE 1996

Abdominal syndrome

Pyrazinamide – Remember as *3 H' s*

► Hepatotoxicity

► Hyperuricemia   UP 1996

► Hyperglycemia

 Ethambutol – Most important side effect **optic neuritis, blue vision**

Streptomycin -

► Vestibulotoxic Cochleotoxic

► Nephrotoxic

✓ Antitubercular Drug which acts intracellularly– pyrazinamide

✓ Antitubercular Drug which **acts at low pH- pyrazinamide**

✓ Antitubercular Drug which **penetrates meninges** – pyrazinamide, INH, Rifampin

✓ Antitubercular Drug which is **contraindicated in renal failure- Ethambutol**

✓ Antitubercular Drug which has maximum resistance in india- **INH**   COMED 2007

➲ First-Line Essential Drugs

⇨ Rifampin

► A semisynthetic derivative of *Streptomyces mediterranei* ✔✔

► Rifampin distributes well throughout most body tissues, including **inflamed meninges**. The fact that rifampin turns body fluids (urine, saliva, sputum, tears) to a **red-orange color**

► Has both intracellular and extracellular bactericidal activity. ✔

► It **blocks RNA synthesis** by specifically binding and **inhibiting DNA-dependent RNA polymerase.**

► Other adverse effects of rifampin include rash, hemolytic anemia, thrombocytopenia, and immune-suppression of unknown clinical importance. Rifampin is a potent inducer of the hepatic microsomal enzymes

► Resistance to rifampin results from spontaneous point mutations that alter the RNA polymerase (*rpoB*) gene

⇨ **Isoniazid**

▶ Its mechanism of action involves **inhibition of mycolic acid cell-wall synthesis** via oxygen-dependent pathways such as the catalase-peroxidase reaction.

▶ **Isoniazid** is <u>bacteriostatic</u> against resting bacilli and <u>bactericidal</u> against rapidly multiplying organisms, both extracellularly and intracellularly. **JKBOPEE 2012**

▶ The two most important adverse effects of **isoniazid** therapy are **hepatotoxicity and peripheral neuropathy.** **KCET 2012**

▶ Other adverse reactions are either rare or less significant and include rash (2%), fever (1.2%), anemia, acne, arthritic symptoms, a systemic lupus erythematosus-like syndrome, optic atrophy, seizures, and psychiatric symptoms. (Pshycosis) **KCET 2012**

— **Isoniazid-associated hepatitis** is **idiosyncratic and increases in incidence with age.**☞ **SGPI 2005**

— The risk of **isoniazid**-associated hepatitis is increased by daily alcohol consumption, concomitant rifampin administration, and slow **isoniazid** acetylation. ☞ **PGI 2000**

— Serum concentrations of aspartate aminotransferase (AST) or alanine aminotransferase (ALT) be determined at baseline in patients over 35 years of age who are receiving **isoniazid** for chemoprophylaxis, with monthly determinations thereafter.

— Discontinuation of **isoniazid** be strongly considered whenever an asymptomatic AST or ALT level exceeds 150 to 200 IU (three to five times the upper limit of normal) in high-risk patients whose baseline values were normal.

— Peripheral neuritis associated with **isoniazid** relates to **interference with pyridoxine (vitamin B$_6$) metabolism.** This can be reduced with the prophylactic administration of 10 to 50 mg of pyridoxine daily.☞ **KAR 2004 AI 1991**

— Almost all isoniazid-resistant strains have amino acid changes in the catalase-peroxidase gene (*katG*) or a two-gene locus known as *inhA*.

⇨ **Pyrazinamide**

▶ Bactericidal drug used in short-course therapy for tuberculosis. **UPSC 2005**

▶ Levels in <u>CSF</u> are high☞ **Kerala 1986**

▶ **Intracellular** action **PGI 1989**

▶ *Mechanism of Action* Pyrazinamide is similar to **isoniazid** ☞

▶ *Adverse* hepatotoxicity, Hyperuricemia ☞ **UP 1996**

⊃ **First-Line Supplemental Drugs**

▶ **Ethambutol:** *Adverse Effects* Retrobulbar optic neuritis is the most serious adverse effect; axial or central neuritis, Hyperuricemia **TN 1989**

▶ **Streptomycin:** An aminoglycoside isolated from *Streptomyces griseus*, streptomycin is available for intramuscular and intravenous administration only.

⊃ Second-Line Drugs

▶ **Capreomycin** Capreomycin, a complex cyclic polypeptide antibiotic derived from *Streptomyces capreolus* After streptomycin, capreomycin is the injectable drug of choice for tuberculosis.

▶ **Amikacin and Kanamycin** These well-known aminoglycosides are bactericidal to extracellular organisms.

▶ **Para-Aminosalicylic Acid** PAS, drug has a short half-life (1 h), and 80% of the dose is excreted in the urine.

▶ Thiacetazone ✳

▶ Viomycin

▶ Ethionamide ✳✳

▶ Cycloserine.

⊃ Newer Antituberculous Drugs

▶ This group includes **rifabutin, rifapentine,** ☞

▶ The newer **fluorinated quinolones,** ☞

▶ Amoxicillin/clavulanic acid,

▶ Clofazimine,

▶ Clarithromycin, and

▶ Rifamycins KRM-1648 (benzoxazinorifamycin). ✳✳

⇨ Resistance is due to:

▪ Isoniazid, Kat G or Inh A gene ☞

▪ Rifampin, rpo B gene ☞

▪ Pyrazinamide, pnc A gene ☞

▪ Ethambutol, emb B gene ☞

▪ Streptomycin 16 s r RNA gene or ribosomal protein S 12 gene

⇨ Antileprotics:

▶ **Multibacillary leprosy: Rifampicin, Dapsone, Clofazamine** ☞☞

▶ **Paucibacillary leprosy: Rifampicin, Dapsone** ☞☞

Rifampicin is the drug **most rapidly acting** and **most potent** against Leprosy bacillius.☞ (R-R)   AI 2003

Dapsone is the "drug of choice".

— Dose is "1-2mg/kg".

— Half life is "24 hrs".☞(D-D)

— Leprrostatic☞

— Acedapsone is repository form used as IM.☞

⊃ Side Effects of Dapsone:

* **Peripheral motor weakness** may occur more frequently.✱

* Fatalities have occurred due to **agranulocytosis**, aplastic anemia, and other blood dyscrasias.

* Serious **cutaneous reactions**, such as **exfoliative dermatitis, toxic erythema, erythema multiforme, toxic epidermal necrolysis, morbilliform and scarlatiniform reactions, and erythema nodosum** may occur.

* A **dose-related hemolysis** is **seen in all patients**, (Most common side effect) (with a slight decrease in hemoglobin and an increase in reticulocyte count. Patients with G6PD-deficiency or a decrease in activity in glutathione reductase are more susceptible to hemolysis. ✱   **PGI 1997**

* A low level of **methemoglobinemia** also occurs in all patients at recommended doses

* **Hepatitis**☞☞

* **Infectious mononucleosis like illness**☞

* **Fixed drug eruptions**☞

⊃ Side effects of clofazamine:

• **Reddish black discoloration of skin**	**PGI 2001**
• **Acneform eruptions**	**AIIMS 1997**
• Enteritis.	

⊃ Antiparasitic Drugs

Parasites	Drug of Choice	
1. Ascariasis	➤ Albendazole	
2. Capillariasis	➤ Mebendazole	
3. Giardiasis	➤ Metronidazole✱	
4. Trichuris trichura	➤ Albendazole	
5. Cysticercosis (T. solium)	➤ Praziquental✱	**PGI 1988**

6. Sheep Liver Fluke (due to Fasciola hepatica)	(a) Triclabendazole-a veterinary fasciolicide is adrug of choice. (b) Biyhionol is alternative drug of choice. (c) Pranziquantel-generally ineffective.	
7. Chinese Liver Fluke (Clonorchis sinensis)	➤ Pranziquantel✽	
8. Intestinal Fluke (Fasciolopsiasis)	➤ Pranziquantel✽	
9. Lung Fluke (Paragonimus westermani)	➤ Pranziquantel✽	
10. Tape worms, dwarf tapeworm	➤ Pranziquantel	
11. Schistosomiasis	➤ Pranziquantel	
12. Trichomonius vaginalis	➤ Metronidazole	
13. Dracunculiasis	➤ Metronidazole.	AIIMS 1984
14. Enterobiasis	➤ Mebendazole✽	
15. Strongyloidiasis	➤ Ivermectin✽	
16. (a) Pnuemocystis carinii	➤ Trimethoprim sulfamethoxazole	
17. (a) Angiostrongyliasis (b) Cutaneous larva migrans	➤ Thiabendazole✽	
18. Amoebic meningoenciphalitis	➤ Amphotericin B	
19. Babesiosis	➤ Quinine plus Clindamycin	
20. Balantidiasis	➤ Tetracycline	
21. Filariasis	➤ Diethyl carbamazine	
22. Leishmaniasis	➤ Stibogluconate sodiumdiazine	
23. Toxoplasmosis	➤ Pyrimethamine plus either trisulfamethoxazole or, sulfadiazine (Sulfonamides).	
24. Trypanosomiasis (a) T.cruzi (Chagas' Disease) (b) T. brucei (Sleeping Sickness) (1) Haemolymphatic stage (2) Late stage (CNS involvement)	➤ Suramin ➤ Melarsoprol ✽	
25. Onchocerciasis (River blindness)	➤ Ivermectin ✽	
26. Hook Worms (a) Ancylostoma duodenale (b) Necator americánus	➤ Mebendazole	
26. Uncomplicated Gonorrhea	➤ Ceftriaxone ✽	
27. Nocardiasis	➤ Trimethoprim-Sulfamethoxazole	
28. Actinomycosis	➤ Penicillin-G	

➲ Antihypertensives

Beta Blockers

> ▶ Half life of esmolol is 10 minutes (**shortest**)   KAR 2003
>
> ▶ Half life of nadolol is 24 hours (**longest**)
>
> ▶ Esmolol is a **class II**antiarrhythmic.
>
> ▶ Cardioselective (beta 1antagonists) **are safer** to use in asthma, diabetics and peripheral vascular diseases.
>
> ▶ Celiprolol has **membrane stabilizing properties**
>
> ▶ Cardioselective Beta Blockers are (B_2EA_2M)   JIPMER 2003

Betaxolol	Bisoprolol	Esmolol	Atenolol	Acebutolol	Metoprolol.

Beta Blockers with both alpha and beta blocking properties are: PGI 2007

Labetalol	Dilevalol	Cardivelol

⇨ Remember:

Agents used in CHF <u>and have proven survival advantage</u>

☐ **Carvedilol**

☐ **Metoprolol**

☐ **Bisoprolol**

Classification of beta-blockers

Non-selective Beta blockers/First generation blockers

✓ Propranolol

✓ Sotalol

✓ Timolol

✓ Nadolol

✓ Penbutalol

BETA1 selective blockers/Second generation blockers

✓ Acebutolol

✓ Atenolol

✓ Bisoprolol

✓ Esmolol

✓ Metoprolol

➔ **BETA 2 selective blockers not clinically used** Butoxamine

➔ **Ca++ entry blockade**—carvedilol, betaxolol, and bevantolol

➔ **Opening of K+ channels :** tilisolol

➔ **Antioxidant action:** carvedilol.

7

⇨ **Used in:**

Cardiovascular

- Angina   **AMU 1995**
- Hypertension
- Myocardial Infarction
- Cardiac Tacchyarythmias
- Hepatic portal hypertension
- Oesophageal variceal bleeding.

Endocrine

- Hyperthyroidism
- Phaechromocytoma

CNS:

- Anxiety
- Migrane Prophhylaxis   **AMU 1995**
- Essential tremor

Eye :

- Glaucoma (Timolol)

■ **ACE inhibitors**   **AIIMS 2009**

- Benazepril
- Captopril
- Cilazapril
- Enalapril
- Enalaprilat
- Fosinopril☞
- Lisinopril☞
- Moexipril
- Perindopril☞
- Quinapril
- Ramipril
- Trandolapril

⇨ **ACE Inhibitors**

✓ Are used for [treatment of malignant, refractory, or accelerated hypertension, and for treatment of renovascular hypertension (except in patients with bilateral renal artery stenoses or renal artery stenosis in a solitary kidney

✓ Are also indicated, in combination with diuretics and digitalis therapy, for treatment of **congestive heart failure** not responding to other measures.

✓ **Congestive heart failure,** ☞

✓ **Post-myocardial infarction** ☞

✓ **Left ventricular dysfunction**

✓ Indicated for the treatment of hemodynamically stable patients within 24 hours of an acute myocardial infarction to improve survival

✓ **Nephropathy in patients with Type 1 insulin-dependent diabetes mellitus (IDDM)**☞

✓ **Hypertension or renal crisis in scleroderma** ☞

✓ **Cause cough because of bradykinin.**   JHRKND 2003

✓ **Ommission of prior diuretic dose decreases risk of postural hypotension.**☞✳   AIIMS 2009

▶ ACE inhibitors are used for reducing proteinuria in **both diabetic as well as non diabetics.**

▶ They are however the **drugs of choice for reducing proteinuria** in Diabetic Renal failure.

▶ ACE Inhibitors delay ESRD in Diabetic Nephropathy. Albuminuria remains stable after ACE Inh Therapy.

▶ However it should be remembered that ACE Inhibitors are **contraindicated in:**

✓ Patients with Single kidney   KAR 1996

✓ B/L Renal artery stenosis↓GFR   KAR 1996

✓ Hyperkalemia

✓ Pregnancy   KAR 1996

✓ NOT used in phaeochromocytoma   AIIMS 2005

⊃ **Angiotensin Receptor Blockers**

— **Losartan**

— **Eprostan**

— **Irbesartan**

— **Candersartan**

— **Olmesartan**

— **Telmisartan**

▶ These drugs have effects similar to those of ACE inhibitors.

▶ However, instead of blocking the production of angiotensin II, they competitively inhibit its binding to the angiotensin II AT_1 receptor subtype.

▶ Their utility and tolerability are similar to those of the ACE inhibitors, but they **do not cause cough or angioedema.**   Calcutta 2000

PHARMACOLOGY

7

➲ Drugs used in Malignant Hypertension: (High yield for 2011-2012)

■ **Nitroprusside** is given by **continuous intravenous infusion.**

It is the **agent of choice** in this condition, since **it dilates both arterioles and veins.**   **KERALA 1995**

It has the advantage over the ganglionic blockers of not being associated with the development of tachyphylaxis and can be used for days with few side effects. The dosage must be controlled with an infusion pump. ✳

▶ ↑Gaunylate cyclase   **AI 2002**

▶ No central effects.   **AI 1991**

▶ ↑NO levels along with hydralazine, nitrates.   **AIIMS 2007**

■ Nitroglycerin

▶ Affects **veins more than arterioles**

▶ It is particularly useful in the treatment of hypertension following coronary bypass surgery, myocardial infarction, left ventricular failure, or unstable angina pectoris.

■ **Diazoxide** is the easiest agent to administer, for no individual titration of dosage is required, However, it is probably less effective than the other agents. It primarily affects arteriolar and not venous tone.

▶ Inhibits labour   **UPSC 1985**

■ **Intravenous labetalol** may be particularly useful in patients with a myocardial infarct or angina because it prevents an increase in heart rate. However, it may be ineffective in patients previously treated with beta blockers and is contraindicated in patients with heart failure, asthma, bradycardia, or heart block.

Indicated in pregnancy   **AIIMS 2007**

■ intravenous hydralazine

Causes drug induced lupus   **AIIMS 1987**

Hydralazine should be used with caution in patients with significant coronary artery disease and should be avoided in patients manifesting myocardial ischemia or aortic dissection. It is effective in preeclampsia. ✳

■ **Esmolol,** a beta blocker with an onset of action of 1 to 2 min, is particularly useful in aortic dissection and for perioperative hypertensive crisis

Enalaprilat, an intravenous form of the ACE inhibitor enalapril, has also proven effective, particularly in individuals with left heart failure. ✳

➲ Diazoxide (High Yield for 2011-2012 AIPGME/AIIMS)

Is related to the **thiazide class of drugs but has no diuretic action.**

It promotes **opening of the potassium adenosine triphosphate (ATP) channel**, which **inhibits pancreatic secretion of insulin, stimulates glucose release from the liver, and stimulates catecholamine release.** (This effect is opposite that of the sulfonylurea drugs used in diabetes mellitus, which close the ATP channel.) **Diazoxide causes sodium and water retention** and should be used cautiously in patients with congestive heart failure or poor cardiac reserve. **Hypertrichosis**, coarsening of the facies, decreased serum immunoglobulin G levels, and hyperosmolar nonketotic comas have been reported with diazoxide, especially with long-term use.

▶ Indapamide: diuretic with vasodilator properties☞

▶ Clonidine, methyl dopa, gaunabenz, gaunafacine, moxonidine, rilmenidine : central sympatholytics☞

▶ Clonidine: α 2 agonist☞

▶ Minoxidil, : potassium channel opener☞   MAHE 2001

⇨ Venodilators:✳✳✳

- ✓ Nitrates
- ✓ Nitroprusside   AIIMS 1993
- ✓ ACE inhibitors

⇨ Arteriolar dilators:✳✳

- ✓ Calcium channel blockers☞☞
- ✓ Minoxidil☞   AIIMS 1993
- ✓ Hydralazine   AIIMS 1993
- ✓ ACE inhibitors☞
- ✓ Nitroprusside☞   AIIMS 1993
- ✓ Alpha blockers
- ✓ Fenoldapam

➲ Don't get confused. Some are both

⇨ Phenoxybenzamine

During perioperative period, Patients require medications that block the excessive amounts of noradrenaline and adrenaline that is secreted by the tumor. A medication called "Phenoxybenzamine" is used to block noradrenaline activity. This medication usually controls the hypertension and also allows an expansion of the blood volume. In patients with pheochromocytoma the blood volume is diminished because of the effects of the catecholamines. After some periods of treatment with phenoxybenzamine, a beta-blocker is added to control the effects of the excessive production of adrenaline from the tumor (P-P)   AIIMS 2002

- ■ Alisikiren:
- ✓ Is a "Renin inhibitor" approved for Hypertension.
- ✓ Prevents conversion of angiotensinogen to angiotensin 1
- ✓ Used especially for primary hypertension.

⊃ Hypertension in Pregnancy

Drugs considered safe in pregnancy are:

► Hydralazine and Methyl dopa.   AI 2010

► The drug of choice for "**Hypertension**" <u>in pregnancy</u> is Methyl dopa.✳✳   AIIMS 1997

► The drug of choice for "**Hypertensive crisis**" in Pregnancy is Hydralazine.✳

► The drug of choice to control "**seizures**" <u>in pregnancy</u> is Magnesium sulfate.✳   AIIMS 2006

► ACE inhibitors are absolutely contraindicated in pregnancy.✳✳   KCET 2012

Magnesium sulfate therapy should be monitored by Tendon reflexes and respiratory rate.	KCET 2012
<u>Loss of deep tendon reflexes</u> is a warning sign for magnesium sufate therapy.	MAH 2012

⊃ Prolonged QT Syndrome (TORSADES DE POINTES)

⇨ Causes:✳✳✳

✓ Quinidine☞☞   AI 2008

✓ Procanamide☞

✓ Disopyramide☞

✓ Terfenadine, astemizole☞☞☞

✓ Cisapride☞☞   AI 2004

✓ Gatifloxacin☞

✓ Sparfloxacin☞

✓ Halofantrine☞

✓ Mefloquine☞

✓ TCA☞

Treatment is by: beta blockers, magnesium sulfate.

⊃ Antiarrythmics:

Class	Example	Mechanism of action	
Ia	Disopyramide, quinidine, procainamide	Block sodium channels☞☞	PGI 2008
Ib	Lidocaine, phenytion, mexilitene	Block sodium channels☞	
Ic	Flecainide, encanide, propafenone	Block sodium channels	
II	Propranolol, esmolol, sotalol☞	Beta-adrenoceptor antagonists	PG1 1994
III	Amiodarone,bretylium, ibutilide☞	Block potassium channels	
IV	Verapamil, dilatazem ☞	Calcium channel blockers	AI 1992

7

➲ Lignocaine

- Lignocaine is one of the **most useful** drugs for **Ventricular arrhythmia.**   AI 1994

- Lignocaine belongs to **Class IB** Antiarrythmic.

- Lignocaine blocks **fast Na⁺** channels.

- Lignocaine **decreases APD** (action potential duration)

- Used in Arrythmias due to:

  1. *Post MI*

  2. *Open Heart Surgery*

  3. *Digoxin Toxicity*

Side effects:

  ▶ Hypotension

  ▶ Convulsions

  ▶ Myocardial depression

Potassium channel blockers used in the treatment of cardiac arrhythmia are classified as **class III antiarrhythmic agents.** Pottasium channel blockers are: JK BOPEE 2007

  ✓ **Dofetilide**

  ✓ **Sotalol**

  ✓ **Ibutilide**

  ✓ **Azimilide**

  ✓ **Bretylium**

  ✓ **Clofilium**

  ✓ **Nifekalant**

  ✓ **Tedisamil**

  ✓ **Sematilide**

  ✓ DOC for ventricular arrhythmias: lidocaine   KAR 2005

  ✓ DOC for AF without Heart failure: beta blockers

  ✓ DOC for Atrial flutter without heart failure : beta blockers

  ✓ DOC for AF <u>with</u> Heart failure: digoxin

  ✓ DOC for Atrial flutter <u>with</u> heart failure : digoxin

  ✓ DOC for PSVT: adenosine   KAR 2006

  ✓ DOC for WPWS: procainamide   AIIMS 2003

  ✓ DOC for ventricular ectopics: beta blockers

  ✓ DOC for sinus bradycardia: atropine

⊃ Drugs used in Heart Failure (HF)

The treatment of <u>HF</u> may be divided into four components:

(1) Removal of the precipitating cause,

(2) Correction of the underlying cause,

(3) Prevention of deterioration of cardiac function, and

(4) Control of the congestive HF state.

Angiotensin-Converting Enzyme Inhibitors The administration of ACE inhibitors has been shown to prevent or retard the development of HF in patients with left ventricular dysfunction without HF, to reduce symptoms, enhance exercise performance, and to reduce long-term mortality when they are begun in such patients shortly after acute myocardial infarction. These beneficial effects are related only in part to the salutary hemodynamic effects, i.e., the reduction of preload and afterload. Their major effect appears to be on inhibition of local (tissue) renin-angiotensin systems.

Lisinopril or enalapril have been shown to be useful in the management of **heart failure**.

Angiotensin Receptor Blockers In patients who cannot tolerate <u>ACE</u> inhibitors (because of cough, angioneurotic edema, leukopenia), an angiotensin II receptor blocker (type AT1) antagonist (e.g., losartan 50 mg qid) may be used instead.

Aldosterone spironolactone, 25 mg/d reduces total mortality, as well as sudden death and death from pump failure. Since spironolactone is also a useful diuretic its widespread use in systolic **heart failure** should be considered.

b-Adrenoceptor Blockers administration of gradually escalating doses of **metoprolol, carvedilol, and bisoprolol** have been reported to improve the symptoms of HF, and to reduce all-cause death, cardiovascular death, sudden death, and pump failure death. In patients with moderately severe HF (classes II and III), their administration of has been shown to be beneficial

THIAZIDE DIURETICS

Thiazide diuretics are effective and useful in the treatment of <u>HF</u> as long as the glomerular filtration rate exceeds approximately 50% of normal.

FUROSEMIDE DOC in acute failure   PGI 1999

BUMETANIDE, ETHACRYNIC ACID, PIRETANIDE, AND TORSEMIDE

These powerful diuretics are useful in all forms of <u>HF</u>, particularly in patients with otherwise refractory HF and pulmonary edema.

ALDOSTERONE ANTAGONISTS

Spironolactone may be administered.   PGI 2007

TRIAMTERENE AND AMILORIDE exert renal effects similar to those of the spironolactones

⊃ Vasodilators

Direct vasodilators may be useful in patients with severe, acute HF who demonstrate systemic vasoconstriction despite ACE inhibitor therapy. The combination of **hydralazine (up to 300 mg qd orally) and isosorbide** may be useful for chronic oral administration.

Enhancement of Myocardial Contractility

Digitalis The improvement of myocardial contractility by means of cardiac glycosides is useful in the control of HF.

Phosphodiesterase, inhibitors: amrinone and milrinone, are noncatecholamine, nonglycoside agents that exert both positive inotropic and vasodilator actions by inhibiting a specific phosphodiesterase.

Other Measures

Anticoagulants Patients with severe HF are at increased risk of pulmonary emboli secondary to venous thrombosis and of systemic emboli secondary to intracardiac thrombi and should be treated with **warfarin.** Patients with HF and atrial fibrillation, previous venous thrombosis, and pulmonary or systemic emboli are at especially high risk and should receive **heparin followed by warfarin.**

Assisted Circulation/Cardiac Transplantation When patients with HF become unresponsive to a combination of all the aforementioned therapeutic measures, are in New York Heart Association class IV, and are deemed unlikely to survive 1 year, they should be considered **for temporary assisted circulation and/or cardiac transplantation.**

⇨ Neseritide:

► Recombinant brain natriuretic peptider BNP   AI 2007
► It acts by reducing preload.
► Has short half life.   AI 2005

⊃ Conivaptan: AIIMS 2011

Conivaptan:

V1a and V 2 (Vasopressin) receptor antagonist used to Treat (Acute heart failure and Hyponatremia and SIADH)
AIIMS 2011

Relcovaptan is a selective *V1 antagonist.*
Selective V2 antagonists.
   ☐ LIXIVAPTAN
   ☐ MOZAVAPTAN
   ☐ TOLVAPTAN

⇨ **Digoxin:**

▶ Theurapetic level: 05 -1.5 ng/ml.	**AIIMS 1987**
▶ Toxic level>2.4 ng/ml.	**Delhi 1989**
▶ Increases ventricular contractile force.	**AIIMS 1982**
▶ Excreted by kidneys.	**JIPMER 1992**
▶ Half life is 40 hours	
▶ Inhibits Na / K ATPase.	**MAH 2005**
▶ Contraindicated in HOCM.	**SGPI 2005**

⇨ **Digoxin Toxicity**

Digoxin toxicity

Features: Generally unwell, lethargy, N/V, confusion, **yellow-green vision**, arrhythmias (e.g. AV block, bradycardia)he

Precipitating factors

▶ Renal disease	**AIIMS 2007**
▶ Classically: hypokalaemia*he	
▶ Myocardial ischaemia	**AIIMS 2007**
▶ Hypomagnesaemia,	
▶ Hypoalbuminaemia	
▶ Hypothermia	
▶ Hypothyroidism	
▶ Hypercalcaemia, hypernatraemia	
▶ Acidosis	
▶ Drugs: amiodarone, quinidine, verapamil, spironolactone (compete for secretion in distal convoluted tubule therefore reduce excretion) he	

Management

• Digibind	
• Correct arrhythmia.	**AMC 1983**
• Phenytoin	**JIPMER 1992**
• Monitor K$^+$	

⮞ **Treatment of Acute Pulmonary Edema:**

It is life-threatening and must be considered a medical emergency

1. **Morphine is administered intravenously** repetitively, as needed, in doses from 2 to 5 mg. This drug reduces anxiety, reduces adrenergic vasoconstrictor stimuli to the arteriolar and venous beds, and thereby helps to break a vicious cycle.

2. Naloxone should be available in case respiratory depression occurs.☞

3. Because the alveolar edema interferes with O_2 diffusion resulting in arterial hypoxemia, **100% O_2 should be administered, preferably under positive pressure.** The latter increases intraalveolar pressure, reduces transudation of fluid from the alveolar capillaries, and impedes venous return to the thorax, reducing pulmonary capillary pressure.☞

4. **The patient should be maintained in the sitting position,** with the legs dangling along the side of the bed, if possible, which tends to reduce venous return.☞

5. **Intravenous loop diuretics, such as furosemide (DOC) or ethacrynic acid or bumetanide**, will, by rapidly establishing a diuresis, reduce circulating blood volume and thereby hasten the relief of pulmonary edema. In addition, when given intravenously, furosemide also exerts a venodilator action, reduces venous return, and thereby improves pulmonary edema even before the diuresis commences.

6. Afterload reduction is achieved with intravenous **sodium nitroprusside** at 20 to 30 ug/min in patients whose systolic arterial pressures exceed 100 mm Hg.☞

7. **Inotropic support should be provided by dopamine or dobutamine.** ☞

8. **Aminophylline (theophylline ethylenediamine),** is effective in diminishing bronchoconstriction, increasing renal blood flow and sodium excretion, and augmenting myocardial contractility.

If the above-mentioned measures are not sufficient, **rotating tourniquets** should be applied to the extremities.

After these emergency measures have been instituted and the precipitating factors treated, the diagnosis of the underlying cardiac disorder responsible for the pulmonary edema must be established, if it is not already known.

⮞ **Acute MI:**

▶ **Aspirin:** Rapid inhibition of cyclooxygenase in platelets followed by a reduction of thromboxane A_2 levels is achieved by buccal absorption of a chewed 160 to 325 mg tablet in the emergency department. This measure should be followed by daily oral administration of aspirin in a dose of 160 to 325 mg.

▶ **Supplemental oxygen.** In patients whose arterial oxygen saturation is normal as estimated by pulse oximetry or measured by an arterial blood gas specimen, supplemental oxygen is of limited. However, when hypoxemia is present, oxygen should be administered by nasal prongs or face mask (2 to 4 L/min) for the first 6 to 12 h after infarction; the patient should then be reassessed to determine if there is a continued need for such treatment.

▶ **Morphine** is a very effective analgesic for the pain associated with AMI.

▶ Before morphine is administered, sublingual nitroglycerin can be given safely to most patients with AMI.

▶ Intravenous beta blockers are also useful in the control of the pain of AMI. These drugs control pain effectively in some patients, presumably by diminishing myocardial oxygen demand and hence ischemia.

7

▶ Tissue plasminogen activator (tPA), streptokinase, anisoylated plasminogen streptokinase activator complex (APSAC) and reteplase (rPA) have been approved by the Food and Drug Administration for intravenous use in the setting of AMI. These drugs all act by promoting the conversion of plasminogen to plasmin, which subsequently lyses fibrin thrombi.

▶ The standard antithrombin agent used in clinical practice is **unfractionated heparin (UFH).**

▶ An alternative to UFH for anticoagulation of patients with AMI that is being used with increased frequency are the low-molecular-weight heparin preparations **(LMWHs)**

▶ **Angiotensin converting enzyme inhibitors**: Angiotensin-converting enzyme (ACE) inhibitors reduce the mortality rate after AMI, and the mortality benefits are additive to those achieved with aspirin and beta blockers.

▶ ACE inhibitors should be prescribed within 24 h to all patients with AMI

⇨ **Other drugs used as maintenance:**

▶ Aspirin, Clopidregel or ticlopidine as antiplatelet drugs
▶ Beta blockers ☞
▶ Nicronadil as pottaium channel opener : ↓preload
▶ Statins: for lipid lowering☞
▶ Heparin, warfarin, GP IIa/ IIIb inhibitors: as antithrombotic ☞

⇨ **Nitrates:**

✓ **Release NO**	
✓ **Cause vasodilation**	
✓ **↓preload and after load**	AI 1997
✓ **↓myocardial oxygen consumption**	AI 1997
✓ **Cause reflex taccycardia, hypotension.**	AI 1999
✓ **Long acting nitrates are not used chronically as tolerance develops (due to SH Group).**	AIIMS 1993
✓ **Amyl nitrite is the shortest acting nitrite.✱**	
✓ **Nitriglycerine is the shortest acting nitrate.✱**	
✓ **Penta erythritol tetra nitrate is longest acting nitrate.✱**	
✓ **Nitrates cause vasodilation, flushing, headache, dizziness, methemoglobunemia✱**	
✓ **Molisidomine: tolerance does not develop to it.**	

⊃ Hypolipidemic Drugs

⇨ Statins

(Also known as HMG CoA reductase inhibitors). Statins are most effective at **lowering the LDL (bad) cholesterol,** but also have modest effects on lowering triglycerides (blood fats) and **raising HDL (good) cholesterol**.

➲ Statins Currently Used:

✓   Atorvastatin
✓   Fluvastatin
✓   Lovastatin ✳   TN 1998
✓   Pravastatin
✓   Rosuvastatin ✳
✓   Simvastatin

✓   ↑LDL receptor levels➝➝   AIIMS 2K
✓   ↓cholesterol synthesis➝
✓   ↓VLDL➝
✓   ↑HDL➝

▶   Most effective hypolipidemics✳
▶   Best tolerated.✳
▶   Statins have
✓   Antioxidant,
✓   Anti inflammatory and
✓   Anti proliferative properties.
▶   Rosuvastatin is longest acting, most potent, greatest ↑↑ HDL.
Selective cholesterol absorption inhibitors:
•   Are most effective at <u>lowering the LDL (bad) cholesterol, but may also have modest effects on lowering triglycerides (blood fats) and raising HDL (good) cholesterol.</u>
•   The first medication of this class, **ezetimibe**

Resins (also known as bile acid sequestrant or bile acid-binding drugs)

•   This class of LDL-lowering drugs works in the intestines by promoting increased disposal of cholesterol.
•   These medicines bind to bile, so it can't be used during digestion.
•   Resins currently available
▶   Cholestyramine ➝
▶   Colestipol ➝
▶   Colesevelam Hcl ➝

Fibrates (fibric acid derivatives)

- Fibrates **are best at lowering triglycerides** and in some cases increasing HDL (good cholesterol) levels.
- These drugs are **not very effective in lowering LDL** (bad) cholesterol.
- That's why fibrates are generally used in people whose triglycerides are high or whose HDL is low, after reaching LDL goal. Fibrates are most effective at lowering triglycerides (blood fats).
- Additionally, they act to raise the levels of HDL (good) cholesterol. **Fibrates** may be used in combination therapy with the statins.

  ► **Gemfibrozil** ☞

  ► **Fenofibrate** ☞

  ► **Clofibrate** ☞

Niacin (nicotinic acid)

This drug works in the liver by affecting the production of blood fats.

Lower triglycerides and LDL cholesterol and raise HDL ("good") cholesterol.	**PGMCET 2007**

- Niacin side effects may include **flushing, itching and stomach upset.**
- Liver functions may be closely monitored, as niacin can cause toxicity.
- Niacin is used cautiously in diabetic patients as it can raise blood sugar levels.

Remember:

- **Niacin is vitamin B3**
- **NAD and NADP are its active forms✱**
- **Deficency of niacin causes pellagra.✱**
- **Deficency occurs in: Maize eaters, Carcinoid syndrome, Hartnups disease.**

Drugs	Adverse effects
► Statins (HMG CoA reductase inhibitors)	► Myositis, deranged LFTs✱
► Ezetimibe	► Headache✱
► Nicotinic acid	► Flushing, myositis✱
► Fibrates	► Myositis, pruritus, cholestasis✱
► Anion-exchange resins	► GI side-effects

➲ **(Very Important) Expect Questions from the Table**

- ■ **Rituximab:** is anti CD 20, Used in **B cell lymphomas with CHOP Regime✱✱**
- ■ **Trastuzumab** is used in **Breast Cancer.✱✱✱**
- ■ **Alemtuzumab** is used in **CLL and T cell Lymphomas✱**
- ■ **Dacluzimab** is used for **Kidney transplant✱**

■ Trastuzumab:

　　HER-2 /neu Breast ca☞☞

■ Alemtuzumab:

　　CD 25 Resistant CLL (seems u have forgotten read just two line above)

　　(Concentration in this book is important)

■ Cetuximab: EGFR

Resistant Colorectal Ca, Head and neck cancer　　　　　　　　　　　　　　AIIMS 2009

■ Bevacizumab: VEGF

Anti <u>angiogenic</u> drug (Colorectal Ca, RCC, Breast Ca)☞

■ Gemtuzumab ozoogamicin: Anti CD33, used for refractory AML. ☞

■ Golimumab: Anti TNF α monoclonal antibody used for psoriatic arthritis, rheumatoid arthritis and ankylosing spondylitis

■ Pavluzimab: is used for Respiratory syncytial virus infections

➲ Cetuximab: (High Yield for 2011-2012)

➡ It is a monoclonal antibody that acts against **EGFR (Epidermal Growth Factor Receptor).**

➡ **EGFR** is a **signaling protein** that normally **controls cell division.**

➡ In some cancers this is **altered** to cause **uncontrolled cell division.**

➡ Cetuximab attaches itself to EFGR and **prevents** the receptor from being activities. This prevents the cancer cells from **uncontrolled cell division.**

➡ Cetuximab is a **chimeric monopclonal antibody.**

➡ Used in combination with radiation therapy for treating **squamous cell carcinoma of the head and neck** or a single agent in patients who had prior platinum based therapy.

➡ Used in treatment of EGFR positive metastatic colorectal cancer as a single agent in patient who could not tolerate irinotecan based therapy or in combination with irinotecan for refractory patient.　　**AIIMS 2009**

■ **Trastuzumab (Herceptin)** is used in Breast Cancer. It is an important drug.　　AIIMS 2009✳✳✳

▶ It is a **humanized monoclonal antibody** to HER2/neu specifically directed to target tumor cells.

▶ HER 2 has been found to be increased in 5-10% of breast cancer patients.

▶ It is associated with larger tumor size, higher tumor grade and positive lymph nodes.

▶ HER 2 is also ↑ in **ovarian, prostate, gastric and bronchial cancer**

▶ **Lepatinib** is HER 2 and EGF receptor antagonist　　　　　　　　　　　　　AI 2010

7

⇨ **(LATEST DRUGS) KNOW ABOUT THEM:**

■ **Aldesleukin:** Is recombinant IL-2 used in treatment of **metastatic renal cell cancer and melanoma.**

Is implicated in causation of **capillary leak syndrome.** ☛☛

■ **Bendamustine:** a **purine alkylator** used in treatment of **CLL** and relapsed indolent **Non Hodgkins lymphoma.** ☛

■ **Xabepilone:** indicated for treatment of patients of **breast cancer.** ☛

■ **Plerixafor:** is a **CXCR4 chemokine receptor antagonist** used in autologous transplantation in patients with **NHL and Multiple myeloma.** ☛

■ **Pegvisomant**

- Highly selective **Growth Hormone Receptor Antagonist**

- Once daily s/c administration he

- Decreases IGF-1 levels in 90% of patients to normal he

- Doesn't reduce tumour volume therefore surgery still needed if mass effect

■ **Temozolamide:**

- Oral **alkylating agent.**

- Derivative of Dacarbazine

- Treatment of **Brain Tumor and Metastatic Melanoma**

■ **Porfimer**

- It is a mixture of oligomers of upto eight porphyrin units.

- It is a **photosensitizing agent** which is used in combination with light and causes cellular damage and cellular death.

- It is used for **esophageal cancer** in patients who cant be treated with Nd: Yag LASER.

➲ Imatinib ☛☛☛

(High Yield for AIIMS/AIPGME/DNB 2012-2013)

- Imatinib is a **magic bullet.** ☛
- Imatinib is effectively used as a **tyrosine kinase inhibitor.** ☛   **AIIMS 2006**
- **Imatinib targets bcr-abl and breaks it.** ✳   **DNB 2011**

It is used in treatment of:

- **CML**   **AIIMS 2008, JK 2008**
- GISTS (Gastrointestinal stromal tumors)   **AI 2010**
- Systemic Mastocytosis
- Hyper eosinophilic Syndrome

Imatinib mesylate is effective in patients with systemic **mastocytosis,**

Drugs in same class:

▶ Imatinib, Dasatanib, Bastinib,nilotinib, : used in CML ☛   **JK 2008**

     ☐ Sunitinib used in renal cell carcinoma ☛

     ☐ Sorafenib used in renal cell carcinoma ☛

     ☐ Pazopanib used in Renal cell carcinoma.

▶ Gefitinib, erlotinib: used in non small cell lung cancer

▶ Bartezomib is a proteosome inhibitor.   **PGI 2007**

▶ **Remember: Ofatumumab is a CD 20 directed monoclonal antibody used in Patients of CML.**

➲ Tyrosine Kinase Inhibitors:

— **Lapatinib** is an orally active chemotherapeutic agent used for treatment of solid cancers. It is considered to be a dual inhibitor of tyrosine kinase enzyme domains. It blocks HER2 and EGFR.

— **Geftinib** is an EGFR domain inhibitor of tyrosine kinase and is used to treat those patients of non small cell lung cancer who have not responded to other drugs.

— **Erlotinib** is also an EGFR domain inhibitor of tyrosine kinase enzyme. It is used for non small cell cancer and cancer of pancreas with cisplatin.   **AIPGME 2010**

Abatacept (Costimultation modulator that inhibits activation of T cells) DMARD FOR **Rhematoid arthritis.**

Gnrh analogues:

Goserlin, Histerlin, Leuporolide, Naferline, Triptorelin

Bromocriptine Cabergoline.(ergot derivatives)

Quinagolide (Is a non ergot agent with high D2 receptor affinity)

Tigecycline is an antibiotic used against drug resistant MRSA.

- ➡ Ciprofloxacin is used in MRSA   **AIIMS 2011**
- ➡ Vancomycin is used in MRSA   **AIIMS 2011**
- ➡ Cotrimaxazole is used in MRSA

➲ Heparin

- ✓ Heparin is a polysaccharide.   **ROHTAK 1997**
- ✓ Heparin causes **alopecia**☞☞
- ✓ Heparin causes **heparin induced thrombocytopenia HIT**☞
- ✓ Heparin causes **osteoporsis**☞   **AI 2007**
- ✓ Heparin causes **hyperkalemia** ☞   **AI 2007**
- ✓ Heparin **does not cross placenta.**☞
- ✓ **Protamine sulfate is used in heparin overdose**   **AIIMS 2009**
- ✓ Anticoagulant of choice in HIT(heparin induced thrombocytopenia) is Argatroban   **AI 2010**
- ▶ **Replace warfarin by heparin prior to conception and through first trimester(organogenesis)**☞
- ▶ **After ist trimester replace heparin by warfarin (heparin causes osteoporosis)**☞
- ▶ **Near term replace warfarin by heparin.**☞
- ▶ **Heparin is anticoagulant of choice in pregnancy.**   **UP 2007**
- ✓ LMW heparins **(enoxaparin, reviparin, nadroparin, ardeparin,)** inhibit factor Xa.✷✷
- ✓ LMW heparins act by inducing conformational change in AT III.✷
- ✓ LMW heparins have slight antiplatelet effect.✷

➲ Danaparoid Sodium

- ➡ It is an anticoagulant **that works by inhibiting** <u>activated factor X</u> (factor Xa).
- ➡ It consists of a mixture **of heparin sulfate, dermatan sulfate and chondroitin sulfate.**
- ➡ It is **a low molecular weight heparinoid derived from** <u>porcine gut mucosa.</u>
- ➡ The major difference between danaparoid and other low moleculer weight heparins (LMWH) is that danaparoid is devoid of heparin or heparin fragments.
- ➡ Danaparoid is primarily eliminated via the kidneys.
- ➡ Cross-reactivity with heparin-induced antibody (In vitro) is seen.
- ➡ <u>Uses: Heparin induced thrombocytopenia (HIT), DVT prophylaxis</u>.
- ➡ Side effects:
- ✓ Bleeding,
- ✓ Low platelet
- ✓ Asthma exacerbation.

➲ **Warfarin:**

✓ Oral anticoagulant.
✓ Causes **inhibition of vitamin K dependent clotting factors. (II, VII, IX, X)**✻✻
✓ Warfarin induced skin necfrosis is because of protein c deficiency.   **PGI 2003**
✓ Is a raecemic mixture.
✓ Monitoring is done by INR monitoring.
✓ Warfarin **crosses placenta.**☞
✓ Warfarin causes **fetal warfarin syndrome**☞
✓ In liver diseases dose of warfarin needs to be decreased.

➲ **Drugs used for ITP are:**

(High Yield for AIIMS/AIPGME/DNB 2012-2013)

• **Platelet infusion** may be administered in an emergency bleeding situation in order to attempt to quickly raise the count
• Removal of the spleen is sometimes undertaken, as platelets targeted for destruction will often meet their fate in the spleen. **Splenectomy** is said to be successful in 60 to 65 percent of cases, less so in older patients
• **Romiplostim** is a new treatment for **stimulating platelet production**. It is a **thrombopoiesis stimulating Fc-peptide fusion protein (peptibody)** that is administered by subcutaneous injection.
• **Eltrombopag** is an **orally-administered agent** with an effect similar to that of romiplostim. It has been demonstrated to **increase platelet counts and decrease bleeding in a dose-dependent manner.**
• **Dapsone** has also proved helpful as a second-line treatment for ITP.
• **Rituximab**, a chimeric monoclonal **antibody against the B cell surface antigen CD20**, has been shown in preliminary studies to be an effective alternative to splenectomy in some patients
• Promising results have been reported in a small phase II study of the experimental kinase inhibitor **Tamatinib**   (R788)

➲ **Common Anticoagulants:**

■ Aspirin (irreversibly inhibits cyclooxygenase)   **JK BOPEE 2011**
■ Clopidregel, ticlopidine
■ GP IIb, IIIa inhibitors: abciximab, eptifibatide, tirofiban☞☞   **JK BOPEE 2012**
■ LMW Heparin: enoxaparin, dalteperin☞
■ Direct thrombin inhibitors:
✓ Lepuridin,
✓ Argatroban,
✓ Bivaluridin,
✓ Ximelagratan,
✓ Dabigatran   **AIIMS 2011**
✓ Melagartan
■ Factor X A inhibitor: **Fondapurinix**☞

⊃ Argatroban:

Anticoagulant of choice in heparin induced thrombocytopenia: Argatroban

— Argatroban or lepirudin which are anticoagulants of direct thrombin inhibitor class and can be started.

— Argatroban is a direct thrombin inhibitor and is specific anticoagulant when heparin has to be stopped in case of HIT. It is an arginine derivative.

— It directly and reversibly bind to thrombin. Itdoes not require antithrombin III unlike heparin. As a result of inhibition of thrombin, fibrin formation, activation of V, VIII, XIII and platelet activation is inhibited.

— Bivalirudin, another DTI can be used when hepatic and renal failure preclude the use of argatroban or lepirudin in treatment of HIT.

Newer Fibrinolytics: **Reteplase, Tenecteplase**

⊃ Treatment of Hypercalcemia ✱✱✱

Treatment	Advantages
▶ Hydration with saline	▶ Rehydration invariably needed
▶ Forced diuresis; saline plus loop diuretic	▶ Rapid action
▶ Bisphosphonates 1st generation: etidronate	▶ First available bisphosphonate; intermediate onset of action
▶ 2d generation: pamidronate	▶ High potency; intermediate onset of action
▶ Calcitonin	▶ Rapid onset of action; useful as adjunct in severe hypercalcemia
▶ Phosphate Oral	▶ Chronic management with hypophosphatemia
▶ Intravenous	▶ Rapid action, highly potent but *rarely used* except with severe hypercalcemia and cardiac and renal decompensation present
▶ Glucocorticoids	▶ Oral therapy, antitumor agent
▶ Dialysis	▶ Useful in renal failure; onset of effect in hours; can immediately reverse life-threatening hypercalcemia

7

➲ Mechanism of Action of Strontium Ranelate

- Increases bone mass throughout the skeleton.
- **It appears to be modestly antiresorptive while at the same time not causing much decrease in bone formation.**
- Strontium is incorporated into **hydroxyappatite** replacing calcium, a feature that might explain some of its fracture benefit.
- It is unique because **it decreases osteoclastosis as well as promotes bone formation.**

➲ SERMs:

(High Yield for AIIMS/AIPGME/DNB 2012-2013)

1. **Raloxifene Hcl:** a potent estrogen agonist in bone. It is approved for the prevention and treatment of osteoporosis in postmenopausal women.
2. **Ormelpxifene:** a potent estrogen antagonist on uterus as well as breast tissue. It is approved for the prevention and treatment of dysfunctional uterine bleeding (DUB) in women.　　　　**KCET 2012**
3. **Tamoxifen:** exhibits anti-estrogenic activity (on uterus and breast tissue), estrogenic activity in bone, liver and the endometrium tissue. It is approved for the treatment and prevention of metastatic breast cancer.　　　　**KCET 2012**
4. **Toremifene:** is chemically related to Tamoxifen, and is approved for the treatment of metastatic breast cancer in postmenopausal women.

Other SERMs :

- Toremifene
- Roloxifene　　　　**KCET 2012**
- Idoxifene
- Raloxifene
- lasofoxifene
- Arzoxifene
- Miproxifene
- Levormeeloxifene

Unlike, Hormone Replacement Therapy (HRT), **SERMs do not produce:**

✓ **Endometrial Cancer**

✓ **Breast Cancer**

✓ **Uterine Cancer**

✓ **Gall Bladder Disease**

✓ **Blood Clots / Hypertension**

✓ **Undiagnosed Vaginal Bleeding**

Bisphosphonates

✓ Are concentrated in areas of high bone turnover and are taken up by and inhibit osteoclast action; the mechanism of action is complex.

✓ Alter osteoclast proton pump function or impair the release of acid hydrolases into the extracellular lysosomes contiguous with mineralized bone. ✱✱

✓ **Pamidronate**, is a potent inhibitor of osteoclast-mediated skeletal resorption ✱

✓ Several additional bisphosphonates **(alendronate, tiludronate, and risedronate)**

✓ Overall, **second-generation bisphosphonates are now the agents of choice in severe hypercalcemia,** particularly that associated with malignancy.

✓ **Zoledronate, a third-generation bisphosphonate,**

Plicamycin (mithramycin), which inhibits bone resorption, has been a useful therapeutic agent but is now little used because of the effectiveness of bisphosphonates. Plicamycin must be given intravenously, either as a bolus injection or by slow infusion. ✱

Gallium nitrate exerts a hypocalcemic action by inhibiting bone resorption and altering the structure of bone crystals. ✱

➲ Osteoporosis : Drugs Used

ESTROGENS (equine)	
Estradiol	
Raloxifene	**AIIMS 2011**
Bisphosphonates ;	
✓ Alendronate	**PGI 2011**
✓ Risedronate	
✓ Ibandronate	
Calcium	

⇨ Rheumatoid arthritis:

▶ First Aspirin and NSAIDS are used.☞

▶ Second line involves use of low dose glucocorticoids☞

▶ Third line involves use of DMARDS (Disease modifying Anti rheumatic drugs)

✓ Methotrexate,

✓ Gold Compounds, (stomatitis, dermatitis, metallic taste)

✓ Pencillamine,

✓ Hydroxychloroquine and

✓ sulfasalazine☞

▶ Fourth line is use of TNF alpha blockers.

▶ (Infliximab and Etarnacept)☛

▶ Fifth line is use of Immunosupressants and Cytotoxic drugs.☛

The immunosuppressive drugs

✓ Azathioprine,

✓ Leflunomide,

✓ Cyclosporine, and

✓ Cyclophosphamide

⊃ Anti TNF Alpha Drugs are used in Treatment of:

(High Yield for AIIMS/AIPGME/DNB 2012-2013)

✓ Crohns disease	AIIMS 2008
✓ Rheumatoid arthritis	
✓ Juvenile rheumatoid arthritis	AIIMS 2008
✓ Psoriasis	AIIMS 2008

Infliximab:☛☛

✓ Chimeric Monoclonal antibody	
✓ Given iv	KAR 2006

Etarnacept:☛☛

✓ Recombinant fusion protein biding TNF α.

✓ Administered sc

Anakinra:☛☛

✓ IL1 receptor antagonist

✓ Adminstered SC

Abatacept: ☛

✓ Fusion protein of CTLA4 and Fc PART of IgG .

✓ Inhibits T cell activation

⊃ GOUT:

▶ Allopurinol is not given in acute gout.☛☛	
▶ Drugs in acute gout: NSAIDS, colchicine, corticosteroids☛	PGI 1988
▶ Uric acid synthesis inhibitors: allopurinol☛	
▶ Uricosuric drugs: probencid, sulfinpyrazone☛	AI 1989
▶ Newer drugs: PEGylated uricase✱✱	
▶ Xanthine oxidase inhibitor: Febuxostat✱✱	

Allopurinol

✓ Decreases the production of uric acid by **inhibiting the action of xanthine oxidase,** ✱✱   **PGI 2004**

✓ Decreases uric acid concentrations in **both serum and urine.** ✱

✓ By lowering both serum and urine concentrations of uric acid below its solubility limits, **allopurinol** prevents or decreases urate deposition, thereby preventing the occurrence or progression of both gouty arthritis and urate nephropathy✱

✓ Decreases tophi formation and chronic joint changes, ✱

✓ Promotes resolution of existing urate crystals and deposits, and, after several months of therapy, reduce the frequency of acute gout attacks

✓ **Allopurinol** inhibits hepatic microsomal enzyme activity.✱

✓ **DOC in chronic gout.**✱

✓ **USED In Lesh nyhan syndrome**   **AI 2010**

✓ Used in urate nephropathy   **AI 2010**

NSAIDs

✓ Are affective in about 90% of patients, and the resolution of signs and symptoms usually occurs in 5 to 7 days. The most effective drugs are **indomethacin, ibuprofen, diclofenac,** ✱

Glucocorticoids

✓ Such as prednisone, a single intravenous dose of methylprednisolone, betametasone, triamcinolone acetonide have been equally effective.✱

✓ <u>ACTH</u> as an intramuscular injection is effective in patients with acute polyarticular refractory **gout** or with a contraindication for using colchicine or NSAIDs.✱

⮑ Colchicine: (High Yield for AIIMS/AIPGME/DNB 2012-2013)

• Colchicine **inhibits microtubule polymerization and stabilizes tubulins in microtubules**

• Neither analgesic nor anti-inflammatory ☛☛   **JK BOPEE 2011**

• Colchicine stimulates the **"Depolymerization"** of microfilaments and <u>not</u> polymerization.

• Availability of tubulin is essential to mitosis, and therefore colchicine effectively functions as a **"mitotic poison" or spindle poison. (metaphase arrestor)**☛

• Colchicine also **inhibits neutrophil motility** and activity, leading to a net **anti-inflammatory effect.**

• Colchicine can act as a cardiac glycoside. ☛

• Colchicine also **inhibits uric acid (urate) crystal deposition**, which is enhanced by a low pH in the tissues, probably by inhibiting oxidation of glucose and subsequent lactic acid production in leukocytes. The inhibition of uric acid crystals is a vital aspect on the mechanism of gout treatment.

• Mc side effect is diarrhoea (bloody)   **PGI 1996**

• Causes aplastic anemia, agranulocytosis, myopathy

• Hair loss

Colchicine as medicine:

- It is prescribed for the **treatment of gout** and also for **familial Mediterranean fever, secondary amyloidosis (AA)**, and **scleroderma**.

- It is also used as an anti-inflammatory agent for long-term treatment of **Behçet's disease**.

- A combination therapy to treat constipation-predominant **irritable bowel syndrome** which combines colchicine with the anti-inflammatory drug olsalazine.

- Now a developing a prodrug of colchicine, **ZD6126** (also known as ANG453) as a treatment for cancer.

- Colchicine has a **relatively low therapeutic index**.

Classes of Antidepressants

⊃ List of TCA's:

✓ Amitryptiline✱✱	KCET 2012
✓ Amoxapine✱	
✓ Cloimipramine✱	KERALA 1996
✓ Desimipramine	
✓ Doxepin	

⊃ Tetracyclic Antidepressants (Second Generation)

✓ Lofepramine✱	
✓ Maprotiline✱	PGI 1988
✓ Mianserin	

⊃ SSRI'S are:

✓ Fluoxetine✱	AI 1991
✓ Fluoxamine✱	
✓ Paroxitene✱	
✓ Sertaline✱	
✓ Citalopram	

Tricyclic overdose

Early features relate to **anticholinergic properties**: dry mouth, dilated pupils, agitation, sinus tachycardia, blurred vision.

AI 1988

Features of severe poisoning include:

- **Arrhythmias**
- **Seizures**
- **Metabolic acidosis**
- **Coma**

  ECG changes include:
- **Sinus tachycardia**
- **Widening of QRS he**
- **Prolongation of QT interval**

Widening of QRS > 100ms is associated with an increased risk of seizures whilst QRS > 160ms is associated with ventricular arrhythmias

Management

- **IV bicarbonate** may reduce the risk of seizures and arrhythmias in severe toxicity

- Arrhythmias: class 1a (e.g. quinidine) and class Ic antiarrhythmics (e.g. flecainide) are contraindicated as they prolong depolarisation. Class III drugs such as amiodarone should also be avoided as they prolong the QT interval. Response to lignocaine is variable and it should be emphasized that correction of acidosis is the first line in management of tricyclic induced arrhythmias

- Dialysis is ineffective in removing tricyclics

⊃ Typical Antipsychotics

Low-potency
- ✓ Chlorpromazine
- ✓ Thioridazine

Mid-potency
- ✓ Trifluoperazine
- ✓ Perphenazine

High potency
- ✓ Haloperidol
- ✓ Fluphenazine
- ✓ Thiothixene

Novel antipsychotics
- ✓ Clozapine ✳
- ✓ Risperidone ✳
- ✓ Olanzapine
- ✓ Quetiapine✳✳

► A serious side effect of long-term use of the classic antipsychotic agents is **tardive dyskinesia,** characterized by **repetitive, involuntary, and potentially irreversible movements of the tongue and lips (bucco-linguo-masticatory triad),** and, in approximately half of cases, choreoathetoid movements of the limbs✷✷

► Antipsychotic agents remain the cornerstone of acute and maintenance treatment of schizophrenia and are effective in the treatment of hallucinations, delusions, and thought disorders, regardless of etiology.

► **Older agents, such as chlorpromazine and thioridazine, are more sedating and anticholinergic and more likely to cause orthostatic hypotension, while higher potency antipsychotics, such as haloperidol, perphenazine, and thiothixene, carry a higher risk of inducing extrapyramidal side effects.**

► Chlorpromazine causes cholestasis. (c-c)   MAH 2012

(Drug-induced cholestasis may be a complication of treatment with a number of therapeutic agents. Chlorpromazine typically produces an acute febrile illness accompanied by elevation of both aminotransferases and alkaline phosphatase.)

► Long-acting injectable preparations (haloperidol decanoate and fluphenazine decanoate) are considered when noncompliance with oral therapy leads to relapses.

► In treatment-resistant patients, a transition to clozapine usually results in rapid improvement, but a prolonged delay in response in some cases necessitates a 6- to 9-month trial for maximal benefit to occur.

► Antipsychotic medications can cause a broad range of side effects, including **lethargy, weight gain, postural hypotension, constipation, and dry mouth.**

► **Rabbit syndrome:** Late onset, drug induced extra pyramidal symptoms is seen.

► **Extrapyramidal symptoms** such as **dystonia, akathisia, and akinesia** ✶are also frequent with traditional agents and may contribute to poor compliance if not specifically addressed.

► Akathisia is **restlessness**   COMED 2008

► May respond to beta blockers. (Propranolol)   JIPMER 2002

► Haloperidol especially causes Akathasia.   AI 2006

► In rare cases, more serious and occasionally life-threatening side effects may emerge, including ventricular arrhythmias, gastrointestinal obstruction, retinal pigmentation, obstructive jaundice, and **neuroleptic malignant syndrome** (characterized by hyperthermia, autonomic dysfunction, muscular rigidity, and elevated creatine phosphokinase levels). ✷✷

► The most serious adverse effects of **clozapine** are **agranulocytosis,** which has an incidence of 1%, and induction of seizures, which has an incidence of 10%. Weekly white blood cell counts are required, particularly during the first 3 months of treatment.   COMED 2008

► **Extra pyramidal side effects are rare with Clozapine.**   AI 2006

➲ Extrapyramidal Side-Effects:

1. Parkinsonism☞☞ (Responds to Leva dopa)   AI 2005

2. Acute dystonia (e.g. torticollis, oculogyric crisis)☞☞

3. Akathisia (severe restlessness)☞   COMED 2008

4. Tardive dyskinesia (late onset of choreoathetoid movements, abnormal, involuntary, may occur in 40% of patients, may be irreversible, most common is chewing and pouting of jaw)☞☞

⇨ Haloperidol

is an antipsychotic drug that has less antimuscarinic side effects than does chlorpromazine, but has more extrapyramidal effects, such as acute dystonia (face, neck, and back spasms-abnormal posture), parkinsonism, neuroleptic malignant syndrome (catatonia, rigidity, stupor, fever, dysarthria, fluctuating BP), and akathisia (restlessness). It can also cause tardive dyskinesia. It does not cause agranulocytosis.

➲ Anti Parkinsonism Drugs

☐ Selegeline: MAO" B" inhibitor.☞

☐ Dopamine Agonists: Bromocriptine, Lysuride, Pergolide, Pramipexole, Ropinirole, Rotigotine

☞☞ JKBOPEE 2012

☐ Rotigotine IS USED AS CRANIAL PATCH.   AIIMS 2011

☐ Levadopa and Dopa Decarboxylase inhibitors☞

☐ Anti viral: Amantidine☞

☐ COMT (Cathecol O Methyl Transferase) Inhibitors: Tolcapone and Entacapone☞   PGMCET 2007

The anti cholinergics/ anti muscarinics are used in Parkinsonism.

Useful in drug induced parkinsonism are: AI 1990

→ Benzhexol

→ Orphenadrine

→ Benztropine

→ Procyclidine

→ Biperiden

→ The addition of the anticholinergic drugs, such as Trihexyphenidyl, may provide additional symptomatic relief, particularly in younger patients and patients in whom tremor predominates. Associated depression, present in many parkinsonian patients, can be treated with tricyclic antidepressants, such as amitriptyline or nortriptylin.   MAH 2012

• They provide moderate improvements in tremor, rigidity, sialorrhea, muscular stiffness and cramps.

• They are more effective as IM/IV in drug induced dystonias.

• Side effects include

• Dry mouth, blurred vision, constipation, urinary retention, glaucoma, hallucinations, memory deficits.

⊃ Antiepileptic and Mechanism of Action:

Barbiturates	✓ Acts on **GABA:BZD receptor Cl channel** complex
Benzodiazepine	✓ **GABA facilitatory**
Carbamazepine	✓ Blocks **Na+ channel**
Ethosuximide	✓ Blocks **Ca²+ mediated T current**
Valproic acid	- **GABAergic** action, by inhibiting GABA transaminase
	- Blocks **Na+ channels** (phenytoin like)
	- Blocks **Ca ²+ mediated T current** (ethosuximide like)

▶ **Inhibition of Na+-dependent action potentials in a frequency-dependent manner** (e.g., phenytoin, carbamazepine, topiramate, zonisamide), ☛☛

▶ **Decrease of glutamate release** (lamotrigine), ☛

▶ **Potentiation of GABA receptor function** (benzodiazepines and barbiturates), and ☛

▶ **Increase in the availability of GABA** (valproic acid, gabapentin, tiagabine). ☛

▶ The two most effective drugs for absence seizures, ethosuximide and valproic acid, probably act by inhibiting
T-type Ca2+ channels in thalamic neurons.

Inducers of cytochrome P450: carbamezapine, phenytoin✻   **AIIMS 2007**

Teratogenic: valproate, phenytoin, carbamezapine✻

Steven johnsons syndrome: phenytoin, lamotrigine, ethoxysuccimide, carbamezapine ✻

Side effects of Phenytoin:✻✻✻

✓ **Hypertrophy of gums.**	**PGI 2003, PGI 2007**
✓ **Hirusitism**	
✓ **Hypersensitivity**	
✓ **Hyperglycemia**	
✓ **Hydantoin syndrome**	**AI 2010**
✓ **Cerebellar atrophy**	**AI 2010**
✓ **Megaloblastic anemia**	**AIIMS 2002**
✓ **Osteomalacia**	
✓ **Opthalmoplegia**	
✓ **Lymphoma**	**AIIMS 2002**
✓ **Hepatocellular damage**	
✓ **Phenytoin follows saturation kinetics**	
✓ **Depresses CNS**	**AI 2010**

➲ Phenytoin (Repeated In 2008, 2009, 2010, 2011)

Phenytoin follows Saturation kinetics Given orally, the drug is well absorbed. It has a saturable metabolism and follows zero order kinetics.

Its antiseizure activity closely resembles blood concentration

Depresses CNS

Cerebellar atrophy occurs on long-term administration

With long-term administration; the drug can cause osteomalacia due to(increase in vitamin D metabolism), Hodgkin's lymphoma like illness (pseudolymphoma), cerebellar atrophy and megaloblastic anemia due to (folic acid deficiency).

Phenytoin is a drug known for causing Osteomalacia after prolonged use. Chronic epileptics on Phentoin are liable to have osteomalacia and should be evaluated for the same.   **AIPGME 2012**

Rare side effects include: interstitial lung disease, gynecomastia, pure red cell aplasia PRCA).

A safer form of phenytoin is **Fosphenytoin**.

➲ Carbamezipine is also used for:✱

➔ Grand mal epilepsy☞☞	
➔ Manic Depressive Pshycosis☞	AI 1997
➔ Trigeminal neuralgia.☞	AIIMS 1997
➔ Atypical pain syndromes.	☞ AIIMS 2008

✓ **Epilepsy:** Carbamazepine is indicated for the treatment of **partial seizures with simple or complex symptomatology (psychomotor, temporal lobe), generalized tonic-clonic seizures (grand mal)** ; mixed seizure patterns that include the above; or other partial or generalized seizures <u>not</u> *absence seizures*

✓ Carbamazepine is a **first-choice anticonvulsant** because of its relatively low behavioral and psychological toxicity and the rarity of serious adverse effects.

✓ Carbamazepine is indicated for relief of pain due to **true "trigeminal neuralgia "(tic douloureux) and glossopharyngeal neuralgia** ☞☞

✓ Carbamazepine is used alone or in combination with lithium and/or antidepressants or antipsychotic agents to treat patients with **"manic-depressive illness"** who are unresponsive to, or cannot tolerate, lithium or neuroleptics alone.

✓ Carbamazepine may also be used in some patients to relieve the lightning pains of **tabes dorsalis; neuralgic pain associated with multiple sclerosis, acute idiopathic neuritis (Guillain-Barre syndrome), peripheral diabetic neuropathy, phantom limb, restless leg syndrome (Ekbom"s syndrome) and hemifacial spasm; post-traumatic neuropathy or neuralgia; and postherpetic neuralgia.**☞

✓ Carbamazepine is used alone or with other agents such as clofibrate or chlorpropamide in the treatment of partial **central diabetes insipidus.**☞

✓ Carbamazepine is used for the **detoxification of alcoholics**. It has been found to be effective in rapidly relieving anxiety and distress of acute alcohol withdrawal and for such symptoms as seizures, hyperexcitability, and sleep disturbances.

✓ Carbamazepine has been shown to be effective in certain psychiatric disorders including **schizoaffective illness, resistant schizophrenia, and dyscontrol syndrome associated with limbic system dysfunction.**

⊃ **Side Effects of Carbamezipine:**

- CNS depression
- Osteomalacia
- Megaloblastic anemia
- Aplastic anemia✳
- Exfoliative dermatitis
- Incresed ADH secretion.✳ Hyponatremia.   COMED 2006
- Teratogenecity (Spina Bifida, cleft lip and cleft palate)✳

⇨ **Topiramate**

- Topiramate is used to treat **epilepsy in both children and adults.**☛
- Topiramate can also be used as an **antidepressant**. In children it is also indicated for treatment of **Lennox-Gastaut syndrome**.
- Topiramate is now frequently prescribed for, the **prevention of migraines**. It has been used by psychiatrists to treat **bipolar disorder**.
- Chemically, topiramate is a sulfamate-substituted monosaccharide, related to **fructose**, a rather unusual chemical structure for an anticonvulsant.
- Topiramate enhances **GABA-activated chloride channels.**
- In addition, topiramate **inhibits excitatory neurotransmission**, through actions on **585hospho and AMPA receptors.**
- It is also an **inhibitor of carbonic anhydrase, particularly subtypes II and IV,** but this action is weak and unlikely to be related to its anticonvulsant actions, but may account for the bad taste and the development of renal stones seen during treatment.
- As topiramate inhibits carbonic anhydrase, the concomitant use of other inhibitors of carbonic anhydrase (e.g. acetazolamide) may lead to an **increased risk of renal stones.** ☛☛   JK BOPEE
- **Acute myopia and secondary angle closure glaucoma**, in a small subset of patients who take topiramate regularly, may cause transient (reversible), or permanent, loss of vision.
- Another serious side-effect is the development of **osteoporosis in adults and children** (bones affected break more easily) and **rickets (**abnormal, deformed growth of bones) in children.
- In other postmarketing research, a risk of **decreased sweating and hyperthermia** was noticed.☛

⊃ DOC for Epilepsy (High Yield for AIIMS/AIPGME/DNB 2012-2013)

☐ **Doc for generalized tonic Ionic seizures:** Valproic acid✱✱

☐ **Doc for absence seizures:** Ethoxsuccimide , valproic acid✱   **JK BOPEE 2012**

☐ **Doc for atonic seizures :** valproic acid✱✱

☐ **Doc for myoclonic epilepsy:** valproic acid✱   **AI 2010, JKBOPEE 2011**

☐ **Doc for partial seizures:** carbamezapine✱   **SGPGI 2005**

☐ **Doc for status epilepticus:** IV lorazepam✱✱

☐ **Doc for febrile seizures:** Rectal diazepam✱

☐ **Doc for eclampsia:** Magnesium sulfate✱

☐ **Doc for infantile spasms:** vigabatrin/ ethoxsuccimide✱✱

Lacosamide: amino acid related peptide used in pain syndromes and partial seizures.

Inactivation of voltage gated sod channels.

Binds to collapsing response mediator protein CRMP 2.

Zonisamide, Rufinamide inactivate sodium plus calcium channels

⊃ Nootropics (High Yield for AIIMS/AIPGME/DNB 2012-2013)

Also referred to as **smart drugs**, **memory enhancers**, and **cognitive enhancers**, are drugs, supplements, nutraceuticals, and functional foods that are purported to improve mental functions such as **cognition, memory, intelligence, motivation, attention, and concentration**

▶ These drugs are used primarily to treat people with cognitive difficulties: **Alzheimer's disease, Parkinson's disease, ADHD**

▶ Although **piracetam** is the most commonly taken nootropic, there are many relatives in the family which have different potencies and side effects.

▶ Other commom racetams include **pramiracetam, oxiracetam, and aniracetam.** There is no generally accepted mechanism for racetams. They generally show no affinity for the most important receptors, although modulation of most important central neurotransmitters, including acetylcholine and glutamate have been reported.

⊃ Stimulants (High Yield for AIIMS/AIPGME/DNB 2012-2013)

Stimulants are often seen as smart drugs, but are actually just productivity enhancers. These typically improve concentration and a few areas of cognitive performance, but only while the drug is still in the blood. Some scientists recommend widespread use of stimulants such as methylphenidate and amphetamines by the general population to increase brain power. Unfortunately amphetamines in particular have well known draw backs and side effects including serious dependency issues. Being repackaged as "safe" treatments for ADHD is resulting in huge up tick in speed use among young adults.

- ❑ Amphetamines (and related drugs)
- ❑ Amphetamine (Adderall) - Dopaminergic
- ❑ Cocaine - Dopaminergic
- ❑ Methamphetamine - Dopaminergic, Serotonergic, Adrenergic
- ❑ Methylphenidate (Ritalin) - Dopaminergic
- ❑ Pemoline - Dopaminergic

➲ Eugeroics ("Wakefulness Enhancers") - Unproven Primary Mechanisms but Proven Efficacy

- ❑ Adrafinil
- ❑ Armodafinil
- ❑ Modafinil
- ❑ Caffeine - reduces fatigue perception
- ❑ Theophylline

➲ PDE Inhibitors (Phosphodiesterase Inhibitors)

(High Yield for AIIMS/AIPGME/DNB 2012-2013)

PDE1 selective inhibitors

- ▪ Vinpocetine

PDE2 selective inhibitors

- ▪ EHNA (erythro-9-(2-hydroxy-3-nonyl) adenine
- ▪ Anagrelide

PDE3 selective inhibitors

- ▪ **Enoximone and milrinone**, used clinically for short-term treatment of cardiac failure. These drugs mimic sympathetic stimulation and increase cardiac output.

PDE4 selective inhibitors

- ▪ **Mesembrine**, an alkaloid from the herb Sceletium tortuosum
- ▪ **Rolipram**, used as investigative tool in pharmacological research
- ▪ **Ibudilast**, a neuroprotective and bronchodilator drug used mainly in the treatment of asthma and stroke. It inhibits PDE4 to the greatest extent, but also shows significant inhibition of other PDE subtypes, and so acts as a selective PDE4 inhibitor or a non-selective phosphodiesterase inhibitor depending on the dose.
- ▪ **Pentoxifylline**, a drug that potentially enhances circulation and may have applicability in treatment of diabetes, fibrotic disorders, peripheral nerve damage, and microvascular injuries

PDE5 selective inhibitors

Sildenafil, tadalafil and vardenafil, udenafil and avanafil selectively inhibit PDE5, which is cGMP-specific and responsible for the degradation of cGMP in the corpus cavernosum. These phosphodiesterase inhibitors are used primarily as remedies for **erectile dysfunction**, as well as having some other medical applications such as treatment of **pulmonary hypertension**.
Dipyridamole also inhibits PDE5.

⟳ Other Drugs Used in Erectile Dysfunction: (ED)

Alprastadil: (PGE1) analogue. Directly injected into corpora cavernosa, powerful vasodilator.✱✱

→ **Papaverine:** non specific **PDE inhibitor.**✱ (Intracavernosal injection)

→ **VIP Analouge (Aviptadil).**✱(Intracavernosal injection)

→ **Ketanserin.**✱ (Intracavernosal injection)

→ **Thymoxamine.**✱(Intracavernosal injection)

→ **Bremelanotide: is an active metabolite of melatonon II.**   AIIMS 2011

Androgens: only used in case of associated androgen deficiency.✱

Apomorphine: sometimes given for ED✱ (Sublingual)

L arginine: (NO Precursor)

Drugs causing Hyperuricemia:

- **Pyrizamide**   PGI 2011
- Ethambutol
- Furosemide
- Cyclosporine
- Clofibrate
- Alcohol
- Levodopa
- **Low dose aspirin**   PGI 2011
- Chlorthalidone
- Nicotinic acid.

⟳ Drugs Causing Hirsutism:

► **Minoxidil**
► **Phenytoin**
► **Cyclosporine**
► **Diazoxide**
► **Androgens**
► **Oral contraceptives - containing progesterone**
► **Penicillamine**
► **Heavy metals**
► **Acetazolamide**
Flutamide is an antiandrogen and is used in treatment of hirsutism

Drugs causing extra pyramidal side effects:

- Haloperidol
- Levodopa
- Methyldopa
- Metocloperamide
- OCP
- Phenothiazines
- TCA

◌ Drug-Induced Hematologic Syndromes:

Immune Hemolytic Anemia

IHA has been described with cephalosporins, nonsteroidal anti-inflammatory agents, levaquin, oxaliplatin, and teicoplanin

Nonimmune Hemolytic Anemias

G6PD deficiency is the most frequent red cell enzymopathy associated with hemolysis. Hemolysis may be precipitated by **infection, fava beans, and drugs. Primaquine, phenazopyridine, nitrofurantoin, and certain sulfas** have been associated with hemolysis

Methemoglobinemia

Phenazopyridine, used for relief of cystitis, can cause oxidative hemolysis.

Dapsone, used for leprosy, dermatitis herpetiformis, and prophylaxis for pneumocystis carinii Primaquine and local anesthetics, benzocaine, prilocaine, Amyl nitrite and isobutyl nitrite.

Megaloblastic Anemia

Drugs that act by interfering with DNA synthesis, such as antimetabolites and alkylating agents, some antinucleosides used against HIV and other viruses [14], can all induce megaloblastic anemia. **Trimethoprim (in high, extended doses) and pyrimethamine,** sulfasalazine and anticonvulsants such as phenytoin

Sideroblastic Anemia

Drug-induced sideroblastic anemia has been associated with isoniazid Linezolide, penicillamine, and triethylene tetramine dihydrochloride

Aplastic Anemia

Aplastic anemia (AA), characterized by pancytopenia with a hypocellular bone marrow, can be inherited or acquired. Drugs implicated in inducing AA include antirheumatic drugs, antithyroid medications, antituberculous drugs, NSAIDs, and anticonvulsants. Specific drugs cited include chloramphenicol, butazone, sulfonamide, gold salts, penicillamine, amidopyrine, trimethoprim/sulfamethoxazole, methimazole, and felbamate.

Pure Red Cell Aplasia

Pure red cell aplasia (PRCA) is characterized by normocytic anemia, reticulocytopenia, and absence of mature marrow erythroid progenitors. PRCA can be acquired through exposure to a number of drugs, including immunosuppressants (azathioprine, FK506, antithymocyte globulin), antibacterials (linezolide, isoniazid, rifampin, chloramphenicol), antivirals (interferon-alpha, lamivudine, zidovudine), fludarabine, anticonvulsants (diphenyldrantoin, carbamazepine, valporic acid), as well as chloroquine, allopurinol, ribavirin, and gold. Additionally, PRCA has been reported to develop after prolonged exposure to recombinant human erythropoietin (rHuEPO)

Immune Thrombocytopenia

Classical causes of drug-induced thrombocytopenia are the quinine and quinine-like drugs, Vancomycin sulfanomides, rifampin, linezolid, anti-inflammatory drugs, antineoplastics, antidepressants, benzodiazepines, anticonvulsants (carbamazepine, phenytoin, valproic acid).

Heparin is well known to be associated with thrombocytopenia, sometimes with arterial or venous thrombosis, which is generally a far greater threat than the risk of bleeding. **Heparin-induced immune thrombocytopenia** is caused by antibodies against complex of heparin and platelet factor 4 (PF4), which can lead to platelet activation and the initiation of thromboses.

One drug commonly implicated in inducing TMA is the immunosuppressant cyclosporine A (CyA). Other drugs associated with TMA include chemotherapeutic agents mitomycin-C, gemcitabine, and cisplatin, as well as α-interferon and tacrolimus.

Hypercoagulability

Erythropoietin has been associated with increased thrombotic risk. Hormonal therapies including oral contraceptives, hormone replacement therapy, and tamoxifen (a selective estrogen receptor modulator with some agonist activity) have all been associated with increased thrombotic risk.

Circulating Anticoagulants

Lupus anticoagulants and antiphospholipid antibodies may be induced by drugs such as chlorpromazine, hydralazine, phenytoin, quinine, and procainamide.

Hypoprothrombinemia

Hypoprothombinemia, with prolongation of the PT/INR, is most commonly due to vitamin deficiency or liver disease. Certain drugs have been linked with hypoprothrombinemia, such as broad spectrum antibiotics, usually in patients who are also malnourished. Reports have linked sulfonamides, ampicillin, chloramphenicol, tetracyclines, and cefoxitin to deficiency in vitamin -dependent clotting factors.

⇨ **Oncology :**

► M phase: Vinblastine, vincristine, paclitaxel JIPMER 2004

► G$_0$ phase: Alkylating agents, doxarubicin, daunorubicin, nitrosoureas, cisplatin

► S phase: Cytarabine, 6 MP, Methotrexate, Hydroxyurea, Etoposide

► G2 phase: Bleomycin

➲ Direct DNA-Interactive Agents

☐ Formation of covalent DNA adducts occurs

☐ **Alkylating agents** as a class break down, either spontaneously or after normal organ or tumor cell metabolism, to reactive intermediates that covalently modify bases in DNA.

☐ This leads to cross-linkage of DNA strands or the appearance of breaks in DNA as a result of repair efforts. "Broken" or cross-linked DNA is intrinsically unable to complete normal replication or cell division.

✓ Nitrogen mustard (mechlorethamine)

✓ Cyclophosphamide ☞☞   AIIMS 2009, 2008

✓ Ifosfamide ☞   AIIMS 2008

✓ Chlorambucil ☞   AIIMS 2009, 2008

✓ Nitrosoureas ☞

✓ Melphalan   AIIMS 2009

✓ Streptozotocin

✓ Lomustine, Carmustine, semustine

✓ Procarbazine, altretamine

✓ Dacarbazine

✓ Cisplatin, carboplatin, oxaliplatin, nedaplatin

➲ Antitumor Antibiotics and Topoisomerase Poisons ☞

✓ Doxorubicin

✓ Daunorubicin

✓ Idarubicin

✓ Bleomycin.

✓ D-Actinomycin

✓ Mitomycin C

✓ Mitoxantrone

✓ Etoposide

✓ Camptothecin

➲ Indirect Effectors of DNA Function: Antimetabolites ☞☞

✓ Methotrexate   AIIMS 2007

✓ 5-Fluorouracil (5FU) excreted by lungs   AIIMS 2008

✓ Cytosine arabinoside (ara-C)

✓ Gemcitabine

✓ Fludarabine

✓ 2-Chlorodeoxyadenosine

✓ Hydroxyurea

☐ Purine antagonists: mercaptopurine, azathioprine, thioguanine, fludarabine, cladarabine

☐ Pyrimidine antagonists: 5 FU, cytosine arabinoside, gemicatibine, capecatabine

☐ Folate antagonist: Methotrexate, premetraxate.

7

➲ Mitotic Spindle Inhibitors

Microtubules are cellular structures that form the mitotic spindle and in interphase cells are responsible for the cellular "scaffolding" along which various motile and secretory processes occur.

- ☐ Vincristine
- ☐ Vinblastine
- ☐ Paclitaxel and Docetaxel
- ☐ Estramustine

➲ Hormonal Agents

- ✓ Glucocorticoids ☞
- ✓ Progestational agents including medroxyprogesterone acetate, androgens
- ✓ Diethylstilbesterol (DES) ☞
- ✓ Aminoglutethimide or ketoconazole☞
- ✓ Retinoids, including tretinoin☞

Topoisomerase I inhibitors:	Irinotectan Topetectan		AI 2005
Topoisomerase II inhibitors:	Teniposide Etoposide Doxorubicin		

➲ Specific Toxicities:

■	Cyclophosphamide:	Haemorrhagic cystitis☞☞	
■	Ifofsamide:	Haemorrhagic cystitis☞	
■	Cisplatin:	Nephrotoxicity, ototoxicity, vomiting(most emetogenic), peripheral neuropathy	
■	Busulfan:	Pulmonary fibrosis, adrenal insufficency, hyperpigmentation☞	
■	Procarbazine:	Disulfuram like reaction, secondary leukemia☞	
■	Cytarabine:	Cerebellar toxicity☞	AIIMS 2009
■	5 FU:	Nausea, vomiting, stomatitis, diarrhoea, hand foot syndrome	
■	Methotrexate, 6 MP:	Hepatotoxicity ☞	
■	Gemicatabine:	Diarrhoea.☞	

➲ Cyclophosphamide:

Is metabolized to **acrolein**, which is excreted in the urine. If the patient's urine is concentrated, the toxic metabolite may cause severe bladder damage. **In severe hemorrhagic cystitis**, large segments of the bladder mucosa may be shed which can lead to prolonged, gross hematuria. The incidence of cyclophosphamide-induced hemorrhagic cystitis can be decreased by ensuring that the patient maintains a high fluid intake. **Cyclophosphamide is an alkylating agent used in the treatment of breast carcinoma, malignant lymphoma, multiple myeloma, and adenocarcinoma of the ovary, as well as various other forms of cancer.** The major toxic reactions commonly seen with this agent include

✓ Mucositis, nausea,

✓ Hepatotoxicity,

✓ Sterile hemorrhagic and non-hemorrhagic cystitis,

✓ Leukopenia, neutropenia, and

✓ Interstitial pulmonary fibrosis.

⇨ **Remember:**

► ATRA (All Trans' retinoic acid) is used in APML. (ACUTE PROMYELOCYTIC LEUKEMIA)

► Virinostat (histone deacylase inhibitor) is used in **cutaneous T cell lymphoma**

► Boartezomib (proteosome inhibitor) is used in **multiple myeloma**

➲ Vinca Alkaloids (Vincristine)

✓ Vincristine is a vinca alkaloid from the **Catharanthus roseus** (Madagascar periwinkle).

✓ It is a **mitotic inhibitor**, and is used in cancer chemotherapy.

✓ Vincristine binds to **tubulin dimers**, inhibiting assembly of microtubule structures. Disruption of the microtubules **arrests mitosis in metaphase.**   DNB 2011

✓ The vinca alkaloids therefore affect all rapidly dividing cell types including cancer cells, but also intestinal epithelium and bone marrow.

✓ Vincristine is delivered via **intravenous infusion** for use in various types of chemotherapy regimens.

✓ Its main uses are in **non-Hodgkin's lymphoma** as part of the chemotherapy regimen CHOP, Hodgkin's **lymphoma as part of MOPP, COPP, BEACOPP, or the less popular Stanford V chemotherapy regimen**, in acute lymphoblastic leukemia, and in treatment for nephroblastoma (Wilms tumor, a kidney tumor common in children).

✓ The main side-effects of vincristine are **peripheral neuropathy, hyponatremia, constipation and hair loss.**

✓ Peripheral neuropathy can be severe, and hence a reason to avoid, reduce, or stop the use of vincristine. **One of the first symptoms of peripheral neuropathy is foot drop**

✓ Accidental injection of vinca alkaloids into the spinal canal (intrathecal administration) is highly dangerous, with a mortality rate approaching 100%.

➲ Immunosuppressants: AIIMS 2008

✓ Cyclosporine✲

✓ Sirolimus✲

✓ Azathioprine✲

✓ Mycophenolic acid✲ (PRODRUG)   AI 2010

✓ Tacrolimus✲

✓ Thalidomide✲

✓ Muromonab CD 3

✓ Antithymocyte globulin

✓ Hydroxychloroquine

7

⊃ Mycophenolate Mofetil (Repeated In 2008, 2009, 2010, 2011)

— Is a **prodrug** and is given as prodrug to improve oral bioavailability of drug. The drug is derived from **Penicillium stoloniferum.**   AIPGME 2010

— It has **Immunosuppressive** properties.

— Used as a **'steroid sparing'** agent in patients with psoriasis, vasculitides, and certain immune mediated disorders such as IgA nephropathy.

— It has **decreased the incidence of acute rejection** in solid transplant recipients

— Mycophenolate mofetil is beginning to be used in the management of autoimmune disorders such as

— Idiopathic thrombocytopenic purpura (ITP), systemic lupus erythematosus (SLE), and pemphigus vulgaris (PV)

— Maintaining remission of C-ANCA positive (Wegener's) granulomatosis.

⊃ Drugs Preventing Toxicities: (High Yield for AIIMS/AIPGME/DNB 2012-2013)

☐ Alopurinol/Rasburicase	♯ *Helps in preventing Hyperuricemia from Tumor Lysis Syndrome*
☐ Mesna	♯ *Prevents Haemorrhagic Cystitis from Cyclophosphamide/Ifofsamide Treatment. Cyclophosphamide is the most widely used alkylating agent and is effective in the treatment of both hematologic malignancies and solid tumors. It does not have significant vesicant effects, as it is a prodrug and must be biotransformed in the liver, which breaks down cyclophosphamide to the active metabolite phosphoramide mustard plus acrolein. Cyclophosphamide is available in both intravenous and oral formulations and is well absorbed by the oral route.*
☐ Granisteron/ Ondansterone	♯ *Prevents vomiting / Nausea after chemotherapy*
☐ Filgastrim/ Sargamostim	♯ *Neutropenia Prophylaxis*
☐ Oprelvekin	♯ *For Thrombocytopenia*
☐ Dexrazoxane	♯ *PREVENTS antharacycline induced Toxicity*

⊃ **Important Drugs Asked and Repeated Frequently:**

Amiadarone:

(High Yield for 2011/2012)   AIIMS 2009

✓ **Class III antiarrhythmic.✶✶**
✓ Has class I, II, III, IV properties.
✓ **Potassium channel blocker✶**
✓ Prevention of atrial and ventricular arrhythmia.✶
✓ Causes:
✓ Pulmonary fibrosis✶   AI 1994
✓ Hepatitis✶
✓ Photodermatitis✶
✓ Grey blue discoloration of skin✶
✓ Corneal microdeposits✶
✓ Bradycardia, heart block
✓ Hyperuricemia   AI 2004
✓ Hypothyroidism/ hyperthyroidism   AI 2004

Cyclosporin :

(High Yield for 2011/2012)

▶ Cyclosporin is an immunosuppressant which decreases clonal proliferation of T cells by **reducing IL-2 release**.   AI 1992
▶ It acts by binding to cyclophilin forming a complex which **inhibits calcineurin**, a phosphotase that activates various transcription factors in T cells
▶ Acts on **CD 4 +T cells**.   AIIMS 1996, AIIMS 1997
Adverse effects of cyclosporin
1. **Nephrotoxicity** (MAJOR limitation)   JK BOPEE 2011
2. **Hepatotoxicity**
3. **Fluid retention** <u>not Dehydration</u>
4. **Hypertension**   PGI 2006
5. **Hyperkalaemia** <u>not Hypokalemia</u>   KERALA 1990
6. **Hypertrichosis** <u>not Alopecia</u>   PGI 2006
7. **Hyperplasia of gum**
8. **Tremor**   KERALA 1990

⇨ **Indications:**

- Crohn's disease
- Rheumatoid arthritis
- psoriasis (has a direct effect on keratinocytes as well as modulating T cell function)
- The primary mode of action of **orilistat** is to **inhibit pancreatic lipases**, which in turn will decrease the absorption of lipids from the intestine

➲ **Tacrolimus: (High Yield for 2011/2012)**

▶ Inhibits <u>IL-2</u> like cyclosporine.	PGI 2004
▶ Acts on <u>T cells</u> mainly	PGMCET 2007
▶ FK 506 is Tacrolimus.	
▶ Used in **organ transplantation**.	PGI 2000
▶ Is a <u>Macrolide</u> antibiotic.	AIIMS 2006
▶ **Glucose intolerance** is a significant side effect.	AI 2004
▶ **Nephrotoxicity** is a well established feature.	AIIMS 2005

Nicergoline

Nicergoline is an "ergot derivative" used in treatment of **Dementias, Raynauds disease, vascular migranes, and retinopathy.**

- It increases mental agility✱✱
- Enhances clarity and perception✱
- Increases arterial blood flow in brain.✱
- Increases activity of nerve growth factor✱
- Improves utilization of oxygen by neurons✱
- <u>Codergocrine</u> is other ergot compound used in dementia. JK BOPEE 2012

Nimodipine

- Vasospasm remains the leading cause of morbidity and mortality following <u>**aneurysmal SAH**</u>
  PGMEE KAR 2006
- Treatment with the calcium channel antagonist **nimodipine** (60 mg orally q6h) has been reported to be beneficial, but the effects seem to be modest.✱✱
- **Nimodipine** can cause significant hypotension in some patients, which may worsen cerebral ischemia in patients with vasospasm. The most widely accepted therapy for symptomatic cerebral vasospasm is to increase the cerebral perfusion pressure by raising mean arterial pressure through plasma volume expansion and the judicious use of vasopressor agents, usually phenylephrine or dopamin
- **Nimodipine** is indicated for improvement of neurological outcome by reducing the incidence and severity of ischemic deficits in patients with **subarachnoid hemorrhage from ruptured congenital intracranial aneurysms who are in good neurological condition post-ictus.** AIPG 2011
  JK BOPEE 2012

⊃ Desmopressin (High Yield for 2011/2012)

- Desmopressin (DDAVP) is a synthetic replacement for vasopressin, the hormone that reduces urine production during sleep. It may be taken **nasally, intravenously, or as a pill.** ✳✳

- Clinical uses

⇨ **Bedwetting**

- Desmopressin is frequently used for treatment of bedwetting. It is usually in the form of Desmopressin acetate, DDAVP. The drug replaces the antidiuretic hormone for a single night with no cumulative effect.✳

⇨ **Coagulation disorders**

- Desmopressin can be used to **promote the release of von Willebrand factor and factor VIII** in patients with coagulation disorders such as type I von Willebrand disease, mild hemophilia A, and thrombocytopenia. It is not effective in the treatment of hemophilia B or severe hemophilia A.✳

⇨ **Diabetes Insipidus**

- Desmopressin is also used to replace missing ADH in central diabetes✳

⊃ Bromocriptine (High Yield for 2011/2012)

✓ It is indicated in the treatment of prolactin-secreting pituitary tumors in men and women

✓ Considered to be the treatment of choice for microadenomas and for macroadenomas including those with visual defects. However, surgery may be required to treat macroadenomas in those patients who either cannot take **bromocriptine** or who exhibit a poor therapeutic response to **bromocriptine**

✓ Inhibits prolactin secretion.   **PGI 1988**

✓ **Treatment of Amenorrhea**, secondary, due to hyperprolactinemia ✳

✓ **Treatment of Galactorrhea** due to hyperprolactinemia ✳   **AIIMS 1997**

✓ **Treatment of Hypogonadism**, male, due to hyperprolactinemia ✳

✓ **Treatment of Infertility** due to hyperprolactinemia ✳   **AI 1989**

✓ **In Acromegaly**   **AI 1989**

✓ It is indicated, usually as an adjunct to levodopa/carbidopa therapy, in the treatment of the signs and symptoms of **idiopathic or postencephalic parkinsonism**✳   **JIPMER 1997**

✓ It is indicated in the treatment of some cases of **acromegaly**, usually as an adjunct to surgery or radiotherapy.   **JIPMER 1997**

✓ It is sometimes used as adjunctive therapy in the treatment of **neuroleptic malignant syndrome** was Used in induction of ovulation, Corpus luteum cyst   **AIIMS 1997**

⊃ Octreotide

- ✓ It is indicated for palliative management of gastrointestinal endocrine tumors, such as:
  Carcinoid tumors to suppress or inhibit the associated severe diarrhea and facial flushing
- ✓ Vasoactive intestinal polypeptide-secreting tumors **(VIPomas)** for the treatment of the profuse watery diarrhea associated with VIPomas.
- ✓ It is indicated to suppress secretion of growth hormone from pituitary tumors and decrease blood concentrations of insulin-like growth factor-I (IGF-I; somatomedin C) in patients with acromegaly
- ✓ It is indicated to reduce the incidence and severity of the **postoperative complications of high-risk pancreatic surgery.** These complications may include abscess formation and subsequent sepsis, acute pancreatitis, pancreatic fistula, and peripancreatic fluid collection.
- ✓ It is indicated in **Varices, gastroesophageal, bleeding** ✳   AI 2007
- ✓ It is indicated to reverse life-threatening **hypotension due to carcinoid crisis** during induction of anesthesia.
- ✓ It is indicated for use as palliative treatment of the symptoms resulting from hyperinsulinemia from severe **refractory metastatic insulinoma.** ✳
- ✓ It is indicated in **AIDS patients with severe secretory diarrhea** who have failed to respond to antimicrobial or antimotility agents.✳✳   AI 2011

⊃ Dantrolene (High Yield for AIIMS/AIPGME/DNB 2012-2013)

- ✓ Intravenous **dantrolene** is indicated to reverse the symptoms of the **Malignant Hyperthermic crisis syndrome** occurring during or following surgery or anesthesia. ☛☛
- ✓ It is also indicated for administration prior to surgery or anesthesia to prevent or attenuate the symptoms of the malignant hyperthermic crisis syndrome in patients known or suspected to be at risk for this complication
- ✓ Oral **dantrolene** is indicated to **relieve spasticity caused by upper motor neuron disorders** such as spinal cord injury, cerebrovascular accident, cerebral palsy, and multiple sclerosis. ☛
- ✓ It is used to relieve the **symptoms of Neuroleptic malignant syndrome**, which are similar to those caused by malignant hyperthermia.
- ✓ Treatment of exercise-induced pain in muscle **phosphorylase deficiency.**☛
- ✓ Oral dantrolene is used in the management of flexor spasms in patients who are confined to bed or a wheelchair.☛

⊃ Riluzole (High Yield for AIIMS/AIPGME/DNB 2012-2013)

- ✓ It is indicated in the treatment of **Amyotrophic lateral sclerosis (ALS)** ☛☛
- ✓ **Riluzole** presynaptically **inhibits glutamate release in the central nervous system (CNS)** and postsynaptically interferes with the effects of excitatory amino acids.☛

⊃ Ivermectin (High Yield for AIIMS/AIPGME/DNB 2012-2013)

Binds selectively and with high affinity to **"glutamate-gated chloride ion channels"** in invertebrate muscle and nerve cells of the **microfilaria**. This binding causes an increase in the permeability of the cell membrane to chloride ions and results in hyperpolarization of the cell, leading to paralysis and death of the parasite.

Ivermectin also is believed to act as an **"agonist of the neurotransmitter gamma-aminobutyric acid (GABA)"**, thereby disrupting GABA-mediated central nervous system (CNS) neurosynaptic transmission.

Oral agent for scabies now.

➲ Thalidomide

- Thalidomide is a **drug, immunomdulator** but **a potent teratogen** as well.✴✴

- It is an **old drug with new uses.**

- Thalidomide is used in **Mutiple Myeloma** due to antiangiogenic activity.(**Thalidomide+Dexamethasone +Melphalan**) is a very effective therapy for MM.✴

- Thalidomide reduces production of TNF alpha and is used for **Rh. arthritis and Crohns disease.** Serious infections including sepsis and tuberculosis cause the level of Tumor necrosis factor-alpha (TNFα) to rise. TNFα is a chemical mediator in the body, and it may enhance the wasting process in cancer patients as well. Thalidomide may reduce the levels of TNFα, and it is possible that the drug's effect on ENL is caused by this mechanism. Thalidomide also has potent anti-inflammatory effects that may help **ENL patients.**

- Thalomide, in conjunction with dexamethasone, is now standard therapy for **multiple myeloma.**

- Thalidomide is also prescribed for its anti-inflammatory effects in **actinic prurigo**, an autoimmune skin disease.

- Thalidomide also inhibits the growth of new blood vessels (angiogenesis), which may be useful in treating macular degeneration and other diseases. This effect helps AIDS patients with **Kaposi's sarcoma**, although there are better and cheaper drugs to treat the condition.

- Thalidomide may be able to fight painful, debilitating **aphthous lesions** in the mouth and esophagus of AIDS patients which prevent them from eating.

- Thalidomide is also being investigated for treating symptoms of **prostate cancer, glioblastoma, lymphoma, arachnoiditis, Behçet's disease, and Crohn's disease.**

Remember: AIIMS 2009

■ Used in leprosy (ENL).➤➤   AI 2010

■ HIV associated ulcer➤➤

■ AIDS related wasting syndrome➤➤

■ Multiple myeloma➤   AI 2010

■ Crohns disease➤

■ Behcets syndrome

■ Rheumatoid arthritis, Ankylosing spondylitis

■ Behcets ulcer

■ Has teratogenicity associated with its use.   AI 2010

7

PHARMACOLOGY

PHARMACOLOGY

⇨ **Cisplatinum:**

✓ **Highly emetogenic**☛	**PGI 2004**
✓ Highly nephrotoxic☛	
✓ Ototoxic☛	
✓ Neuropathy ++☛	
✓ Hyperuricemia ☛	

⇨ **Amifostine**

- Amifostine is a **thiophosphate (Cytoprotective agent).**☛☛
- It is used for **reduction of** <u>renal toxicity of Cisplatin</u>. Cisplatin **causes mitochondrial injury** and apoptosis plus necrosis of renal tubular cells.☛
- **Amifostine** is indicated to **reduce cumulative nephrotoxicity** associated with cisplatin therapy in patients with advanced ovarian,non-small cell lung carcinoma (NSCLC) or advanced solid tumors of non-germ cell origin.
- **Amifostine** is indicated to **reduce acute and cumulative hematologic toxicities** associated with a cisplatin and cyclophosphamide (CP) regimen in patients with advanced solid tumors of non-germ cell origin. **Amifostine** is also indicated to decrease bone marrow toxicity during treatment with high-dose cisplatin alone for head and neck carcinoma.
- **Amifostine** is also indicated to **decrease the frequency or severity of cisplatin-induced peripheral neuropathy** ☛☛
- It also **reduces xerostomia** in patients undergoing therapy for head and neck cancer.
- It is **administered iv** after reconstitution with normal saline.
- Hypersensitivity to mannitol is a **contraindication** to its use.

⊃ **Gallium Citrate (High Yield for AIIMS/AIPGME/DNB 2012-2013)**

- ✓ Is indicated to demonstrate the **presence and extent of lymphoma, bronchogenic carcinoma,** [acute myelocytic leukemia], [chronic myelocytic leukemia], [hepatoma], and [bone sarcoma]. ☛
- ✓ Gallium citrate Ga 67 is indicated for the <u>localization of focal inflammatory lesions</u>, such as abscess, osteomyelitis, pneumonia, pyelonephritis, and granulomatous diseases (sarcoidosis). May also be useful in the detection of active tuberculosis; and for assessing the activity of the inflammatory process in certain interstitial pulmonary diseases, including sarcoidosis and fibrosing alveolitis.
- ✓ In combination with thallous chloride Tl 201 imaging, gallium citrate Ga 67 imaging may be **useful in the diagnosis of myocardial sarcoidosis** and in predicting the response to corticosteroid therapy.
- ✓ Useful in the diagnosis and monitoring of *Pneumocystis carinii* pneumonia, **tuberculosis, and other infections in acquired immunodeficiency syndrome (AIDS) patients.** ☛☛
- ✓ Is useful as a **diagnostic screening test in cases of** <u>prolonged fever (PUO)</u>, when physical examination, laboratory tests, and other imaging studies have failed to disclose the source of the fever☛

⊃ Obesity and Orlistat

▶ **Orlistat** is an **inhibitor of intestinal lipase** that causes modest weight loss due to drug-induced fat Malabsorption.☞   AI 2007

▶ **Orlistat** is indicated for the **management of obesity in persons** with an initial body mass index (BMI)[3] 30 kg per square meter of body surface area (kg/m^2), or a BMI [3] 27 kg/m ^{2} when other risk factors (such as hypertension, diabetes, or dyslipidemia) are present. ☞

▶ **Orlistat** is a <u>reversible inhibitor of intestinal lipases</u>. In the lumen of the stomach and intestine, it bonds covalently with active serine residues of gastric and pancreatic lipases, making them unavailable to hydrolyze dietary triglycerides into absorbable fatty acids and monoglycerides.

▶ **Other drugs used in obesity are:**
- ☐ **Sibutarmine**   AI 2007
- ☐ **Olestra (Sucrose Polyesters)**   AI 2007
- ☐ **Fenfluramine**
- ☐ **Neuropeptide Y antagonists**
- ☐ **Beta 3 agonists**

⊃ Important Questions: AIPGME/ AIIMS/MAH 2011/2010/2009

- ☐ **Alkalinisation of urine ameliorates the toxicity of** Methotrexate   **AIPGME 2011**
- ☐ **Digitalis toxicity causes:** Ventricular bigeminy, Paroxysmal atrial tachycardia with variable AV Block, Biventricular tachycardia   **AIPGME 2011**
- ☐ **Drugs used to treat alcohol dependence :** <u>Naltrexone, Acamprostate, Disulfiram</u>   **AIPGME 2011**
- ☐ **Regarding** <u>Aprepitant</u> **True is :** Crosses Blood Brain Barrier, Ameliorate Nausea vomiting of chemotherapy, Metabolized by CYP450   **AIPGME 2011**
- ☐ **Diuretic drugs precipitate lithium toxicity**   **AIPGME 2011**
- ☐ **True about are:** Used in Non Small Cell Carcinoma, is a tyrosine kinase inhibitor, causes skin rash   **AIPGME 2011**
- ☐ <u>**Ramelton**</u> is antagonist of **MT1 and MT2** melatonin receptors, causes rapid sleep induction.   **AIIMS 2010**
- ☐ **A woman treated with lithium during pregnancy, should betested for:** Cardiac malformations   **AIIMS 2010**
- ☐ **Drugs causing SLE like syndrome** <u>INH, Hydralazine, Sulphonamide</u>   **AIIMS 2010**
- ☐ **Child with phocomelia is due to which drug taken by mother:** Thalidomide   **AIIMS 2010**
- ☐ **Drug used in estrogen dependant breast cancer:** Tamoxifen   **AIIMS 2010**
- ☐ <u>**Hemorrhagic cystitis**</u> **is caused by** Cyclophosphamide   **AIIMS 2010**
- ☐ **Prolonged testosterone treatment to a man results in:** Azoospermia   **AIIMS 2010**
- ☐ **Methotrexate resistance is due to:** Overproduction of DHFR   **AIIMS 2010**

PHARMACOLOGY

☐ **Mechanism of EDTA in carbonic anhydrase inactivation:** Chelation of metal in enzyme   AIIMS 2010

☐ <u>SERM</u> used for osteoporosis: Raloxifene   AIIMS 2010

☐ **Thalidomide** causes <u>phocomelia.</u>   AIIMS 2010

☐ **TAMOXIFEN is used in estrogen dependent breast cancer.**   AIIMS 2010

☐ **Prolonged Testosterone treatment causes Azoospermia.**   AIIMS 2010

☐ **Methotrexate resistance is due to overproduction of DHFR.(Dihydrofolate reductase), Changes in transport of MTX,**   AIIMS 2010

☐ <u>Raloxifene</u> is a SERM used in osteoporosis.   AIIMS 2010

☐ <u>Retapamulin:</u> Is a semisynthetic derivative effective in treatment of skin infections caused by group A β hemolytic streptococci and staph aureus.

☐ **Alefacept:** Is an immunosupressive dimeric fusion protein (extracellular CD2 binding portion of HLA antigen 3 linked to Fc portion of human IgG_1. Used in Psoriasis

☐ **Pralidoxime** is ineffective or fails against treatment of carbamate poisoning because: **Anionic**

☐ Ropinirole, Pramipexole, are **Dopamine agonists** used in treatment of parkinsonism

    MH 2010, JK BOPEE 2012

☐ **Ondansetron** acts on **$5HT_3$ receptors:**   **MH 2010**

☐ The adrenergic drug <u>**Sibutramine**</u> is used as:**Anorectic**   **MH 2010**

☐ <u>Ezetimibe</u> **is an** anti-lipidemic drugs reduces cholesterol levels by reducing the cholesterol absorption in intestine by acting on NPCILI receptors: **MH 2010**

☐ **Thiazolidinediones** anti-diabetic drugs acts by inhibiting **PPAR gamma:**   **MH 2010**

☐ Fluticasone, Budesonide, Ciclesonide are not effective in treatment of acute exacerbation of asthma and status asthmaticus   **MH 2010**

☐ <u>Mifepristone</u> is glucocorticoid receptor blocker   **MH 2010**

☐ <u>Eplerenone</u> is aldosterone antagonist: **MH 2010**

☐ <u>Reversible</u> hearing loss can be see (as side-effect) with: **Clarithromycin**   **MH 2010**

☐ Abciximab is: **Gp IIb/IIIa antibody**   **MH 2010 JKBOPEE 2012**

Important questions from 2009

■ **Thalidomide** is used in: ENL, Behchets syndrome, HIV associated ulcer.   AIIMS 2009

■ Omission of prior diuretic dose ↓**risk of postural hypotension by ACE inhibitors.**   AIIMS 2009

■ **Cerebellar toxicity** is a feature of <u>cytarabine.</u>   AIIMS 2009

■ **MDR gene** causes <u>efflux of drug</u>.   AIIMS 2009

■ **Cetuximab** is used in <u>**palliation of head and neck cancer + colorectal cancer**</u>.   AIIMS 2009

■ Pharma**co<u>vigilance</u>** is used for **monitoring <u>drug toxicity.</u>**   AIIMS 2009

■ **Tolazoline** is used as a <u>vasodilator</u> during coronary angiography   AIIMS 2009

■ **Protamine sulfate** is used in **heparin overdosage.**

➲ Tolazoline: (High Yield for AIIMS/AIPGME/DNB 2012-2013)

- **It is a competitive α receptor antagonist** and has similar affinities for α1 and α2 receptors. Tolazoline has **moderate α blocking property** and has histamine agonistic activity.
- It is a **vasodilator** and is quite similar to phentolamine but less potent. Vasodilatory action is due to increase in histamine secretion.
- Tolazoline is used the treatment of **persistent pulmonary hypertension** in the newborn when systemic arterial oxygenation cannot be maintained by supplemental oxygen/ and or mechanical ventilation.

AIIMS 2009

⇨ Naloxone (Remember while using Naloxone for MI)

- Naloxone is short acting
- Naltrexone used to lower craving in alcoholics
- Nalmefene can also be used in alcohol dependence
- IS USED IN OPOID DEPENDENCE TO PREVENT RELAPSE. **JK BOPEE 2012**
- Naloxone is LESS potent than naltrexone **AIPGME 2010**

➲ True About Thalidomide:

- Used in pregnancy as sedative but withdrawn due to teratogenicity **AIPGME 2010**
- Can be used in MM as primary as well as in refractory MM
- Used in ENL

Amphotericin B toxicity can be lowered by incorporating it in liposomal complex **AIPGME 2010**
Pharmacologically, both amphotericin A and B are known. However, clinically, amphotericin
B is most commonly used. Isolated originally from *streptomyces*.
It has been shown that Amp B (liposomal), is more effective and safer compared to usual Amp B

➲ Go Through Newer Drugs: High Yield for 2011-2012 AIPGME/AIIMS

☐ Surfactants used for Neonatal RDS	➜ Poractant /Beractant
☐ VIP analouge for Erectile Dysfunction	➜ Aviptadil
☐ μ Opoid receptor antagonist for Paralytic ileus	➜ Alvimopan
☐ PAF antagonists for Acute Pancreatitis	➜ Lexipafant/Apafant
☐ Recombinant Dnase used for hydrolysing Pulmonary Secretions in Cystic fibrosis	➜ Dornase Alpha
☐ IL-1 antagonist used as Disease Modifier in Osteoarthritis	➜ Diacerin
☐ Disease modifier for osteoarthritis(COX-LOX inhibitor)	➜ Licofelone
☐ Used in CML	➜ Imatinib, Dasatanib , Bastinib, Nilotinib
☐ Used in renal cell carcinoma	➜ Sunitinib ➜ Pazopanib
☐ NMDA Antagonist for ALS (Amyotrophic Lateral Sclerosis)	➜ Riluzole
☐ NMDA Antagonist for Alzhiemers Disease	➜ Memantine

Used in non small cell lung cancer	→ Efitinib, Erlotinib
Vasopeptidase inhibitors used for CHF treatment	→ Omapatrilat, Sampatrilat
PDE 4 inhibitors for Asthma	→ Roflumilast, Tofimilast,
CD 20 directed monoclonal antibody used in Patients of CML	→ Ofatumumab
Kallikerin Inhibitor used in Acute attack of Hereditary Agioneurotic edema	→ Ecallantide
An Ach release inhibitor and Neuromuscular blocker used for Dystonias /Torticollosis	→ Abobotulinomtoxin
Glucagon Like Peptides used in Type 2 Diabetes Mellitus	→ Exenatide, Liraglutide
Anti TNF agent used in Crohns Disease /Rheumatoid arthritis	→ Certoluzimab
5 Lipooxygenase inhibitor for Actinic Keratosis	→ Mesoprocol

Fidaxomicin: as a treatment for patients with <u>Clostridium difficile infection</u> (CDI).

Racecadotril: an oral enkephalinase inhibitor for use in the treatment of acute diarrhoea. Prevents the degradation of endogenous enkephalins plus reducing hypersecretion of water and electrolytes into the intestinal lumen. Racecadotril treatment results in significant reductions in stool output.

Ioflupane I 123 injection: is a radiopharmaceutical indicated for striatal dopamine transporter visualization using single photon emission computed tomography (SPECT) brain imaging to assist in the evaluation of adult patients with suspected Parkinsonian syndromes.

Leukotriene-receptor antagonists (**pranlukast, zafirlukast, montelukast**) and synthesis-inhibitors (zileuton) reduce the severity of bronchial hyperresponsiveness in asthma.

Suplatast tosilate is a novel <u>oral anti-asthma compound</u> that, in vitro, selectively inhibits IL-4 and IL-5 production from allergen-stimulated human Th2 lymphocytes, but not IFN-γ production from human Th1 lymphocytes. Suplatast may also prevent allergen-induced goblet-cell metaplasia and attenuates inflammatory mediators-induced eosinophil chemotaxis and eosinophil adhesion to endothelial cells.

Icatibant is a <u>selective B2 bradykinin receptor antagonist</u> indicated for the treatment of acute attacks of hereditary angioedema.

Ticagrelor is a <u>P2Y12 platelet inhibitor</u> indicated to reduce the rate of thrombotic cardiovascular events in patients with acute coronary syndrome.

Rivaroxaban is a <u>factor Xa inhibitor</u> indicated for the prophylaxis of deep vein thrombosis (DVT) in patients undergoing knee or hip replacement surgery, and to reduce the risk of stroke in people who have abnormal heart rhythm (non-valvular atrial fibrillation).

Tamsulosin is a **subtype-selective alpha (1A)- and alpha (1D)-adrenoceptor antagonist.** alpha(1)-Receptors **predominate in the prostate gland, prostatic capsule, prostatic urethra and bladder, and the relaxation of prostate and bladder smooth muscles** is associated with improved maximal urine flow (Q(max)) and alleviation of lower urinary tract symptoms (LUTS) in patients with benign prostatic hyperplasia (BPH). Tamsulosin, a sulfamoylphenethylamine-derivative alpha-adrenoceptor blocker with enhanced specificity for the alpha- adrenoceptors of the prostate, is commonly **used to treat benign prostatic hyperplasia (BPH)**. The drug is commercially available in a racemic mixture of 2 isomers, and is pharmacologically related to doxazocin, prazosin, and terazosin. **Used in the treatment of signs and symptoms of benign prostatic hyperplasia (reduction in urinary obstruction and relief of associated manifestations such as hesitancy, terminal dribbling of urine, interrupted or weak stream.** MAH 2012

Indacaterol inhalation powder is a **long-acting beta2-agonist** (LABA) for the long-term maintenance treatment of airflow obstruction in patients with chronic obstructive pulmonary disease (COPD).

Fentanyl is an **opioid analgesic nasal spray** for the management of breakthrough pain in cancer patients.

Ezogabine is a **potassium channel opener** indicated for the adjunctive treatment of adults with partial-onset seizures.

Varenicline is a prescription medication used to **treat smoking addiction**. This medication is the first approved **nicotinic receptor partial agonist**. Specifically, varenicline is a partial agonist of the **alpha4/beta2 subtype of the nicotinic acetylcholine receptor**. In addition it acts on alpha3/beta4 and weakly on alpha3beta2 and alpha6-containing receptors. Varenicline is a partial nicotinic acetylcholine receptor agonist, designed to partially activate this system while **displacing nicotine at its sites of action in the brain**. The drug competitively inhibits the ability of nicotine to bind to and activate the alpha-4 beta-2 receptor. The drug exerts mild agonistic activity at this site, though at a level much lower than nicotine; it is presumed that this activation eases withdrawal symptoms. MAH 2012

Tesamorelin: It is a synthetic **analog of growth hormone-releasing factor** — a hypothalamic peptide that acts on pituitary cells in the brain to stimulate the production and release of endogenous growth hormone. Treatment indicated to reduce excess abdominal fat in HIV-infected patients with lipodystrophy.

Denosumab: human **monoclonal antibody** which is being studied in the treatment of **osteoporosis**, treatment induced bone loss, Denosumab targets **RANKL** (**RANK** ligand), a protein that acts as the primary signal to promote bone removal. In many bone loss conditions, RANKL overwhelms the body's natural defense against bone destruction. Used in postmenopausal women with risk of osteoporosis.

Retapamulin - A pleuromutilin antibiotic ointment for **topical treatment of impetigo.**

Ropinirole: Antiparkinsonian drug also approved by FDA for treatment of Restless leg Syndrome. MAH 2012, JK BOPEE 2012

Doripenem - A carbapenem antibiotic for intra-abdominal and **urinary tract infections.**

Raltegravir - An integrase inhibitor for treatment of **HIV-1.** AIIMS 2011

Eribulin mesylate: unique **inhibitor of microtubule dynamics** binding predominantly to a small number of high affinity sites at the plus ends of existing microtubules. Eribulin exerts its anticancer effects by triggering apoptosis of cancer cells following prolonged and irreversible mitotic blockade. Has a role in breast cancer

Ixabepilone A microtubule inhibitor for metastatic or advanced **breast cancer.**

Sapropterin - An enzyme enhancer for treatment of **phenylketonuria (PKU).**

Fidaxomicin: as a treatment for patients with Clostridium difficile infection (CDI).

Dazoxiban: Direct thrombin inhibitor AIMS 2011

Ambrisentan -An endothelin receptor antagonist for **pulmonary arterial hypertension.**

Ioflupane I 123 injection: is a radiopharmaceutical indicated for striatal dopamine transporter visualization using single photon emission computed tomography (SPECT) brain imaging to assist in the evaluation of adult patients with suspected Parkinsonian syndromes.

Rotigotine - A transdermal dopamine agonist for **Parkinson's disease.**

Maviroc - A CCR5 antagonist, antiretroviral for treatment of **HIV-1 infection.**

Lanreotide - A depot injection for treatment of **acromegaly.**

Nilotinib - A kinase inhibitor for a specific type of **chronic myelogenous leukemia.**

Aliskiren - A direct renin inhibitor for treatment of **hypertension.**

Temsirolimus- A kinase inhibitor for advanced **renal cell carcinoma.**

Lisdexamfetamine A prodrug of dextroamphetamine for **ADHD.**

Atopaxar, voropaxar: Antiplatelet agents which are reversible protease-activated-receptor 1 (PAR-1) thrombin-receptor antagonist that targets thrombin-induced platelet activation.

Rivaroxaban:

It is a highly selective **direct Factor Xa inhibitor** with oral bioavailability and rapid onset of action.oral, direct acting inhibitors of Factor Xa include **rivaroxaban, apixaban, betrixaban.**

Alfimeprase

It is **a fibrolase derivative with thrombolytic activity produced by recombinant DNA technology.** Fibrolase is a zinc-containing metalloendopeptidase that was first isolated from the venom of the Southern copperhead snake, Agkistrodon contortrix. Alfimeprase degrades fibrin directly and entrapped blood cells are freed. Excess alfimeprase is rapidly inactivated by alpha-2 macroglobulin through an irreversible, covalent interaction.

⊃ Monoclonal Antibodies and their uses: (High Yield for AIIMS/AIPGME/DNB 2012-2013)

☐ Abciximab	→ Antiplatelet	JK BOPEE 2012
☐ Adalimulab (<u>HUMANIZED ANTIBODY</u>)	→ Rheumatoid arthritis	
JK BOPEE 2012		
☐ Canakinumab		
☐ Infliximab JK BOPEE 2012		
☐ Belimumab	→ SLE	
☐ Epratuzumab		
☐ Toclizumab		
☐ Agbagovomab	→ Ovarian cancer	
☐ Cetuximab	→ Colorectal cancer	
☐ Naclozomab	→ Colon cancer	
☐ Edrocolomab		
☐ Ustekinumab	→ Multiple sclerosis	
☐ Stamulumab	→ Muscular dystrophy	
☐ Palivizuimab	→ RSV infection (Resp Syncytial virus)	
☐ Trastuzumab	→ Breast cancer	
☐ Ertumaxomab		

➲ Filgrastim: (High Yield for AIIMS/AIPGME/DNB 2012-2013)

— It is a **granulocyte colony-stimulating factor (G-CSF)** analog used to stimulate the proliferation and differentiation of granulocytes.

— It is produced by recombinant DNA technology.

— Filgrastim is used to treat neutropenia stimulating the bone marrow to increase production of neutrophils.

AI 2007

— Filgrastim is also used to increase the number of hematopoietic stem cells in the blood before collection by leukapheresis for use in hematopoietic stem cell transplantation.

➲ Calcitonin (High Yield for AIIMS/AIPGME/DNB 2012-2013)

— **Inhibits bone reabsorption** by osteoclasts.

— It is important to know that although calcitonin inhibits reabsorption of calcium and phosphate in renal tubule, hypocalcemia which occurs, overrides this direct action by decreasing the total calcium filtered at glomerulus; urinary calcium is actually reduced

USES OF CALCITONIN:-

✓ **Hypercalcemia**

✓ **Osteoporosis**

✓ **Paget's disease**

➲ Denosumab: (High yield for 2011/2012)

— It is a fully human monoclonal antibody which is being studied in the treatment of osteoporosis, treatment induced bone loss, bone metastases, rheumatoid arthritis, multiple myeloma and giant cell tumor of bone.

— Denosumab is designed to target **RANKL** (RANK ligand), a protein that acts as the primary signal to promote bone removal. In many bone loss conditions, RANKL overwhelms the body's natural defense against bone destruction.

AIIMS 2006

— It was approved by FDA for use in postmenopausal women with risk of osteoporosis.

➲ Entacapone

— It is a drug that functions as a catechol-O-methyl transferase (COMT) inhibitor.

— It is used in the treatment of Parkinson's disease.

BHU 2006

— Entacapone is a member of the class of drugs known as nitrocatechols.

➲ Letrozole : (High Yield for AIIMS/AIPGME/DNB 2012-2013)

— It is an **oral non-steroidal aromatase inhibitor** for the treatment of hormonally-responsive breast cancer after surgery.

BHU 2006

— Estrogens are produced by the conversion of androgens through the activity of the **aromatase** enzyme. Estrogens then bind to an estrogen receptor, which causes cells to divide.

— Letrozole prevents the aromatase from producing estrogens by competitive, reversible binding to the heme of its cytochrome P450 unit. The action is specific, and letrozole does not reduce production of mineralo- or corticosteroids.

7

➲ **Thymosin alfa: TA1**

✓ TA1 is a **synthetic polypeptide.**
✓ The drug is in Phase III trials for the **treatment of hepatitis C** and in Phase II trials for **hepatitis B.** Additional possible indications are **malignant melanoma, hepatocellular carcinoma, drug-resistant tuberculosis, and Di George's syndrome.**
✓ TA1 is thought to **modulate the immune system by augmenting T-cell function.**
✓ TA1 may affect thymocytes by stimulating their differentiation or by converting them to active T cells.

➲ **Bevirimat: (High Yield for AIIMS/AIPGME/DNB 2012-2013)**

✓ It is an **anti-HIV drug** believed to inhibit HIV by a novel mechanism, so-called **maturation inhibition.**
✓ Like protease inhibitors, bevirimat and other maturation inhibitors **interfere with protease processing** of newly translated HIV polyprotein precursor, called **gag.**
✓ This molecule contains a number of HIV proteins in a single polypeptide which is then cleaved by the enzyme protease to produce functional structural proteins.
✓ However, unlike the protease inhibitors, **bevirimat binds the gag protein,** not protease.
✓ Once bound to gag, bevirimat **prevents a critical cleavage at a site called the capsid-SP1 junction.**
✓ The resulting virus particles lack functional capsid protein and have structural defects, rendering them incapable of infecting other cells.

➲ **Raltegravir: (High yield for 2011/2012)**

— It is an antiretroviral drug, the first of a new class of HIV drugs, the <u>integrase inhibitors, to receive such approval</u>.   **AIIMS 2011**
— **Integration occurs** following production of the double-stranded viral DNA by the viral RNA/DNA-dependent DNA polymerase, <u>reverse transcriptase</u>.
— *<u>The main function of Integrase is to insert the viral DNA into the host chromosomal DNA, a step that is essential for HIV replication.</u>*
— Integration is a point of no return for the cell, which becomes a permanent carrier of the viral genome (provirus).
— Integration is in part responsible for the persistence of retroviral infections. After integration, the viral gene expression and particle production may take place immediately or at some point in the future.

➲ **Tigecycline: (High Yield for AIIMS/AIPGME/DNB 2012-2013)**

— It is a **glycylcycline antibiotic.**
— It was developed in response to the growing prevalence of antibiotic resistance in bacteria such as **Staphylococcus aureus and Acinetobacter baumannii.**
— Tigecycline is **bacteriostatic and is a protein synthesis inhibitor by binding to the 30S ribosomal subunit** of bacteria and thereby blocking entry of Aminoacyl-tRNA into the A site of the ribosome during prokaryotic translation.
— Tigecycline is **active against many Gram-positive bacteria, Gram-negative bacteria and anaerobes -** including activity against methicillin-resistant Staphylococcus aureus (**MRSA**), Stenotrophomonas maltophilia, Haemophilus influenzae, and Neisseria gonorrhoeae

➔ Iclaprim: (High Yield for AIIMS/AIPGME/DNB 2012-2013)

It is a <u>diaminopyrimidine</u> <u>dihydrofolate reductase</u> <u>inhibitor</u> being developed for the treatment of complicated skin and soft tissue infections caused by <u>antibiotic-resistant</u> bacteria.

It is structurally related to <u>trimethoprim</u> <u>intravenously</u>-administered iclaprim was found to be as effective in skin and soft tissue infections, many caused by <u>methicillin-resistant</u> *Staphylococcus aureus* (MRSA).

Melatonin is used for:

- Jet lag
- Insomnia

Ramelteon:

— Is agonist of **MT1 and MT2** melatonin receptors.causes rapid sleep induction.

— Metabolized by CYP1A2.

— Has less addiction liability.   AIIMS 2010

— Minimal rebound.

— Minimal withdrawl symptoms.

➔ Methanol:

- It is a component of shellacs, varnishes, paint removers, canned fuel windshield-washer solutions, and copy machine fluid. It is also used to denature ethanol and render it unfit for consumption.
- It is a CNS depressant with a potency about half of that of ethanol.
- **Methanol is initially metabolized by alcohol dehydrogenase to formaldehyde, with subsequent oxidation to formic acid, and then to carbon dioxide and water.**
- **Formic acid is responsible for metabolic acidosis and retinal toxicity.** Its detoxification utilizes tetrahydrofolate as a cofactor.
- Ophthalmologic manifestations occur 15 to 30 hour after ingestion and include clouding and diminished vision, dancing and flashing spots, dilated or fixed pupils, hyperemia of optic disks, retinal edema, and blindness.

➔ Rave drugs: (High Yield for 2011/2012)

There are a variety of substances that have been connected with **Rave Clubs**. This is a brief list of some of the drugs by slang names and some of their effects:

1. **Ecstasy** - (Hallucinogen/stimulant)
2. **Ephedrine** - (Stimulant)
3. **Ketamine** - (Hallucinogen)
4. **GHB** - (Depressant)
5. **Methcathinone** - (Stimulant)
6. **LSD** - (Hallucinogen)
7. **Magic Mushrooms** -
8. **Methamphetamine** - (Stimulant) Methamphetamine affects many areas of the central nervous system.

⊃ **New Drugs: Frequently Asked and High Yield Topic. They will be asked**

■ **Natalizumab:** Is a **humanized IgG$_4$ monoclonal antibody** shown to be effective in patients with moderate to severe Crohns Disease.

■ **Neurokinin 1 (NK 1) receptor antagonists** have antiemetic properties.   **AIPGME 2011**
   Already highlighted last year Platinum notes.

→ **Aprepitant** is a highly selective NK 1 receptor antagonist that permeates Blood Brain Barrier.

→ Not an Agonist But Antagonist at NK1

→ Crosses Blood Brain Barrier

→ Ameliorate Nausea , vomiting of chemotherapy

→ Metabolized by **CYP 450**

• **Fosaprepitant** is an IV formulation

■ **Alosteron** is a **5HT 3 antagonist** approved for treatment of patients with **"Severe IBS with diarrhoea".** (Diarrhoea predominant IBS)

• **Prucalopride** has high affinity **5 HT $_4$ agonist. (Motility promoter)**

• **Tegaserod** is a partial **5HT $_4$ partial agonist** affinity. **(Motility promoter)**

■ **P FOX inhibitors**

• (Partial inhibitors of fatty acid oxidation pathway):

• **Ranolazine** (Metabolism Modifiers).

• **Used for treatment of chronic angina.**   **AIPGME 2012**

Newer Drugs acting used in CVS, Respiratory Medicine

Alisikiren:

✓ is a **"Renin inhibitor"** approved for Hypertension.

✓ Prevents conversion of angiotensinogen to angiotensin 1.

✓ Used especially for **primary hypertension.**

Bosentan and Tezosentan: **MAH 2012**

   • Are orally active competitive **"inhibitors of endothelin"**

   • Used for pulmonary hypertension.

   • Both are non selective acts on ET$_A$, ET $_B$

Sitasextan and ambrisentan : are selective ET $_A$ **ANTAGONISTS**

Conivaptan:

   V1a and V2 (Vasopressin) receptor Treat (Acute heart failure and Hyponatremia)

Neseritide:

- Activates BNP receptors, increases cGMP.
- Used to treat acutely decompensated congestive heart failure.
- It promotes vasodilation, natriuresis and diuretics.

■ **Epoprpostenol, Iloprost, Trepostinil** are Used in Pulm Hypertension.

Bartezomib: Proteasome inhibitor used for Multiple Myeloma✱✱✱   **PGI 2007**

Revlimid: inhibits TNF alpha, Effective in Multiple Myeloma✱✱

Rimonabant: Cannabinoid CB 1 receptor antagonist helpful in **alcohol abstinence.**

Myeloid growth factors (Recombitant human Colony stimulating factrtors)

- **Filgastrim**

- **Sargramostim**

- **Pefilgastrim**

▶ **Sargramostim is GM-CSF used in treatment of neutropenia.**

▶ **Epoetin alpha and Darpoetin alpha are recombinant erythropoetin used in treatment of anemia.**

▶ **Oprelvekin (Recombinant IL-2) is used in thrombocytopenia.**

⮑ Erythropoietin /EPO

It is produced mainly by **peritubular fibroblasts of the renal cortex.**

It is synthesized by renal peritubular cells in adults, with a small amount being produced in the liver

- Regulation is believed to rely on a **feed-back mechanism measuring blood oxygenation.**
- It binds to the **erythropoietin receptor (EpoR)** on the red cell surface and activates a **JAK2 cascade.** This receptor is also found in a large number of tissues such as bone marrow cells and peripheral/central nerve cells
- **Erythropoietin has its primary effect on red blood cells by promoting red blood cell survival through protecting these cells from apoptosis. (But not increasing life span)**
- It also cooperates with various growth factors involved in the development of precursor red cells. Specifically, the colony forming unit-erythroid (CFU-E) is completely dependent on erythropoietin. The burst forming unit-erythroid (BFU-E) is also responsive to erythropoietin.
- Under hypoxic conditions, the kidney will produce and secrete erythropoietin to increase the production of red blood cells by targeting CFU-E.
- It has a range of actions including vasoconstriction-dependent hypertension, stimulating angiogenesis, and inducing proliferation of smooth muscle fibers.
- It has also been shown that erythropoietin can increase iron absorption and induce haemoglobin formation.

● **Drugs and Syndromes: (High Yield for 2011/2012)**

⇨ **Ebsteins Anamoly:**

* **Lithium given in pregnancy results in:** Cardiac malformation.
* Lithium given in early pregnancy; the drug causes cardiac and vascular abnormalities.
* **"Atrialization of right ventricle"** is known as **Ebstein's anomaly.**
* It results into displaced and malformed tricuspid valves.

● **Serotonin syndrome (High Yield for 2011/2012)**

Remember important facts:	**AIPGME 2010**

➡ It is a complication of two drugs with serotonergic activity is combined together.
➡ This is often the case when **tricyclic antidepressants + monoamineoxidase inhibitors.**
➡ This interaction is potentially life threatening and has features similar to that of neuroleptic malignant syndrome.
➡ These include a variety of **autonomic, somatic and cognitive symptoms.**
➡ Symptoms include :   **MAH 2008**
✓ **Rigidity+**
✓ **Hyperthermia+**
✓ **Autonomic instability+**
✓ **Myoclonus+**
✓ **Confusion+**
✓ **Delirium and**
✓ **Coma.**
Serotonin syndrome caused by:
* Phenelzine
* Imipramine
* Fluoxetine
* Treated by Dantrolene.   **AIPGME 2012**

● **Fetal-Hydantoin Syndrome/Phenytoin Embryopathy: (High Yield for AIIMS/ AIPGME/DNB 2012-2013)**

Features: Growth and mental deficiency in fetal hydantoin with/without heart defects and cleft lip syndrome. Folic acid is essential for protein synthesis and growth, and since hydantoin interferes with intestinal transport of folic acid, it has been postulated that part of the fetal hydantoin syndrome may be due to inhibition of placental folic acid by maternal hydantoin.

● **Gray Baby Syndrome (High Yield for AIIMS/AIPGME/DNB 2012-2013)**

— It is a rare but serious side effect that occurs in newborn infants (especially premature babies) following the intravenous administration of **chloramphenicol.**
— This condition is due to a **lack of glucoronidation reactions** occurring in the baby, thus leading to an accumulation of toxic chloramphenicol metabolites.
— The **UDP-glucuronyl transferase enzyme** system of infants, especially premature infants, is immature and incapable of metabolizing the excessive drug load.

➲ Fetal Hydantoin Syndrome, (High Yield for AIIMS/AIPGME/DNB 2012-2013)

— Also called **Fetal Hydantoin Syndrome, Dilantin Embryopathy,** or **Phenytoin Embryopathy.**

— About one third of children whose mothers are taking this drug during pregnancy typically have children who **have intrauterine growth restriction with microcephaly and develop minor dysmorphic craniofacial features and limb defects including hypoplastic nails and distal phalanges.**

➲ Red Man Syndrome (High yield for 2011/2012)

— **Vancomycin** can cause two types of hypersensitivity reactions, the **red man syndrome and anaphylaxis.**
— Red man syndrome has often been associated with **rapid infusion of the first dose** of the drug which **stimulates histamine** release results in red man syndrome.

➲ Purple-Toe Syndrome: (High yield for 2011/2012)

It is one of the **thromboembolic complications of warfarin therapy.**
These problems are much less common than bleeding complications, they nevertheless demand a prompt diagnosis and treatment.   **BHU 2006**

➲ Fetal Warfarin Syndrome: (High Yield for AIIMS/AIPGME/DNB 2012-2013)

- **Warfarin given in early pregnancy** increases birth defects especially skeletons abnormalities
- **Foetal warfarin syndrome,**
  - Hyperplasia of nose, eye, socket, hand bones and
  - Growth retardation.
- **Given later in pregnancy it causes:-**
  - CNS defects,
  - Foetal death and
  - Accentuates neonatal hypothrombinemia

➲ Dress Syndrome (High yield for 2011/2012)

— Drug Reaction with Eosinophilia and Systemic Symptoms.

— It is a syndrome, caused by exposure to certain medications, that may cause a rash, fever, inflammation of internal organs, lymphadenopathy, and characteristic hematologic abnormalities such as eosinophilia, thrombocytopenia, and atypical lymphocytosis.

— Treatment consists of stopping the offending medication and providing supportive care.

➲ Fanconi Syndrome: (High yield for 2011/2012)

- It is a generalized **defect in proximal tubule transport** involving amino acids, glucose, phosphate, uric acid, sodium, potassium, bicarbonate, and proteins.
- **Idiopathic Fanconi syndrome** may be inherited as an autosomal dominant, autosomal recessive, or X-linked trait. Sporadic cases are also seen.
- A variety of inherited systemic disorders are also associated with **Fanconi syndrome** including Wilson's disease, galactosemia, tyrosinemia, cystinosis, fructose intolerance, and Lowe's oculocerebral syndrome. The syndrome may be acquired in multiple myeloma, amyloid, and heavy metal toxicity.
- Kindly remember to distinguish it from *Fanconis <u>Anemia</u> which is a different entity*.

PHARMACOLOGY

7

7

Ɔ **Pharmacologically useful Competitive Inhibitors (High Yield for AIIMS/AIPGME/DNB 2012-2013)**

Drug	Enzyme inhibited
▪ Allopurinol	☐ Xanthine oxidase
▪ 6-mercapto-purine	☐ Adenylosuccinate synthetase
▪ 5-fluorouracil	☐ Thymidylate synthase
▪ Azaserine	☐ Phosphoribosyl-amidotransferase
▪ Cytosine arabinoside	☐ DNA polymerase
▪ Acyclovir	☐ DNAP of virus
▪ Neostigmine	☐ ACh-esterase
▪ Alpha-methyl dopa	☐ Dopa-decarboxylase
▪ Lovastatin	☐ HMGCoA-lowering
▪ Oseltamiver	☐ Neuraminidase
▪ Dicoumarol	☐ Vit.K-epoxide-reductase
▪ Penicillin	☐ Transpeptidase
▪ Sulphonamide	☐ Pteroid synthetase
▪ Trimethoprim	☐ FH2-reductase
▪ Pyrimethamine	☐ FH2-reductase
▪ Methotrexate	☐ FH2-reductase

Ɔ **Remember "Mechanism of Action" of: (High Yield for AIIMS/AIPGME/DNB 2012-2013)**

- **Sucralfate:** Aluminum sucrose sulfate polymerizes in the acid environment of the stomach and selectively binds necrotic peptic ulcer tissue. Acts as a barrier to acid, pepsin, and bile.

- **Celecoxib, Rofecoxib:** Selectively inhibit cyclooxygenase (COX) isoform 2, which is found in inflammatory cells nad mediates inflammation and pain; spares COX-1 which helps maintain the gastric mucosa.

- **Cromolyn:** Prevents release of mediators from mast cells. Effective only for the prophylaxis of asthma. Not effective during an acute attack.

- **Flutamide:** is a nonsteroidal competitive inhibitor of androgens at the testosterone receptor, used in prostate carcinoma.

- **Ketoconazole and Spironolactone:** Inhibit steroid synthesis, used in the treatment of polycystic ovarian syndrome to prevent hirsutism.

- **Acetaminophen:** Reversibly inhibits cyclooxygenase, mostly in CNS. Inactivated peripherally.

- **Allopurinol:** Inhibits xanthine oxidase, decresing conversion of xanthine to uric acid.

- **Aspirin:** Acetylates and irreversibly inhibits cyclooxygenase (COX I and COX II) to prevent the conversion of arachidonic acid to prostaglandins.

- **Clomiphene:** It is a partial agonist at estrogen receptors in the pituitary gland. Prevents normal feedback inhibition and increses release of LH and FSHfrom the pituitary, which stimulates ovulation.

- **Colchicine:** Depolymerizes microtubules, impairing leukocyte chemotaxis and degranulation.

- **Cyclosporine:** Binds to cyclophilins (peptidyl proline cis-trans isomerase), blocking the differentiation and activation of T cells mainly by inhibiting the production of IL-2 and its receptor.

- **Heparin:** Heparin catalyzes the activation of antithrombin III.

- **Mifepristone (RU486):** Competitive inibitor of progestins at progesterone receptors.

- **Misoprostol:** It is a PGE1 analog that increases the production and secretion of the gastic mucous barrier.

- **Omeprazole, Lansoprazole:** Irreversibly inhibits H+/K+ ATPase in stomach parietal cells.

- **Probenacid:** Inhibits reabsorption of uric acid.

- **Sildenafil:** Inhibits cGMP phosphodiesterase, casuing increased cGMP, smooth muscle relaxation in the corpus cavernosum, increased blood flow, and penile erection.

- **Alpha-glucosidase inhibitors:** Inhibit intestinal bursh border Alpha-glucosidases; delayed hydrolysis of sugars and absorption of sugars leading to decresed postprandial hyperglycemia.

- **Glucocorticoids:** Decrease the production of leukotrienes and protaglandins by inhibiting phospholipase A2 and expression of COX-2.

- **H2 Blockers:** Reversible block of histamine H2 receptors

- **Thrombolytics:** Directly of indirectly aid conversion of plasminogen to plasmin which cleaves thrombin and fibrin clots. (It is claimed that tPA specifically converts fibrin-bound plasminogen to plasmin.)

- **Ticlopidine, Clopidogrel:** Inhibits platelet aggregation by irreversibly inhibiting the ADP pathway involved in the binding of fibrinogen.

- **Warfarin (Coumadin):** Warfarin interferes with the normal synthesis and gamma-carboxylation of vitamin K-dependent clotting factors II, VII, IX, and X, Protein C and S via vitamin K antagonism.

- **Azathioprine:** Antimetabolite derivative of 6-mercaptopurine that interferes with the metablolism and synthesis of nucleic acid.

- **Leuprolide:** GnRH analog with agonist properties when used in pulsatile fashion and antagonist properties when used in continuous fashion, causing a transient initial burst of LH and FSH

- **Tacrolimus (FK506):** Similar to cyclosporine; binds to FK-binding protein, inhibiting secretion of IL-2 and other cytokines.

⊃ Drug Causing (High Yield for AIIMS/AIPGME/DNB 2012-2013)

- Drug(s) causing **Adrenocortical Insufficiency:** Glucocorticoid withdrawal

- Drug(s) causing **Agranulocytosis:** Cloazapine -carbamazapine -colchicine -Propylthiouracil

- Drug(s) causing **Aplastic anemia :** Chloramphenicol -benzene -NSAIDS -PTU –phenytoin

- Drug(s) causing **Cardiac toxicity:** Daunorubicin & Doxorubicin

- Drug(s) causing **Cinchonism:** Quinidine, quinine

7

PHARMACOLOGY

7

- Drug(s) causing **Cough**: ACE inhibitors

- Drug(s) causing **Cutaneous flushing** : Niacin -Ca^{++} channel blockers -adenosine -vancomycin

- Drug(s) causing **Diabetes insipidus**: Lithium   **JK BOPEE 2012**

- Drug(s) causing **Disulfram-like reaction** :Metronidazole -certain cephalosporins -procarbazine -sulfonylureas

- Drug(s) causing **Drug induced Parkinson's** :Haloperidol -chlorpromazine -reserpine –MPTP

- Drug(s) causing **Extrapyramidal side effects** :Chlorpromazine -thioridazine -haloperidol

- Drug(s) causing **Fanconi's syndrome**:Tetracycline

- Drug(s) causing **hepatic necrosis** :Halothane -Valproic acid -acetaminophen -Amantia phalloides

- Drug(s) causing **G6PD hemolysis**: Sulfonamides -INH -ASA -Ibuprofen -primaquine -nitrofurantoin / -pyrimethamine -chloramphenicol

- Drug(s) causing **Tubulointerstitial Nephritis** :Sulfonamides -furosemide -methicillin -rifampin

- Drug(s) causing **Osteoporosis** : Corticosteroids -heparin

- Drug(s) causing reaction: **Oto and Nephrotoxicity** : aminoglycosides -loop diuretics -cisplatin

- Drug(s) causing **P450 induction**:Barbiturates -phenytoin -carbamazipine -rifampin -griseofulvin -quinidine

- Drug(s) causing **P450 inhibition**:Cimetidine -ketoconazole -grapefruit juice -erythromycin -INH - sulfonamides

- Drug(s) causing :**Photosensitivity**:Tetracycline -amiodarone -sulfonamides

- Drug(s) causing: **Pseudomembranous colitis**: Clindamycin

- Drug(s) causing **Pulmonary fibrosis**:Bleomycin -amiodarone -busulfan

- Drug(s) causing : **SLE-like syndrome**: Hydralazine -Procainamide -INH -phenytoin

- Drug(s) causing **Stevens-Johnson syndrome**: Ethosuxamide -sulfonamides -lamotrigine

- Drug(s) causing **Tardive dyskinesia**: Antipsychotics

- Drug(s) causing **Tendonitis** : Fluoroquinolones

- Drug(s) causing **Thrombotic complications**: Oral Contraceptives

- Drug(s) causing **Torsade de pointes**: Class III antiarrhythmics (sotalol) -class IA (quinidine)

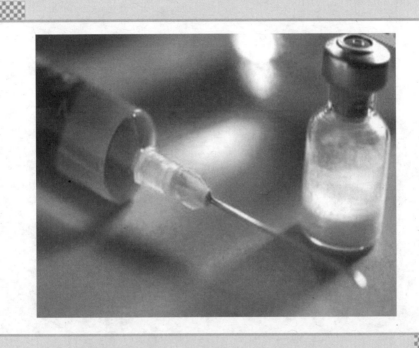

SOCIAL AND PREVENTIVE MEDICINE

⊃ Important Contributors

☐ John Snow	Cholera **epidemiology**		
☐ Robert Koch	V. cholera **identification**		
☐ Pettenkoffer	Concept of **Multi factorial Causation**		
☐ Lious Pausteur	**Germ Theory** of Disease		
☐ Fracostorius	Theory of **Contagion**	**JK BOPEE 2008**	
☐ Mc Mahon and Pugh	**Web of Causation** concept of Disease		
☐ Jules Guerin	**Social medicine**	**UPSC 01**	
☐ Road to Health Chart	David Morley	**MAHE2007**	

Remember:

➡ Father of **Medicine**	Hippocrates
➡ Father of **Epidemiology**	John Snow
➡ Father of **Genetics**	Mendel
➡ Father of **Pshycoanalysis**	Frued
➡ Father of **Anatomy**	Vesalius
➡ Father of **Bacteriology**	Loius Pausteur
➡ **Father of public health : John Snow**	
➡ Thank god that there are not mothers of medical sciences	

➡ Medical systems truly indian in origin are: **Ayurveda and Siddha**
➡ Ayurveda is practiced **throughout India**
➡ **Aterya** was the first acknowledged Indian physician and teacher. **JK BOPEE 2012**
➡ Siddha is practisced in **Tamil speaking areas of South India.**
➡ **Atharveda** (one of the four Vedas) gradually developed into science of Ayurveda.

⇨ "Sociology of Health"

Theory	Model of society	Cause of the Disease	Role of the Medical Profession
☐ Marxist	✓ Conflictual and exploitative	**Putting profit ahead of health**	✱ To discipline and control the working class; and provide individualized explanations of disease
☐ Parsonian	✓ Basically harmonious and stable set of interlinked social roles and structures	**Social strain caused by meeting the demands of social roles**	✱ Rehabilitate individuals to carry out their social roles
☐ Focucauldian	✓ A net of power relations, with no one dominant source-administered surveillance	**'Disease' are labels used to sort and segregate the population to make it easier to control**	✱ To enforce compliance with 'normal' social roles; and to ensure that we internalize these norms.
☐ Feminist **AIIMS 2009**	✓ Exploitative and repressive of women through patriarchy	**Carrying out the social role enforced on women by patriarchal men; the medicalization of a woman around her reproductive life cycle.**	✱ To enforce conformity with patriarchal norms of femininity and motherhood.

8

- ➡ **State Medicine:** implies provision of **free medical services** to people <u>at Governments expenses.</u> **(UPSC 99)**

- ➡ **Socialized Medicine:** provides provision of medical services and professional education by the state but programme is operated and regulated by <u>**professional groups rather than government**</u>. The concept was first introduced by **Neumann and Virchow** **(Kerala 2K)**

- ➡ **FREE** medical care supported by state is a feature.

- ➡ Ensures social equity, universal coverage of health services. **AIIMS 2011**

- ➡ Eliminates competition among physicians in search of clients. **AIIMS 2011**

Physical Quality of Life index: consists of: P(ILL)   MAHE 2007, SGPI 2005, AI 2006, KCET 2012

- ➡ Infant mortality rate

- ➡ Life expectancy at age <u>one</u>

- ➡ Literacy rate

➲ **Important Indices:**

Human poverty index (HPI)	Sullivan's index	HALE (Health adjusted life expectancy)	Disability adjusted life year (DALY)
➡ Introduced in 1997 ➡ Measures <u>average achievements in basic dimensions of human development</u> ➡ Formula for calculating HPI for **developing countries is HPI1** ➡ Formula for calculating HPI for **developed countries is HPI2** **(Karnataka 06)**	➡ Expectation of <u>**life free of disability**</u> ➡ Is calculated by subtracting from life expectancy the probable duration of bed disability and inability to perform major activities. **(MAHE 01)**	➡ Is based <u>on life expectancy at birth</u> but includes an <u>adjustment for time spent in poor health</u>. **(Karnataka 06)**	➡ Is a measure of <u>**burden of disease**</u> in defined populations and effectiveness of the interventions ➡ DALY express **years of life lost to premature death** and years lived with disability adjusted for the severity of disability. ➡ <u>**One DALY is one lost year of healthy life.**</u> **AIPGME 2012**

⇨ **Human Developmental Index**   **(UPSC 97)**

- ➡ Education   **PGI 2011**
- ➡ Life expectancy and
- ➡ Purchasing power   **PGI 2011**

⊃ Socioeconomic Indicators   JK BOPEE 2012

✓ FAMILY SIZE	
✓ LITERACY RATE	
✓ LEVEL OF UNEMPLOYEMENT	

⇨ **Kuppuswamys Index:**   AIIMS 1999

➡ Income	JK BOPEE 2012
➡ Education	JK BOPEE 2012
➡ Occupation	JK BOPEE 2012

⊃ Levels of "Prevention"

Primordial Prevention	Primary prevention	Secondary Prevention	Tertiary prevention
Prevention of the emergence or development of risk factors in populations in which they have not yet appeared.	Action taken prior to onset of disease which removes possibility that disease will occur. It includes ➡ Health promotion ➡ Specific protection — Immunization — Chemoprophylaxis MAHE 2007	Action halting the progress of disease at early stage and prevents its complications. It includes — Early diagnosis and Treatment	It includes Disability limitation Rehabilitation

⇨ Examples

✳ Salt restriction and smoking cessation in non communicble diseases are examples of: primordial prevention.	PGI 2005
✳ Source reduction in malaria is an example of primordial prevention.	
✳ Defloridation of water is an example of primary prevention.	AIIMS 1994
✳ Marriage conselling and immunization are examples of: primary prevention.	PGI 2005
✳ Pap smear is an example of secondary level of prevention.	
✳ IOL implantation in catract is an example of secondary level of prevention.	
✳ Physiotherapy to a case of poliomyelitis is an example of teritary level of prevention.	
✳ Spectacle use in refractive errors is an example of teritary prevention.	

⇨ Mass chemoprophylaxis is used in

— Yaws	AI 2010
— Filariasis	
— Trachoma	

8

SPM

Impairment	Any loss or abnormality of Psychological , physiological or anatomical structure or function e.g. loss of foot, defective vision, mental retardation
Disability	Because of impairment, affected person may be unable to carry out certain activities considered normal for his age, sex. etc. Listed as ICIDH II AIPGMEE 2009 e.g. Cannot Walk
Handicap	As a result of disability, person experiences certain disadvantages in life and is not able to discharge the obligations required of him and play the role expected of him in society e.g. Unemployed

Remember Kaplan Meier method is used for survival.   AIIMS 2008

Disease Eradication:

- Objective is to eliminate the disease to the extent that no **new case occurs in future.**
- **Complete extermination** of an organism.
- **"Tearing out by roots"** of a disease.
- Exhibits **All or None Phenomenon.**
- **Smallpox** has been eradicated. Next target diseases for eradication are:
- Polio
- Measles
- Guinea worm

Investigation of Epidemic: High Yield for 2011-2012

A.	Confirm/verify diagnosis
B.	Confirm existence of epidemic
C.	Define population at risk
D.	Rapid search of cases
E.	Data analysis
F.	Formulate hypothesis
G.	Test hypothesis
H.	Evaluate ecological factors
I.	Investigate population at risk
J.	Write report

- **Generation time** is the interval of time between receipt of infection by a host and **maximal infectivity** of that host, eg. **In leprosy it is about: 10-14 days**   AIPGME 2010, DNB 2011
- Generation time is roughly equal to the incubation period BUT incubation periodcan only be applied to infections that result in manifest disease whereas **generation time refers to transmissions of infection whether clinical or sub- clinical**

8

- **Incubation period:** The time interval between invasion by an infectious agent and appearance of **the first sign or symptom** of the disease in question.

- **Lead time:** is the advantage gained by screening that is period between diagnosis by early detection and diagnosis by other means. JKBOPEE 2005, KCET 2012

➲ **Important Indicies**

MMR=

Number of female deaths due to complications of pregnancy, child birth or within 42 days of delivery from "Puerperal causes" in an area during a given year × 1000

Total no. of live births in the same area and year

Indicators of MCH care where live births are used in the denominator:

STILL BIRTH RATE =

Foetal deaths weighing over 1000grams at birth × 1000

Total live births + still births weighing over 1000grams at birth

PERINATAL MORTALITY RATE =

Late foetal deaths + early neonatal deaths in one year × 1000

Live births in the same year

NEONATAL MORTALITY RATE =

Number of deaths of children under 28 days of age in a year × 1000

Total live births in the same year

POST NEONATAL MORTALITY RATE=

Number of deaths of children between 28 days and 1 year of age in a given year × 1000

Total number of live births

INFANT MORTALITY RATE =

Number of deaths of children less than one year of age in a year × 1000

Number of live births in the same year

UNDER 5 MORTALITY RATE (child mortality rate) =

Number of deaths of children less than 5 years of age in a given year × 1000

Number of live births in the same year

Indicators of MCH care where Live births are not used in the denominator:

1-4 YEAR MORTALITY RATE (CHILD DEATH RATE) =

Number. of deaths of children aged 1-4 years during a year × 1000 Total no. of children aged 1-4 years at the middle of the year

CHILD SURVIVAL RATE = 1000 -$\frac{\text{Under 5 mortality rate}}{10}$

It gives the percentage of those who survive to the age of 5 years.

Midyear population is used in the denominator of Crude Death Rate and Birth Rate.

➲ Health Care Delivery Indicators

- Doctor -population ratio
- Doctor-nurse ratio
- Population – bed ratio
- Population per health/sub centre multipurpose health worker works at sub centre. **AIIMS 2007**
- Population per traditional birth attendant

Infectivity	Pathogenecity	Virulence
— Ability of infectious agent to invade and multiply in a host	— Ability to induce **clinically apparent illness**	— Proportion of **clinical cases** resulting in severe clinical manifestations

- **Illness:** Is a **subjective state** of the person who feels aware of not being well.
- **Sickness:** Is a state of **social dysfunction** ie a role an individual assumes when one is ill.
- **Incidence rate:** number of **new cases** occurring in a defined population during a specific period of time. **MAHE 2005**
- **Secondary attack rate: number of exposed persons developing disease** within a **range of incubation period** following exposure to primary case.
- **Prevalance:** All current cases **(old and new)** total number of all individuals who have an attribute or disease at a particular time divided by population at risk of having disease at this point in time. Prevalence is product of incidence and duration
- **Prevalence is a ratio** **AIIMS 1997**
- **P=I x D (incidence × duration)** **UPSC 1996**

- ☐ **Crude death rate:**
- ☐ The number of deaths per 1000 population per year in given community **KCET 2012**
- ☐ **Expectation of life:**
- ☐ Life expectancy at birth is **"the average number of years that will be lived** by those born alive into a population if the current-age specific mortality persists.
- ☐ **Infant mortality rate:**
- ☐ **Ratio of deaths under 1 year of age** in a given year to the total number of live births in the same year.
- ☐ **Child mortality rate: Number of deaths at ages 1-4 years** in a given year per 1000 children in that age group at the mid point of the year concerned.

Birth rate: = (no of livebirths during year/mid yr population) × 1000
- — Is a **ratio.**
- — Is a fertility indicator. Still borne is not included. **AIPGMEE 2009**

▶ Crude death rate=: (no of deaths during year/mid year population) × 1000.   KCET 2012

▶ General fertility rate=: (no of live births during year/mid yr female population **aged 15 to 44**) × 1000

▶ General marital fertility rate=: (no of live births during year/mid yr **married female** population) × 1000

▶ Case fatality rate=: (no of deaths due to a disease/no of cases due to same disease) × 100

DETERMINES Virulence   KAR 2005

Best indicator of short duration acute disease.   AIIMS 2004

ⓞ **Primary case:**

First case of communicable disease <u>introduced into population</u> being studied.

ⓞ **Index case**

First case to come <u>to attention of investigator.</u>

ⓞ **Secondary case:**

Are those **developing from contact with primary case after incubation period.**

ⓞ **Serial interval:**   JK BOPEE 2011

Gap in time between onset of primary case and secondary case.   SGPGI 2005

Measures incubation period of disease.   KERALA 1997

ⓞ **Generation time:**

Interval of time between host receiving infection and <u>maximum infectivity</u> of that host.   KAR 2004

➲ Different Types of Bias

Proficiency Bias occurs when the intervention under consideration is delivered with unusual skill (or incompetence) so that it cannot be reproduced in typical settings.

Ascertainment Bias occurs when patients with the suspected outcome are most extensively probed about their symptoms and histories than are patients without the suspected outcome.

Detection Bias occurs when more information is solicited from the treatment group than from the placebo group.

Recall Bias occurs in retrospective studies. Patients may not remember the severity of their symptoms or how much intervention occurred over the specified course of time.

Referral Bias occurs when the sample of patients used in a study is not typical of the general population. For example, if an academic medical center sees the most acutely ill patients admitted for bypass mortality rates will appear extraordinarily high.

Suseptibility Bias occurs when patients receive one intervention or another on the basis of the severity of their disease. For example, since sicker patients would be less likely to survive a coronary bypass operation, they might be designated to receive medical therapy instead. This, however, might result in poorer outcomes for the medical therapy group. Susceptibility bias can be avoided by randomizing subjects to different study groups.

Attention bias (Hawthorne effect) occurs when subjects under study may alter their behaviour when they know they are being observed.

Berkensionian bias: admission rates to hospital differ

Purpose of **randomization** is to reduce bias.

In clinical trials reduces selection bias in allocation to treatment.   AIPGMEE 2007

⇨ **Analytical Studies Are**

Case control study	AIPGMEE 2009
Retrospective study	AIPGMEE 2009
Cross sectional study	

Case control study		Cohort Study	
Proceeds from effect to cause (retrospective)		Usually Proceeds from cause to effect	
Starts with disease		Starts with people exposed to risk	
Easy to carry			
Involves fewer subjects		Involves larger number of subjects	
Gives quick results	AIMS 2011	Gives delayed results	
Suitable for rare diseases	AIIMS 2000	Suitable for common diseases	
Yields odds ratio		Yields	
Yields casual association	AIIMS 2000	• Incidence,	AIPGMEE 2009
Risk factor can be identified		• Attributable risk,	
		• Relative risk	
Inexpensive		Expensive	
► Attrition not a problem		Attrition can be a problem	
► Minimal ethical problems			
► No risk to subjects			
► Rapid	AIIMS 2000		
► Inexpensive	AIIMS2000		

⇨ **Nested Case Control Studies**

- Is a type of case control study that **draws its cases and controls from population that has been followed** for a pretty long period of time
- **Potential recall bias and temporal ambiguity are reduced**
- Likelihood of **selection bias is also reduced**
- It is considered to be a **strong observational study**
- It is **cost effective** as well.

⇨ **Cross-Sectional Study**

- Based on single examination of a cross section of population at one point of time.
- Provides information about prevalence of disease.
- Gives snap shot of a population.
- More useful for chronic diseases.
- Does not establish time sequence.

⇨ **For Screening Following Criterion Should be Met**

→ Prevalence of condition should be **high**

→ A **recognizable latent symptomatic stage** should be present

→ There **should be a test** that can detect the disease prior to onset of signs and symptoms

→ **Facilities for confirmation of disease** should be available

→ There should be **effective treatment**

→ Expected benefits of **early detection** should exceed the risks and costs

→ There should be **good evidence that early detection and treatment reduces morbidity and mortality**

Single Blinding:

➡ Study subjects are not aware of treatment they are getting.

Double Blind Study:

➡ Both observer and group/person being studied is blind about study.   RJ 2006

➡ The patient does not know which treatment they are receiving.   AIPGME 2006

➡ The investigator also is not aware of treatment they are giving.

Triple Blind Study:

➡ Analyzer, observer and group/person being studied is blind about study.

⇨ **Screening Tests**

Screening test(s)	Disease screened
✳ Papanicolaou (pap) smear test	→ Cervical cancer
✳ Breast self examination test (BSE)	→ Breast cancer
✳ Mammography	→ Breast cancer
✳ Bimanual oral examination	→ Oral cancer
✳ ELISA, RAPID, SIMPLE	→ HIV (National AIDS Control Program)
✳ Urine for sugar, random blood sugar	→ Diabetes mellitus
✳ AFP (alpha feto protein)	→ Development anomalies in fetus
✳ Digital rectal examination (DRE)	→ Prostrate cancer
✳ Prostrate specific antigen (PSA)	→ Prostrate cancer
✳ Fecal occult blood test	→ Colorectal cancer

➡ **Disinfectant:** substance destroying harmful microbes (not spores)

➡ **Antiseptic:** substance which destroys or inhibits growth of microorganisms

➡ **Deodorant:** substance suppressing/neutralizing bad odors

➡ **Sterilization:** destroying organisms and spores

⇨ **Terms Commonly Asked**

➡ **Quarantine:** limitation of freedom of movement of such <u>healthy persons</u> exposed to communicable disease for a period of time not longer than longest incubation period.

➡ **Isolation:** separation for a period of communicability of <u>infected persons</u> to prevent spread of infections.

- ➡ Incubatory carriers: those carriers <u>who shed infectious agents during incubation period of disease.</u>

- ➡ Convalescent carriers: those carriers <u>who shed infectious agents during convalescence</u>.

- ➡ Healthy carriers: those carriers <u>who shed infectious agents without themselves suffering from overt disease.</u>

- ➡ Temporary carriers: those carriers who <u>shed infectious agents for short periods of time</u>

- ➡ Chronic carriers: those carriers who <u>shed infectious agents for indefinite periods of time</u>

- ➡ Pseudo carriers: carriers of <u>avirulent carriers</u>

- ➡ Carriers are not important in measles.   AIPGMEE 2007

➲ "Quarantable" Diseases: High Yield for 2011-2012

- ➡ Diphtheria
- ➡ Yellow fever
- ➡ Plague
- ➡ Smallpox
- ➡ Infectious TB
- ➡ Viral haemmorhagic fevers
- ➡ Severe acute respiratory syndrome

➲ "Isolation" Has a Definitive Value in

- ☐ Diphtheria
- ☐ Cholera
- ☐ Pneumonic Plague
- ☐ Streptococcal respiratory disease

➪ Isolation May be Attempted but Unlikely to Prevent Spread of Infection are:

- ✳ Polio
- ✳ Hepatitis A
- ✳ Typhoid
- ✳ Mumps

- — Active surveillance: Worker visits every house hold in the area to find out cases.

- — Passive surveillance: Search of cases by <u>local health agencies</u>.

- — Sentinel surveillance: Method of identifying <u>missing cases.</u>   MAH 2012

Surveillance: "It is continuous scrutiny of all aspects of occurrence and spread of disease that are pertinent to effective control." It can be various types:

- ➡ Sentinel surveillance – used to find hidden cases
- ➡ Individual surveillance – done for infected persons until they are no longer a risk
- ➡ Local population surveillance, e.g. surveillance of malaria
- ➡ National population surveillance, e.g. surveillance of smallpox after disease has been eradicated International surveillance, e.g. for malaria, polio, influenza

- ➥ <u>Concurrent Disinfection:</u>
- ➥ Disinfection as <u>soon as possible after discharge</u> of infectious material from body of an infected person or after soiling of articles with such infectious discharges
- ➥ <u>Terminal Disinfection:</u>
- ➥ Application of disinfective measures after patient has been removed by death or has ceased to be a source of infection
- ➥ <u>Prophylactic Disinfection:</u>
- ➥ Such as disinfection of water by chlorine, pasteurization of milk and hand washing

➲ Pasteurization: High Yield for 2011-2012

- — The process of pasteurization is named after **Louis Pasteur** who discovered that spoilage organisms could be inactivated in wine by applying heat at temperatures **below its boiling point.**
- — The process was later applied to milk and remains the most important operation in the processing of milk. Pasteurization uses temperatures **below boiling point** since at temperatures above the boiling point for milk, casein micelles will irreversibly aggregate (or "curdle").
- — Pasteurization **kills nearly 90 % of the bacteria in milk** including the more heat-resistant tubercle bacillus and the Q fever organisms.
- — **It does not kill thermoduric bacteria nor the bacterial spores.** Therefore, despite pasteurization, with subsequent rise in temperature, the bacteria are bound to multiply. In order to check the growth of microorganisms, pasteurized milk is rapidly cooled to 4 deg C. It is kept cold until it reaches the consumer. Hygenically produced pasteurized milk has a keeping quality of **not more than 8 to 12 hours at 18 deg C.**
- — Note that unlike sterilization, pasteurization is not intended to kill all pathogenic micro-organisms in the food or liquid.

- ▶ **Disinfectant** kills <u>all pathogenic organisms</u>   AIIMS 1984
- ▶ **Sterilization:** destruction of <u>all living organisms</u>
- ▶ **Antisepsis:** prevention of infection by inhibiting growth of bacteria in wounds/tissues.   AI 1990
- ▶ Agent on addition to a colony inhibiting growth and on removal colony regrows is said to be **Bacteriostatic**   AI 1996
- ▶ Pausterization by **Holder method**: 63^0c for 30 minutes
- ▶ Pausterization by **Flash method**: $72\ ^0$c for 15-20 seconds   PGI 1986
- ▶ **Prions** are <u>most resistant</u> **to sterilization.**   AI 2008
- ▶ **Hot air oven** is used for sterilization of: MP 1998
- ✓ Glass ware
- ✓ Liquid paraffin
- ✓ Dusting powder
- ✓ Forceps, scissors, scalpels

8

SPM

▶ Endoscopes are strelized by glutaraldehyde.	AIIMS 1986
▶ Cidex is 2% glutaraldehyde.	AIIMS 1987
▶ Disposable syringes are sterilized by gamma rays.	AIIMS 1989
▶ Vaccines are sterilized by heat inactivation.	AI 1989
▶ Hospital dressing is best disinfected by inceneration.	TN 1991
▶ Efficacy of disinfectant is measured by Phenol coefficient.	
▶ Riedal walker coefficient determines germicidal efficiency of disinfectant as compared to phenol.	PGI 1987
▶ Intermittent sterilization is Tyndalization.	KAR 1995
▶ Bacterial spores are destroyed by autoclaving.	TN 1998
▶ Cold sterilization is by gamma rays.	AIIMS 1984

⊃ Types of Development

⇨ Propagative Development:

A.	Organism multiplies only	
B.	Plague bacilli in rat flea	CUPGEE 1996
C.	Yellow fever in mosquito	

⇨ Cyclo Propagative Development:

A.	Organism multiplies +undergoes change in form	
B.	Malaria P in mosquito	AIIMS 1997
C.	Leishmania donovani	

⇨ Cyclo Development:

A.	No multiplication, only development of organism	
B.	Microfilaria in mosquito	AIIMS 2009, MAH 2012
C.	Guinea worm in Cyclops	

⊃ Mother to Child Transmission (MTCT)

— RUBELLA : Any trimester; MC and most serious in I trimester
— VARICELLA : Any trimester; MC and most serious in I trimester
— SYPHILIS : any trimester, more common in late II trimester or III trimester
— TOXOPLASMOSIS : Any trimester; MC in III trimester; more serious in I trimester
— HERPES SIMPLEX : During delivery (from infected genital secretions)
— HIV: during delivery, breast feeding (16%)
— HEPATITIS B : MC in III trimester and through breast feeding

⊃ Cleans of Safe Delivery

Five cleans (practices) under strategies for elimination of neonatal tetanus include,

- ☐ <u>Clean delivery surface</u>   AI 2004
- ☐ <u>Clean hands (of birth attendants)</u>   AI 2004
- ☐ <u>Clean cord cut (blade or instrument)</u>
- ☐ <u>Clean cord tie</u>
- ☐ <u>Clean cord stump (no applicant)</u>

Some times these practices are called '3 cleans':

- ☐ Clean delivery surface
- ☐ Clean hands
- ☐ Clean cord care(cut, tie and stump)

Suggested 'seven cleans' include 5 cleans and

- ☐ **Clean water and Clean towel**, for handwashing

3 CLEANS	7 CLEANS	5 CLEANS
✳ Clean Hands	✳ Clean Hands	✳ Clean Hands
✳ Clean Delivery Surface	✳ Clean Delivery Surface	✳ Clean Delivery surface
✳ Clean Cord Care	✳ Clean Cord cut/blade	✳ Clean cord cut/blade
	✳ Clean cord tie	✳ Clean cord tie
	✳ Clean cord stump	✳ Clean cord stump
	✳ Clean towel	
	✳ Clean water	

VACCINE	STRAIN(s)
☐ BCG	▶ **Danish 1331 strain** (WHO recommended)
☐ OPV/IPV	➡ P1,P2,P3 strains (mono or trivalent)
☐ Measles vaccine	▶ **Edmonston Zagreb strain (MC)**
	➡ Schwartz strain
	➡ Moraten strain
☐ Mumps vaccine	➡ Jeryll lynn strain
☐ Rubella vaccine	▶ **RA 27/3**
☐ Yellow fever vaccine	▶ **17D strain**
☐ Varicella vaccine	▶ **OKA strain**
☐ JE vaccine	▶ **Nakayama strain (MC)**
☐ (Japanese encephalitis)	➡ Beijing P3 strain
	➡ SA 14-14-2
☐ Malaria vaccine	➡ SPf 66 strain(lytic coktail)
	➡ Pf 25 strain

☐ HIV vaccine	➠ mVA (modified ankara) strain
	➠ rAAV (recombinant adeno associated viral vaccine) strain
	➠ CTL (Cytotoxic T- lymphocytic) strain
	▶ AIDSVAX strain
	▶ Subunit vaccine strain

⇨ **BCG**

- ➠ WHO has recommended the **'Danish 1331' Strain** for the production of BCG vaccine
- ➠ **Normal saline** is recommended as diluent for BCG vaccine.
- ➠ The reconstituted vaccine should be used **within 3 hours** and left over vaccine should be discarded.
- ➠ The Vaccine must **not be contaminated** with any antiseptic or detergent.
- ➠ If alcohol is used to swab the skin, it must be allowed to evaporate before the vaccine is given.
- ➠ **Mantoux test normally** because positive **after 8 weeks** of vaccination, but sometimes it takes **about 14 weeks.**
- ➠ BCG vaccines are stable for several weeks at ambient temperature in tropical climate, and for **up to 1 years** if kept away from direct light and stored in a cool environment. The vaccine must be protected from exposure to light during storage (wrapped up in double layers of red or black cloth).
- ➠ Dosage:Usual strength is **0.1 mg in 0.1 ml** volume: Dose to newborn aged below 4 weeks is **0.05 ml**
- ➠ **Administration: Intradermal** with tuberculin syringe.
- ➠ **Site of injection:** Just above the insertion of the deltoid muscle.
- ➠ **Duration of protection:** 15 to 20 years.

⇨ **Phenomenon after Vaccination**

- ✳ A papule develops at the site of injection 2 to 3 weeks after vaccination.
- ✳ It increases in size and reaches a diameter of 4 to 8 mm in about 5 weeks.
- ✳ The papule then ulcerates
- ✳ Healing occurs spontaneously to leave a tiny scar (4 to 8 mm in diameter) within 6 to 12 weeks.

Immunization

➠ WHO launched **EPI** (Extended Programme of Immunization) in **1974**	
➠ EPI was launched <u>in India</u> in **1978**	
➠ UIP (Universal Immunization Programme) was launched in India in **1985.**	
➠ **BCG, polio, DPT, are included in UIP**	AIIMS 1988
➠ **Measles aims at preventing blindness.**	AIIMS 1998
➠ **MMR is not included in EPI.**	AI 2007
➠ **Ring vaccination is given around 100 yards of a case detected.**	MAHE 2005

⇨ **National Immunization Schedule**

At Birth	— BCG and OPV-0 dose
6 weeks	— DPT 1, OPV1, Hep B 1
10 weeks	— DPT2, OPV2, Hep B 2
14 weeks	— DPT3, OPV3,Hep B 3
9 months	▶ Measles
16-24 months	— DPT and OPV
5 years	▶ DT
10 and 16 YEARS	— Tetanus Toxoid

⇨ **Live Vaccines are**

⓪	BCG	JKBOPEE 2012
⓪	Measles	PGI 2006, JKBOPEE 2012
⓪	Mumps	
⓪	Rubella	
⓪	Oral Typhoid	
⓪	Oral polio (sabin)	JKBOPEE 2012
⓪	Influenza	
⓪	Yellow fever (17 D)	PGI 2006

⇨ **Killed Vaccines**

Rabies	
Plague	
Salk polio	AI 1998
KFD	
Typhoid	
Cholera	
Japanese encephalitis	
Pertussis	DELHI 1989

⇨ **Fragment Vaccines**

➡ Diphtheria	
➡ Tetanus	
➡ Meningococcus, pneumococcus, haemophilus	
➡ Hepatitis B	JK BOPEE 2011

8

SPM

⇨ **Hepatitis B Vaccine**

✓	The original hepatitis vaccine consisted of purified, inactivated, alum-adsorbed, 22-nm hepatitis B surface antigen (HBsAg) particles obtained from human plasma.	
✓	Is a DNA Vaccine.	PGI 2011
✓	Currently produced vaccines are derived from inserting the gene for HBsAg into Saccharomyces cerevisiae.	
✓	Hepatitis B vaccine is the first vaccine that can prevent cancer	

Freeze dried vaccines:

►	BCG,	
►	Yellow fever,	JIPMER 2005
►	Measles	JIPMER 2005
►	OPV	PGI 1985

Vaccines to be stored in cold compartment but not freezer:

► Typhoid,

► DPT,

► Tetanus Toxoid,

► Diluents

⊃ **Newer Tests in Typhoid: High Yield for 2011-2012**

Test of Diagnosis	Remarks
✓ IDL tubex test	✓ Detects IgM antibodies
✓ TYPHI DOT	✓ Detects IgM and IgG antibodies
✓ TYPHI DOT-M	✓ Detects IgM antibodies
✓ DIPSTICK TEST	✓ Detects IgM antibodies

The **Vi capsular polysaccharide vaccine** (or **ViCPS**)

— Is one of two vaccines recommended by the World Health Organisation for the prevention of typhoid (the other is Ty21a).

— It was first licensed in the US in 1994 and is made from the purified Vi capsular polysaccharide from

The Ty2 Salmonella Typhi strain; it is a subunit vaccine.

— Indications: The vaccine may be used in endemic areas in order to prevent typhoid. It is also commonly used to protect people who are traveling to parts of the world where typhoid is endemic.

— Dosing: The vaccine is injected either **under the skin or into a muscle** at least seven days before traveling to the typhoid-affected area. It is given to children 2 years or older, ideally one month before travel, as a single dose (0.5 ml) with a booster every year.

Oral vaccine, Ty21a, is given to children 6 years of age or older. It is given as 4 doses over 1 week, with repeat every 5 years.

8

SPM

Characteristics	Killed vaccine	Live vaccine	
Doses	▶ Multiple	▶ Single	
Adjuvant	▶ Needed	▶ Not needed	
Duration of immunity	▶ Short	▶ Long	AIPGMEE 2008
Effectiveness of protection	▶ Lower	▶ Greater	
Reversion of virulence	▶ No	▶ Possible	
Stability at room temperature	▶ High	▶ Low	
Immunity Mucosal immunity Cell mediated immunity	 ▶ Poor ▶ Poor	 ▶ High ▶ High ▶ Contain major and minor antigens. ▶ Booster doses not required. ▶ Immunoglobulin's can be given 2 weeks after live vaccine.	 AIPGMEE 2008 UPSC 2002

⇨ **Again Remember Vaccines and Strains Used:**

— Measles	▶ Edmonston Zagreb Strain	
— BCG	▶ Danish 1331	AIPGMEE 2007
— Rubella	▶ RA 27/3	
— IPV	▶ Salk Strain	
— OPV	▶ Sabin Strain	PGI 2004
— Chickenpox	▶ Oka Strain	PGI 2004

➲ **Thermolability of Vaccines (Sensitivity to Heat):**

— Reconstituted BCG, YF,OPV, Measles	JK BOPEE
➡ Most thermo labile vaccine :Reconstituted BCG	
➡ Most thermostable vaccine :TT	
➡ Vaccines contraindicated in pregnancy: All live vaccines (except yellow fever) and meningococcal vaccine	
➡ Vaccines not to be given in pregnancy: MMR.	APPG 2006
➡ Preservative in measles vaccine is kanamycin.	
➡ Preservative in OPV vaccine is MgC_{l2}.	
➡ Thiomersal is preservative in BCG.	AIIMS 2008

⇨ **Classification of Adverse Events Following Immunization (AEFIs)**

▶ Vaccine reaction	— Event due to **inherent property of vaccine**
▶ Programme error	— Event due to **vaccine preparation error**
▶ Coincidental	— Event after vaccination not caused by vaccine
▶ Injection reaction	— Event from anxiety /pain from injection rather than vaccine
▶ Unknown	— Events cause cannot be determined

| **Anaphylactoid reaction after immunization** | Acute allergic reaction occurring within 2 hours after immunization characterized by:
 Wheezing and shortness of breath due to brochospasm
 Laryngospasm/laryngeal edema
 Skin manifesatation/s |
| **Anaphylaxis after immunization** | Severe immediate (within 1 hour) allergic reaction leading to circulatory failure with or without bronchospasm and/or laryngospasm/laryngeal edema |

Vaccine	Contraindications
▶ All vaccines	Previous anaphylaxis
▶ Live vaccines	Pregnancy, Radiation Therapy
▶ Yellow fever	Egg allergy Immunodeficiency
▶ BCG	Symptomatic HIV infection
▶ Influenza, Yellow fever	anaphylaxis following egg ingestion

| — Ring vaccination is given around 100 yards of a case detected. | **Delhi 93** |
| — **DPT should not be given to a child suffering from Convulsions.** | |

▬ BCG is a live attenuated vaccine given intradermal.	**RJ 2002**
▬ TY21 A is vaccine for typhoid.	**MP 2005**
▬ There is no vaccine for Dengue fever yet.	**MP 2009**
▬ Influenza vaccine is adminstered as nose drops.	**UP 2006**
▬ Ring vaccination is given around 200 yards of a case detected.	**DNB 2006**
▬ HPV vaccine is both bivalent and quadrivalent.	**AIIMS 2009**

⊃ **Diseases to be Known**
⇨ **Chickenpox:**

| ▶ Also called Varicella (HHV 3) |
| ▶ IP: 7-21 days |
| ▶ Secondary attack rate 90% |
| ▶ Rash **centripetal** |

8

- ▶ Palms and soles seldom affected
- ▶ Rash on **Flexor aspect**
- ▶ Rash is **superficial**
- ▶ Temperature rises with each fresh crop of rash.
- ▶ Infectivity lasts for 6 days after onset of rash.

Smallpox	Chickenpox
— IP: 7-17 days	— IP: 7-21 days
— Rash Centrifugal	— Rash **centripetal**
— Palms and soles frequently involved	— Palms and soles seldom affected
— Rash on extensor aspect	— Rash on **Flexor aspect**
— Rash is deep seated	— Rash is **superficial**
— Fever subsides with appearance of rash	— Temperature rises with each fresh crop of rash.
	— Infectivity lasts for 6 days after onset of rash. AIPGMEE 2002

⊃ Measles

- — Measles is also called as **Rubeola.**
- — It is caused by measles virus **(RNA Paramyxovirus group).**   JK BOPEE 2011
- — **Kopilik spot is a feature of Measles.**   (COMED 07)
- — **Incubation period is 10-14 days.**   MAHE 2007
- — Source of infection is only a **case** of measles.
- — Rash appears on **fourth day.**   KAR 1989
- — Measles is highly infective during "**prodromal**" **period.**
- — Infection confers **life long immunity.**
- — Measles is **severe in malnourished children.**
- — Measles is a **winter disease.**
- — Transmission is through **droplet infection.**
- — Measles can lead to **blindness** and **Vitamin A is** given in high doses.

- ➡ SSPE is not a common but __rare__ complication of measles. (**Febrile convulsions, Encephalitis and SSPE are rare complications**)   (COMED 2008)
- ➡ **Diahorrea, pneumonia, Otitis** are the **common complication**
- ➡ Measles vaccine in india is produced by **Serum Institue Pune**   (MAHE 98)
- ➡ Reconstituted measles vaccine is used within **1 hour**
- ➡ Measles vaccine given to contact of measles case exerts protective influence within **7 days.**   (Delhi 96)
- ➡ **Measles vaccine has high efficiency.**   AIPGMEE 2009
- ➡ **Contamination of measles vaccine can cause TSS (Toxic Shock Syndrome)**   AIPGMEE 2009

⇨ **Rubella**

— Caused by RNA virus of toga virus family	
— Incubation period <u>2-3 weeks</u>	
— **Risk to fetus is maximum if mother gets infected in 6-12 weeks of pregnancy.**	AIIMS 2005
— Congenital rubella syndrome is <u>deafness, cardiac malformations, cataracts</u>.	AI 2005
— Glaucoma, retinopathy, microcephalus, IUGR, Hepatospleenomegaly are a feature.	
— RA 27/3 is given as a single dose of 0.5 ml SC.	
— **Pregnancy is a contraindication** to its use.	
— Recepients of vaccine should be advised not to remain pregnant over next 3 months.	
— **Rubella vaccine is given in girls 11-14 years of age.**	JIPMER 2002
— **Recommended vaccination strategy is to vaccinate women 15-49 years.**	AIPGMEE 2007

⇨ **Mumps**

— Mumps is caused by RNA virus of **paramyxovirus family.**
— Only **one serotype** is present.
— One attack gives **life long immunity**.
— Incubation period varies from 2-3 weeks.
— **Pain and swelling of parotids (ear ache) is a feature.**
— Orchitis, ovaritis, pancreatitis, meningoencephalitis, thyroiditis, neuritis, hepatitis, myocarditis are a feature.
— **Control of mumps is difficult because disease is infectious before a diagnosis is made.**

Bacterial Zoonosis:
➥ Anthrax
➥ Brucellosis
➥ Q fever
➥ Tuberculosis
➥ Plague
Viral Zoonosis:
➥ Cow pix
➥ Monkey pox
➥ Yellow fever
➥ Lassa Fever
➥ Japenese Encephalitis
➥ Rabies
Protozoan Zoonosis
➥ Leishmaniasis
➥ Toxoplasmosis
➥ Trypanosomiasis
➥ Babeiosis

Helminthic Zoonosis

- Clonorchiasis
- Taeniiasis
- Trichenellosis

Rabies

- Caused by **Bullet shaped, RNA Virus** of Rhabdoviridae family. (<u>**Lyssa virus type 1**</u>)
- Rabies is a **zoonosis**.
- Rabies is a **dead end** infection.
- Symptoms appear in about **10 days**. (4 DAYS -8 WEEKS)   **MANIPAL 2004**
- **Most animal bites except human and rat bites can cause rabies**
- A **"Fixed"strain of virus** is defined as one that has a **short, fixed and reproducible incubation period** (4-6) days when injected intracerebrally. Vaccine prepared from it.   **COMED 2006**
- Animal bites, Licks, Aerosols, Person to person are modes of transmission.
- **Fixed virus** is used for preparation of **vaccine.**
- Virus recovered from **naturally occurring cases** of Rabies is called **"Street" virus.**
- Incubation period **depends on**: Site of bite, severity of bite, number of wounds, amount of virus injected, species of bitting animals.
- **"Hydrophobia and Aerophobia"** are seen in Rabies.
- **"Rabies free area"** is one in which no case of indigenously acquired rabies has occurred in man or any animal species for 2 years.
- **Immunoflorescence is used for diagnosis.**   **AI 1991**
- **Rabies vaccine was developed by Pauster.**
- **HDCV vaccine is recommended by WHO.**   **TN 1995**
- **Vaccine uses Pitman Moore L503 Strain**
- The **Post exposure** schedule of cell culture vaccines consist of 6 doses on days **0, 3,7,14 and 28** and a booster on day 90   **AI 1998**
- The **Pre exposure** prophylaxis is given on days <u>**0,7 and 28**</u>

Yellow Fever

- Example of **Exotic disease** in India.
- IP=<u>**3-6 days.**</u>
- Caused by **flavi** virus.   **UPSC 1988**
- Transmitted to man by **culicine** mosquito.
- One attack gives **life long immunity.**
- **Absent in India. (VIRUS ABSENT)**   **COMED 2008**

8

— Quarantine is for 6 days. AI 1988

— Vaccination is by: **17 D vaccine.**

— Airports and sea ports are kept free from breeding of insect vectors over **400 meters.**

⊃ Should Remember

* **Yellow fever** is a typical **Haemmoragic fever accompanied by prominent hepatic necrosis.**

* A period of viremia, typically lasting 3 or 4 days, is followed by a period of **"intoxication."** During the latter phase in severe cases, the characteristic jaundice, hemorrhages, black vomit, anuria, and terminal delirium occur, perhaps related in part to extensive hepatic involvement.

* Urban **yellow fever** can be prevented by the control of A. aegypti.

* Immunity By vaccine is provided **within 10 days and lasts for at least 10 years.**

⇨ Dengue Fever

✓ MC **Arboviral** disease. PGI 2011

✓ Both **endemic and epidemic** PGI 2011

✓ It usually sually starts with sudden onset of high fever and the signs and symptoms of dengue fever, which include facial flush, anorexia, headache, nausea, and pains in the muscles and joints. Hepatic tenderness, epigastric or generalized abdominal pain, and sore throat are frequent. The liver is usually palpable, and the spleen is characteristically prominent on radiographs. The temperature continues high for 2 days to a week.

✓ There is no specific treatment. The object of therapy is to maintain hydration, to combat acidosis, and to correct coagulation abnormalities. Salicylates may contribute to bleeding and acidosis and are contraindicated. Paracetamol may be used. Steroids should not **be used. (self limiting)** PGI 2011

⇨ Dengue Hemorrhagic Fever DHF

Features: Fever:

➧ Acute onset

➧ High

➧ Continuous

➧ Lasting 2-7 days

Haemorrhagic manifestations:

Petechiae, purpura,ecchymosis,epistaxis, gum bleeding, haematemesis, melena including positive tourniquet test with > 20 petechaie/2.5 sq cm.

Hepatomegaly

⇨ Polio Virus

▶ Commonest presentation is **sub clinical infection. (Inapparent)**

▶ Abortive or minor illness (4-8%)

▶ Only·<1 % cases are of Paralytic type.

Features are

➥ Assymetric,

➥ Descending,

➥ Flaccid Paralysis without any sensory loss

— <u>Sabin vaccine</u> is **attenuated**, oral vaccine useful in epidemics.

— <u>Salk</u> is a **killed formalized vaccine used** subcutaneously or intramuscularly not useful in epidemics

— **Tonsillectomy and IM injections should be avoided** in polio epidemic because risk of paralytic polio increases. UPSC 01

— **Death** in polio is due to **respiratory paralysis.** AI 92

— **"Vaccine induced polio"** is usually due to <u>Type 3 virus</u>.

— **"Most common** "type of virus in epidemics is <u>Type 1.</u>

— **"Pulse polio"** was introduced in **1995.** MAHE 07

— **Pulse polio is given to children below 5 years.** CUPGEE 1999

— A country is certified for polio eradication if no case of polio has been confirmed for last <u>5 years</u>. MAHE 05

— In acute flaccid paralysis examination for residual palsy should be done after 60 days AI 2010

Day carriers contain = 6 - 8 vials vaccine **and 2 fully frozen ice packs**

Also Remember:

➥ **Vaccine carries** contain 16 - 20 vials vaccine **and 4 fully frozen ice packs**

➥ **Ice packs** - ice packs contain water and **no salt** should be added.

➥ The risk of cold chain failure is greatest at **sub-centre and village level.** For this reason, vaccines are not stored at the sub centre level and must be supplied on the day of use.

Avian Flue Influenza Virus

RECENT TOPIC I have tried to prevent it detailed as we can expect questions in any examination.

➥ <u>H5 N1</u> IS THE "AVIAN FLUE INFLUENZA VIRUS" ALSO CALLED AS "THE BIRD FLU VIRUS."

➥ H5N1 **was** previously believed to cause outbreak in birds only. **(enzootic)**

➥ H5N1 is a **highly pathogenic** virus.

➥ Risk factor is handling of infected **poultry.**

➥ H stands for **Haemaglutinin** and **N** in H5N1 Stands for **Neuraminidase.**

➥ Virus can pass **vertically** from mother to fetus.

8

SPM

Swine Flu

- "Swine flu" also occurred in Mexico in may 2009 with threat of a pandemic spreading as far as New zeland, Australia, Asia, UK, etc.
- Caused by swine influenza virus(SIV)
- SIV usually infects pigs.
- Undercooked pork is a common cause.
- When infection spreads to humans, it is called zoonotic flu.
- Clinical features: chills, fever, sore throat, headache, coughing weakness.
- SIV subtype: H1N1 CAUSED 2009 OUTBREAK.
- This strain has human to human transmission.
- The U.S. Centers for Disease Control and Prevention recommends the use of "Tamiflu" (oseltamivir) or (zanamivir) for the treatment and/or prevention of infection with swine influenza viruses.
- However, the majority of people infected with the virus make a full recovery without requiring antiviral drugs.
- The virus isolates in the 2009 outbreak have been found resistant to amantadine and rimantadine.

- Antigenic shifts are because of genetic reassortments (Major changes)
- Antigenic drifts are because of Point mutations. (Minor changes)
- Pandemics are caused by Influenza type A.
- Epidemics are caused by Type A and Type B.

Influenza

- Influenza viruses are members of the Orthomyxoviridae family.
- Influenza A and B viruses constitute one genus, and influenza C viruses make up the other.
- The designation of influenza viruses as type A, B, or C is based on antigenic characteristics of the nucleoprotein (NP) and matrix (M) protein antigens.
- Influenza A viruses are further subdivided (subtyped) on the basis of the surface hemagglutinin (H) and neuraminidase (N) antigens
- The most extensive and severe outbreaks are caused by influenza A viruses.
- In part, this predominance is a result of the remarkable propensity of the H and N antigens of influenza A virus to undergo periodic antigenic variation.
- Major antigenic variations are referred to as antigenic shifts, which may be associated with pandemics and are restricted to influenza A viruses. Minor variations are called antigenic drifts. These antigenic changes may involve the hemagglutinin alone or both the hemagglutinin and the neuraminidase.
- In human infections, three major antigenic subtypes of hemagglutinins (H1, H2, and H3) and two of neuraminidases (N1 and N2) have been recognized.

➲ Influenza Virus

► Antigenic variation seen as	PGI 2004
► Antigenic drift (minor change) seen. Small mutations in H and N.	MAHE 2007
► Antigenic shift (major change) seen.	

► Influenza has most frequently been described as an illness characterized by the **abrupt onset of systemic symptoms, such as headache, feverishness, chills, myalgia, or malaise, and accompanying respiratory tract signs, particularly cough and sore throat.**

► Respiratory complaints often become more prominent as systemic symptoms subside.

► The most common complication of influenza is pneumonia: "primary" influenza viral pneumonia, secondary bacterial pneumonia, or mixed viral and bacterial pneumonia.

► Secondary bacterial pneumonia follows acute influenza. The most common bacterial pathogens in this setting are Streptococcus pneumoniae, Staphylococcus aureus, and Haemophilus influenzae.

► The most common pneumonic complications during outbreaks of influenza have mixed features of viral and bacterial pneumonia.

➥ Laboratory diagnosis is accomplished during acute **influenza** by **isolation of the virus from throat swabs, nasopharyngeal washes, or sputum.** Virus is usually detected in tissue culture or less commonly is found in the amniotic cavity of chick embryos within 48 to 72 h after inoculation.

➥ **The rapid viral diagnostic tests** detect **viral nucleoprotein or neuraminidase** with high specificity and sensitivities.

➥ Viral nucleic acids have been detected in clinical samples by **reverse transcriptase polymerase chain reaction.**

➥ Serologic methods for diagnosis require comparison of antibody titers in sera obtained during the acute illness with those in sera obtained 10 to 14 days after the onset of illness and are useful primarily in retrospect. **Fourfold or greater titer rises as detected by Haemaglutination inhibition or Complement fixation or significant rises as measured by ELISA are diagnostic of acute infection.**

➥ **Severe leukopenia** has been described in overwhelming viral or bacterial infection, while leukocytosis with more than 15,000 cells/uL raises the suspicion of secondary bacterial infection.

➲ Treatment

In uncomplicated cases of influenza, **symptom-based therapy** with acetaminophen for the relief of headache, myalgia, and fever may be considered, but the use of salicylates should be avoided in children below 18 years of age because of the possible association of salicylates with Reye's syndrome.

Amantadine and Rimantadine for influenza A and the **neuraminidase inhibitors zanamivir and oseltamivir for both influenza A and influenza B.**

Zanamivir, inhaled orally at a dose of 10 mg twice a day for 5 days, or **oseltamivir, ingested orally at a dose of 75 mg twice a day for 5 days,** has reduced the duration of signs and symptoms of influenza by 1 to 1.5 days if treatment is started within 2 days of the onset of illness.

Therapy for primary influenza pneumonia is directed at maintaining oxygenation and is most appropriately undertaken in **an intensive care unit**, with **aggressive respiratory and hemodynamic support as needed**.

Antibacterial drugs should be reserved for the therapy of bacterial complications of acute influenza, such as secondary bacterial pneumonia.

PROPHYLAXIS

The major public health measure for prevention of influenza has been the **use of inactivated influenza vaccines derived from influenza A and B viruses** that circulated during the previous influenza season. Although the **1976 swine influenza vaccine appears to have been associated with an increased frequency of Guillain-Barre syndrome**, influenza vaccines administered since 1976 generally have not been

Vaccines currently available:

- Inactivated whole-virus vaccine
- Subvirion vaccine and
- Purified surface-antigen vaccine

The neuraminidase inhibitors zanamivir and oseltamivir have also been reported to be highly effective in the prophylaxis of influenza A and offer the advantage of efficacy against influenza B as well.

➲ HIV/AIDS

▶ **Subtype A is most prevalent worldwide.**	
▶ **Subtype C is most prevalent in india**	**JK 2011**
▶ Seroconversion takes **4 weeks**	**JIPMER 1993**

▶ Heterosexual mode is the mc mode of transmission of HIV.	**SGPGI 2004**
▶ Male -female transmission>female-male.	**PGI 2000**
▶ **Accidental needle prick for health worker is 1%.**	**PGI 1999**
▶ **RNA-DNA-RNA is the retroviral sequence in host cell.**	**AI 2002**
▶ **p 24 is used for early diagnosis.**	
▶ **p 24 antigen disappears 6-8 weeks after HIV infection.**	**AMU 2005**
▶ **CD 4 cells are attacked. CD4: CD 8 ratio is reversed.**	**AI 2002**
▶ **Macrophages serve as reservoir of infection.**	**AI 2002**
▶ **Window period of AIDS: infection to appearance of antibodies in serum.**	**JIPMER 2004**
▶ **Both ELISA and western blot are negative in window period.**	**NIMHANS 1996**

▶ People living with **HIV/AIDS (PLHA)** in world : 40 million
▶ 3 by 5 target : announced by **WHO** and **UNAIDS** on December 1, 2003
▶ **Interim target** : providing anti retroviral treatment **(ART)** to '3million people living with **HIV/AIDS (PLHA)**', in developing countries (low and middle income), by end of 2005
▶ **Ultimate goal** : universal access to ART to anyone who needs it

Focus Areas: (FIVE PLANS)

- Simplified standard tools to deliver ART
- A new service to ensure effective, reliable supply of medicine and diagnosis
- Dissemination and application of new knowledge and successful strategy
- Urgent, sustained support to countries
- Global leadership backed by strong partnership

⇨ **Role of Laboratories in 3 by 5 Initiatives:**

Peripheral lab	Intermediate lab	Central lab
Rapid HIV test	Peripheral lab tests	Intermediate lab tests
Hb – estimation	Total blood count	CD4 count (FC)
TB microscopy	2nd HIV detection test	EQAS for FC
Pregnancy test	Total lymphocyte counts	Viral load
	CD4 count (NFC)	Clinical chemistry markers
	Liver and renal function tests	Resistance studies
	Opportunistic infections diagnosis	

Hb – hemoglobin
NFC – non flow cytometry
FC flow cytometry

⇨ **WHO Clinical Staging System for HIV Infection in Adults and Adolescents >13 Years**

Clinical Stage I	Clinical Stage II
• Asymptomatic • Persistent generalized lymphadenopathy (PGL) **Performance scale I:** **Asymptomatic, normal activity**	• **Weight loss, <10% Of body weight** • Minor mucocutaneous manifestations **(seborrheic detmatitis, prurigo, fungal nail infections, recurrent oral ulcerations, angular cheilitis)** • **Herpes zoster,** within the last five years • **Recurrent upper** respiratory **tract infections** (i.e. bacterial sinusitis) and/or performance scale 2. Symptomatic, normal activity.

Clinical Stage III

- ✓ Weight loss, **>10% of body weight**
- ✓ Unexplainedchronicdiarrhe>1month   MAHE 2007
- ✓ Unexplained prolonged fever > 1 month
- ✓ Oral candidiasis (thrush)
- ✓ Oral hairy leukoplakia
- ✓ Pulmonary tuberculosis, within the past years.
- ✓ Severe bacterial infections
- ✓ **And/or performance scale 3: bedridden, < 50% of the day during the last month.**

8

SPM

Clinical Stage IV	
— HIV wasting syndrome, as defined by CDC	— Any disseminated endemic mycosis
— Pneumocystic carinii pneumonia	— Candidiasis of the oesophagus, trachea bronchi or lungs
— Toxoplasmosis of the brain	— Atypical mycobacteriosis, disseminated
— Cryptococcosis, extrapulmonary	— Non-typhoid salmonella septicemia
— Cytomegalovirus (CMC) disease of an liver, spleen or lymph nodes	— Extra pulmonary tuberculosis
— Herpes simplex virus (HSV) infection, mucocutaneous >1 month, or visceral any duration	— Lymphoma
	— Kaposi's sarcoma (KS)
— Progressive multi focal leukoence phalopathy (PML)	— HIV encephalopathy, as defined by CDC b and/or performance scale $: bedridden, >50% of the day during the last month.

➠ **HIV wasting syndrome:** Weight loss of >10% of body weight, plus eitherunexplained chronic diarrhea (>1 month), or chronic weakness andunexplained prolonged fever (>1 month).

➠ **HIV encephalopathy:** Clinical findings of disabling cognitive and/or motordysfunction interfering with activities of daily living, progressing over weekto months, in the absence of a concurrent illness or condition other than HIVinfection that could explain the findings.

⇨ **WHO Clinical Staging System for HIV Infection and Related Disease in Children**

Stage 1:
✓ Asymptomatic
✓ Persistent generalized lymphadenopathy

Stage 2:	
✓ Unexplained chronic diarrhea	
✓ Serve persistent or recurrent candidiasis outside the neonatal period	DNB 2007
✓ Weight loss or failure to thrive	
✓ Persistent fever	
✓ Recurrent serve bacterial functions	

Stage 3:
✓ AIDS-defining opportunistic infections
✓ Severe failure to thrive
✓ Progressive encephalopathy
✓ Malignancy
✓ Recurrent septicemia or meningitis

Hepatitis

⇨ **Incubation Period**

▶ Hepatitis A 2- 6 weeks

▶ Hepatitis B 4 - 8 weeks

▶ Hepatitis C 2 - 22 weeks

▶ Hepatitis D 4 - 8 weeks

▶ Hepatitis E 2 - 9 weeks

❑ Hepatitis B is a **DNA virus** ; all others are RNA virus

❑ Spreads by <u>faeco oral</u> route - **hepatitis A and E**

❑ Spreads by <u>percutaneous</u> route - **Hepatitis B,C and D**

❑ Hepatitis B also spread by vertical and sexual route

❑ Oncogenicity present in Hepatitis B especially after neonatal infection.

❑ **Carrier state** present in Hepatitis B only

❑ Hepatitis B virus may present in blood and other body fluids and excretions such as saliva, breast milk, semen, vaginal secretions, urine, bile, etc.

❑ Feces not known to be infectious

❑ HBs Ag is the **first viral marker to appear in blood** after infection; it remains in circulation throughout icteric course of disease. In a typical case it disappear within roughly 2 months but may last for 6 months.

❑ HB C Ag is not demonstrable in circulation but antibody, antiHBe appear in serum a week or two after appearance of HbSAg

❑ So **anti-HbeAg** is the **antibody marker** to be seen in blood.

❑ HBeAg (HB envelop antigen) appears in blood concurrently with HBsAg.

❑ **HbeAg** is an indicator of intrahepatic viral replication and its presence in blood indicates **high infectivity.**

❑ For diagnosis of HBV infection, simultaneous presence of IgM, HBC indicates **recent infection** and presence of **IgG; anti H-Be** indicates **remote** infection.

❑ **Type E hepatitis:** enterically transmitted.

❑ Non A – non B hepatitis caused by Hep. C virus

— **MC cause of chronicity:** hepatitis C

— **MC cause of carriers:** hepatitis B

— **MC cause of cancers:** hepatitis C

— **MC cause of maternal mortality: hepatitis E.**   PGI 1986

8

SPM

⇨ **Risk of Transmission to Doctors**

- Doctors can readily acquire **hepatitis B** virus from patients. The risk of acquiring hepatitis B is significantly higher than the risk for HIV, and somewhat higher than the risk for hepatitis C. Thus, it is essential that health care workers be immunized against the hepatitis B virus. Thimmunization schedule is for administration of the vaccine at 1, 2, and 6 months. It is recommended that postvaccination testing for antibodies be performed to identify an adequate response to the immunization. Individuals who do not demonstrate the formation of antibodies after the immunizations should be tested for hepatitis B surface antigen to ensure that they haven't already been infected. With immunization, the risk of acquiring hepatitis B from a needle stick injury is significantly lessened.

- **HIV** can be transmitted through needle-stick injury. However, the risk of this transmission is less than that of hepatitis B in individuals who have not been immunized.

- **Hepatitis C** appears to be more transmissible through needle-stick injury than HIV, but less transmissible than hepatitis B. However, because there is no immunization for hepatitis C available yet, and because the infection is so widespread in the population, the risk of transmission is of grave concern.

- **Scabies** is a skin parasite that is transmitted through physical contact. Syphilis is a sexually transmitted disease that is most often transmitted through sexual contact. Transmission through needle-stick injury is not a primary route.

⊃ **Cholera**

- John Snow is associated with cholera.
- Called father of public health.
- Acute diahorreal disease caused by vibrio cholera.
- Rice water stools/pea soup diarrhoea.
- Produces enterotoxin acting on c AMP.
- IP= 1-2 days.
- DOC:
  ✓ Doxycycline in adults. **AIPGMEE 2005**
  ✓ Cotrimaxozole in children.
  ✓ Furazolidine in pregnant.
  ✓ Tetracycline for prophylaxis.

⇨ **Remember Classification**

▶ Chikungunya:	alpha virus	PGI 2003
▶ Japanese encephalitis	flavi virus	
▶ West nile Fever	flavi virus	
▶ Yellow fever	flavi virus	
▶ Dengue	flavi virus	PGI 2006
▶ Kyanasaur forest disease	flavi virus	

SPM

▶ Sandfly fever	➡ bunya virus
▶ Rift valley fever	➡ bunya virus
▶ Hanta virus	➡ bunya viridae

⇨ **Gems About Bordetella Pertussis**

▶ Gram negative cocco bacillus	
▶ Capsulated	
▶ Bordet gengou media used	PGI 1994
▶ Causes whooping cough	
▶ Incubation period 1-2 weeks	AIIMS 2005
▶ Thumb printing appearance in culture films.	KAR 1999
▶ Erythromycin prevents spread of disease in children,	

Gems about Brucellosis

➡ Is a zoonosis.	PGI 2002
➡ NO person-person transmission.	AIIMS 2007

⇨ **Causative Organisms**

▶ B. militensis from goat, sheep, cattle (most common) ➡➡➡
▶ B. abortus from cattle➡➡➡
▶ B. suis from hogs➡➡
▶ B. canis from dogs➡➡

➡ Brucella survive in unpasteurized milk for up to 8 weeks.	
➡ Brucella is **transmitted most commonly through un pasteurized milk/milk products, raw meat and bone marrow. ➡**	
➡ It can also be contracted through **inhalation** in farm houses, slaughter houses, labs. Other routes are skin abrasion, inoculation, Conjuctival splashing. ➡➡	
➡ Rose Bengal Card test used.	ROHTAK 1986
➡ Milk Ring test used.	JIPMER 1999
➡ Diagnosis is by culture, Phage typing, DNA Characteristics, Metabolic profiling(BACTEC)	

⇨ **Some Arboviruses known to be Prevalent in India are:**

Group 'A' (Alpha viruses)	Group 'B' : (Flavi viruses)
✳ Sindbis	✳ Dengue
✳ Chikungunya	✳ KFD
	✳ Japanese encephalitis
	✳ West Nile

⊃ Japanese Encephalitis

(JE) is a **mosquito borne encephalitis** caused by **group B arbovirus** and transmitted by <u>Culex</u> mosquito.

- JE is transmitted to man by **bite** of mosquito.
- Man is **a dead end host.**
- Man to man transmission **does not** occur.
- **Pigs** are the **major vertebrate hosts** and **don't** manifest the disease.
- **Culex tritaeniorrhyncus, Culex Vishnuvi, Culex gelidus** are known vectors for JE.
- Incubation period of JE is **5-15** days.
- **Remember Group B flaviviruses** also cause (revise)

  > Dengue
  > JE
  > KFD (Vector: haemaphsalis tick in india)   JK BOPEE 2011
  > West Nile Fever

⇨ Malaria

- MPO for Malaria was launched in April **1977.**
- In this operation, areas are classified according to **API (Annual parasite incidence).**
- **API** is based on active, passive surveillance and cases are confirmed by blood examination.
- **National Malaria Control Programme (NMCP)** was launched in India in April **1953.** It was in operation for 5 years (1953-58).
- **National Malaria Eradication Progamme (NMEP)** launched in **1958.**
- **Roll back malaria programme was launched in 1998.**   JK BOPEE 2012
- New approach to malaria control was approved by WHO in 1978, i.e. Implementation of malaria control in the context of the primary health care strategy.
- **An Enhanced Malaria Control Project** with world bank support launched on 30th September 1997.
- In 1999, the government of India decided to drop the term "National Malaria Eradication Progamme" and renamed it **"National anti-malaria programme"**

Type of Mosquito	Disease
Anopheles	▶ Malaria
	▶ Filaria
Culex	▶ Bancroftarian filariasis
	▶ Japanese encephalitis
	▶ West nile fever
	▶ Viral arthritis

Aedes			
▶ Recurrent day time biters.	▶ Yellow fever		
▶ Stagnant water preferred.	▶ Dengue	AIPGMEE 2009	
	▶ Dengue hemorrhagic fever		
	▶ <u>Chikungunya</u>		
	▶ Chikungunya hemorrhagic fever	MAH 2012	
	▶ Rift valley fever		
Mansonoides	▶ Malarian filariasis		
	▶ Chikungunya <u>fever</u>		

▶ Urban Malaria is caused by **Anopholes Culcifacies**

▶ <u>Type of malaria **not** seen in India is: **ovale**.</u>

However lately only a few cases were reported from Indian states of:

Orissa PGI 2011 Delhi and Gujrat PGI 2011

Remember:

The gems:

✓ Most patients with malaria have recurrent fever and chills (**at 48-hour intervals for P. vivax and P. ovale and at 72-hour intervals for P. malariae**).

✓ **Giemsa stain is preferable to Wright's stain**, especially for persons with P. vivax or P. ovale infection, because the Schüffner's dots characteristic of those infections are often not visible with Wright's stain. Thick smears are more sensitive than thin smears because the red cells have been lysed

✓ Patients with **P. vivax or P. ovale infection should be tested for glucose-6-phosphate dehydrogenase deficiency** before treatment with primaquine, which is used to eradicate persistent hypnozoites in the liver to prevent relapse.

✓ Patients with P. vivax, P. ovale, or P. malariae **infection respond well to chloroquine** and make an uneventful recovery.

▶ **Most sensitive index** of malaria is **Infant parasite rate.**	
▶ Size of RBC is increased in vivax malaria	AI 1996
▶ The infective agent of malaria is **sporozite.**	PGI 1990
▶ **Gametocytes** are seen in PBF of falciparum malaria.	PGI 2005
▶ Shizont is **not seen** in PBF.	PGI 1999

Relapse of malaria is seen in P. ovale and P. malariae

⇨ ## Important Features of P. Falciparum

▶ **Spleenic rupture** is commonest with P. falciparum	AIIMS 1978
▶ **Parasitemia is highest** with P. falciparum	JIPMER 1981
▶ Most virulent form. P.falciparum.	JK 2005
▶ **Exoerythrocytic stage is absent** in P. falciparum	PGI 1996

| ► Multiple infection of RBC,S is seen in P. falciparum | KAR 2005 |
| ► Most Virulent plasmodium species is P. falciparum | AI 1997 |

8

SPM

⊃ Severe Malaria is Indicated by

- ✓ **Coma.** Coma (cerebral malaria) is the most feared complication of P. falciparum infection and has a substantial fatality rate. Although it has been attributed to the blockage of capillaries with parasitized red cells, both hypoglycemia and the effects of cytokines such as TNF-a are important factors. **PGI 2011**
- ✓ **Hypoglycemia**
- ✓ **Renal Failure.** Patients with massive parasitemias may have dark urine from the free hemoglobin produced by hemolysis (blackwater fever) and may later develop renal failure.
- ✓ **Pulmonary Edema.** This complication also occurs in patients with high P. falciparum parasitemias. Hemodynamic measurements indicate that this is a noncardiogenic form of pulmonary edema with normal pulmonary arterial and capillary pressures.
- ✓ **Hypotension /shock** **PGI 2011**
- ✓ **DIC**
- ✓ **Convulsions**

Mosquito control measures may be divided into 3 steps.
- ✳ Anti-larval measures
- ✳ Anti-adult measures
- ✳ Protection against mosquito bites

⊃ Anti-Larval Measures

a. Environmental Control (Source ruction)

- ➡ Source reduction means elimination of the breeding places of mosquitoes. This is the most important step in controlling mosquitoes.
- ➡ Source reduction methods include:
- — Minor engineering methods such as filling, leveling and drainage of breeding places
- — Water management (such as **intermittent irrigation**)
- — Changing the salinity of water (this makes water unsuitable for mosquito breeding)

b. Chemical Control

- ➡ Chemical control methods are:
- i. **Mineral oil—** Oil spreads on water forming a thin film, which cut off the air supply to the mosquito larvae and pupae
- ii. **Paris Green—** It is a stomach poison (that is it must be ingested in order to work). It mainly kills the Anopheles larvae because they are surface feeders. Bottom feeding larvae are also killed when Paris green is applied as a special granular formulation.
- iii. **Synthetic insecticides—** The common synthetic larvicidàs used are: **Abate, Malathion, Fenthion, and Chloropyrifos.** The organochlorine compounds, e.g. DDT, HCII are izot used for larviciding operations because of their long residual effect, water contamination and increased risk of developing resistance in the vector mosquitoes.

c. Biological control- it includes larva eating fishes such as Gamnbusia affinis and Lebister reticulates

Anti-adult measure

a. **Residual sprays**- e.g. DDT, Lindane, Malathion, OMS – 33. DDT is the insecticide of choice.

b. **Space sprays**- Space sprays are those that are sprayed into the atmosphere in the form of a mist or fog to kill mosquitoes. e.g. pyrethrum, Malathion, Fenitrothion

c. **Genetic control**

These include sterile male technique, cytoplasmic incompatibility, chromosomal translocations, sex distortion, and gene replacement. These methods are still in research phase.

Protection against mosquito bites

✓ Mosquito net

✓ Screening- screening of buildings with copper or bronze gauze is costly but excellent method

✓ Repellant

⊃ DDT (Dichlorodiphenyltrichloroethane)

* DDT is an **organochlorine**, highly hydrophobic, nearly insoluble in water but has a good solubility in most organic solvents, fats, and oils.
* Commercial DDT is actually a mixture of several closely related compounds.
* The major component (70-80 %) is a para-para (p, p) isomer.
* This isomer is also present in significant amounts (15%). Dichlorodiphenyldichloroethylene (DDE) and dichlorodiphenyldichloroethane (DDD) make up the balance.
* The term "total DDT" is often used to refer to the sum of all DDT related compounds (p, p-DDT, o, p-DDT, DDE, and DDD) in a sample.
* It is primarily a **contact poison**. It acts on the nervous system of insects and causes paralysis. It dissolves into the waxy covering of the feet and causes paralysis of the feet and wings and finally death. It does not cause immediate death but takes several hours to kill. The **residual action** of DDT may last as long as 18 months depending upon the treated surface. Mud walls however by absorption cause decreased duration of action.
* DDT has no repellant action on insects.
* **Pyrethrum** and DDT have synergistic action; hence most sprays contain a combination of them.

⇨ Kala-azar

KALA-AZAR (Visceral Leishmaniasis; Dumdum Fever)

☐ Kala-azar occurs in **India, China, southern USSR, Africa, the Mediterranean basin**, and several South and Central American countries.

☐ **Leishmania donavani** is the cause of kala azar.

☐ Life cycle involves **sandfly.**

☐ **Amastigote forms** are seen in macrophages, bone marrow, spleen, liver and bone marrow.

☐ Sandfly ingests macrophages containg amastigotes which then form promastigotes.

☐ **Children and young adults** are particularly susceptible.

☐ The protozoa (L. donovani) invade the bloodstream and localize in the **reticuloendothelial system**, causing fever, pronounced **hepatosplenomegaly, emaciation, and pancytopenia.**

☐ The fever is seldom sustained and recurs irregularly.

☐ **Hypergammaglobulinemia** is present.

☐ The parasite may be found in needle biopsy of the liver, spleen, bone marrow, skin lesions, or lymph nodes or in cultures from these tissues or from blood.

☐ **Pentavalent antimony** compounds and **pentamidine** are the drugs of choice.

☐ **Sodium stibogluconate** (sodium antimony gluconate) is given.

⊃ Tuberculosis

⇨ Gems about Mycobacterium Tuberculosis

Mycobacterium Tuberculosis:

▶ Discovered by **Robert Koch.**	TN 2004
▶ **Obligate aerobe**	
▶ **Acid fast**	
▶ Acid fastness is due to **mycolic acid and cell wall.**	AIIMS 1993
▶ **Lung** is the mc organ involved.	
▶ <u>Kochs phenomenon</u> is seen in Tuberculosis.	
▶ TB is the <u>barometer of social welfare in india</u>	
▶ Tuberculin test is assess prevalence of TB in community	AIPGMEE 2004
▶ **Rural and urban population do not differ in TB incidence.**	AI 2010

Primary Oulmonary Tuberculosis

➡ Results from an initial infection with tubercle bacilli.

➡ This form of disease is **often seen in children** and is frequently localized to the **middle and lower lung zones.**

➡ The lesion forming after infection is usually **peripheral** and **accompanied by hilar or paratracheal lymphadenopathy**, which may not be detectable on chest radiography. In the majority of cases, the lesion heals spontaneously and may later be evident as a small calcified nodule **(Ghon lesion).**   **AIIMS 1998**

➡ **Fibrocaseous lesion or phylenticular conjunctivitis can be a part of primary TB.**   **AIIMS 1988**

➡ In children and in persons with impaired immunity, such as those with malnutrition or HIV infection, primary pulmonary **tuberculosis** may progress rapidly to clinical illness.

Category I	▶ New smearpositive ▶ Seriously ill ▶ Extra pulmonary	$2 H_3R_3Z_3E_3/4H_3R_3$	
Category II	▶ Previously treated smear positive (relapse, failure, Default)	$2H_3R_3Z_3E_3S_3/ 1H_3R_3Z_3E_3$ $5H_3R_3E_3$	**AIIMS 2004**
Category III	▶ New smear negative ▶ Extrapulmonary not ▶ seriously ill	$2H_3R_3Z_3/4H_3R_3$	

If the patient	Then Identify him as
Was registered as pulmonary smear Positive, completed treatment and had negative smear results on 2 occasions one of which was at the end of treatment	Cured
Was registered as pulmonary smear Positive, completed treatment and had negative smear at the end of intensive phase but none at end of treatment Or was registered as pulmonary smear negative or extrapulmonary and completed treatment	Treatment completed
Was known to have died from any cause while on treatment	Died
Was Registered as pulmonary smear positive CAT I and smear positive at five months or later Or Was Registered as pulmonary smear positive CAT II and smear positive at five months of treatment. Or Was Registered as pulmonary smear Negative or extra pulmonary on CAT III but was smear positive at any time during treatment	Failure
Has not taken drugs for more than <u>2 months</u> consecutively any time after starting treatment.	Defaulter **JK BOPEE 2011**
Was transferred to another district with transfer form sent and treatment outcome not available	Transferred out

▶ Case finding in RNTCP is based on: <u>sputum microscopy</u>.	**AI 2007**
▶ Standard dose for PPD for Mantoux test is: **5 TU.**	**COMED 2007**
▶ DOTS means: **short term treatment under supervision.**	**KAR 2006**
▶ Alternate day treatment used.	**AIIMS 2001**
▶ Compliance is improved.	
▶ Continuation phase drugs are administered in multi blister pack.	
▶ BCG vaccine: Dannish 1331 strain used.	**KAR 2006**

8

SPM

* Sputum microscopy is the **method of choice** as a case finding tool.

* Sputum culture is the **second most important** case finding tool

* Mass Miniature radiography has been **stopped** as a case finding tool

* Tuberculin Testing has little value but is still used.

➲ Leprosy

⇨ Gems about M. Leprae

▶ **Gram positive**	
▶ Generation time **12 days.**	**MANIPAL 2006**
▶ **Acid fast bacilli.** Less acid fast than M. tuberculosis.	
▶ **Globi and cigar bundle appearance** are a feature.	
▶ Cultivated in <u>Armadillo</u>	
▶ Can be grown in **foot pad of mice.**	**AIIMS 1994**
▶ Spreads by <u>skin -skin contact</u>.	**KERALA 1995**
▶ **Lepra cells are <u>histiocytes</u>**	**DELHI 1993**

— Leprosy is also called as **Hansens Disease.**	
— The sensation to be lost earliest in Leprosy is **Touch.**	
— **Leprosy is a public health problem when prevalence is 1: 10,000.**	**AIPGMEE 2003**
— **Rifampicin** is the drug **most rapidly acting** and **most potent** against Leprosy bacillius.	
— **Dapsone is the "drug of choice". Dose is "1-2mg/kg". Half life is "24 hrs".**	

— Leprosy bacillus is a **gram positive, acid fast bacillus.**	
— **Lepra cells** are also called as **foamy cells** are actually Histiocytes within which globi are found.	
— Generation time of lepra bacillus is **12 days.**	
— Only source of infection is the **patient.**	
— Incubation period of leprosy is **2-5 years.**	
— Most common nerve involved is **ulnar nerve** followed by post. Auricular nerve.	
Schwann cells are involved first of all	
Leprosy is not transmitted vertically.	**AIPGME 2004**
CNS, ovaries, lungs are **"not commonly" involved** in leprosy.	
Lepromin test is important for determining prognosis.	**AIPGME 2003**
TT is the most common type of leprosy in India	
Dharmendra index and Joplings classification deal with leprosy.	**AIPGMEE 2007**

➲ Plague

- Black sickness
- Causative agent: **Yersenia Pestis**   UPSC 1988
- Reservior of infection: Wild Rodents
- Commonest vector: Rat Flea (Xenopsylla cheopsis)
- Waysons staining is done in a case of plague.   AIPGMEE 2006
- Types:
- **Pneumonic plague(MOST CONTAGIOUS)**   TN 2003
- Bubonic plague
- Septicemic plague
- Drug of choice for Treatment: **Streptomycin.**
- Drug of choice for prophylaxis: **Tetracycline**
- Average number of fleas of each species per rodent is <u>specific flea rate</u>.   UPSC 2007
- **Best indicator of potential explosiveness of plague outbreak is <u>total flea index</u>.**   UPSC 2006
- **Isolation is strictly needed.**   AIPGMEE 2008

➲ Rickettsesial Diseases:

Species	Disease	Vector
❐ R. Prowazeki	Epidemic typhus Brill Zinser Disease(delayed manifestation of <u>epidemic</u> typhus) **JK BOPEE 2011**	<u>Louse</u> PGI 1986
❐ R.Typhi	Endemic Typhus	Rat Flea AI 2007
❐ R.Rickettsie	Rocky Mountain Spotted fever	Tick
❐ R.Conori	Indian tick typhus Relapsing fever	Tick Soft tick
❐ R.Akari	Rickettsial pox	Mite
❐ R.Tsutugmashi	Scrub Typhus	Mite AI 2010

Leptospira icterohaemmorhagica	Anaerobic	Weils disease☛☛
Leptospira canicola	Anaerobic	Canicola fever☛☛☛
► Rickettsia prowazeki ► Ricketssia mooseri ► Ricketssia burnetti ► Ehrilichia chafeensis	► Obligate intracellular bacteria	► Epidemic typhus☛☛ ► Endemic typhus☛☛ ► Q fever☛☛☛ ► Ehrilichiosis☛☛

8

SPM

Remember:

▶ Trepenoma pallidium	✓ Anaerobic, spiral, motile	▶ Syphilis
▶ Trepenoma pertenue	✓ Anaerobic	▶ Yaws
▶ Trepenoma carateum	✓ Anaerobic	▶ Pinta

Man -arthopod-man	Malaria
Mammal-arthopod -man	Plague
Man-snail-fish-man	Clonorchis sinesis
Man -snail-crab-man	Paragonimiasis

⇨ **Scrub Typhus**

- The causative agent of scrub typhus is **Rickettsia tsutsugamushi.**
- The **true reservoir** of infection is the trombiculid mite (**Leptotrombidium delinese and L. akamushi**).
- The infection is maintained in nature transovarially from one generation of mite to the next.
- The nymphal and adult stages of the mite are free-living in the soil; they do not feed on vertebrate hosts. It is the larva (chigger) that feed on vertebrate hosts and picks up the rickettsiae.
- The larval stage serves both as a reservoir, through ovarian transmission, and as a vector for infecting humans and rodents.
- **Typical feature is the punched-out ulcer covered with a blackened scab (eschar)** which indicates the location of the mite bite.
- The Weil Felix reaction is strongly positive with the Proteus strain OXK.
- **Treatment:** Tetracycline is the drug of choice   AIPGME 2010

⇨ **Coronary Heart Disease**

Modifiable risk factors:
- ✓ **Cigarrate smoking**
- ✓ ↑bp
- ✓ ↑cholesterol
- ✓ **Diabetes**
- ✓ **Obesity**

Non modifiable risk factors:
- ✓ **Age**
- ✓ **Sex**
- ✓ **Family history**
- ✓ **Genetic factors**
- ✓ **Type A Personality**

- ▶ Avoid alcohol
- ▶ ↓fat intake
- ▶ ↑complex carbohydrate intake
- ▶ ↓salt intake
- ▶ Smoking cessation.   AIPGMEE 2005

⇨ **Hypertension**

- ▶ Is an ice berg disease.
- ▶ Mc cardiovascular disease.
- ▶ Single most test useful to identify coronary disease is Hypertension.
- ▶ Systolic BP is a better indicator than diastolic bp.

⇨ **Obesity**

Remember:

- ❑ Obesity is BMI>30 in males.☞☞
- ❑ Obesity is BMI>28.6 in females.☞
- ❑ **Hyperplastic obesity** is ↑ size of fat cells.✳
- ❑ **Hypertrophic obesity** is ↑ number of fat cells.✳
- ❑ **Brocas index, Ponderal index, Lorentz Formula, Fat fold Thickness** assesses obesity✳
- ❑ **Gyanoid obesity** is deposition of fat predominantly in <u>gluteal/femoral</u> regions☞☞
- ❑ **Android obesity** is deposition of fat predominantly in <u>trunk/ abdomen</u> regions.☞☞☞

➲ **Obesity is Often Expressed in Terms of Body Mass Index (BMI)**

High Yield for 2011-2012

✳ BMI < 16.00	✳ Indicates grade 3 thinness
✳ BMI 16.0 - 16.99	✳ Indicates grade 2 thinness
✳ BMI 17.0 - 18.49	✳ Indicates grade 1 thinness
✳ **BMI 18.5 - 24.99**	✳ **Is the normal range for an individual**
✳ BMI 25.0 - 29.99	✳ Indicates grade 1 overweight
✳ BMI 30.0 - 39.99	✳ Indicates grade 2 overweight
✳ BMI >/ = 40.00	✳ Indicates grade 3 overweight

⇨ **Various other Indicators used are**

- ✓ Body mass index (Quetelet's index)
- ✓ Ponderal index
- ✓ Broca index
- ✓ Lorentz's formula
- ✓ Corpulence index

✳ Body mass index is weight (kg)/height ^{2} (metres)   MH 2005

✳ Abdominal fat accumulation is assessed by waist to hip ratio.   MP 2005

✳ Body mass index is Quetlets index.   UP 2007

✳ Corpulence index measures obesity.   DNB 2008

➲ "STEP"

— "STEP is a **sequential process of gathering comparable and sustainable NCD (non-communicable disease) risk factor information at the country level.**

— By using the same standardized questions and protocols, all countries can develop surveillance systems containing quality information about NCD risk factors in their unique settings.

— This information can, in turn, be used to plan for and implement currently available interventions to address the disease patterns caused by these risks factors."-   AIIMS 2008

STEP wise approach to surveillance (STEPS)

➥ The WHO STEP wise approach to Surveillance (STEPS) is a **simple, standardized method for collecting, analyzing and disseminating data in WHO member countries.**

➥ By using the same standardized questions and protocols, all countries can use STEPS information not only for monitoring within-country trends, but also for making comparisons across countries. The approach encourages the collection of small amounts of useful information on a regular and continuing basis.

➥ Quality health information is essential for planning and implementing health policy in all countries. Risk factor data are especially important as predictors of future disease or injury.

➥ Country level data is sparse for many of these major non-communicable diseases (NCD) risk factor data is needed to promote the usefulness of this data both for country health policy development and also for comparison across countries and regions. WHO is promoting the use of the STEP wise approach to enable countries to set up surveillance system for NCD risk factors?

➥ There are **currently two primary STEPS surveillance systems**, the Step wise approach to chronic disease risk factor surveillance and the STEP wise approach to stroke surveillance.

STEP wise approach to chronic disease risk factor surveillance (STEPS)

✳ The STEPS approach focuses on obtaining core data on the established risk factors that determine the major disease burden.

✳ The STEPS instrument covers three different levels of "steps" of risk factor assessment. These steps are:-

✳ Questionnaire

✳ Physical measurements

✳ Biochemical measurements

STEP wise approach to stroke (cerebrovascular disease) surveillance

— In response to the need for improvements in stroke data collection, prevention and treatment, WHO has developed an international stroke surveillance system: the STEP wise approach to stoke surveillance (STEPS-stoke) which forms a framework for surveillance and data collection and aims to provide data for all WHO Member States.

➲ Intrauterine Contraceptive Device (IUCD)

Act by ovulation inhibition, causing aseptic endometritis	JIPMER, AIIMS
Act by prevention of fertilization	AI 2006
Act by interfering with implantation	AI 2006
Contraindications:	

- ✓ PID
- ✓ Diabetes mellitus
- ✓ Congenital uterine anomalies
- ✓ Heart disease
- ✓ Pelvic TB
- ✓ HIV Positive
- ✓ Suspected pregnancy
- ✓ Previous ectopic
- ✓ menorrhagia

Commonest side effect is bleeding.

Nova T has a silver core but contains both copper and silver	PGI 2005

- ► In CuT_{200}, 200 means 200 mm^2 of copper.
- ► CuT_{200} is inserted postnatally after 8 weeks — **Kar 2005**
- ► If CuT_{200} is implanted in Myometrium treatment is hysteroscopic removal — **CUPGEE 2K**
- ► CuT_{200} should be replaced after every 10 years. — **COMED 2008**

Contraceptive TODAY	APPG 2006

- ► Contains 9 NON OXYNOL
- ► Is a barrier contraceptive
- ► Effective for 24 hours after insertion
- ► Spermicidal in nature.

- ► NORPLANT contains levonorgesterol.
- ► **Centrochroman** is anti estrogenic, anti progestogenic non teratogenic, long acting pill.
- ► **Mifeprestone** is an anti progestogen.
- ► **MINERA** is progesterone IUCD. — **AIIMS 2007**

➲ Uses of OCP

- ► **Contraception, emergency postcoital (prophylaxis)** A combination of levonorgestrel 50 or norgestrel with ethinyl estradiol is used as emergency contraception (also called intraception, morning-after treatment, or postcoital contraception) for postcoital birth control, after pregnancy has been ruled out. The dosing method using high doses of estrogen-progestin hormones is commonly called the **Yuzpe method.**

- Acne vulgaris
- Amenorrhea
- Dysfunctional uterine bleeding (DUB)
- Dysmenorrhea
- Hypermenorrhea
- Endometriosis (prophylaxis and treatment)
- Hirsutism, female
- Hyperandrogenism, ovarian
- Polycystic ovary syndrome

- ▶ OCPS protect against **endometrial cancer; Ovarian cancer.**
- ▶ OCP of choice in Lactating females is Mini Pill.   **COMED 2008**
- ▶ Fertility returns 6 months after OCP use.   **UPSC 2007**

⇨ **Drugs Decreasing Effectiveness of OCP**

Barbiturates
Carbamezapine
Phenytoin
Rifampicin

⇨ **Levonorgestrel**

- Levonorgestrel is a **synthetic progestogen** used as an active ingredient in hormonal contraception.
- **Makes endometrium unreceptive.**   **UPSC 2007**
- **Makes cervical mucus thick.**
- It is used effectively in emergency contraception both **in combined form with estrogens as well as levonorgestrel only method.**
- Levonorgestrel only method uses **"1500µgm single dose"** or **"750µ gm"** doses **twelve hours** apart within 3 days of unprotected sexual activity.

⇨ **Progastasert:**

- ✓ Third generation IUCD containing progestrone.
- ✓ Decreases blood loss.
- ✓ Decreases dysmenorrhea.
- ✓ BUT ↑ risk of ectopics

⇨ **Choices of Contraception**

➤ Newly married	Pill
➤ Post abortal	Pill
➤ Post partum Non lactating	Pill
➤ Diabetic	IUCD
➤ Pulm. TB	Barrier
➤ Emergency	LNG

SPM

⇨ **Lifespan**

- Nova T: 5 YEARS
- Cu T 380A: **10 YEARS**
- Progastasert: 1 YEAR
- Cu T 200B: 4 YEARS
- LNG IUCD: 5 YEARS

⇨ **Third Generation OCP**

Contain 3rd generation progesterone

✓ Desogestrel

✓ Norgestimate

✓ Gestodene

Lower risk of arterial thrombosis

Higher risk of venous thrombosis

Lipid friendly   UPSC 2002

⊃ **OCP**

Helps in protection against:

→ Uterine ca   AIIMS 2002
→ Ovarian ca   AIIMS 2002
→ Ovarian cysts
→ Endomteriosis
→ PID
→ Ectopics (Indirectly)
→ Menorrhagia
→ Polymenorrhea
→ Rheumatoid arthritis   AI 2007
→ Endometriosis   AI 2007

⇨ **Natural Family Planning Methods**

- Basal body temperature method
- Cervical mucus method/ Billing method   AIPGME 1994
- Symptothermic method. (Most effective).   MH 2008

⇨ **Barrier Methods**

- Diaphragm
- Foam tablets
- Vaginal sponge.   UP 2006

- ▶ NORPLANT contains levonorgesterol.

- ▶ Centrochroman is anti estrogenic, anti progestogenic non teratogenic, long acting pill.

- ▶ Mifeprestone is an anti progestogen.

- ▶ MINERA is Progesterone IUCD. **AIIMS 2007**

⇨ **Criterion for Sterilization** **UPSC 2006**

Age of female >22 years
Age of male<60 years.
Couple should have at least 2 children.

⊃ **Minilap Methods**

Pomeroys method
Madlener method
Fimbriectomy

⇨ **Laproscopic Sterilization**

- ▶ Here fallopian tube is identified and clipped by Fallope ring, Hulka clip, Filsche clip.

- ▶ Most common site for female sterilization is Isthmus. **AIIMS 2007, AI 2007**

- ▶ In Pomeroys method of female sterilization, isthimo ampullary porition is ligated. **UPSC 2007**

⇨ **Emergency Contraception is by** **UPSC 2006**

✓ OCP
✓ CuT
✓ Levonorgestel

⊃ **Indications for Emergency Contraception**

➡ In protected sex
➡ Condom rupture
➡ Missed pill
➡ Sexual assault
➡ Rape

⇨ **Life-Table Analysis for Contraception**

- ➡ Life-table analysis calculates a failure rate for each month of use. A cumulative failure rate can then compare methods for any specific length of exposure.

- ➡ Use of life table methods eliminates time-related biases (i.e. the most fertile couples getting pregnant and dropping out of the study early, and couples becoming more skilled at using the method as time goes on), and in this way is superior to the Pearl Index. This method using decrement tables calculates the probability of pregnancy in successive months, which are then added over a given interval.

⇨ **Pearl Index**

$\underline{\text{Total accidental pregnancies}} \times 1200$
Total months of exposure.

- Pearl index is called so as it was developed by **Raymond Pearl.**
- It is used for studing the **effectiveness of a contraceptive**   MP 2005
- The number of pregnancies includes all pregnancies whether this has terminated as live births, still births or absotions or has not yet terminated.

⊃ WATER

⇨ **Chlorination**

- ❑ Normal chlorination **does not affect polio virus.**
- ❑ Action of chlorine to kill the germs at maximum at - **pH 7.**
- ❑ **Break point chlorination** -point at which residual cl appears in the water
- ❑ **Cheapest and effective** method of disinfection water sources - **bleaching powder.**
- ❑ The 60 minutes period kept after bleaching - **contact period.**
- ❑ **WHO standards of drinking water** - less than **10 coliform bact per 100 ml.**
- ❑ When **Nitrites** are present in water - **recent** contamination
- ❑ **Nitrates** in water indicate **old** contamination.
- ❑ **Temporary hardness** is due to - **Ca, Mg, Bicarbonate.**
- ❑ **Hypochlorus acid is the most effective form of chlorine for water disinfection.**   JK BOPEE 2012
- — **Permanent hardness** is due to -**Chlorides. Nitrates. Sulphates**
- — **Flourine concentration recommended is: 1.5 ppm.**   PGMCET 2007
- — **Hardness level of soft water is: 50.**   PGMCET 2007
- — **Tube well water does not require disinfection.**   COMED 2005

Temporary hardness is removed by:
- Boiling
- Addition of lime
- Addition of sodium carbonate
- Permutit process

Permanent hardness is removed by:
- Addition of sodium carbonate
- Base exchange process

- Minimum recommended concentration of free chlorine is 0.5 mg/litre.
- Pt at which chlorine demand of water is met: **Break point**
- Chlorine added beyond break point: **free chlorine**
- Least amount of time for which free chlorine should be present: **one hour**
- Orthotoluidine test determines both free and combined chlorine.   COMED 2007
- Horrocks apparatus measures Chlorine demand of WATER.   AIIMS 2007

8

SPM

Who Recommendations for Drinking Water Quality

- Color <15 true color units (**TCU**)
- TURBIDITY <5 nephlometric units (**NTU**)
- Hardness < **100-300** mg/liter
- pH : 6.5-8.5
- Total dissolved solids (**TDS**) <600 mg/liter
- Zero pathogenic microorganisms
- Zero infectious viruses
- Absence of pathogenic protozoa and infective stages of helminthes
- Fluorine < 1.5 ppm (0.5-0.8 ppm: optimum level)
- Nitrates <50 mg/liter
- Nitrites <3 mg/liter
- Gross alpha radiological activity < 0.1 Bq/liter
- Gross beta radiological activity < 1.0 Bq/liter

Remember: in pure water **coliforms should not be detected** in 100 ml sample.   **AIPGMEE 2009**
Not more than 5% samples should have coliforms.

Classification of Hardness in Water

Classification	Level of hardness (mEq/litre)
(a) Soft water	Less than 1 (< 50 mg/L)
(b) Moderately hard	1-3 (50-150 mg/L)
(c) Hard water	3-6 (150-300 mg/L)
(d) Very hard water	over 6 (> 300 mg/L)

SOFTENING IS RECOMMENDED AT HARDNESS LEVEL EXCEEDING 3mEq/L   **JK BOPEE 2012**

Purification of Water is done by:

- Bleaching powder
- Chlorine solution
- Iodine
- Potassium permanganate
- Sand filter
- Ozonation
- UV Radiation

Endemic Flourosis

- Endemic Flourosis is prevalent in Punjab, Haryana, Karnatka, Tamil Nadu.
- Flourine follows <u>double edged sword pattern</u>.   **PGI 1989**
- Fluoride levels are>3 mg/dl in drinking water
- Mottling of dental enamel with chalky white appearance is a feature(Caries)   **AIIMS 2008**

- Permanent teeth are almost always involved.
- Genu valgum is a feature
- "Osteoporosis in lower limbs" is a feature.
- Skeletal flourosis occurs after chronic ingestion
- Crippling flourosis occurs at10mg/l or greater levels.

Interventions:

- Change of water source
- Nalgonda technique developed by National Environmental Engineering Institute Nagpur   PGI 1985

⊃ Important Diseases:

Panicum miliare is contaminated with seeds of Crotalaria which contain **Pyrazzolidine alkaloids** which are hepatotoxins causing **Endemic ascites**.

Lathyrism is spastic paralysis of lower limbs due to toxin present in lathirus sativa called **BOAA** (Beta oxalyl amino alanine).

Epidemic Dropsy is contamination of mustard oil with argemone oil containing sanguirine which interferes with oxidation of pyruvic acid and causes swelling of legs, diarrhea, cardiac failure and convulsions.

KCET 2012, AIIMS 2007

Mexican Prickly poppy is the common name of the plant.

Sanguirine causes inhibition of Na+ K+ ATPase activity in heart.

ASSOCIATED WITH:

Erythematous mottling	PGI 2011
Raised hemangiomas	PGI 2011
Glaucoma	

It is tested by

- Nitric acid test and
- Paper chromatography.

⇨ Essential Fatty Acids are:

— Linoleic acid	JK 2001
— Linolenic acid	PGI 1986, AIIMS 1986
— Ecosopantanoic acid	
— Docosa Hexanoic acid	
— Arachidonic acid.	PGI 1986

- Most essential is linoleic acid.
- Safflower oil, Sunflower oil is a rich source of linoleic acid.   AI 1993
- Breast milk is a rich source of Docosa Hexanoic acid
- Vegetable oils have high concentration of unsaturated fatty acids.   AI 1989
- Mustard oil, ground nut oil, fish oil are sources of omega 3 PUFA acids.   AIIMS 2007
- Soya bean has high concentration of PUFA.   AI 2007

⊃ PUFA Contents of different Fats (% out of Total Fat Content)

1. Safflower oil-75%
2. Sunflower oil-65%
3. Corn oil-65%
4. Soyabean oil-62%
5. Cotton seed oil-50%
6. Margarine-50%
7. Ground nut-31%
8. Palm oil-10%
9. Cocconut oil-2%

⇨ Indicators for Epidemilological Assessment of Iodine Deficency

- Prevalence of goiter
- Prevalence of cretinism
- Urinary iodine excretion
- Measurement of thyroid function (T4,TSH)
- Prevalence of neonatal hypothyroidism
- Most sensitive indicator for monitoring iodine deficiency disorders in control programmes is neonatal hypothyroidism

                                                                                              AIPGMEE 2007

The spectrum of **"Iodine – deficiency disorders"** in approximate order of increasing severity are:

- ✓ Goitre
- ✓ Hypothyroidism
- ✓ Subnormal intelligence
- ✓ Delayed motor milestones
- ✓ Mental deficiency
- ✓ Hearing defects
- ✓ Speech defects
- ✓ Squint
- ✓ Nystagmus
- ✓ Spasticity
- ✓ Neuromuscular weakness
- ✓ Endemic cretinism
- ✓ Intra uterine death (abortion, miscarriage)

Essential trace elements are

- Iodine
- Zinc
- Selenium
- Copper
- Molybdenum
- Chromium

Indian Reference Male

Weight	60kg	AIPGMEE 2009
Age	20-39 years	AIIMS 2008
Occupation	moderate	
Working hours	8	AIIMS 2008
BMR	35.5	
Surface area	1.62	
Energy needed	1380	MAH 2012
Protein requirement	1 gm/kg/day	

➲ "Dietary Goals" Recommended by WHO are

* Reduction of fat intake to **20 - 30% of total energy intake**
* Consumption of Satuarted fats must be limited to less than 10%
* Reduction of dietary cholesterol to below 100mg per 1000Kcal per day
* Increase in complex carbohydrate consumption
* Protein should account for approximately 15-20% of the daily intake
* Avoidance of alcohol consumption, **reduction** of **salt intake to 5g daily or less.**
* Junk foods such as colas that supply empty calories should be reduced.

➲ Some Note worthy Daily Requirements

Nutrient	Recommended daily requirement
Calcium	400-500 mg
Iron	28 mg (males) :30 mg (female)
Iodine	150 mg
Fluorine	0.5-0.8 mg/liter

Vitamin A (acts as hormone)	▶ Deficency: ▶ Conjuctival xerosis. (Earliest sign) — COMED 2008 ▶ Night blindness — AIIMS 1997 ▶ Xeropthalmia ▶ Follicular Hyperkeratosis ▶ Daily requirement in children is 1500 UNITS. — SGPGI 2005 ▶ FAT enhances absorption of Vitamin A. — UPSC 2007 ▶ Child health problem if prevalence of night blindness in children aged 6m- 6 years is 1% — AIIMS 2006
Vitamin D	▶ Rickets ▶ Osteomalacia
Vitamin E **Prevents lipid peroxidation.** (ORISSA 2005)	▶ Hemolysis ▶ Retinitis pigmentosa ▶ Neurological problems

VitaminK	▶ Bleeding tendency with ↑PT normal BT
▶ (Gamma carboxylation) AIIMS 2008, AIIMS 2007	

During pregnancy, iron and folic acid tablets (IFA) containing 100 mg of elemental iron and 500 microgram of folic acid are given daily.	AIPGMEE 2003
Paediatric tablets given under RCH contain iron and folic acid 20 mg of elemental iron and 100 microgram of folic acid are given daily.	AIPGMEE 2003
Iron and folic acid supplementation is specific protection.	AIPGMEE 2002

Haemoglobin	Total IFA Tablets taken
Greater than 11 gms/dl	100
≤ 11gms/dl	200

➲ Food Items as Poor Sources of Nutrients

⇨ Egg

* Egg is poor in carbohydrates and vitamin C.	AIIMS 1998
* NPU of egg is 96.	
* Egg yields 70 k Cal	RJ 2004
* Egg white contributes 58% of egg.	RJ 2003

⇨ Milk and other Products

▶ Milk is poor source of vitamin C and iron.	KERALA 1994
▶ Meat is poor source of calcium	
▶ Fish is poor source of iron and carbohydrates	AIIMS 2008
▶ Egg is poor source of vitamin C and carbohydrates	
▶ Mothers milk has more lactose.	AI 2007
Pausterization is precurrent disinfection.	ORISSA 2005
Pausterization of milk kills:	TN 1990
— Brucella	
— Streptococcus	
➡ TESTS FOR Pausterized milk:	UPSC 2007
▶ Phosphatase test	
▶ coliform test	
▶ Standard plate count.	
➡ Methylenes blue test in milk is done to detect: activity of milk.	UPSC 1988

⇨ Milk Borne Diseases are

✓ Tuberculosis	
✓ Salmonellosis	PGI 2011

✓	Q fever	
✓	Streptococcal infections	PGI 2011
✓	Brucellosis	
✓	Enteropathogenic e.coli	PGI 2011
✓	Cholera	
✓	Cow pox	
✓	Anthrax	
✓	Foot and mouth disease	
✓	Leptosporiosis	

⊃ Human Milk has:

✓	Less fat than cows milk	
✓	Less calcium than cows milk	PGI 2011
✓	Less sodium than cows milk	
✓	More protein than cows milk	
✓	More carbohydrate than cows milk	PGI 2011

⇨ Baby Friendly Hospital Initiative

▶	Guidelines:	AIPGMEE 2009
▶	Mother and infant to be kept together for 24 hours a day	
▶	Initiate breast feeding immediately after delivery	
▶	Give new borne infants nothing except breast milk	
▶	Encourage breast feeding on demand	

⇨ Egg

Eggs lack carbohydrate.	APPGEE 2005
Eggs lack vitamin C.	PGI 1983
Energy value of egg: 70 K cal	

Food Items as Rich Sources of Nutrients	
➡ Halibut liver oil is richest source of vitamin A and Vitamin D	
➡ Indian gooseberry (amla) is richest source of vitamin C	
➡ Jaggery has high concentration of iron	PGI 1986
➡ Gingelly seeds are richest source of vitamin B1 (Thiamine)	
➡ Sheep liver is richest source of vitamin B2 (riboflavin)	
➡ Ragi, Dates (millet) is rich source of calcium	APPGE 2004
➡ Pistachio is the richest source of iron	

8

SPM

— Pulses are deficient in <u>methionine.</u>	SGPGI 2005, KCET 2012
— Cereals are deficient in **lysine.**	SGPGI 2005
— Wheat is deficient in **threonine**	
— Maize is deficient in **tryptophan/lysine**	SGPGI 2005
➡ Eggs have the highest biological value.	TN 1990

⇨ **Soyabean**

— **is richest among pulses**
— It contains **43.2% proteins,**20% fats and 4% minerals
— Proteins of Soya bean are of high nutritive value
— Soya bean is also relatively richer in Lysine, calcium, iron and vitamin B as compared to other pulses.
JK 2001
— Limiting amino acid in Soya bean is **methionine.**   ALLHPH 2001
— NPU of Soya bean is **55.**

⊃ **Energy Yeild of Macro Nutrients (Proximate Principles)**

NUTRIENT	ENERGY YEILD
Carbohydrates	✓ 4 Kcal per gram
Proteins	✓ 4 Kcal per gram
Fats	✓ 9 Kcal per gram

⊃ **Net Protein Utilization (NPU)**

➡ NPU is a **method of assessing protein quality.**   AIIMS 2009
➡ It is the ratio of amino acid converted to proteins to the ratio of amino acids supplied.
➡ Experimentally, this value can be determined by determining dietary protein intake and then measuring nitrogen excretion.
➡ As a value. NPU can range from **1 to 0,** with a **value of 1 indicating 100% utilization of dietary nitrogen as protein and a value of 0 an indication that none of the nitrogen supplied was converted to protein.**
➡ Certain foodstuffs, such as eggs or milk, rate as 1 on an NPU chart.
➡ The NPU gives a more complete expression of protein quality than the amino acid score.
➡ The protein requirement varies with the NPU of dietary protein. If NPU is high, the protein requirement is low and vice versa.

⊃ **Amino Acid Score**

➡ Other method of assessing protein quality is amino acid score.
➡ Amino acid score is a measure of the concentration of each essential amino acid in the test protein expressed as a percentage of that amino acid in the reference protein (usually egg protein)

⊃ Protein Digestibility Corrected Amino Acid Score (PDCAAS)

- ⇒ Protein Digestibility Corrected Amino Acid Score is a method of evaluating the protein quality based on the amino acid requirements of humans.
- ⇒ It has been **adopted by FAO/WHO** as the **preferred method** for the measurement of the protein quality in human nutrition.
- ⇒ The method is **based on comparison of the concentration of the first limiting essential amino acid** in the test protein with the concentration of that amino acid in a reference (scoring) pattern.
- ⇒ This scoring pattern is derived from the essential amino acid requirements of the **preschool-age child.**
- ⇒ The chemical score obtained in this way is corrected for true fecal digestibility of the test protein.
- ⇒ A PDCAAS value of **1 is the highest,** and 0 the lowest as the table demonstrates the ratings of common foods

- ✳ Egg white   1.0
- ✳ Casein   1.0
- ✳ Milk   1.0

- ⇒ The Protein Digestibility Corrected Amino Acid Score (PDCAAS) is **superior** to other methods for evaluating the protein quality of food proteins for humans because it measures the quality of a protein based on the amino acid requirements of a 2- to 5-year old child (the most demanding age group), adjusted for digestibility.
- ⇒ PDCAAS is based on a food protein's amino acid content, its true digestibility, and its ability to supply indispensable amino acids in amounts adequate to meet the amino acid requirements of a 2- to 5-year old child, the age group used as the standard.

⊃ Protein Content of Some Foods

Food item	Protein content (gm % per 100 gms)
Soya bean	43
Pulses	22.25
Fish	21
Meat	20
Egg (hen)	13
Wheat	12
Rice	7
Milk (Cow)	3

▶ Richest source of vitamin A:	⇒ fish liver oil
▶ Richest source of vitamin D:	⇒ cod liver oil
▶ Richest source of vitamin K:	⇒ cows milk
▶ Richest source of vitamin B_{12}:	⇒ liver
▶ Richest source of folic acid:	⇒ green leafy vegetables
▶ Richest source of iron:	⇒ jaggery
▶ Richest source of iodine:	⇒ sea food

▶ Recommended daily allowance RDA is used to assess nutritional status on basis of adequate intake.

AIPGME 2009

▶ RDA caters to dietary requirements of all people.

AIPGME 2008

	Energy (Cal)	Protein	Calcium	Iron	Folic acid
▶ Adult female	2225	50	400	30	100
▶ Pregnant	+300	+15	1000	40	400
▶ Lactating					
▶ 0-6 months	+550	+25	1000	50	150
▶ 6-12 months	+400	+18			

➲ Protein Content of Some Foods

Food item	Protein content (gm % per 100 gms)
✱ Soya bean	✓ 43
✱ Pulses	✓ 22.25
✱ Fish	✓ 21
✱ Meat	✓ 20
✱ Egg (hen)	✓ 13
✱ Wheat	✓ 12
✱ Rice	✓ 7
✱ Milk (Cow)	✓ 3

➲ Recommended Daily Requirements

Vitamin	Recommended daily requirement
✱ Vitamin A	600 mcg retinol
✱ Vitamin B1 (Thiamine)	0.5 mg per 1000 Kcal of energy intake
✱ Vitamin B2 (Riboflavin)	0.5 mg per 1000 Kcal of energy intake
✱ Vitamin B3 (Niacin)	6.6 mg per 1000 Kcal of energy intake
✱ Vitamin B5 (Pantothenic acid)	10 mg
✱ Vitamin B6 (Pyridoxine)	2 mg
✱ Vitamin B9 (Folic acid)	100 mcg
✱ Vitamin B12 (Cobalamin)	1 mcg
✱ Vitamin D	100 IU (2.5 mcg calciferol)
✱ Vitamin E (Tocopherol)	0.8 mg per gm of essential fatty acids
✱ Vitamin K	0.03 mg per kg

⤳ Screening Tests

Screening test(s)	Disease screened
▶ Papanicolaou (pap) smear test	✓ Cervical cancer
▶ Breast self examination test (BSE)	✓ Breast cancer
▶ Mammography	✓ Breast cancer
▶ Bimanual oral examination	✓ Oral cancer
▶ ELISA, RAPID, SIMPLE	✓ HIV (National AIDS Control Program)
▶ Urine for sugar, random blood sugar	✓ Diabetes mellitus
▶ Alpha feto protein	✓ Development anomalies in fetus
▶ Digital rectal examination (DRE)	✓ Prostrate cancer
▶ Prostrate specific antigen (PSA)	✓ Prostrate cancer
▶ Fecal occult blood test	✓ Colorectal cancer

STEPS is a WHO recommended tool for surveillance of non communicable diseases and their risk factors:

AIPGMEE 2009

⤳ Blindness

- ➡ **Legal blindness:** visual acuity <6/60 (<20/200) or visual field <20 degree in better eye with best possible correction
- ➡ **Work vision:** <6/60 (economic blindness)
- ➡ **Walk vision:** <3/60 (social blindness)
- ➡ Under NPCB, school teachers are supposed to conduct vision screening for children.   AIPGMEE 2006

Blindness (WHO)	<3/60 in BEBPC
Blindness (NPBC, India)	<6/60 in BEBPC
Low vision (NPCB, India)	<6/18 -6/60 in BEBPC
Economic blindness (NPCB, India)	<6/60-3/60 in BEBPC
Social blindness (NPCB, India)	<3/60-1/60 in BEBPC
Manifest blindness (NPCB, India)	<1/60 -PL+ in BEBPC
Absolute blindness (NPCB, India)	<PL- in BEBPC
Legal blindness (NPCB, India)	<6/60 (<20/200) or vf <20degree in BEBPC
Work vision	<6/60 in BEBPC (economic blindness)
Walk vision	<3/60 in BEBPC (social blindness)
Referral in school eye screening	<6/9 in either eye

8

SPM

⇨ **National Program for Control of Blindness (NPCB, India) Defined**

- **WHO** defined blindness: 'visual acuity of <3/60 in **better eye with best possible correction'** (BEBPC) blindness: AIPGMEE 2006

- **Blindness in India :** 'visual acuity of less 6/60 in better eye with best possible correction'

- **Blindness in India :**

  ▶ India is single largest contributor to global blind pool
  ▶ **Catract is the mc cause in India**   JK BOPEE 2012
  ▶ Measured according to : NPCB criterion (<6/60 in BEBPC)
  ▶ Total estimated number of blind person : 15 million
  ▶ State with highest prevalence of blindness : Jammu and Kashmir
  ▶ Sate with lowest prevalence of blindness : Meghalaya
  ▶ Prevalence after correction : 0.56%(2001-02)
  ▶ Prevalence of blindness in age :> 50 years : 8.5 %
  ▶ Prevalence of one eyed blindness: 0.8% (MCC: cataract-73%)
  ▶ India is overestimating the number of blinds as per WHO definition if WHO cut off (<3/60 in BEBPC) is employed in India , estimated prevalence of blindness would be : 0.7%
  ▶ Blindness in India includes : economic blindness, social blindness, manifest blindness and absolute blindness(**WHO** blindness includes: social, manifest and absolute blindness)
  ▶ MCC of blindness in (India): cataract (63%)   AIPGMEE 2006
  ▶ **Remember Diseases in global vision 2020**   AIIMS 2007
  ▶ **WHO, Orbis International and International Agency for Prevention of Blindness are involved in Vision 2020**   AIIMS 2011
  ▶ Given below:

Global Vision 2020	Indian Vision 2020
— Cataract	— Cataract
— Refractive errors	— Refractive errors
— Childhood blindness	— Childhood blindness
— Trachoma	— Glaucoma
— Onchocerciasis	— Diabetic retinopathy
	— Color blindness

⇨ **Occupational Exposures and Cancers**

AGENT	CANCER(s) CAUSED
Asbestos	Mesothelioma
Arsenic	Skin. lung, liver
Benzene	Leukemia
Benzidine	Urinary bladder
Beryllium	Lung
Cadmium	Lung

Chromium	Nasal sinus, lung
Ethylene oxide	Leukemia
Ionizing radiation	Skin, thyroid, lung
Nickel	Nasal sinus, lung
Polycyclic aromatic hydrocarbons	Skin, scrotum, lung
Radon	Lung
Silica	Lung
Vinyl chloride	Liver
Wood dust	Nasal sinus

✓ **Oropharyngeal cancer** is the mc cancer in adult males in India. AIPGMEE 2004
✓ **Cervical cancer** is the mc cancer among females in India.
✓ **Breast cancer** is the mc cancer in urban Indian females. AIPGMEE 2005
✓ **Lung cancer** is the mc cancer in males/females in world. AIIMS 2005

➲ Diseases Due to Physical Agents

► Heat Heat hyperpyrexia, heat exhaustion, heat syncope, cramps, burns and local effects such as prickly heat
► Cold Trench foot, frostbite, chilblains
► Light Occupational cataract, miner's nystagmus
► Pressure Caisson disease, air embolism, blast (explosion)
► Noise Occupational deafness
► Radiation Cancer, leukaemia, aplastic anaemia, pancytopenia
► Mechanical factors Injuries, accidents
► Electricity Burns

⇨ Hearing

— **Human ear is sensitive to frequency of: 20-20,000 Hz.**
— **Maximal tolerable sound level daily: 85-90 dB.** MH 2010
— **Tympanic membrane rupture: ≥ 150dB.**

➲ Noise level:

Acceptable Noise Levels (In Decibels): High Yield for 2011-2012

⇨ **Measuring unit for loudness is: Decibel.** JK BOPEE 2012

Residential	Bed room	25
	Living room	40
Commercial	Office	35-45
	Conference	40-45
	Restaurants	40-45
Industrial	Workshop	40-60
	Lab	40-50

Educational	Classroom	30-40
	Library	35-40
Hospitals	Wards	20-35

⇨ **Other Important Things to Remember are**

- No classroom should accommodate more than **40 students**
- Desks should be of **minus type.**
- Combined door and window area should **be at least 25% of floor space**
- Inside color of classroom should be **white** and periodically white washed.
- Classrooms should have sufficient natural light, preferably from the **left and** not from the front.

⇨ **Standards of Ventilation**

- Minimal fresh air supply: 300-3000 cubic ft/hr/person
- 2-3 air changes in one hour in a **living room.**
- 4-6 air changes in one hour in **work rooms and assemblies**
- 50-100 sq feet is optimum floor space per person. JK 2010

⇨ **Diseases Due to Chemical Agents**

(1) Gases: CO_2, CO, HCN, CS_2, NH_3, N_2, H_2S, HCI, SO_2 - these cause gas poisoning.

(2) Dusts (Pneumoconiosis):

(i) Inorganic Dusts :

▶ **Coal dust Ahthracosis**

▶ **Silica Silicosis**

▶ **Asbestos Asbestosis, Cancer Lung**

Iron Siderosis

▶ **Cane fibre Bagassosis**

▶ **Cotton dust Byssinosis**

▶ **Tobacco Tobacossis**

▶ **Hay or grain dust Farmers'lung**

✳ Inhalation of sugar cane dust causes: bagassosis.	MH 2010
✳ Thermoactinomyces causes: bagassosis.	AIPGME 1998
✳ Micropolyspora faeni causes farmers lung.	AIPGME 1996
✳ Textile industries favour development of bysinosis	DNB 2003
✳ Monday fever is associated with bysinosis.	TN 2003
✳ Snow storm appearance is seen in silicosis.	UP 2006

⇨ **Indicators of Air Pollution Monitored on Daily Basis are: (S3)**

► Sulfur dioxide	JK BOPEE 2012
► Soiling index	JK BOPEE 2012
► Suspended particles (grit and dust)	JK BOPEE 2012

► General level of air pollution is estimated by SO_2 only.

► Smoke index or soiling index is an index of air pollution and "not water or land pollution."

Remember:

Comfort Zones	Corrective Effective Temperature
Pleasant and cool	20°C
Comfortable and cool	20-25°C
Comfortable	25-27°C
Hot and uncomfortable	27-28°C
Extremely hot	Greater than 28°C
Intolerably hot	30°C

⇨ **Wastes:**

Sewage - solid waste containing liquid as well as solid excreta.

Garbage - waste substances of food and vegetables.

Refuse - solid waste of the cities.

Sullage - kitchen waste water

➢ Most satisfactory method of refuse disposal is - **Controlled tipping.**

➢ Hospital refuse is best disposed off by - **Incineration.**

➢ Most effective in a sanitation barrier is - Segregation of faeces and its proper disposal

⇨ **Purification of Water is done by**

* ✳ Bleaching powder
* ✳ Chlorine solution
* ✳ Iodine
* ✳ Potassium permanganate
* ✳ Sand filter
* ✳ Ozonation
* ✳ UV Radiation

➲ **Methods of Refuse Disposal**

Methods of refuse disposal	
In sanitary methods	Sanitary methods
✳ Hog feeding	✳ Compositing
✳ Stacking	✳ Sanitary land fill
✳ Salvaging	✳ Incineration
✳ Dumping	

Remember:

- In **service type**, night soil is collected from pail or bucket type of latrines by human agency and later disposed of by burying or compositing.

- A **sanitary latrine** is one which fulfils the following criteria.

- Excreta should not contaminate the ground or surface **water**.

- Excreta should not pollute the **soil**.

- Excreta should not be accessible to flies, rodents, animals and other vehicles of transmission.

- Excreta should not create a nuisance due to odor or unsightly appearance.

⊃ Waste Management

Color coding	Waste Catageory	Treatment
Yellow	■ Human Anatomical waste AIPGMEE 2005 ■ Animal waste ■ Solid waste (items contaminated with blood, body fluids including cotton dressings, casts, linen, beddings, etc.	Incineration Deep Burial
Red	■ Solid waste (generated from disposable items other than sharps (tubings, catheters, blood sets, glucose bottles)	Autoclaving Microwaving Chemical Treatment
Blue	■ Waste sharps (Needles, blades, glass) ■ Solid wastes which are disposable	Autoclaving Microwaving Chemical Treatment
Black	■ Discarded medicine, ■ Plastic wrapers. AIIMS 2008 ■ Cytotoxic drugs ■ Incineration ash ■ Chemical wastes used in disinfection, as insecticides ■ General non infective wastes	Chemical Treatment and disposal in secured land fills

⊃ Biomedical Waste Management

⇨ Categories of Bio Medical Wastes (BMW) (Schedule I)

Cat	BMW	Wastes Included
1	Human anatomical waste	Human tissues, organs, body parts
2	Animal waste	Animal tissues, body parts, organs, carcasses, fluids, blood
3	Microbiology and biotechnology waste	Waste from lab cultures, stocks, specimens of microorganisms, live or attenuated vaccines, cell cultures (human/animal), wastes from production of biological, toxins.

4	Waste sharps	Needles syringes, blades, scalpels, glass.
5	Discarded medicines and cytotoxic drugs	Outdated contaminated and discarded medicines.
6	Soiled waste	Items contaminated with blood and fluids including cotton, dressings, soiled plaster casts, linen, beddings.
7	Liquid waste	Waste generated from lab and washing, cleaning, housekeeping and disinfecting activities.
8	Solid waste	Disposable items (except sharps) including tubing's, catheters, intravenous sets.
9	Incineration ash	Ash from Incineration of any BMW
10	Chemical waste	Chemical used in disinfection(insecticides) or in production of biological

⇨ **Color Coding and Type of Container for BMW Disposal (Schedule II)**

Color Coding	Type of Container	BMW Category	Treatment Option
Yellow	Plastic bag	1,2,3,6	Incineration/deep burial MAH 2012, JK BOPEE 2012
Red	Disinfected container/ plastic bag	3,6,7	autoclave/microwave
Blue/White translucent	Plastic bag	4,7	autoclave/microwave/chemical treatment and destruction/shredding
Black	Plastic bag	5,9,10	Secured landfill

Big tables but they are asked. Try your level best to memorize most

➲ **Instruments of Importance in Public Health**

Instrument	Use
▶ Ice lined refrigerator	Cold chain temperature maintenance
▶ Dial thermometer	Cold chain temperature monitoring
▶ Horrock's apparatus	Chlorine demand estimation in water
▶ Chlorinator,chloronome	Mixing/regulating the dose of chlorine in water
▶ Chloroscope	Measuring level of residual chlorine in drinking water
▶ Winchester quart bottle	Assess physical and chemical quality of drinking water
▶ Kata thermometer	Assess cooling power of air and air velocity UPSC 1986
▶ Anemometer	Assess air/wind velocity
▶ Hygrometer	Assess air humidity (moisture content of air)
▶ Mercurial barometer	Atmospheric pressure
▶ Aneroid barometer	Atmospheric pressure

▶ Sling pshycometer	Humidity	COMED 2008
▶ Wind vane	Assess air/wind direction	
▶ Salter's scale	Field instrument of **low birth weight(LBW)**	
▶ Infantometer	**Length** of infants	
▶ Stadiometer	**Height** of adults	
▶ Shakir's tape	Mid arm circumference(MAC)	
▶ Sound level meter	Measures **intensity** of sound	
▶ Audiometer	Hearing ability assessment	
▶ venturimeter	Measuring **bed strength in slow sand filter.**	UPSC 2002

Goal is a set point framed for long term plans but can't be measured or quantified yet.	AIPGMEE 2009

⊃ National Health Policy

Goals to be achieved by 2015

⓪ Eliminate Kala-azar		2010
⓪ Eliminate Lymphatic Filariasis 2015		AI 2010
⓪ ↓mortality by 50% on account of TB, Malaria and water borne diseases		2010
⓪ ↓prevalence of blindness to 0.5%		2010
⓪ ↓IMR to 30/100 and MMR to 100/lakh		2010 AIIMS 2008
⓪ ↑Utilization of public health facilities to 75%		2010
⓪ ↑Health expenditure as a % of GDP to 2%		2010
⓪ ↑ share of central grants to at least 25% of total health spending		2010
⓪ 100% registration of birth, death, pregnancy		AIIMS 2008

⇨ Remember Various Committees

Chadah Committee:

➡ PHC at block level.	
➡ Concept of multipurpose worker.	RJ 2007
➡ VIGILANCE operation of NMEP by general health servces	PGI 2011

Kartar Singh Committee:

➡ Multipurpose health worker.	RJ 2006

Bhore Committee:

➡ PHC (Primary health centre) Concept.	RJ 2006
➡ Three million plan	

Mudailiar Committee

➡ Constitution of All India Health Service	PGI 2011

Srivastava Committee

➡ Creation of Health Assistant cadre	PGI 2011

○ Primary Health Care

▶ Primary health care came into existence at Alma Ata in 1978	MAH 2012
▶ Best advocacy for PHC was done in alma ata	AI 2010
▶ Primary health care was proposed by Bhore Committee.	
▶ Principles of Primary Health care are:	
➡ Equitable distribution	
➡ Community participation	
➡ Intersectoral coordination	
Qualitative enquiry is a new concept in PHC.	AI 2010

○ Primary Health Care Systems: High Yield for 2011-2012

	Sub centre	PHC	CHC
✳ Level of care	Primary	Primary	Secondary
✳ Population norm			
✳ Plains	5000	30,000	1,20,000
✳ Hilly/tribal areas	3000	20,000	80,000
✳ Staff	3	15	30
✳ Maintenance	Central govt.	State govt.	State govt.
✳ Rural area covered	21 sq. km	140 sq. km	770 sq. km
✳ Radial distance covered	2.6	6.6	15.6
✳ Average no. of villages covered	4	29	158

⇨ Panchayati Raj

Is a three tier system of rural local self government, linking village to a district. The three institutions are:

➡ Panchayat: at village level

➡ Panchayat samiti: at block level

➡ Zilla parishad: at district level

Primary Health Care	Secondary Health care	Tertiary Health Care
Provided by agency of **multipurpose health worker, village health guide** or dias	Provided by **District hospitals and community health centres**	Provided by **regional/central level** institutions
JOB OF FEMALE HEALTH WORKER IS: PGI 2011		Medical college hospitals, Regional hospitals
➡ Monitoring growth and development of infant		
➡ Maintaining cleanliness of sub centre		

⊃ Latest Suggested Norms for Health Personnel

Personnel	Norms suggested	
► Doctors	► 1: 3500	
► Nurses	► 1: 5000	
► Health worker	► 1: 1000 (Plains),1:3000(hilly, tribal area)	
► Trained Dai	► 1 per village	AIIMS 1987
► Health Assistant	► 1: 30,000 (plains),1:20,000 (hilly, tribal area)	
► Pharmacist	► 1: 10,000	
► Lab Technician	► 1: 10,000	
► ASHA(village level)	► 1: 1000	AI 2010

⇨ ASHA

- **Is posted at the:** Village level
- Under the **National Rural Health Mission (NRHM)** one of the important component of plan of action to strengthen the primary health care is by creation of a cadre of **Accredited Social Health Activist** (ASHA) at the village level.
- **ASHA:** Must be a resident of the village in the age group of **25-45 years** with formal education up to **VIII class and having communication and leadership skills.**
- 1ASHA for 1000 population; in tribal, hilly and desert areas I ASHA for every habitation

Role and Responsibility: AIPGME 2010

✓ Counsel women on birth preparedness, Importance of safe delivery, breastfeeding and other aspects of child care
✓ Mobilize community to access health care provided under primary health care
✓ Work with village health and sanitation committee to develop a comprehensive healthplan
✓ Escort pregnant women and children who require referral
✓ Act as depot holder for ORS, IFA, DDK, contraceptives and some essential drugs
✓ Promote construction of household toilets
✓ Inform the Sc and Create awareness and provide information to the community on determinants of health
✓ PHC about births, deaths or any unusual heath occurrence or outbreak in her village.

⇨ Remember:

■ One village health guide caters to population of 1000.	DNB 2000
■ One PHC caters a population of 30,000	
■ Population covered by PHC in hilly region is 20,000	RJ 2006
■ One sub centre caters to population of 5000.	DNB 2000
■ An ideal sub centre caters to population of 5000.	DNB 2005
■ Recommended numbers of PHC and sub centres for tribal area: 20, 000 and 3000 respectively.	MH 2003
■ A trained dai caters to a population of 1000.	RJ 2003
■ Village health guide caters to a population of 1000	RJ 2004

Village health guide	Local dais	Anganwadi workers
► Not a full time government functionary ► A person with aptitude for social services ► 1 per village	Trained for **30 days** Functions : ► Conduct Delivery ► Health education ► Registration	► 1: 1000 population ► Trained for **4 months**

⇨ **Anganwadi Worker:**

They come under ICDS scheme. There is one Anganwadi worker for a population of 1000. Beneficiaries are esp. nursing mothers, other women (15 - 45 years) and children below 6 years. Their function includes:
✓ Health checkup
✓ Immunization
✓ Supplementary nutrition
✓ Health education
✓ Non-formal pre-school education and referral
✓ Anganwadi worker does not take part in sentinel surveillance

⇨ **Principles of Primary Health Care are**

► Equitable distribution
► Community participation
► Intersectoral coordination

► Primary Health care concept came into existence in **1978 in Alma Ata.**
► Primary Health Care delivery was first proposed by **Bhore in 1946.**
► Primary Health care is a **concept by WHO** and adopted by India.
► Primary care is provided by agency of **Multi purpose health workers, Village Health Guides, Trained Dais.**
► Includes:
► **IMMUNIZATION against major infectious diseases**   AI 2010
► **Provision of essential drugs**   AI 2010
► **Health education**
► **Maternal and child health including family planning.**
► **Promotion of food supply and proper nutrition.**

⇨ **Primary Health Care**

— Has undergone a lot of architectural and qualitative improvement under the (NRHM) National Rural Health Mission with the formulation of **Indian Public health standards for the subcentres, PHC, CHC and up to the sub district hospital level.**

— **"Indian Public Health Standards"** are means of describing the level of Quality that health care organizations are expected to meet or aspire to.

8

SPM

For achieving desired targets, first step is to lay down norms and standards.

— To provide optimal health care to the community

— To achieve and maintain an acceptable standard of quality care

— To make services more receptive and sensitive to the needs of community

IPHS: Components

* Assured services
* Manpower
* Physical Infrastructure
* Equipments
* Drugs
* Support Services: diagnostic, electricity, water, telephone, kitchen, laundry, sanitation, waste disposal, referral service, record maintenance
* Quality assurance and accountability
* Standard Operative Procedures and other guidelines
* Rogi Kalyan Samiti/Hospital Management Committee: Involving PRI/Community in management
* Charter of Patients Rights
* Monitoring Mechanism: Internal and External
* Service facility survey check-list

➲ National Health Policy Implementations

➥ To establish one **sub centre** for every **5000** rural population/population in plains.	
➥ To establish one **sub centre** for every **3000** tribal/hilly population.	AIPGMEE 2001
➥ To establish one **PHC** for every **30,000** rural population.	
➥ To establish one **PHC** for every **20,000** hilly/tribal population.	
➥ To establish **CHC** for **one Lakh** Population.	UP 2007
Remember as per RCH, CHC is a first referral unit.	AIPGMEE 2008
Under NTCP, PHC is said to be PHC R if microscopy+radiology facilities exist	AIPGMEE 2001

⇨ Guidelines for FRU, Ministry of Health and Family Welfare, Govt of India

1. Avalibility of surgical interventions **High yield for 2011-2012**.
2. Avalibilty of new borne care
3. Avalibilty of blood storage facility on 24 hour basis

Facilities required but not Critical are:

* Minimum bed strength of 20-30.
* Fully functioning operation theatre
* Fully functional labour room
* Blood storage facility
* Functional laboratory
* 24 hour water and electricity supply
* Arrangements for waste disposal
* Ambulance facility

➲ Practice of Health Education Includes

(i) Individual and family health education

(ii) Group health education

- ➠ Lectures
- ➠ Group discussions
- ➠ Panel discussions
- ➠ Symposium
- ➠ Workshop
- ➠ Institute
- ➠ Role playing
- ➠ Demonstrations
- ➠ Programmed instruction
- ➠ Simulation exercises

iii) Education of the general public: It includes radio, press, posters museum, etc.

"Practice" is a habit or accustomed way of doing things. It is the usual way of action or an act performed without thinking. There should be a strong emotional stimulus and motivation to practice certain habits like taking a vow, reward, recognition, etc.

Practice requires "motivational encouragement and emotional stimulus"

"Attitudes" are acquired characteristics of an individual. They are more or less permanent ways of behaving. Attitudes are not learnt from books, they are acquired by social interaction, e.g. attitude towards persons, things, situations and issues. Once formed attitudes are difficult to change.

"Belief" is the psychological state in which an individual holds a proposition or premise to be true. Beliefs are permanent, stable and almost unchanging.

Beliefs are the assumptions we make about ourselves, about others in the world and about how we expect things to be. Beliefs are also how we think things really are.

When belief is backed by experience and experimentation it becomes "knowledge"

Opinions

— Are views held by people on a point of dispute.

— They are based on evidence available at the time.

— Opinions by definitions are temporary and provisional. They can be looked on as beliefs for the time being.

➲ Attitude

— An attitude has been defined as a relatively enduring organization of beliefs around an object, subject or concept which pre-disposes one to respond in some preferential manner.

— An Attitude represents an individual's degree of like or dislike for an item.

— Attitudes are generally positive or negative views of a person, place thing, or event.

— Attitude is acquired characteristics of an individual.

8

- They are **more or less permanent** ways of behaving.

- Attitudes **are not learned from text-books**, they are **acquired by social interaction**, e.g. attitude towards.

- Persons, things, situations and issues. **"Attitudes are caught and not taught."**

- Once formed, **attitudes are difficult to change.** The responsibility to develop healthy attitudes depends upon parents, teachers, religious leaders, and elders. Ones success and failure in life depend upon one attitude.

▶ **Primordial prevention:** Prevention of emergence of risk factors

▶ **Primary prevention:** Includes health promotion and specific protection

▶ **Secondary prevention:** includes early diagnosis and treatment.

▶ **Teritary prevention:** Includes diability limitation and rehabilitation.

⊃ **Important Facts**

▪ Chairman of **Health survey and planning committee** was Dr A.L. Mudaliar

▪ Chairman of **Health survey and Development committee** was Sir Joseph Bhore.

▪ Chairman of committee on **Integration of health services** was Dr Jungalwalla

▪ Chairman of Committee on **Multipurpose Health Worker** was Kartar Singh.

⊃ **BIOSTATICS**

⇨ **Normal Curve**

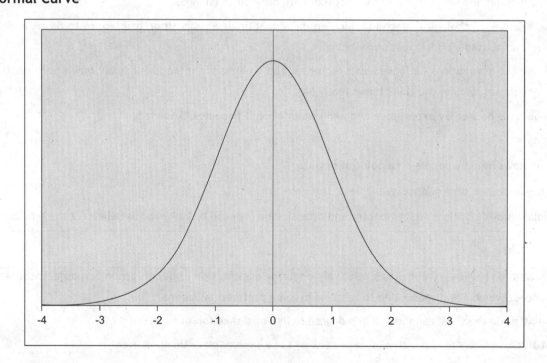

Normal curve is **smooth, bell shaped symmetrical curve with**	ASSAM 1995

- Total area under curve =1
- Mean of curve =0
- Standard deviation=1
- Mean, Median and Mode coincide
- Normal standard deviation has variance =1   AIPGMEE 2005
- Standard deviation is a <u>measure of deviation from mean</u>.   AIPGMEE 2008

"A graph representing the density function of the Normal probability distribution is also known as a Normal Curve or a Bell Curve.   AIIMS 1997

To draw such a curve, one needs to specify two parameters, the mean and the standard deviation.

The graph above has a mean of zero and a standard deviation of 1.

ISD=68% of values

2SD=95% of values.   AI 1996

3SD=99.7% of values.

<u>Z score</u> determines how many standard deviations an observation is above or below the mean.

Z score is done for normal distribution   AI 2010

Standard error= SD/root of sample size

⇨ **Tests Used in Biostatics**

— The student t-test is used to compare **two means derived from two samples.**

— **Analysis of variance** is used when the means of a continuous variable are being **compared in three or more groups** or when the independent variable responsible for a difference in means is being sought.

— The chi-square test is commonly used to compare <u>non continuous data</u> in two groups.
  Both samples should be mutually exclusive.   UPSC 2K

— The **Fisher Exact Test and the Pittman Welch Permutation Test** considers all possible permutations of the data and compares them with the values actually observed.

— **Multiple Linear Regression** is used to consider the impact of more than one independent variable on the dependent variable.

— The **Paired t-test** is typically used when an **observation is made twice on a sample.**

— The **Pearson Correlation Formula** can be used for ranked data that have no intrinsic numeric value, where the ranking system represents equal intervals between measurement units.

— **Simple Linear Regression** is a process by which the data collected are fitted to the best straight line.

— The **Spearman Rank Order Formula** produces a **correlation coefficient** - a numeric way of describing the direction and strength of the linear relationship between two variables. This particular formula is used for data that are continuous and based on ranking.

8

SPM

- To compare the results obtained by a new test and a gold standard test, **Bland and Altman test** is used.

  AIIMS 2007, AIIMS 2011

- Sensitivity and specificity are used for **assessing criterion validity.**   AIPGMEE 2003

➤ **Correlation indicates degree of association between two variables.**   AIIMS 1997

➤ **Correlation coefficient of 1 means two variables expresses linear relationship.**

➤ **Causation implies correlation.**

▶ **True positive (TP)** = A positive test result in the presence of the disease   AI 1997

▶ **True negative (TN)** = A negative test result in the absence of the disease

▶ **False positive (FP)** = A positive test result in the absence of the disease   KERALA 1997

▶ **False negative (FN)** = A negative test result in the presence of the disease

▶ **Sensitivity** = the ability of the test to identify the disease in those who have it

Equals TP / (TP + FN)

▶ **Specificity** = the ability of the test to exclude the disease in the absence of the disease

Equals TN / (TN + FP)

▶ Sensitivity and specificity determine validity of screening test.   AIIMS 1996

▶ **Screening is useful when incidence of disease in community is high.**   KERALA 1994

▶ **The reliability** of a measurement refers to the **ability of other researchers to reproduce the results.**

▶ **The accuracy** of a measurement refers to the **"trueness" of the measurement,** i.e., how close the measured value is to the true value

▶ **LJ chart** measures accuracy.   AIIMS 2007

▶ **The power of a study** is best conceptualized as the probability of rejecting a null hypothesis that is in fact false. This is equal to **1 minus the probability of a type II error**

▶ **The validity** of a measurement is an index of **how well the test measures what it purports to measure.**

  COMED 2007

▶ **Tests in parallel :** sensitivity↑, specificity↓, PPV↓, NPV↑

▶ **Tests in series:** sensitivity↓, specificity↑, PPV↑, NPV↓

- Screening is not effective in lung cancer detection.

- Sensitivity is affected by **interobserver variation.**   UPSC 2007

- True positivity is sensitivity.   MAHE 2005

- True negativity is specificity.   MAHE 2005

- **False positive= 1-specificity**

- **False negative=1-sensitivity**

- **Likelihood ratio** for a negative test=1-sensitivity/specificity

- **Likelihood ratio** for a positive test=sensitivity/ 1-specificity

- True positive is **directly related to sensitivity.**

- True negative is **directly related to specificity.**   JKBOPEE 2012

- False positive is **inversely related to specificity.**

- False negative is **inversely related to sensitivity**

- Prevalence= **Incidence x duration.** (prevalence ↑duration)   AIPGMEE 2009

- Diagnostic power of a test to correctly exclude a disease is negative predictive value: AIPGMEE 2005

- Diagnostic power of a test to correctly diagnose a disease is positive predictive value:

- Bayes theorem gives relationship between PPV, Sensitivity, specificity, prevalence of a screening test.

⇨ **Evaluation of Screening Tests**

Criteria	Numerator	Denominator
Sensitivity	True positive (a)	True positive + false negatives (a + c)
Specificity	True negatives (d)	True negatives + false positives (b + d)
PPV	True positives (a)	True positive + false positives (a + b)
NPV	True negatives (d)	True negatives + false negatives (b + d)
% False positives	False positives (b)	True negatives + false positives (b + d)
% False negatives	False negatives	True positives + false negatives (a + c)

- Positive skew: Mean>Median>Mode

- Negative Skew: Mean<Median<Mode

- Type I error: null hypothesis true but rejected

- Type II error: null hypothesis wrong but accepted

- Cross sectional studies:
- Cohort studies:
- Case control study:

  - Chi square test
  - Relative risk, Attributable risk, <u>Incidence rate</u>.   AIPGMEE 2009
  - Odds ratio

- Odds ratio >1 = Risk

- Odds Ratio<1= Protective

- Odds Ratio=0 = No effect

- Odds= probability/1-probability

- Chi square test: Compare <u>proportions</u>

- Two sample <u>Z</u> test: Compare <u>populations</u>

- Two sample <u>t</u> Test: Compare <u>samples</u>

- Anova: <u>Three or more variables</u>

- Meta Analysis: <u>Pooling of data from several studies. Gives most accurate results.</u>   AIIMS 2011

8

SPM

- ▶ Usefulness of **screening test: Sensitivity**
- ▶ **Statistical index** of diagnostic accuracy: **Sensitivity**
- ▶ Power of a test = **1-β**

- ➡ **Relative risk:** incidence **among exposed/ incidence among non exposed**
- ➡ **Attributable risk:** incidence among exposed **minus** incidence among non exposed/ incidence among exposed multiplied by 100.
- ➡ **Eg A study showing 80% of lung cancers are due to smoking is an attributable risk.** AIPGMEE 2007
- ➡ **Population attributable risk:** Incidence of disease (or death) in total population minus incidence of disease (or death) among those who were not exposed to suspected casual factor.

- ➡ **Relative risk:** Incidence **among exposed/ incidence among non exposed**
- ➡ **Attributable risk:** Incidence among exposed **minus** incidence among non exposed/ incidence among exposed multiplied by 100. **E.g.: A study showing 80% of lung cancers are due to smoking is an attributable risk.**
- ➡ **Population attributable risk:** Incidence of disease (or death) in total population minus incidence of disease (or death) among those who were not exposed to suspected casual factor.

P Value: AIPGME 2012

- ▪ The likelihood that an observed difference or an even more extreme difference is due to chance alone is called the p-value. In our study, if a certain difference between mean values in treatment say BP in treatment and control groups was observed, $p < 0.05$ would mean: given that the null hypothesis is true, **there is a < 5% likelihood that this difference or a larger difference is due to random sampling.**
- ▪ **Thus, if the p-value is small, it is unlikely that an observed difference is due to random sampling, the null hypothesis is rejected, and it is inferred that real population differences or a real association exists between treatment and response.**
- ▪ **A small p-value (the conventional level for "small" has been traditionally accepted as 0.05)** safeguards against chance leading us to reject a null hypothesis which is true.
- ▪ **A very low p-value strongly suggests** that the observed data are inconsistent with the null hypothesis.
- ▪ The error of rejecting a true null hypothesis is called **type I error**. This occurs when chance leads to inferring differences or associations that do not exist.
- ▪ In contrast, **type II error** occurs when a large p-value leads to the incorrect conclusion that a difference does not exist (incorrectly not rejecting a null hypothesis).

Chi square test is the most important test measuring **association between two variables.** AIPGME 2003

- ▶ It measures the **probability of association** between two variables.
- ▶ The chi square test assumes that no association exists between two events.
- ▶ Chi square test is a **non parametric** test.
- ▶ Tests significance of asssociation between two or more qualitative variables.

Correlation
▶ Describes the **strength of linear relationship** between two variables.
▶ It is denoted by **Correlation coefficient or Pearsons Coefficent**
▶ Its Value ranges from **— 1 to +1**

⊃ **Coorelation: High Yield for 2011-2012**

Types of coorelation	Coorelation coefficent	Examples
Perfectly positive	r = +1	Height and age
Perfectly negative	r = —1	Pressure and volume of gas
Moderately positive	0<r<+1	Temperature and pulse rate
Moderately negative	—1< r <0	Age and vital capacity
No coorelation	r = 0	Husbands skin colour and fertility
Spurious coorelatio n		Skin colour and IQ

" Z score" is done for normal type of distribution
Z score is calculated using a standard normal distribution curve The distance of a value (x) from the mean (x) of the curve in units of standard deviation is called "relative deviate or standard normal variate" and is usually denoted by Z.
"Binomial Distribution" The probability that a specific combination of mutually exclusive independent events will occur can be determined by the use of the binomial distribution. A binomial distribution is one in which there are only two possibilities, such as yes/no, male/female, healthy/sickly. A typical medical use of the binomial distribution is in genetic counseling.
"Comparison of Proportions": Proportions are compared when the data is measured on a nominal or ordinal scale. The test, which is commonly used, is the chi square test. It is a non-parametric test. The test is done by constructing 2 × 2 contingency table and calculating the expected frequency of the variable from the observed frequency. The test can be applied in two or more independent groups and a paired group.

⊃ **Cronbach's α (Alpha): High Yield for 2011-2012**

✳ Cronbach's α (alpha) is a measure of internal consistency reliability.
✳ Internal consistency reliability is used when one wants to know whether the items on a test are consistency with one another in that they represent one, and only one, dimension, construct, or area of interest.

⇨ **Correlation Coefficient**

✳ A correlation simply express the strength and direction of the relationship between two variables in terms of a correlation coefficient.
✳ It does not tell about causation.
✳ It does not tell about the risk of diseases.

➲ Probability

✓   Is the chance that a particular event will occur.probability range is **zero-hundred**
Percent (0-1)Probability can never be zero
✓   Probability cannot exceed one.
✓   Probabilities are added for mutually exclusive events
✓   Probabilities are multiplied for independent events

⇨ Quantitative Continuous Data is Represented by

Histogram
Bar Diagram
Frequency polygon
Pie chart

➲ Division of Distribution

	Divides distribution into	No. of intercepts
Tertile	3 equal parts	2
Quartile	4 equal parts	3
Pentile	5 equal parts	4
Hextile	6 equal parts	5
Heptile	7 equal parts	6
Octile	8 equal parts	7
Ductile	10 equal parts	9
Centile(percentile)	100 equal parts	99

⇨ Variables

▶   **Quantitative**: can be measured directly. Height, weight
▶   **Qualitative**: cannot be measured directly. Weather, gender
▶   **Discrete variable**: has few possible values, no inbetween values. Blood group, gender
▶   **Continuous variable**: large number of possible values and several in between values. Weight, height
▶   **Dichotomous variable**: only two possibilities exist. Eg Blood group A + or—
▶   **Polyotomous variable**: more than 2 possibilities exist. Weight, Height

⇨ So

▶   Height is a quantitative, polyotomous variable.
▶   Gender is a qualitative, discrete, dichotomous variable.

⇨ **Variable:**

Is a "charactertistic or attribute" that varies from person to person

Quantitative:
Variable that can be measured directly
— Height
— Weight
— Haemoglobin
— Blood urea
Qualitative:
Variable that cannot be measured directly
— Weather
— Obesity
— Gender

➡ Discrete variable:

Is a variable that has few possible values and no in between values

Examples:

✓ Parity
✓ Gender
✓ Obesity

➡ Continuous variable

Is a variable that has large number of possible values and few in between values

Examples:

✓ Weight
✓ Height
✓ Blood sugar level

➡ Dichotomous variable

Is a variable that has only two possible values

Examples:

✓ Blood group A present or absent
✓ Gender: male/female

➡ Polyotomous variable

Is a variable that has more than two possible values

Examples:

✓ Weight
✓ Height
✓ Serum cholesterol

➲ Scales of Measurement: High Yield for 2011-2012

	Categorical Scales		Dimensional Scales
	Nominal Scale	**Ordinal Scale**	**Metric Scales**
Definition	Based on NOM (names): No specific order	Based on ORD (order): Grading into categories	Based on ME (measurement): in terms of quantities
Variables	Qualitative	Qualitative	Quantitative
Examples	↪ Race ↪ Religion ↪ Country of birth ↪ Clinical features ↪ Sites of lymphadenopathy ↪ Sex of child ↪ Type of anemia ↪ ABO blood group ↪ Site of malignancy	✳ TNM staging (cancers) ✳ Severity of a disease ✳ Social classes	➲ Blood glucose ➲ Hemoglobin level ➲ Serum cholesterol ➲ Weight ➲ Height ➲ Mid arm circumference ➲ Blood pressure ➲ Pulse rate ➲ Temperature (C, F,K)scale Ratio scale : Geometric mean Harmonic mean, coefficient of variation

➲ Sampling

➥ **Simple random sampling** is done by assigning a number to each of units in a sample.

Sample is drawn in such a way that each unit has an equal chance of being drawn in a sample   **AIPGMEE 2009**

➥ **Systemic random sampling** is done by picking every **5th or 10th** unit at regular intervals.

➥ **Stratified random sampling** is deliberately drawn in such a way that each portion of a sample represents a

Corresponding strata of the universe eg: age groups, classifying according to religion.

Quota sampling is **not** a random sampling method.   **AIIMS 2000**

Non random sampling is seen in:

► Convenience sampling

► Clinical trial sampling

► Quota sampling

► Snow ball sampling.

➥ **Cluster Sampling**

► This method is basically used for assessing immunization status of children under immunization. It is done by three cluster technique.   **AIIMS 2008**

► Error rate is low.   **AIIMS 2008**

➲ Sampling

⇨ Snow Ball Sampling

- ✓ It is a non probability sampling where existing study subjects recruitfuture subjects from theikir acquaintances.
- ✓ The sample growing like a roling snow ball.
- ✓ It is used for hidden population. **PGI 2011**

⇨ Sampling Methods

Simple Random Sampling:

- This is done by **assigning a number to each unit in the population to be sampled and then using lottery method or a table of random numbers** to select units to be included in the sample.
- The principle here is that **every unit of the population has an equal chance of being selected.**
- This method is applicable **when the population is small** Homogenous and readily available such as patients coming to hospital or lying in wards.

Systematic Sampling:

- In this method the first unit of the sample is selected at random and the subsequent units are selected in a systematic way i.e **every fifth or tenth unit at regular intervals.**
- For example in a malaria survey to take a 5 percent sample, all the houses are numbered first. Then the first house is selected at random 1tween 1 and 5, then every 5th house is selected from that point on.
- This method is popularly used in those cases when a complete list of population from which samples is to be drawn, is available. It is more often applied to field studies when the population is large, scattered and not homogenous.

Stratified Sampling:

- This method is used when the **population is heterogenous with regards to characteristic under study.** The population under study is first divided into homogenous groups or classes called strata and then the sample is drawn from each stratum at random in proportion to its size.
- This method of sampling gives representation to all strata of society or population such as selecting sample from defined areas, classes, religions, ages or sexes.
- **For example a population to be sampled consists of people of different religions like Hindus, Muslims, Sikhs, Christians etc. In stratified sampling the population is first divided into religious groups and then samples are drawn from each group in proportion to its size.**
- This method is particularly useful where one is interested in analyzing the data by certain characteristics of the population, viz Hindus, Muslims, Christians, age-groups etc.

Cluster Sampling:

- A **cluster is a randomly selected group.** This method is used when units of population are natural groups or clusters such as villages, wards, blocks, slums, schools etc.
- In this technique clusters are chosen at random from the entire population, and then these clusters are sampled.

- Each cluster should be a small scale representation of the total population. In **single-stage cluster sampling**, all the elements from each of the selected clusters are used. In **two-stage cluster sampling**, a random sampling technique is applied to the elements from each of the selected clusters.
- The main difference between cluster sampling and stratified sampling is than in cluster sampling the cluster is treated as the sampling unit so analysis is done on a population of cluster (at least in the first stage). In stratified sampling, a random sample is drawn from each of the strata, whereas in cluster sampling only the selected cluster is studied. The main objective of cluster sampling is to reduce costs by increasing sampling efficiency. This contrasts with stratified sampling where the main objective is to increase precision.
- Cluster sampling is most often used to evaluate vaccination coverage in Expanded Programme of Immunization (EPI) and Universal Immunization Programme (UIP), where only 210 children, taking 7 from each of the 30 clusters are examined.
- Cluster sample gives a **high standard error** but data collection in this method is simpler and involves less time and cost than in other sampling techniques.

Multistage Sampling:-

- In this method sampling procedure is carried out in several stages using random sampling techniques.
- Multistage sampling is used when the population units arranged in hierarchal groups. For examples farmers in India may be grouped into various states, then into districts, then into talukas, further into villages within the talukas and then farmers within the villages.

Multiphase Sampling:

- In this method, part of information is collected from the whole sample and part from the subsample. For example in a tuberculosis survey, in the first phase, physical examination or mantoux test may be done in all the cases; in the second phase X-ray of the chest may be done in Mantoux positive cases and in those with clinical symptoms; finally the sputum may be examined in X-ray positive cases. Thus number of sample in the second and third phases would become successively smaller and smaller. Survey by multiphase sampling would involve less cost and labour and would be more purposeful.

Cluster Random Sampling

- This method is basically used for assessing immunization status of children under immunization.
- It is done by three cluster technique.
- Applicable when units of population are natural groups or clusters.
- **WHO Technique** used in CRS: 30 × 7 (TOTAL = 210) i.e. 30 clusters each containing 7 children (12-23 months of age)

  AIIMS 2005
- **Low error rates** are seen in this type of sampling.
- Limitation is that **clusters cannot be compared** with each other.
- Sampling interval is also calculated.

➲ Lot Quality

- ▶ Lot Quality assurance sampling (**LQAS**) was introduced in the manufacturing industry for quality control purposes.

- ▶ Rather than checking each item in the lot to determine the number of defects, it is decided to take up sample of items and define the level of risks we are willing to take for not inspecting each and every item.

- ▶ Based on these risks, they would decide to **accept or reject the entire lot.**

- ▶ The only outcome is "**acceptable**" or "**not acceptable**".

- ▶ There is no measure to define different levels of unacceptability.

- ▶ The sample size and decision values for Lot Quality sampling are based on risks the investigators are willing to take.

- ▶ There are two different types of risks that need to be accounted for:

- ▶ "**The risk of accepting a bad Lot**" (Type I error).

- ▶ "**The risk of not accepting a good Lot**" (Type II error).

- ▶ It was extended to **Coverage evaluation survey for immunization.**

- ▶ "**In terms of immunization assessment, acceptability is usually determined by whether the Lot meets some desired proportion of immunization coverage.**"

⇨ Health Management

Consists of

- ➡ Planning
- ➡ Organization
- ➡ Communicating
- ➡ Monitoring (Controlling)

⇨ Quantitative Methods

- ➡ **Cost benefit analysis** (income benefits compared with **costs of programme**)

- ➡ **Cost effective analysis** (similar to above but benefit is **expressed in terms of results achieved**)

- ➡ **Cost accounting** (provides basic data on cost structure of any programme) financial records kept in a manner **permitting costs to be associated with the purpose for which they incurred**

- ➡ **Input output analysis** (shows how much input is needed to produce a unit of output

- ➡ **Model** (basic concept of management science)

- ➡ **Systems analysis** (helps decision maker to choose an appropriate course of action(finding the cost effectiveness of available alternatives)

- ➡ **Network analysis** (graphic plan of all events and activities to be completed in order to reach an end objective. Two types used are:

PERT (Programme Evaluation and Review Technique): makes possible more detailed planning and more comprehensive supervision

CPM(Critical Path Method): **Longest path of network**   MAHE 2007

- ➡ **Planning-programming budgeting system (PPBS)** Helps decision makers to allocate resources in most effective way to achieve objective
- ➡ **Work sampling** systemic observation and recording of activities of one or more individuals carried out at different intervals.   **UPSC 2007**

Systemic observation and recording activities carried out at intervals.   **COMED 2006**

Comparison of a value obtained and a predetermined objective is done by <u>evaluation</u>.   **AIPGMEE 2009**

➲ Preventive and Social Measures Which Influence Genetics

⇨ Health Promotional Measures

- ➡ Eugenics
- ➡ Euthenics
- ➡ Genetic counseling
- ➡ Other genetic preventive measures

EUGENIC:

- ➡ Galton proposed the term eugenics for the science which **aims to improve the genetic endowment of human population.**
- ➡ It has both negative and positive aspects.

➲ Negative Eugenics

The aim of negative eugenics is to **reduce the frequency of hereditary diseases and disability in the community to as low as possible** e.g; Hitler sought to improve german race by killing the weak and defective: this was negative eugenics. Inspite of negative eugenics, new cases of hereditary diseases continue to arise in the population because of

- ➡ Fresh mutation
- ➡ Marital alliances between hidden carriers (heterozygotes) of recessive defects

➲ Positive Eugenics

It seeks to **improve the Genetic composition of the population by encouraging the carriers of the desirable genotypes to assume the burden of parenthood.** It has very little application. It does not yield direct results because of 2 reasons:

- ➡ The majority of socially valuable traits e.g. intelligence have complex, multifactorial, determinants, both genetic and environmental and are not inherited in a simple way as, say blood groups.
- ➡ It is difficult to determine which gene we transmit to our children.

➲ Euthenics

(1) AIM: The solution of improving the human race does not lie in contrasting hereditary and environment, but rather in the mutual interaction of hereditary and environmental factors. **This environmental manipulation is called EUTHENICS**

(2) It has a considerable broader prospects for success. e.g; Studies with mentally retarded (mild) children indicated that exposure to environmental stimulation improved their IQ.

⮑ Genetic Counseling

May be Prospective or Retrospective

(1) PROSPECTIVE GENETIC COUNSELING

AIM: If heterozygous marriage can be prevented or reduced, the prospects of giving birth to affected children will diminish.

APPROACH:

- Identifying the heterozygous for any particular defect by screening procedures
- Explaining to them the risk.
- This allows for the true prevention of disease.
- The application in this field, for example, is sickle cell anemia, Thalassemia.

(2) RETROSPECTIVE GENETIC COUNSELING:

Most genetic counseling at present. Hereditary disorder has already occurred in family. Methods:

- **Contraception**
- **Pregnancy termination**
- **Sterilization**

Other Genetic Preventive Measures:

- Avoiding consanginous marriages
- Avoiding late marriages

⮑ Sample Registration System

- Estimates **birth and death rates** at national and state levels.
- Covers entire country.
- **Source of Health information.**
- It is a **dual record system.**
- Enumerator: assessment of births/deaths continuously.
- Independent survey: survey every 6 months by an investigator.
- ▶ Census: taken at intervals of 10 years.
- ▶ Civil registration system: Not evolved in India fully.

Chalk and Talk:

Carefully prepared oral presentation of facts organized thoughts and ideas by a qualified person.

Group should not be more than **30 and talk should not exceed 15-20 minutes.**

Group Discussion:

Aggregation of people interacting in face to face situation. a group **should not have less than 6 and more than 12 people.**

Panel Discussion:

Here **4-8 qualified people** talk about a topic and discuss a given problem in presence of an audience.

UPSC 2007

Symposium:

Is a **series of speeches on a selected subject**

Workshop:

It is a series of meetings usually four or more with emphasis on individual work, within a group with the help of consultants and resource personnel.

Role Playing:

► Situation dramatized by a group. Effective communication

Demonstration:

► Carefully prepared presentation to show how a particular skill/ procedure is performed.

— **Lectures** is a one way communication.   AI 1988

— Best method of health instruction is **setting an example.**   AIIMS 1984

— **Demonstrating** is the best teaching opportunity.   AIIMS 1984

— **Most common and effective channel of communication is** <u>Interpersonal Communication</u>   JK BOPEE 2012

⮫ Disaster High Yield for 2011-2012

Is any occurrence that causes damage, ecological disruption, loss of human life or deteroration of health and health services on a scale sufficient to warrant an extraordinary response from outside the affected community or area

Disaster Cycle:

✓ Impact

✓ Response

✓ Rehabilitation

✓ Mitigation

Triage System:

✳ Red: highest priorty   (MH2010)

✳ Yellow: high priority

✳ Green: low priority

✳ Black: least priority

⮫ Social Mobility

Movement in socio-economic level is **Social mobility**

➡ Indian society is rigidly based on caste system. There is **little social mobility,** i.e. people do not change their caste or religion. In other words, **Indian society is a "closed-class"** system.

➡ There are societies known as the **"open class societies"** where **movement of the social ladder is unrestricted, on the basis of achievement or gaining wealth.**

➡ Open class societies are therefore more progressive where people according to their ability can go up the social ladder. In closed - class systems, it is difficult to make reforms without meeting resistance of the people.

⊃ Some Important Health Programmes of India

- National Rural Health Mission (NRHM), 2005 —
- National Tuberculosis Programme (NTP),1962
- Revised National Tuberculosis Control Programme (RNTCP),1992
- National Planning Programme 1951
- Child Survival and Safe Motherhood (CSSM) Programme.1992
- Reproductive and Child Health Programme I:1997
- Reproductive and Child Health Programme II: 2004-09
- National AIDS Control Programme I (NACP I):1992 -97
- National AIDS Control Programme II (NACPII):1999-2004
- National AIDS Control Programme III (NACPIII):2006-11
- National Malaria Control Programme (NMCP):1953
- National Malaria Eradication Programme (NMEP):1958
- Urban Malaria Scheme (UMS):1971
- Modified Plan Of Operation (MPO):1977
- Enhanced Malaria Control Project (EMCP): 1997
- National Anti Malaria Programme (NAMP):1999
- Kala Azar Control Programme:1977
- Lymphatic Filariasis Control Programme:1955
- Revised Lymphatic Filariasis Control Programme: 1996-97
- National Vector Borne Disease Control Programme (NVBDP): 2003-04
- Yaws Eradication Programme:1996 -97
- National Leprosy Control Programme:1955
- National Leprosy Eradication Programme (NLEP): 1983
- Modified Leprosy Elimination Campaigns (MLEC):1998-2004
- Swajaldhara Community programme. 2002 — JK BOPEE 2012
- National Guinea worm Eradication Programme: 1983-84 — KERALA 2004
- Integrated Disease Surveillance Project (IDSP): 2004 -09
- Integrated Child Development Services (ICDS) Scheme: 1975

8

SPM

- National Trachoma Control Programme: 1963

- National Programme For Control Blindness (NPCB):1976

- National Goitre Control Programme (NGCP):1962

- National Iodine Deficiency Disorders Control Programme (NIDDCP): 1992

- National Mental Health Programme:1982

- National Cancer Health Programme: 1975 - 76

- National Oral Health Project: 1999

⮂ Some Important Health Legislations Passed In India

- ▶ The Employees State Insurance Act (ESI) 1948

- ▶ The Factories Act:1948

- ▶ The Prevention of Food Adulteration (PFA) Act,1954

- ▶ The Maternity Benefit Act,1961

- ▶ Medical qualifications awarded by institutions outside India and registered by MCI are registered in part II of third schedule of Indian Medical Council Act 1956   **AIPGMEE 2006**

- ▶ The Registration of Births and Deaths Act,1969

- ▶ The Medical Termination of Pregnancy (MTP) Act ,1971

- ▶ The Narcotic Drugs and Psychotropic Substances Act ,1985

- ▶ The Consumer Protection Act (COPRA) ,1986

- ▶ The Environmental Protection Act (EPA) ,1986

- ▶ Information technology act.: 2000   **AIPGMEE 2005**

- ▶ The Mental Health Act.1987

- ▶ The Infant Milk Substitute, Feeding Bottles and Infant Food (Regulation of Production, Supply and Distribution) Act,1992

- ▶ The Protection of Human Rights Act, 1993

- ▶ The biomedical waste (management and handling) rules,1998

- ▶ The national rural employment guarantee act (NREGA), 2005

- ▶ The right to information (RTI) act, 2005

- ▶ The transplantation of human organs act. 1994   **AIPGMEE 2006**

➲ Targeted Interventions for AIDS

Targeted interventions for AIDS

- Targeted interventions are, one of the most important components of the **National AIDS Control Programme.**
- The basic purpose of the Targeted Intervention programme is to reduce the rate of transmission among the high- risk behavior practicing population such as
  - ✓ sex workers,
  - ✓ intravenous drug users,
  - ✓ men having sex with men,
  - ✓ trackers, migrant laborers and
  - ✓ Street children.
- One of the ways of controlling the disease from further spread is to carry out direct intervention programmes among these groups through multi-prolonged strategies, beginning from behavior change, communications, and counseling, providing health care support, treatment for STDs and creating an enabling environment that will facilitate behavior change.
- In order to plan for implementation of this programme, NACO (National AIDS Control Organization) has evolved the following strategy.
- **Decentralization of implementation to the State AIDS Control Society.**
- **Transparent and streamlined procedures for selection of NGOs.**
- **Capacity building of SACS (State AIDS Control Societies) and NGOs for implementing and monitoring targeted intervention projects.**
- The **State AIDS Control Societies (SACS)** are fully empowered to provide funding support to the NGOs for Targeted Interventions. Every State AIDS society has appointed an NGO Advisor, who is professional in the field of social work, to manage and guide the Targeted Intervention Programme.

Millennium Development Goals

- Goal 1: eradicate extreme poverty/ hunger
- Goal 2: universalize primary education
- Goal 3: gender equality: women enpowerment
- Goal 4: reduce child mortality
- Goal 5: improve maternal health
- Goal 6: combat HIV/AIDS, malaria, other diseases
- Goal 7: ensure environmental sustainability
- Goal 8: develop global partnerships for development

◔ New Initiatives Undertaken Under RCH- II Program

1. Training of MBBS doctors in anaesthetic skills for emergency obstetric care at FRUs.

2. Training of MBBS doctors in obstetric management skills.

3. Setting up of blood storage centres at FRUs.

4. Development of cadre of community level skilled birth attendants.

5. Janani Suraksha Yojana (National Maternity Benefit Scheme)   **MAH 2012**

6. Vandemataram Scheme.

◔ Integrated Management of Neonatal and Childhood Illness (IMNCI)

The Indian version of IMCI has been renamed as integrated management of neonatal and childhood illness (IMNCI). It is the central pillar of child health interventions under the RCH II strategy. The majorhighlights of the Indian adaption are:

a. Inclusion of 0-7 days age in the programme

b. Incorporating national guidelines on malaria, anemia, vitamin A supplementation and immunization schedule.

c. Training of the health personnel begins with sick young infants up to 2 months.

d. Proportion of training time devoted to sick young infant and sick child is almost equal.

◔ Health Agencies and the Location of their Headquarters

Health Agencies	Headquarters	
WHO (World Health Organization)	Geneva, Switzerland	
UNICEF (United Nations Children Fund)	New York, USA	**JIPMER 1988**
UNDP (United Nations Development Program) UNESCO	New York, USA, Paris.	**UPSC 1999**
FAO (Food and agricultural organization)	<u>Rome, Italy</u>	**KCET 2012**
ILO (International Labor Organization)	Geneva, Switzerland	

◔ UNICEF

UNICEF was **previously named** as United nations international childrens emergency fund but now its emergency functions are over since 1953 and is called as United nations childrens fund.

➡ The United Nations Children's Fund (or UNICEF) was created by the **United Nations General Assembly on December 11, 1946,** to provide emergency food and healthcare to children in countries that had been devastated by World War II.

➡ In 1953, UNICEF became a permanent part of the United Nations System and **its name was shortened** from the original United Nations International Children's Emergency Fund but it has continued to be known by the popular acronym based on this old name. Headquartered in New York City.

➡ UNICEF is currently focused on three main priorities: **Child Survival and Development, Basic Education and Gender Equality** (including girls' education), Child protection from violence, exploitation, and abuse, HIV/AIDS and children, and Policy advocacy and partnerships for children's rights.

⊃ Voluntary Organizations

- Indian Red Cross Society
- Hind Kushtnivaran Sangh
- Indian council for Child Welfare
- Tuberculosis association of India
- Bharat Sevak Samaj
- Central social welfare board
- Kasturba memorial fund
- Family Associasion of india
- All India womens conference
- All India blind relief society
- Professional bodies

⇨ JSY (Janani Suraksha Yojana)

- It is a **safe motherhood intervention** implemented with the **objective of reducing maternal and neo-natal mortality by promoting institutional delivery among the poor pregnant women.**   MAH 2012
- 100% **centrally sponsored** scheme
- Integrates **cash assistance with delivery and post-delivery care**
- The success of the scheme would be determined by the increase in institutional delivery among the poor families
- **Pregnant women, aged >19 years, 1st and 2nd live births** (3rd in case ready for sterilization) are eligible
- Uttar Pradesh, Uttaranchal, Bihar, Jharkhand, Madhya Pradesh, Chhattisgarh, Assam, Rajasthan, Orissa and Jammu and Kashmir. While these states have been named as **Low Performing States (LPS)**
- The remaining states have been named as **High performing States (HPS)**   AIPGME 2010

⊃ International Red Cross: High Yield for 2011-2012

The Red Cross is a non-political non-official international humanitarian organization devoted to the service of mankind in peaceand war. It was founded by Henry Dunant.

Role of Red Cross: In the beginning, the role of the Red Cross, as conceived by Dunant, was largely confined to humanitarian service on behalf of the victims of war. Soon thereafter, it was realised that natural disasters too bring in their wake great human suffering and that on such occasions there is equally great need for help among nations "as good neighbours". Later on the work of the Red Cross was extended to:

- Service to armed forces,
- Service to war veterans,
- Disaster service,
- First aid and nursing,
- Health education and maternity and child welfare services.

8

SPM

⇨ **Red Cross Sign**

✓	First approved in Geneva
✓	Cannot be used by UNO officials
✓	Using Red Cross sign by others is a criminal offence
✓	Is being conventionally used by doctors all over the world

WHO	UNICEF	UNESCO	FAO	Indian Red Cross
Headquarters at Geneva Was set in 1948	Headquarter at New York Established in 1946	Headquarter at Paris	(Food and Agricultural Organization) Headquarter at Rome	Founded by Henry Dunant Red cross was approved in geneva. Red cross is conventionally being used by doctors all over the world. Using red cross sign by others is a criminal offence. AI 2010

Important Days in SPM	

▶	7th April	World Health day
▶	31st May No	Tobacco day
▶	1st July	Doctors day
▶	9th October	World sight day
▶	1st December	World AIDS day
▶	24th March	Anti TB day
▶	30th January	Anti Leprosy day
▶	Theme for WORLD HEALTH DAY 2012: Ageing and Health	JK BOPEE 2012

⊃ **Important Facts**

➥	Chairman of **Health survey and planning committee** was Dr A.L. Mudaliar
➥	Chairman of **Health survey and Development committee** was Sir Joseph Bhore. (1943) **PGI 1984**
➥	Chairman of committee on **Integration of health services** was Dr Jungalwalla
➥	Chairman of Committee on **Multipurpose Health Worker** was Kartar Singh.
➥	ROME scheme+ village health guide is a result of Srivastava committee. **KERALA 2K**
➥	Health care by specially trained workers. **Srivastava committee** **JK BOPEE 2012**

⊃ **GOBI Campaign**

⇨ **Launched by UNICEF**

✓	Growth
✓	Oral rehydration
✓	Breastfeeding
✓	Immunization

GOBI -FFF Campaign:

✓ Female education

✓ Female spacing

✓ Food supplements

2005	▶ Road safety is no accident
2006	▶ Make every mother and child count
2007	▶ Working together for health
2008	▶ Protecting health from climate change
2009	▶ Health facilities in emergencies
2010	▶ Urbanization and Health

➲ **Questions in**   **AIPGME 2011**

❑ **Denominator in Maternal Mortality Rate is:** Total number of live births	**AIPGME 2011**
❑ **Most common cause of maternal mortality in India is Haemerrhage.**	**MAH 2012**
❑ **People are separated into certain sub groups and then some are selected randomly from sub-groups. This type of sampling** Stratified random sampling	**AIPGME 2011**
❑ **Arthropod transmitted disease not found in India:** Yellow fever	**AIPGME 2011**
❑ **Most useful to predict the virulence of acute illness is:** Case fatality rate	**AIPGME 2011**
❑ **Orthotolidine test is used for detecting:** Chlorine	**AIPGME 2011**
❑ **Human Development Index includes:** Life expectancy at birth. Education, GDP	**AIPGME 2011**
❑ **Pasteurised milk is most commonly tested by:** Phosphatase test	**AIPGME 2011**
❑ **Insect not resistant to DDT is** Phlebotomus	**AIPGME 2011**
❑ **Carrier state is not important in transmission of:** Measles	**AIPGME 2011**

➥ In November 1974, government of India started, Medical Education and Support Manpower under the group of people called: **Shrivastav committee**	**(MH 2010)**
➥ "Poverty line" is defined as energy expenditure of at least **2400 KCAL** or more required for daily activities per person in rural area:	**(MH 2010)**
➥ India is in which phase of demographic cycle: **Late expanding**	**(MH 2010)**
➥ Low birth weight for Indian babies is defined (by Indian scientists) as the birth weight less than: **2.0 kg**	**(MHPGMCET 2007) (MH 2010)**
➥ Under Millennium Development Scheme which year is set as "Target year" to achieve the goal **2015**	**(MH 2010)**
➥ Nalgonda technique is used for: **Defluorination of water**	**(MH 2010)**
➥ Sorghum is pellagrogenic due to excess content of: **Leucine**	**(MHPGMCET 2006) (MH 2010)**

8

SPM

8

SPM

- Claviceps fusiformis is active ingredient in **Ergot alkaloid** (MH 2010)

- Only indicator that considers fertility as well as mortality situation in the society **Net reproduction rate** (MH 2010)

- The interval of time between receipt of infection by a host and maximum infectivity is known as: **Generation time** (MH 2010)

- The percentage of people examined showing microfilaria in blood and/or disease manifestation is known as: **Filaria endemicity rate** (MH 2010)

- The lung disease caused by inhalation of sugarcane dust is known as: **Bagassosis** (MH PGM CET 2001, 2005)

"Vitamin A prophylaxis" is an example of **Specific protection** AI 2009

⇨ **Criteria Suggesting Causality in Non Communicable Diseases** AI 2009

A.	Strength of association
B.	Dose response relationship
C.	Specificity of association

⇨ **Following Studies are 'Analytical'** AI 2009

A.	Case control studies
B.	Cohort studies
C.	**Ecological studies**

Is a study in which the units of analysis are populations or groups of people rather than individuals AIIMS 2011

The most suitable method for presenting frequency distribution of data gathered from continuous variables is: **Histogram** AI 2009

Late Expanding Phase of Demographic Cycle' is **Death Rate declines more than Birth rate.** AI 2009

The guidelines according to **Baby friendly hospital** initiative includes: AI 2009

A.	Mothers and infant to be together for 24 hrs a day
B.	Giving newborn infants no food or drink other than breast milk
C.	Encouraging breast - feeding on demand

'STEPS' is recommended by WHO as a method for: **Surveillance of risk factors for non communicable diseases.** AI 2009

A.   Components of 'IDEAS' include Self care

B.   Communication and Understanding

C.   Performing in work

Part of targeted intervention in preventive strategy in spread of AIDS   AI 2009

A.   Treating Sexually Transmitted Diseases (STD)

B.   Providing Condoms

C.   Behavior change communication

Toxic shock syndrome is caused by: **Infected measles vaccine**   AI 2009

⊃ Lead Poisoning

* Populations are exposed to lead **chiefly via paints,** cans, plumbing fixtures and leaded gasoline.

* The intensity of these exposures remains high because of the deterioration of lead paint used into the past and the entrainment of lead from the paint and vehicle exhaust into soil and household.

* Greatest source of **environmental (Non-occupational) is gasoline**

* Most common mode of absorption in case of **occupational** lead poisoning is **inhalation** of flumes and dust of lead and its compounds.   **AIIMS 2009**

Clinical findings: the clinical findings of lead poisoning are different in the inorganic and organic lead exposures.

Inorganic lead poisoning- abdominal colic, constipation, loss of appetite, blue line on the gums, stippling of red cells, anemia, wrist drop and foot drop.

Organic lead poisoning- the toxic effects of organic lead poisoning are mostly on the CNS causing insomnia, headache, mental confusion, delirium, etc.

⇨ Investigations:

* Epiphyseal plate" **lead lines**" on long bone x-rays.   **JKBOPEE 2005**

* **Normocytic, normochromic** anemia

* Coproporphyrin in urine (CPU)

* Amino levulinic acid in urine (ALAU)

* Lead in blood and urine

8

SPM

❏ Most **common mode** of lead poisoning is **inhalation.**	**AIIMS 2009**
❏ A temporary provisional view <u>held by people on a point of view</u> is **opinion.**	**AIIMS 2009**
❏ **Inner subjective though**t of a person towards an individual or situation is <u>**attitude.**</u>	**AIIMS 2009**
❏ **Specificity of test** determines <u>**true negatives.**</u>	**AIIMS 2009**
❏ **Prevalence** of any disease at one point of time is determined by **cross sectional study**	**AIIMS 2009**
❏ **Association** is measured by **P value, odds ratio, correlation coefficient.**	**AIIMS 2009**
❏ Putting **profit ahead of health as a cause of disease** is provided by theory: <u>**Marxist theory.**</u>	**AIIMS 2009**
❏ <u>**Confounding factor**</u> is a risk factor for disease.	**AIIMS 2009**
❏ **Best** contraceptive for newly married healthy couple is **OCP.**	**AIIMS 2009**
❏ **Nested case control study** is a type of <u>**prospective study.**</u>	**AIIMS 2009**
❏ Person is in isolation for typhoid for a period till: **three bacteriologically negative stool and urine culture**s. **AIIMS 2008**	
❏ **NPU**=ratio of total nitrogen retained by total nitrogen intake multiplied by 100.	**AIIMS 2008**
❏ **Post pasteurized** milk quality is tested by <u>**phosphatase test.**</u>	**AIIMS 2008**
❏ **Best** index of contraceptive efficacy: <u>**life Table analysis.**</u>	**AIIMS 2008**
❏ **Kaplan Meier method** is used for <u>**survival**</u>.	**AIIMS 2008**
❏ **Fish** is deficient in <u>iron</u>.	**AIIMS 2008**
❏ **Incidence** can be calculated from <u>**prospective study**</u>.	**AIIMS 2008**